Baseball Sports Medicine

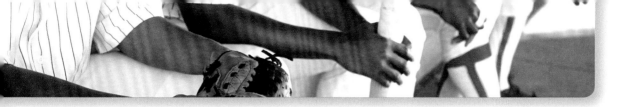

Baseball Sports Medicine

FIRST EDITION

Christopher S. Ahmad, MD
Professor of Orthopedic Surgery
Columbia University Medical Center
Attending Physician, New York-Presbyterian Hospital
Vice Chair of Research, Department of Orthopedic Surgery
Head Team Physician, New York Yankees
Head Team Physician, New York City Football Club (NYCFC)
New York, NY

Anthony A. Romeo, MD
Chief of Orthopaedics
Rothman Orthopaedic Institute
Shoulder and Elbow Surgery, Sports Medicine
President, American Shoulder and Elbow Surgeons
New York, NY

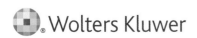. Wolters Kluwer

Philadelphia • Baltimore • New York • London
Buenos Aires • Hong Kong • Sydney • Tokyo

Acquisitions Editor: Brian Brown
Development Editor: Sean McGuire
Editorial Coordinator: Alexis Pozonsky and Jeremiah Kiely
Marketing Manager: Rachel Mante Leung
Production Project Manager: Barton Dudlick
Design Coordinator: Teresa Mallon
Manufacturing Coordinator: Beth Welsh
Prepress Vendor: TNQ Technologies

Copyright © 2019 Wolters Kluwer

9 8 7 6 5 4 3 2 1

Printed in China

Library of Congress Cataloging-in-Publication Data

ISBN-13: 978-1-4963-8146-0

Cataloging-in-Publication data available on request from the Publisher.

shop.lww.com

I found the structure, ideas, and significance for this book in the teachings of
Frank W. Jobe, MD, and Lewis A. Yocum, MD, who mentored me in the field of baseball
sports medicine and to whom I am forever grateful.
My parents Shafi and Judy have been a guiding light for me for my entire life.
My wife Beth and children *Charlie, Sofie, and Brady encourage, challenge, and support me with
love each and every day.*
–*Christopher S. Ahmad*

Baseball is a sport that runs through the fabric of American life. While the athletes have
reached mythical abilities in terms of how fast the ball can be thrown, how fast they can run
to steal a base or catch a ball, or how far the ball can be hit, the fans get the opportunity to
relax and watch the spectacle at a pace that allows exuberant conversation about the current
team and team strategies, the players, the history of the game, and even time for family
communication or developing a new relationship.
From the athlete's side of the experience, it is an incredibly challenging sport, requiring
focus, training, strength, speed, hand–eye coordination, and the ability to find the zone
where they reach their full potential. As someone dedicated to the health and well-being of
these players, it is devastating to see the effort put in to achieve success and then to have it
taken away from an injury. This motivates those of us in *Baseball Sports Medicine* to search
for answers and find new methods of preventing problems that keep them off the field.
Sharing these ideas helps us all, both the athlete and the fan.
My drive for finding answers and pursuing excellence was developed at an early age, with
my father Sam setting high expectations and my mother Pat nurturing our entire family,
which continues even today with their six children and 22 grandchildren.
My parent's example was invaluable when raising my five daughters (Brianna, Alyssa,
Danielle, Christin, Sabrina), who were also an inspiration, as they participated in multiple
sports and had injuries that prevented their participation, challenging not only their athletic
success but also social and academic interactions.
And, a special thanks to my wife Kate, who provides love and nourishment that continue to
support my efforts every day.
–*Anthony A. Romeo, MD*

Contributors

Christopher S. Ahmad, MD
Professor of Orthopedic Surgery
Columbia University Medical Center
Attending Physician, New York-Presbyterian
Hospital
Vice Chair of Research, Department of
Orthopedic Surgery
Head Team Physician, New York Yankees
Head Team Physician, New York City Football
Club (NYCFC)
New York, NY

Frank J. Alexander, MS, ATC
Physician Extender to Dr. Christopher Ahmad
Department of Orthopaedic Surgery
Columbia University Medical Center
New York, NY

Robert B. Anderson, MD
Director, Foot & Ankle
Titletown Sports Medicine and Orthopaedics
Bellin Hospital
Green Bay, Wisconsin

James R. Andrews, MD
Medical Director
The Andrews Institute
Baptist Health care
Gulf Breeze, FL

Christopher A. Arrigo, MS, PT, ATC
Owner/Clinical Director
Advanced Rehabilitation
Tampa, FL

Donald S. Bae, MD
Associate Professor
Department of Orthopaedic Surgery
Harvard Medical School
Boston, MA

Eamon D. Bernardoni, MS
Research Fellow
Midwest Orthopaedics at Rush
Chicago, IL

Meghan Bishop, MD
Clinical Fellow
Department of Sports Medicine and
Shoulder Surgery
Hospital for Special Surgery
New York, NY

Patrick S. Buckley, MD
Resident
Department of Orthopaedic Surgery
Rothman Institute at Thomas Jefferson
University Hospital
Philadelphia, PA

Charles A. Bush-Joseph, MD
Professor
Department of Orthopedic Surgery
Rush University Medical Center
Chicago, IL

E. Lyle Cain Jr, MD
Fellowship Director
American Sports Medicine Institute
Birmingham, AL

Christopher L. Camp, MD
Assistant Professor of Orthopedic Surgery
Department of Orthopedics/Sports Medicine
Mayo Clinic
Rochester, MN

Peter N. Chalmers, MD
Clinical Instructor
Department Orthopaedic Surgery
University of Utah
Salt Lake City, UT

Gregory Chertok, MEd, CMPC
Lecturer in Sport Psychology
Division of Social Sciences
Dominican College
Orangeburg, NY

Joseph L. Ciccone, PT, DPT, FAAOMPT, CSCS, OCS, SCS, Cert. DN/SMT, CIMT
Associate Director
Department of Orthopaedic Surgery
Columbia University
New York, NY

Michael C. Ciccotti, MD
Resident Physician
Department of Orthopaedic Surgery
Thomas Jefferson University and the
Rothman Institute
Philadelphia, PA

Michael G. Ciccotti, MD
The Everett J. and Marian Gordan Professor of
Orthopaedic Surgery
Chief, Division of Sports Medicine Fellowship
and Research
Department of Orthopaedic Surgery
The Rothman Insititute
The Sydney Kimmel Medical College at
Thomas Jefferson University
Head Team Physician, Philadelphia Phillies and
Saint Joseph's University
Philadelphia, PA

Philip N. Collis, MD
Sports Medicine Fellow
Department of Orthopaedics
University of Miami
Miami, FL

David Colvin, PT, DPT, MS, ATC
Physical Therapist
Department of Player Development
New York Yankees
Tampa, FL

Stan Conte, PT, DPT, ATC
Assistant Director of Sports Medicine
Department of Sports Medicine
Santa Clara University
Santa Clara, CA

Gregory L. Cvetanovich, MD
Assistant Professor
Orthopedic Surgeon
Department of Sports Medicine
The Ohio State University Wexner
Medical Center
Columbus, OH

Alek Z. Diffendaffer, MS
Sports Biomechanist
American Sports Medicine Institute
Birmingham, AL

Steve Donohue, ATC
Head Athletic Trainer
New York Yankees
Yankees Stadium
Bronx, NY

Brittany Dowling, MS
Director
Department of Research and Validation
Motus Global
Rockville Centre, NY

Jeffrey R. Dugas, MD
Fellowship Director
Andrews Sports Medicine
American Sports Medicine Institute
Birmingham, AL

Neal S. ElAttrache, MD
Chairman
Kerlan Jobe Orthopaedic Foundation
Kerlan Jobe Institute
Los Angeles, CA

Brandon J. Erickson, MD
Attending Surgeon
Sports Medicine and Shoulder
Rothman Institute
New York, NY

Rafael F. Escamilla, PhD, PT, CSCS, FACSM
Professor
Physical Therapy
California State University, Sacramento
Sacramento, CA

Glenn S. Fleisig, PhD
Research Director
American Sports Medicine Institute
Birmingham, AL

Megan Flynn, MD
Resident Physician
Department of Orthopaedic Surgery
Cleveland Clinic
Cleveland, OH

Samuel E. Galle, MD
Hand and Upper Extremity Fellow
Department of Orthopaedic Surgery
Columbia University Medical Center
New York, NY

Thomas J. Graham, MD
Chief Strategic Alliance &
Partnership Officer
Northwell Health
Lenox Hill Hospital
New York, NY

Gary Green, MD
Clinical Professor
UCLA Division of Sports Medicine
UCLA School of Medicine
Los Angeles, CA

Justin W. Griffin, MD
Orthopaedic Surgeon, Shoulder & Sports
Medicine Specialist
Jordan-Young Institute
Virginia Beach, VA

Justin L. Hodgins, MD
Staff Consultant
Department of Orthopaedic
Surgery
Rouge Valley Centenary Hospital
Toronto, ON

James Irvine, MD
Orthopaedic Sports Medicine
Fellow
Department of Orthopaedic Surgery
Columbia University Medical Center
New York, NY

Timothy Kahn, MD
Resident Physician
Department of Orthopaedic Surgery
University of Utah
Salt Lake City, UT

Lee D. Kaplan, MD
Chief, Sports Medicine
Department of Orthopaedics
University of Miami
Coral Gables, FL

W. Ben Kibler, MD
Medical Director
Shoulder Center of Kentucky
Lexington Clinic
Lexington, KY

Nathan Krebs, DO
Orthopaedic Surgery Resident
McLaren Macomb Medical Center
Mount Clemens, MI

Ronald A. Lehman Jr, MD
Professor, Tenure
Department of Orthopedics
Columbia University
New York, NY

Professor of Orthopaedic Surgery
Department of Orthopaedic Surgery
The Daniel and Jane Och Spine Hospital
NewYork-Presbyterian/The Allen Hospital
New York, NY

Timothy Lentych, MS, ATC/L
Assistant Athletic Trainer
Sports Medicine Department
New York Yankees
Bronx, NY

Bernard Li, DPT, OCS, SCS, LAT
Adjunct Instructor of Clinical Physical Therapy
USC Division of Biokinesiology and
Physical Therapy
University of Southern California
Los Angeles, CA

James D. Lin, MD
Resident in Orthopaedic Surgery
Department of Orthopaedic Surgery
The Daniel and Jane Och Spine Hospital
NewYork-Presbyterian/The Allen Hospital
New York, NY

Joseph M. Lombardi, MD
Resident
Department of Orthopaedic Surgery
Columbia University Medical Center
New York, NY

Gary M. Lourie, MD
Chief of Hand Surgery
Division of Orthopedics
Atlanta Medical Center
Head Orthopedic team Physician
Georgia Tech Baseball
Head Team Physician
Atlanta Braves

T. Sean Lynch, MD
Assistant Professor
Director, Center for Athletic Hip Injuries
and Hip Preservation
Department of Orthopedic Surgery
Columbia University, Vagelus College of
Physicians and Surgeons
New York, NY

Leonard C. Macrina, MSPT, SCS, CSCS
Co-Founder and Director of Physical Therapy
Champion Physical Therapy & Performance
Waltham, MA

Eric C. Makhni, MD, MBA
Orthopedic Surgeon
Department of Orthopedic Surgery
Henry Ford Health System
Detroit, MI

Melvin C. Makhni, MD
Fellow
Department of Orthopaedic Surgery
Columbia Medical Center
New York, NY

Joe Metz, MS, ATC, CSCS
Minor League Medical Coordinator
Atlanta Braves
Jacksonville, NC

John T. Nickless, MD
Associate Professor
Department of Orthopedic Surgery
Rush University Medical Center
Chicago, IL

Fiona E. Nugent, NP
Nurse Practitioner
Orthopedic Surgery
Columbia University
New York, NY

Djuro Petkovic, MD
Orthopedic Surgeon
Illinois Bone and Joint Institute
Morton Grove, IL

Anthony A. Romeo, MD
Chief of Orthopaedics
Rothman Orthopaedic Institute
Shoulder and Elbow Surgery, Sports Medicine
President, American Shoulder and Elbow
Surgeons
New York, NY

Melvin P. Rosenwasser, MD
Robert E. Carroll Professor
Department of Orthopedic Surgery
Columbia University
New York, NY

Paul M. Rothenberg, MD
Resident Physician
Department of Orthopaedics
University of Miami
Miami, FL

Marcus A. Rothermich, MD
Orthopedic Surgeon
Department of Orthopedics
American Sports Medicine Institute
Birmingham, AL

Michael K. Ryan, MD
Orthopaedic Surgeon & Sports Medicine Specialist
Andrews Sports Medicine
Birmingham, AL

Mark Schickendantz, MD
Professor of Surgery
Cleveland Clinic Lerner College of Medicine at case
Western Reserve University
Cleveland, OH

Michael Schuk, PT, DPT, ATC
Assistant Athletic Trainer
Physical Therapist
New York Yankees
Bronx, NY

Aaron Sciascia, PhD, ATC, PES
Assistant Professor
Department of Exercise and Sport Science
Eastern Kentucky University
Richmond, KY

Jamal N. Shillingford, MD
Resident in Orthopaedic Surgery
Department of Orthopaedic Surgery
The Daniel and Jane Och Spine Hospital
NewYork-Presbyterian/The Allen Hospital
New York, NY

Brian Shiu, MD
Orthopedic Surgeon
University of Maryland St. Joseph Medical Center
Towson, MD

J. Alex Sielatycki, MD
Fellow in Spine Surgery
Department of Orthopaedic Surgery
The Daniel and Jane Och Spine Hospital
NewYork-Presbyterian/The Allen Hospital
New York, NY

Heidi Skolnik, MS, CDN, FACSM
Sports Nutritionist
Women Sports Medicine Center
Hospital for Special Surgery
New York, NY

Founder
Nutrition Conditioning, LLC
Englewood Cliffs, NJ

Jonathan S. Slowik, PhD
Sports Biomechanist
American Sports Medicine Institute
Birmingham, AL

Stephen J. Thomas, PhD, ATC
Assistant Professor
Department of Kinesiology
Temple University
Philadelphia, PA

Robert W. Thompson, MD
Professor
Department of Surgery
Washington University
St. Louis, MO

David P. Trofa, MD
Department of Orthopaedic Surgery
Columbia University Medical Center
New York, NY

Alex Valadka, MD
Professor and Chair
Department of Neurosurgery
Virginia Commonwealth University
Richmond, VA

Nikhil N. Verma, MD
Professor, Fellowship Director Division
of Sports Medicine
Department of Orthopedics
Rush University Medical Center
Chicago, IL

Steven Wakeman, MD
Resident
Department of Neurosurgery
Virginia Commonwealth University
Richmond, VA

Kathleen M. Weber, MD
Director, Primary Care Sports Medicine
Department of Orthopedic
Rush University Medical Center
Chicago, IL

Stephen White, MD
Foot & Ankle Institute
OrthoCarolina
Charlotte, NC

Kevin E. Wilk, PT, DPT, FAPTA
Associate Clinical Director
Champion Sports Medicine
Birmingham, AL

AJ Yenchak, PT, DPT, CSCS
Director Sports Therapy
Columbia Orthopedics
Columbia University of Medical Center
New York, NY

Foreword by Dr. James Andrews, MD

Baseball sports medicine has definitely come a long ways since the 1970's and 1980's when there was very little clinical and scientific information on baseball injuries. During those times football was "king" and baseball injuries took a back seat. Very little was known about these injuries until Frank Jobe and Bob Kerlan began to investigate shoulder and elbow baseball injuries. They studied and described the throwing motion at their biomechanical laboratory at Centinela Hospital in Los Angeles.

Those studies definitely ushered in the modern era and many centers began to develop what has since been called "baseball medicine."

This book is certainly a fine reference for anyone interested in this subject. It will become a must read and reference for all of us. It is very comprehensive to include epidemiology, biomechanics, and all of the clinical entities and disorders associated with baseball. Also this book is unique by design to include concussion and spine injuries as well as specific medical issues in baseball.

As with all aspects of sports medicine, rehabilitation, and conditioning covered in this book play such an important role in the overall care of a baseball player whether treated conservatively or surgically for an injury.

I am also proud to see that this book devotes an entire section on "youth baseball injuries." This has become a crucial area of concern by all of us particularly, as there is an approximate 10-fold increase in youth baseball injuries since 2000.

This book brings us up to date on some of the new theories in baseball mechanics and injury such as the scapular thoracic component to the shoulder and the importance of the core and its set of specific injuries.

Overall this book not only covers the tried and true areas of baseball injuries but also covers some of the newer and less known theories and specific areas related to the sport of baseball that are more challenging now than ever. To conclude, this book is certainly comprehensive and includes all of the expanded breath of knowledge related to baseball medicine. It is again a must read for all of us!

Dr. James Andrews, MD

Foreword by Jeff Passan

When I decided to write *The Arm*, a book that I hoped would demystify the act of throwing a baseball and the deep damage it is capable of unleashing on the human body, I did not fully understand the act of hubris I was about to undertake. Here I was, a layman, armed with a thimbleful of medical knowledge, endeavoring to explain in explicit detail the fallibility of ligaments and tendons and muscles and fascia and bones—to decode a language I barely spoke.

What kept me afloat throughout the nearly four-year process—what allowed the book to exist in any salient form—was the wisdom of those who didn't simply know those explicit details but lived them. The doctors whose steady hands repaired arms broken by the ignorant coaches. The biomechanists who hunted for inefficient movement patterns. The athletic trainers who nurtured those with inborn frailties. All of the people who dedicated their lives to the just cause of preventing injury before its birth or fixing it upon its delivery of devastation. If I could not be them, I could be the next-best thing: their translator.

It is from that perch I speak today, to coaches gathered at conferences, to kids on dusty fields around America, and even to the medical professions to whom I owe so much, and my message is constant and resolute. For all of our fragility, I say, the dark feeling of inevitability that so many baseball players shove to the deepest recesses of their minds, for all of that, there is a group of dedicated men and women who spend day and night in laboratories, in workout facilities, in operating rooms, and in all the familiar places, whose goal in life is to never again tell someone his ulnar collateral ligament gave out or his rotator cuff succumbed to the rigors of what he dreamed possible.

That these men and women—whose work you'll read in the forthcoming pages, whose intellect demands respect and whose principle warrants acclaim and whose fastidiousness has delivered innovation after innovation—are there for you. I may just be a voice, but I want to be the loudest one imaginable, and I want to shout the following.

I believe in medicine. I believe in its nobility. I believe we are entering a golden age, where technology will allow curiosity to grow beyond our imaginations. I believe the single-mindedness of this pursuit will reap great dividends. I am neither smart enough nor presumptuous enough to say we can end arm injuries; I am quite certain that a combination of innovation and education can minimize the number of people, particularly children, affected by them.

If all of this makes me sound like a Pollyanna, that is a title I'll wear proudly. Because the moment we stop believing, we've taken the greatest gift of our forebears and spoiled it. That endowment is the notion that there is no ceiling on our ability to learn and achieve wondrous things.

It is the job of doctors, athletic trainers, physical therapists, physician assistants, nurses, biomechanists, and all other medical personnel not just to widen that base of understanding but to collaborate and form a network of know-how—to convince those who can fund research that the efforts are worthy and to understand the responsibility does not end with footnoted papers but extends to the explanation of what they mean and why they're important.

The most I can do is evangelize, so evangelize I will, about the professionals who desire nothing more than the good health of every person playing baseball. I want more books like this, more conferences that broaden the web of those dedicated to the cause, and more of the joint efforts among brilliant minds that can produce something as seminal as what exists in these pages.

Does that make me greedy? Yes. And if that means these words come from a glutton in rose-colored glasses, so be it. I'm not a doctor, so I'll settle for being the next-best thing. A believer.

Jeff Passan

Preface

Baseball, America's pastime, is an incredible sport that defies the capabilities of the human body and fascinates everyone it touches. Unfortunately, we are in the midst of a crisis of ever increasing injuries to those playing this beloved sport.

Baseball Sports Medicine textbook is the product of an educational platform that facilitates the interaction of the world's experts in baseball medicine. The Baseball Sports Medicine: Game-Changing Concepts conference has been held at the Major League Baseball (MLB) offices on Park Avenue in New York City and has been sold out every year since its introduction. The audience and participants consist of diverse individuals connected through the united care of baseball players. Attendees include athletic trainers, physical therapists, strength and conditioning coaches, performance science specialists, nurse practitioners, physicians, and physician assistants. An extensive spectrum of topics addresses the complexities of the professional MLB player and also the troubling injury issues in our youth athletes. The course content has proven powerful, and we were compelled to create a textbook that would serve as a constant available resource for anyone who participates in the care of baseball players or simply cares about baseball medicine.

The textbook chapters are constructed in typical fashion with history, physical examination, imaging, and treatment, but also includes 46 inspirational baseball quotes, side bar explanations called "Trip to the Mound," and chapter summaries called "Manager's Tips." The latest advancements in baseball technology and care are included with remarkable illustrations and clear explanations.

We believe this book will serve all those who care for baseball athletes across the country and around the world. Ultimately, our goal is to keep our athletes at all levels of competition on the field of play. We accomplish this through proper training and coaching, developing strategies for injury prevention, maximizing the value of nonoperative treatment, and developing sophisticated surgical techniques to treat injuries without compromising the healthy tissues so that return to play can be safely expedited. We have captured these principles in our *Baseball Sports Medicine* textbook and live conference, with the hope that education and interaction will help us better serve our athletes, parents, coaches, and fans.

Christopher S. Ahmad
Anthony A. Romeo

Contents

Baseball Epidemiology and the Biomechanics of Baseball Specific Movements

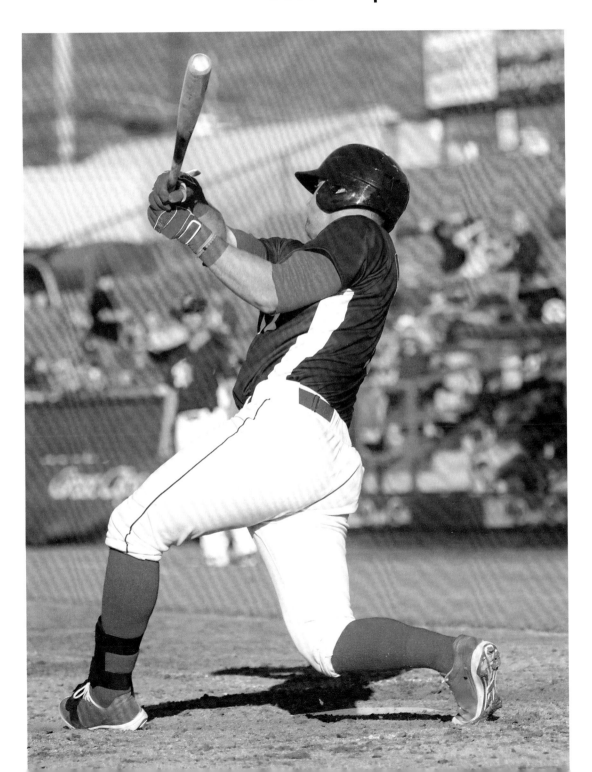

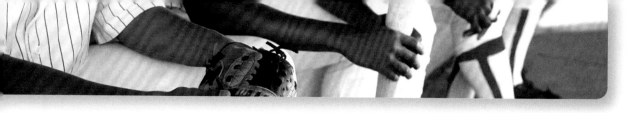

CHAPTER 1

Epidemiology of Baseball Injuries: From Adolescents to the Pros

Stan Conte, PT, DPT, ATC | Christopher L. Camp, MD | Marcus A. Rothermich, MD

You can observe a lot by watching.

—*Yogi Berra*

INTRODUCTION

Although the exact origins of the game of baseball are commonly debated, one thing is certain: statistics have been an integral part of the game since its existence. With new and more advanced technology and data collection systems available, there is little that occurs on the baseball field that is not recorded, counted, and compared analytically. This has been true since the advent of the box score and now is expanded into an entire new field of study: Sabermetrics.[10,24,25] Although much of these data have historically been used to evaluate player performance, they have recently fueled increased interest in the epidemiology of injuries in baseball. Accordingly, the amount of research dedicated to baseball injuries has seen a rapid rise in recent years.

Overall, baseball is a relatively safe sport, and it has been shown to have lower injury rates per athlete-exposure (a-e) than what is observed in other sports.[13] When comparing 2 "nonimpact" professional sports leagues: Major League Baseball (MLB) and the National Basketball Association (NBA), injury rates were only 3.6 injuries per 1000 athlete-exposures in MLB compared with 21.4 injuries per 1000 exposures in the NBA. Despite the overall low rates of injury in baseball, there are a number of unique injury patterns observed in baseball players. These patterns generally vary by position, age of the player, and level of play. In this work, we will discuss the general epidemiology of injuries that occur across 3 major groups: adolescent and high school, collegiate athletes, and professional baseball players.

ADOLESCENT AND HIGH-SCHOOL AGED ATHLETES

An important element in understanding the epidemiology of baseball injuries includes the amateur levels of adolescent and high school baseball. With a rapid increase in injuries to professional baseball athletes[10,11,31]—particularly ulnar collateral ligament (UCL) elbow injuries in pitchers[6,10]—there has recently been significant media attention to baseball injuries in younger players. Over the past decade, an effort has begun to both educate the public about baseball injuries in amateur athletes and establish guidelines to prevent these injuries at the high school, collegiate, and professional levels of play. As with any injury prevention program, the foundation is a thorough understanding of the epidemiology of injuries at that level.

Baseball is consistently ranked as one of the most popular sports played by boys in high school, with estimates of nearly 500 000 athletes each year according to the National Federation of State High School Associations.[27,28] As this number of athletes continues to rise each year, the number of injuries related to baseball in high school athletes is increasing in a similar fashion. Recent epidemiologic studies have described baseball injuries in this specific population of adolescents and have investigated differential injury rates for different positions, the common body locations injured, the severity of the injuries, and the timing of the injuries in relation to the baseball season.[2,7,23,34,36] The results of this literature help to identify opportunities for prevention of these injuries.

Although there are only a few reports that describe injury rates in high school baseball players by position, the findings are fairly consistent.[7,23,36] Collins et al[7] described the results of a National High School Sports-Related Injury Surveillance Study from 2005 to 2007. This study reported the total number of injuries in baseball players in all body locations over 2 baseball seasons. The highest overall incidence of injury was demonstrated by a combination of the infield positions (30% of the injuries), followed by outfielders (22% of injuries) and pitchers (20% of the total injuries). Position players were also found to have a higher overall incidence of injury in a study by Shanley et al[36] in 2011. Krajnik et al[23] described injuries specifically to the shoulder from 2005 to 2008. In this work, they demonstrated that 38% of shoulder injuries occurred in pitchers, compared with 26% in outfielders, and 18% in infielders. However, interpretation of these data is difficult at the high school level, where pitchers more commonly play field positions compared with the collegiate or professional levels. This could confound the results of injury rates by position.

Although these studies consistently report that position players have the highest overall incidence of injury and that pitchers have the highest proportion of shoulder injuries, reports of the most commonly injured body regions vary significantly.[2,7,32,33,34,36] Rechel et al[34] investigated the differential rates of injury between practice and competition and concluded that in high school baseball competition, lower extremity injuries were actually more common than upper extremity injuries. Other studies have consistently shown that the upper extremity is the most commonly injured body location. Bonza et al[2] reported that shoulder injuries represent 17.7% of the total injuries among baseball players, which was the highest of any specific body region. Similarly, Collins et al[7] reported that 17.6% of injuries occurred in the shoulder, and the ankle was the next highest at 13.6%. Powell et al[32,33] reported that 24.6% of injuries occurred in the forearm, wrist, and hand, compared with 19.7% in the shoulder and arm. Although some discrepancy exists, the vast majority of the limited literature describing high school baseball injuries reports the upper extremity as the most common location of injury.

Other epidemiologic factors have been reported regarding high school baseball injuries, including exposure setting, injury severity, and temporal variation in injuries. The literature is mixed in its reports of exposure setting of injury, with Rechel et al[34] reporting a slightly higher incidence during game competition, whereas Knowles et al[22] demonstrated a greater number of injuries occurring during practice. Reports on injury severity are uniform, however, with multiple epidemiologic studies demonstrating that most baseball injuries are ligamentous sprains or tendinous strains.[7,23,36] Shanley et al[36] also investigated temporal variations, and they reported that most injuries occurred during the first month of the roughly 3-month high school baseball season. This is the only known study in the literature to report a variation of injury rates in high school baseball by month, and they suggested that this differential injury rate could likely be attributed to a short preseason and lack of sport-specific off-season training programs at the high school level.

As participation in high school baseball continues to increase annually, an understanding of the epidemiologic factors related to baseball injuries is critical. The literature is sparse and not entirely consistent, but several specific trends can be ascertained from the various reports. The upper extremity appears to be the most commonly injured body region in both position players and pitchers. Injuries occur both during practice and in game competition, and ligamentous sprains and tendinous strains are the most common types of injury. Attention to these epidemiologic commonalities, introduction of structured conditioning programs during the off-season, and guidelines for avoiding overuse injuries may be potential means with which to reduce injury rates in high school baseball.

COLLEGIATE BASEBALL

Of the nearly 500 000 high school athletes who participate in baseball, approximately 25 000 eventually go on to play collegiate baseball each year.[16] The National Collegiate Athletic Association (NCAA) is divided into 3 divisions, with baseball existing as a sponsored sport at most of the nearly 1000 schools in Division I, Division II, and Division III. Although the literature on college baseball injuries is surprisingly sparse, recent reports have investigated the common body locations injured, overall severity of the most common injuries, and the setting in which most injuries occur.[13,18,19,26,28]

In the most comprehensive evaluation of injury epidemiology in collegiate baseball, Dick et al[13] analyzed injuries recorded in the NCAA Injury Surveillance System findings from 16 consecutive college baseball seasons. Of the 5 identified body regions (head/neck, upper extremity, trunk/back, lower extremity, and other/system), the upper extremity accounted for 44.6% of game injuries and 46.4% of practice-related injuries. The next most common location was the lower extremity, with 35.2% of game injuries and 31.7% injuries during practice. Interestingly, when subdivided into specific body parts, upper leg and ankle injuries predominated over shoulder injuries in live game play, whereas shoulder injuries were more common during the practice setting. In a single-institution study by McFarland and Wasik,[26] the upper extremity accounted for 51% of the recorded injuries over 3 seasons of play, with the shoulder comprising nearly half of those upper extremity complaints.

The mechanism and severity of collegiate baseball injuries have been described for different exposure settings such as practice and games. Dick et al[13] reported that 63.9% of injuries that occurred during practice were noncontact injuries. Conversely, 56.1% of game injuries were contact injuries. These data are logical, and the contact injuries in game situations commonly occur as a result of base-running, base-sliding, and ball-contact injuries during live play.[18,19,28] Most injuries in both practices and games are described as tendinous strains and ligamentous sprains, similar to those in high school baseball athletes. However, severe injuries (those requiring 10+ days of activity time loss) do occur, and they accounted for 25.2% of injuries during games and 25.0% of practice injuries in the NCAA Injury Surveillance System data.[13]

The collegiate baseball literature has demonstrated that most injuries incurred in the practice setting occur during the preseason, similar to high school baseball injuries.[13] The majority of game injuries occurred during the regular season, and no data exist on the temporal variation of in-season game injuries by month. However, the trend of preseason or early regular season injuries in collegiate baseball emphasizes the critical importance of adequate off-season conditioning and preseason training to prevent overuse injuries in collegiate student athletes.

INJURIES IN PROFESSIONAL BASEBALL

The Disabled List

The only database that tracked injuries occurred in professional baseball before 2010 was the MLB Disabled List (DL). The DL has existed since 1916; however, the rules on placement have changed over the years. Despite the different forms the DL has taken since its inception, the rules and regulations of the DL have actually remained relatively constant since 1989,[10,11] allowing reasonable comparisons of injury data and trends across this time span. During most of the season, an MLB team is allowed no more than 25 players on its team roster. In the month of September, the rosters can be expanded up to a maximum of 40. MLB rules allow injured players to be placed on a disabled list for a minimum of 15 days (with a few recent exception); and during this time, the injured player may be replaced on the active roster. Although the active roster cannot exceed 25 players (or 40 in September), there is no maximum limit to the number of players allowed on the DL at any one time. For a player to be assigned to the DL, the nature and extent of injury must be certified by a physician.[11] Since 1989, once a player is designated for the DL, he cannot return to the major league team for a minimum of 15 days (although this minimum was reduced to 10 days in 2017). Since 2011, a player diagnosed with a concussion may be placed on the DL for a minimum of 7 days rather than 15 days. If the injury is severe, the player can remain on the DL for the remainder of the season or until he is deemed healthy enough to return to play by a physician.[10,11]

The DL becomes valuable because of its consistency and magnitude, and it is the only historical database of injuries. Despite these strengths, there are a number of significant limitations to DL data. First and foremost, it is primarily designed as a roster management tool (to allow substitutions for injured players) rather than as an injury database. The medical data contained in it are primarily the anatomic regions involved in the injury. Although injury "types" are sometimes noted, the categories are not mutually exclusive and are often vague (for example, strain, surgery, "tear," or weakness), making meaningful analysis very difficult.[10] The data presented in the DL lack significant granular info on player's injuries. Also, in some instances, factors other than medical information may be used in making disabled list decisions. For example, a relatively trivial injury might prompt a disabled list designation if there is a "better" minor league player available to come in as a substitute. On the other hand, a "star" with a more severe injury might be kept off the disabled list if there is an outside chance he can return in fewer than 15 or 10 days. In addition, there is no information on the over 6000 players in Minor League Baseball (MiLB).[1]

To date, there have been only 3 studies that have used the DL to perform robust, multiyear epidemiologic studies of injuries in baseball.[10,11,31] The first study was published in 2001 by Conte et al[11] They studied DL assignments over an 11-year period from 1989 to 1999. During this time, there were 3282 injuries resulting in 195,671 lost days (ie, DL days). The average number of disabled list days per team was 640.6 per season. Note that in 1992 the league expanded from 26 to 28 teams, and in 1998 it expanded to its current size of 30 teams. The number of games reduced in 1994 and 1995 because of a labor strike. Table 1.1 contains the disabled list statistics for the 11 years of study.

TABLE 1.1 Disabled List Days per Team and by Player by Season

Year	Disabled List Reports	Average Disabled List Reports/Team	Disabled List Days	Average Disabled List Days/Team	Average Days/ Disabled List Report
1989	266	10.2	14 869	571.9	55.9
1990	231	8.9	12 603	484.7	54.6
1991	260	10.0	15 830	608.8	60.9
1992	283	10.9	17 656	679.1	62.4
1993	300	10.7	17 810	636.1	59.4
1994[a]	259	9.2	15 724	561.6	60.7
1995[a]	295	10.5	15 552	555.4	52.7
1996	321	11.5	19 432	694.0	60.5
1997	351	12.5	20 454	730.5	58.3
1998	349	11.6	22 127	737.6	63.4
1999	367	12.2	23 614	787.1	64.3

[a]Strike years.

Reprinted with permission from Conte S, Requa RK, Garrick JG. Disability days in major league baseball. Am J Sports Med. 2001;29(4):431-436. Copyright © 2001 SAGE Publications.

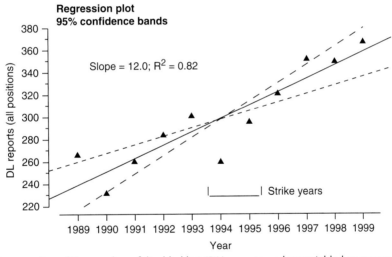

FIGURE 1.1 • A regression of the number of disabled list (DL) reports and year yielded an average increase per year (slope) of 12.0 DL reports. (Reprinted with permission from Conte S, Requa RK, Garrick JG. Disability days in major league baseball. *Am J Sports Med.* 2001. ;29(4):431-436. Copyright © 2001 SAGE Publications.)

The results showed that the number of players on the DL (Figure 1.1) and total DL days (Figure 1.2) increased annually over the study period (P < .05 for both). The increase was still present when the total days were adjusted for the increasing number of players by examining the average disabled list days per team per year.

The study also broke down the number of DL placements by position. Not surprisingly, pitchers were responsible for the greatest number of DL assignments (48.4%). In this work, the shoulder and elbow injuries were responsible for 27.8% and 22.0% of all lost days, respectively. In total, shoulder and elbow injuries represented 49.2% of all DL days between 1995 and

1999. Ultimately, this was the first study to demonstrate rising injury rates in professional baseball.

Posner et al[31] published the second DL-based league epidemiologic study in 2011, analyzing seasons from 2002 to 2008 (Figure 1.3). Their findings indicated a continued rise in the number of players placed on the DL when compared with the previous study. A total of 3072 MLB players were placed on the DL during the study period for an annual average of 438.9 players per season. The highest number of assignments was seen in 2008 (516 injuries) and the lowest occurred in 2005 (388 injuries). The previous high in the Conte study was only 367.[11]

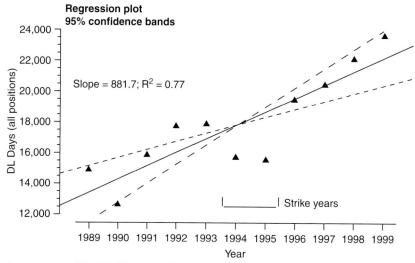

FIGURE 1.2 • A regression of disabled list (DL) days and year yielded an average increase (slope) of almost 882 days per year. (Reprinted with permission from Conte S, Requa RK, Garrick JG. Disability days in major league baseball. *Am J Sports Med.* 2001;29(4):431-436. Copyright © 2001 SAGE Publications.)

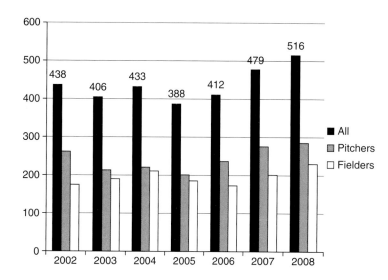

FIGURE 1.3 • Total number injuries to all players, pitchers, and fielders by year. (Reprinted with permission from Posner M, Cameron KL, Wolf JM, Belmont PJ Jr, Owens BD. Epidemiology of major league baseball injuries. *Am J Sports Med.* 2011;39(8):1675-1691. Copyright © 2011 SAGE Publications.)

The study was one of the first to report on injury rates based on athlete-exposures in MLB. The overall incidence of DL designations was 3.61 per 1000 athlete-exposures. In these calculations, injury risk and exposures were estimated by assuming a 25-man roster for each team for the entire 162-game season with each game defined as 1 athlete-exposure. This finding is similar to collegiate studies that indicated a 4.7 to 5.8 injury rate per 1000 exposures.[13]

The study also reported a greater number of players placed on the DL in April, with an average decrease in injury rates of 0.81 per 1000 exposures as the season progressed ($P = .012$). However, these data should be interpreted with caution as injuries reported in April may have occurred in Spring Training (February and March). The opposite problem is seen at the end of the season when roster limits expand to 40 in September, and DL assignments decline because there is additional room of the roster for replacement players. This limitation of the study is discussed in the paper.

Among all player injuries, upper extremity injuries accounted for 51.4%, whereas lower extremity injuries accounted for 30.6%. Injuries to the spine and core musculature accounted for 11.7%, whereas other injuries and illnesses were 6.3% of the total disabled list entries. Pitchers had a higher rate of upper extremity injuries at 67%, whereas nonpitchers had a higher number of lower extremity injuries at 47.5% (Table 1.2).

TABLE 1.2 Body Region Percentage of Injuries Broken Down by Pitchers and Fielders, as well as National League (NL) and American League (AL)

	AL (%)	NL (%)	Total (%)
All Players			
Upper extremity	51.1	51.7	51.4
Lower extremity	30.5	30.7	30.6
Spine and core	12.3	11.2	11.7
Others	6.0	6.5	6.3
Pitchers Only			
Upper extremity	66.9	67.0	67.0
Lower extremity	17.0	17.0	16.9
Spine and core	10.3	10.9	10.6
Others	5.8	5.1	5.5
Fielders Only			
Upper extremity	32.3	32.0	32.1
Lower extremity	46.7	48.2	47.5
Spine and core	14.7	11.6	13.0
Others	6.3	8.2	7.4

Reprinted with permission from Posner M, Cameron KL, Wolf JM, Belmont PJ Jr, Owens BD. Epidemiology of major league baseball injuries. Am J Sports Med. 2011;39(8):1675-1691. Copyright © 2011 SAGE Publications.

TABLE 1.3 Average Injuries by Body Part—All Players

Rank	Body Part	Percentage
1	Shoulder	21.0%
2	Elbow	16.4%
3	Hand/wrist	10.0%
4	Hamstring	8.0%
5	Knee	7.7%
6	Back/spine	7.6%
7	Foot/ankle	5.5%
8	Other lower extremity	4.5%
9	Core	4.3%
10	Groin	3.8%

Reprinted with permission from Posner M, Cameron KL, Wolf JM, Belmont PJ Jr, Owens BD. Epidemiology of major league baseball injuries. Am J Sports Med. 2011;39(8): 1675-1691. Copyright © 2011 SAGE Publications.

The average number of injuries by body part demonstrated that shoulder and elbow injuries represented 37.4% of number of injuries to all players. Pitchers who went on the DL had more shoulder and elbow injuries than any other body parts (30.7% and 26.3%, respectively). The top 10 body parts on the DL by percentage of the total are shown in Table 1.3.

The most comprehensive study utilizing the DL was published in 2016 by Conte et al[10] This retrospective review of DL assignments from 1998 to 2015 reported number of placements and lost days and, for the first time, estimated cost of salaries due to these injuries. Between 1998 and 2015, there were 8357 placements, for a mean of 464 designations per year. This resulted in 460,432 days lost to injury, with a mean of 25,186 days out of play per season. The mean length of DL assignments per year was 55.1 days per injury, with a low of 49.1 days in 2011 and a high of 59.2 days in 2001. As with the 2 previous studies, placements and DL days lost showed a statistically significant increase over time. Placements ranged from a low of 387 in 1998 to a high of 536 in 2015 ($P < .001$;

$R^2 = 0.59$) (Figure 1.4). DL Days lost ranged from a low of 21,132 in 1998 to a high of 30 302 days in 2015 ($P < .003$ and $R^2 = 0.44$).

Shoulder injuries were responsible for the highest percentage of injuries and days lost (20.6% and 26.2%, respectively); however, the elbow injuries were a close second representing 19.6% injuries and 28.2% days lost. This represents an increase in elbow injuries from Posner's study.

Conte further examined the relationship between shoulder and elbow injuries over the 18 seasons, showing that while the overall percentage of injuries occurring to the upper extremity remained stable, the rate of shoulder injuries steadily decreased ($P = .023$) as the rate of elbow injuries increased ($P = .015$) (Figure 1.5). This inverse relationship was similar for the annual number of DL days for shoulder ($P = .033$) and elbow ($P = .005$) injuries.

Not only do injuries have a substantial impact on player performance, career longevity, and team success, but the financial impact can also be profound. In this study, dollars lost were calculated by prorating the injured player's daily salary and multiplying by the number of days missed on the DL. For example, if a player's annual salary is $1,820,000, his daily salary for the 182-day season is $10,000. If assigned to the DL for 15 days, a player who fills the roster spot is paid $150,000. For this work, the replacement player's prorated, daily salary was assumed to be the league minimum for that specific year. For example, if the league minimum for a given season is $182 000, and the season is 182 days long, a replacement player earns a minimum of $1000 per day while he is on the 25-man active roster. Thus, the dollars paid to the replacement would be $15,000. In this scenario, that brings the team's total cost to $165,000 ($150,000 plus

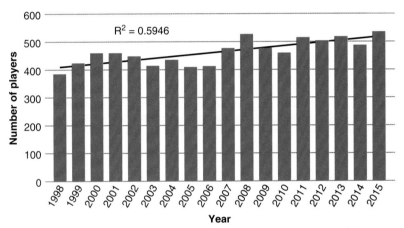

FIGURE 1.4 • Number of players assigned to the disabled list based on year. (Reprinted from Conte S, Camp CL, Dines JS. Injury trends in major league baseball over 18 seasons: 1998-2015. *Am J Orthop. (Belle Mead, N.J.)* 2016;45(3):116-123. Copyright © 2016 The American Journal of Orthopedics. All rights reserved.)

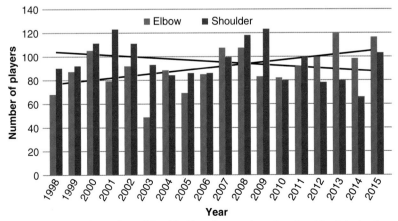

FIGURE 1.5 • Although the annual number of disabled list designations for shoulder injuries is on the decline ($P = .023$), the number of elbow injuries continues to rise ($P = .015$). (Reprinted from Conte S, Camp CL, Dines JS. Injury trends in major league baseball over 18 seasons: 1998-2015. *Am J Orthop. (Belle Mead, N.J.)* 2016;45(3):116-123. Copyright © 2016 The American Journal of Orthopedics. All rights reserved.)

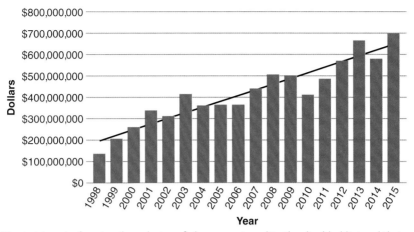

FIGURE 1.6 • The total cost of paying the salaries of players assigned to the disabled list and their replacements. (Reprinted from Conte S, Camp CL, Dines JS. Injury trends in major league baseball over 18 seasons: 1998-2015. *Am J Orthop. (Belle Mead, N.J.)* 2016;45(3):116-123. Copyright © 2016 The American Journal of Orthopedics. All rights reserved.)

$15,000). Because the league minimum salary changes year to year, salaries specific to the year of injury were used in this analysis.[11]

The results showed that an average of over $423 million was paid out by teams per year because of players on the DL plus minimum salaried replacement players. This ranged from $136 to $694 million (Figure 1.6). In total, $6,732,167,180 was paid to players assigned to the DL and $886,650,228 was spent to fill their positions. The total cost of DL assignments was $7,618,817,407 for the study period.

MLB's Health and Injury Tracking System

Most professional sports have now established injury surveillance databases including the National Football League, NBA, and the National Hockey League. In 2010, MLB and the Major League Baseball Players Association (MLBPA) reached an agreement to develop and implement a new electronic medical record (EMR). MLB's EMR was linked to injury data with the development of the Health and Injury Tracking System (HITS). This can be queried to produce deidentified data on injured players. All records were assigned a computer-generated, unique identifier to preserve confidentiality and maintain player anonymity. In addition, all individually identifiable information was stripped based on Health Insurance Portability and Accountability Act guidelines.[30]

HITS was created in 2009, pilot tested during the 2010 season, and fully implemented for injury surveillance during the 2011 season. For research studies, injuries are defined as those that are work related,

did not occur in the off-season (ie, occurred only in spring training, the regular season, or the postseason), and resulted in at least 1 day out of play (practice or game).[30]

With the advent of the HITS database, the majority of limitations associated with DL data could now be overcome.[4,30] HITS added the following categories: level of play, body side, injury mechanism, injury activity, injury location on field, SMDCS description, ICD-9 Code, reinjury, and surgery required, among others.[30] One of the biggest significance is that with the HITS system it also followed injuries occurring in MiLB players. This increased the sample size of the population from 1200 MLB players to well over 6000 players per year.

There have been an increasing number of papers published using HITS data in recent years.[1,4,5,6,12,15] The first publication using the HITS data was a descriptive epidemiologic study of hamstring injuries that occurred during the 2011 season by Ahmad et al.[1] They found that a total of 268 hamstring injuries occurred across MLB (n = 50) and MiLB (218). Hamstring injuries represented the top category of total injuries by body part, with a 0.7 per average exposure rate. When delineated by time loss by body part and injury, hamstring strains again were the most frequent and highest percentage of the total (Table 1.4).

Reinjury rates were reported at 20% for MLB and 8% for MiLB. This was significantly higher than other strains such as the abdominal obliques and adductor/groin muscles. It was similar to recurrence rates reported in other sports, which ranged from 12% to 31%. In addition, when injuries were ranked by body region, thigh, shoulder/clavicle, and hand/fingers were the top 3 categories.

TABLE 1.4 Top 10 Time-Loss Injuries by Body Part and Injury Type: Major and Minor Leagues, 2011

Injury Diagnosis	Major League			Minor League	
	No.	%		No.	%
Hamstring strain	50	5.7		218	5.9
Adductor groin strain	36	4.1		85	2.3
Oblique muscle strain	36	4.1		88	2.4
Hand contusion	32	3.7		203	6.5
Leg contusion	26	3.0		124	3.4
Knee contusion	26	3.0		88	2.4
Quadriceps strain	25	2.9			
Foot contusion	22	2.5		104	2.8
Concussion	18	2.1		101	2.7
Paralumbar muscle strain	18	2.1			
Other shoulder injury				78	2.1
Elbow contusion				73	2.0

Reprinted with permission from Ahmad CS, Dick RW, Snell E, et al. Major and minor league baseball hamstring injuries: epidemiologic findings from the major league baseball injury surveillance system. Am J Sports Med. 2014;42(6):1464-1470. Copyright © 2014 SAGE Publications.

The authors were also able to determine that base running was the top activity associated with hamstring strains, responsible for two-thirds of injuries. They further identified that the majority of base-running hamstring strains in both leagues were associated with running specifically to first base.

Oblique injuries appear to be nearly exclusive to baseball players (although they have been reported in elite level Australian cricketers). These oblique injuries in baseball are unilateral in nature and affect both hitters and pitchers. In cricket, these are almost exclusively sustained by fast pace bowlers. These are distinguished from lower rectus abdominus strains and sports hernias, which occur in multiple sports. This is not surprising as the contralateral internal oblique shows the highest EMG (electromyography) activity of the abdominal muscles during the hitting and pitching motions.[4,9]

In professional baseball, there have been 2 published studies on oblique injuries (one using the DL and the other from HITS data).[4,9] Camp et al[4] in 2017, detail 996 oblique injuries over 5 seasons in professional baseball that resulted in 22,064 total missed days. The annual injury trend remained steady in MiLB; however, injury rates actually declined for MLB. The average lost time was 22.2 days per injury, with pitchers losing more time than hitters. The leading side was injured in 77% of cases and took 5 days longer to recover from than trailing side injuries. This was similar to findings by Conte et al in 2011.[9]

Recurrence rates for oblique injuries (8.15%) were lower than those for hamstring strains (20%). Of those that did recur, 37.8% were sustained in the same season, whereas 61.2% recurred in a subsequent season. In regard to timing of the injuries, there was a downward trend in the number of injuries as the season progressed. Of the 897 oblique strains that occurred over the 6-month period from March to August, 491 occurred in the first 3 months of full activity (March to May), whereas 406 occurred in the last 3 months (June to August) ($P = .005$) (Figure 1.7). This was similar to the findings in hamstrings where the month of May had a statistically significant higher frequency of hamstring injuries than any other month in the season ($P = .0153$).[1,4]

Concussions in sports have been an important topic of study in recent years. Based on athlete-exposure rates, sports such as football, wrestling, ice hockey, and soccer have been shown to have high incidence of concussions. Baseball, however, shows one of the lowest concussion rates of all sports.[15]

At the professional level, Green et al[15] published the first report on concussions using HITS data. They reported on 307 diagnosed concussions in MLB (13.3%) and MiLB (87.7%) over 2 seasons. The median time loss per concussion was 9 days. This represented only 1% of all injuries resulting in time lost from play during that time, and the exposure rate was only 0.42 per 1000 athlete-exposures.

In examining concussions by position, catchers experienced a higher injury rate than any other position. Catchers accounted for 40.8% of concussions in

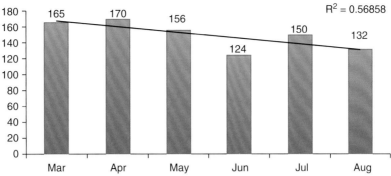

FIGURE 1.7 • Number of oblique injuries by month of the year. (Reprinted with permission from Camp CL, Conte S, Cohen SB, et al. Epidemiology and impact of abdominal oblique injuries in major and minor league baseball. *Orthop J Sports Med.* 2017;5(3):2325967117694025. Copyright © 2017 SAGE Publications.)

MiLB and 47.6% in MLB. In MLB 40% of concussions in catchers were due to collision with another player and 60% from a batted ball. In MiLB 41.4% were caused by collision with another player and 31.0% were secondary to a batted ball. In addition, a study by Rosenbaum et al[35] demonstrated that catchers sustained a higher rate of concussion because of home plate collisions than plays at other bases. These facts help MLB to develop a new rule change to protect catchers from certain slides at home plate.[15]

ELBOW ULNAR COLLATERAL LIGAMENT INJURIES

UCL Injuries

No other baseball injury has generated as much attention by researchers and media than injuries to the UCL. This increased attention and rising injury rates led the MLB and the media to declare a "Tommy John Epidemic" in 2014. Although there are multiple papers written on outcomes, surgical techniques, risk factors, and performance changes, there is a paucity of studies on incidence and prevalence of UCL reconstructions (UCLr's). Many of the epidemiologic studies have focused on MLB pitchers, and there is a void of incidence and trends in the minor league, collegiate, or high school throwers.

Frank Jobe performed the first UCLr in 1974 on the now infamous pitcher, Tommy John.[20] Interestingly, Dr Jobe did not report his series of reconstructions until 12 years later in 1986. He documented 16 reconstructions that were performed during that time, indicating that initially, there was was slow acceptance of the procedure by the orthopedic community. Jobe reported that all 16 athletes were throwers, and the majority were professional pitchers. Although the reported success rate of 62.5% would have been considered less the optimal in today's standards, he

revolutionized a condition that was previously considered to be career ending.[20]

In a more recent, single center study, Cain et al[3] reported on a large population of athletes undergoing UCLr. Although this is not a pure epidemiologic study of UCLr in baseball players, it does represent one the first published accounts that demonstrated an increasing annual number of reconstructions. The study included a total of 1266 UCLr's performed by a single surgeon over a 19-year period from 1988 to 2006. Of these, 1210 (95%) were baseball players, and 89% of the baseball players were pitchers. Broken down by level of play, 32% were professional baseball players, 48% collegiate, and 20% were either at the high school or at the recreational level. The study did not report specific trends in all of baseball: it did report on the trends within the single institution. Over the course of the study, the annual number of surgery more than doubled. They also demonstrated a significant increase in youth surgeries, theorizing that year-round baseball may be an underlying cause (Figure 1.8).

Only one study has been done on the prevalence of reconstructions across all levels of professional baseball. In 2012, an online questionnaire was distributed to the certified athletic trainers of all 30 MLB organizations.[8] They then administered the survey to all of their MLB and MiLB affiliates. It was completed by a total of 5088 players (722 major and 4366 minor league players) for an overall response rate of 89%. Consistent with other works, this study demonstrated that pitchers were undergoing reconstructions more frequently than position players. Prevalence was 10% of all players and 16% among pitchers. 25% of major league pitchers had a history of reconstruction, whereas 15% of minor league pitchers had undergone the procedure at some point during their career. Interestingly, the majority of major league pitchers underwent the UCLr as a professional (86%), in contrast to minor league pitchers who

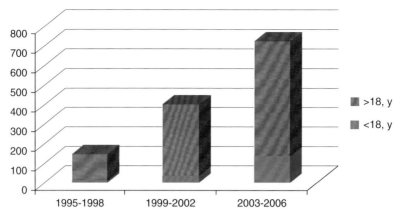

FIGURE 1.8 • Increased number of total ulnar collateral ligament (UCL) reconstructions performed at our institution during consecutive 4-year periods. Note the relative increase in percentage of UCL reconstructions performed in adolescent patients. (Reprinted with permission from Cain EL, Andrews JR, Dugas JR, et al. Outcome of ulnar collateral ligament reconstruction of the elbow in 1281 athletes: Results in 743 athletes with minimum 2-year follow-up. *Am J Sports Med*. 2010;38(12):2426-2434. Copyright © 2010 SAGE Publications.)

TABLE 1.5 Prevalence of Ulnar Collateral Ligament Reconstructions in Pitchers

	Prevalence, % (n)	P
Current level		<.001
Major league	25 (96 of 382)	
Minor league	15 (341 of 2324)	
Current age, y		<.001
21-25	14 (235 of 1698)	
26-30	27 (132 of 484)	
31-35	36 (39 of 108)	
Current role		.002
Starting pitcher	14 (161 of 1176)	
Relief pitcher	18 (276 of 1530)	
Throwing hand		.26
Right-handed	17 (328 of 1969)	
Left-handed	15 (109 of 737)	
Country of origin		
United States	16 (322 of 2007)	
Not United States	16 (115 of 699)	.81
Latin America	16 (91 of 577)	.87
Dominican Republic	16 (54 of 343)	.89

P value based on comparison with "United States."

Reprinted with permission from Conte S. Prevalence of ulnar collateral ligament surgery in professional baseball players. Am J Sports Med. 2015;43(7):1764-1769. Copyright © 2015 SAGE Publications.

were more likely to have had surgery in high school or college (61%). This study also was one the first to delineate between country of birth and UCLr status. Some media outlets had surmised that pitchers from Latin-American countries had a lower prevalence rate than US-born pitchers; however, this study did not show a difference between the two populations[8] (Table 1.5).

In another study, using public data on major league players, Conte et al[10] compiled the incidence of players undergoing the surgery since its inception in 1974 to 2015.[10] Of the 400 MLB players with a history of UCLr, pitchers accounted for 90.3% followed by outfielders (4%), infielders (3.5%), and catchers (2.3%). The data indicate a statistically significant increase in the annual number of procedures (+<0.001), and nearly one-third (32.75%) of UCLr's were performed in the final 5 years (2011-2015) of the 42-year study period (Figure 1.9).

Two recent studies using public and private databases have reaffirmed that youth injuries and resultant UCLr are on the rise. Hodgins et al[17] reviewed a 10-year period in a New York state database that contained records on ambulatory discharges. They identified all UCLr performed in the state from 2002 to 2011 (Figure 1.10). Their findings showed a 195% increase in the number of surgeries during the period with an increase in injury rate from 0.15 to 0.45 per 100,000. Importantly, the greatest increase in the rate of in UCLr was in the 17- to 18-year-old and 19- to 20-year-old age groups.

In a retrospective review of a large, privately insured patient population, Erickson et al[14] evaluated UCLr's performed between 2007 and 2011. They identified 790 surgeries resulting in an incidence of 3.96 per 100,000 patients. They reported that 15- to 19-year-olds were responsible for the greatest number of surgeries compared with any other age group. This finding was similar to the findings of Hodgins et al. Again, Erickson found that there was a statistically significant increase in the annual number of surgeries during the study period ($P = .039$). This finding mirrors other previous epidemiologic studies on an increased incidence.[21,29]

In professional baseball, most reports on UCLr in the medial and lay press rely on publically available data and focus solely on MLB athletes. Although important and informative, these studies have substantial limitations.

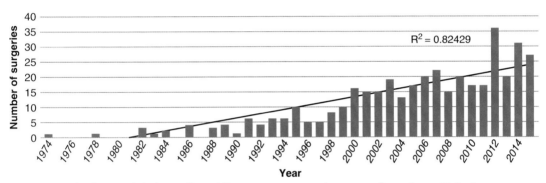

FIGURE 1.9 • The first medial ulnar collateral ligament reconstruction was performed on a Major League Baseball player in 1974. Since that time, the rate of surgery has increased to a significant degree ($P < .001$). (Reprinted from Conte S, Camp CL, Dines JS. Injury trends in major league baseball over 18 seasons: 1998-2015. *Am J Orthop (Belle Mead NJ)*. 2016;45(3):116-123. Copyright © 2016 The American Journal of Orthopedics. All rights reserved.)

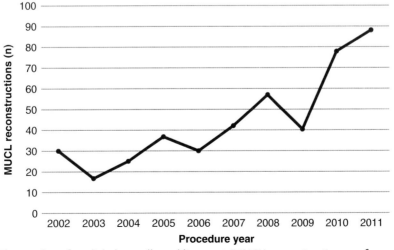

FIGURE 1.10 • The number of medial ulnar collateral ligament (MUCL) reconstructions performed in New York State by year. There is a significant trend for a greater number of reconstructions performed over time ($P < .001$). (Reprinted with permission from Hodgins JL, Vitale M, Arons RR, Ahmad CS. Epidemiology of medial ulnar collateral ligament reconstruction: a 10-year study in New York state. *Am J Sports Med*. 2016;44(3):729-734. Copyright © 2016 SAGE Publications.)

One major limitation is that they are void of minor league players, which represent a population at least 5 times as large as MLB. In 2017, Camp et al[6] reported on the largest group of professional players undergoing UCLr. The study resourced 3 different databases that included MLB HITS system, baseballheatmaps.com, and an online search, which yielded 1429 pitchers who had undergone the surgery from 1974 to 2016. This is the largest sample size of any study on professional pitchers. Of these, 1334 (93.4%) were primary surgeries, whereas 95 (6.7%) were revisions, 490 (34.3%) were MLB level pitchers, and 939 (65.7%) were in the minor leagues at the time of surgery (Figure 1.11). This is the first article to describe results in the minor league players. Ultimately, 83.7% of pitchers were able to return to play at any level, and 72.8% were able to return to their previous level of play (ie, A, AA, AAA, or MLB). The mean time to return to play was 435 days (14.3 months) to return to any level and 506 days to return to their prior level (16.6 months).

The upward incident trends in previous studies were reaffirmed in this study. They further show that there is an increase in UCLr in the period from 2010 to 2016. Notably, this increase is even more pronounced at the minor league level as minor league pitchers made up a steadily increasing proportion of all professional players undergoing UCLr (Figure 1.12). These findings are consistent with other studies that have demonstrated a rising incidence in younger pitchers.[14,17]

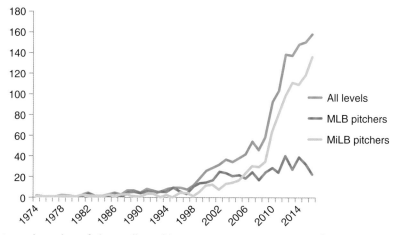

FIGURE 1.11 • Annual number of ulnar collateral ligament reconstruction in professional baseball, from 1974 to 2016. (Reprinted from Camp CL, Conte S, D'Angelo J, Fealy SA. Epidemiology of ulnar collateral ligament reconstruction in Major and Minor League Baseball pitchers: comprehensive report of 1,429 Cases. *J Shoulder Elbow Surg*. 2018;27(5):871-878. Copyright © 2018 Journal of Shoulder and Elbow Surgery Board of Trustees. With permission.)

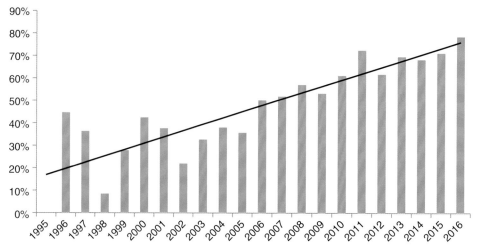

FIGURE 1.12 • Percentage of cases that were performed on minor league pitchers, 1995-2016. (Reprinted from Camp CL, Conte S, D'Angelo J, Fealy SA. Epidemiology of ulnar collateral ligament reconstruction in Major and Minor League Baseball pitchers: comprehensive report of 1,429 Cases. *J Shoulder Elbow Surg*. 2018;27(5):871-878. Copyright © 2018 Journal of Shoulder and Elbow Surgery Board of Trustees. With permission.)

REFERENCES

1. Ahmad CS, Dick RW, Snell E, et al. Major and minor league baseball hamstring injuries: epidemiologic findings from the major league baseball injury surveillance system. *Am J Sports Med*. 2014;42(6):1464-1470. doi:10.1177/0363546514529083.

2. Bonza JE, Fields SK, Yard EE, Dawn Comstock R. Shoulder injuries among United States high school athletes during the 2005-2006 and 2006-2007 school years. *J Athl Train*. 2009;44(1):76-83. doi:10.4085/1062-6050-44.1.76.

3. Cain EL, Andrews JR, Dugas JR, et al. Outcome of ulnar collateral ligament reconstruction of the elbow in 1281 athletes: results in 743 athletes with minimum 2-year follow-up. *Am J Sports Med*. 2010;38(12):2426-2434. doi:10.1177/0363546510378100.

4. Camp CL, Conte S, Cohen SB, et al. Epidemiology and impact of abdominal oblique injuries in major and minor league baseball. *Orthop J Sports Med*. 2017;5(3):2325967117694025. doi:10.1177/2325967117694025.

5. Camp CL, Curriero FC, Pollack KM, et al. The epidemiology and effect of sliding injuries in major and minor league baseball players. *Am J Sports Med*. 2017:363546517704835. doi:10.1177/0363546517704835.

6. Camp CL, Dines JS, van der List JP, et al. Summative report on time out of play for Major and Minor League Baseball: an analysis of 49.955 injuries from 2011 through 2016. *Am J Sports Med*. 2018.

7. Collins CL, Comstock RD. Epidemiological features of high school baseball injuries in the United States, 2005-2007. *Pediatrics*. 2008;121(6):1181-1187. doi:10.1542/peds.2007-2572.

8. Conte SA, Fleisig GS, Dines JS, et al. Prevalence of ulnar collateral ligament surgery in professional baseball players. *Am J Sports Med*. 2015;43(7):1764-1769. doi:10.1177/0363546515580792.

9. Conte SA, Thompson MM, Marks MA, Dines JS. Abdominal muscle strains in professional baseball: 1991-2010. *Am J Sports Med*. 2012;40(3):650-656. doi:10.1177/0363546511433030.

10. Conte S, Camp CL, Dines JS. Injury trends in major league baseball over 18 seasons: 1998-2015. *Am J Orthoped*. 2016;45(3):116-123.

11. Conte S, Requa RK, Garrick JG. Disability days in major league baseball. *Am J Sports Med*. 2001;29(4):431-436. doi:10.1177/03635465010290040801.

12. Dahm DL, Curriero FC, Camp CL, et al. Epidemiology and impact of knee injuries in major and minor league baseball players. *Am J Orthoped*. 2016;45(3):E54-E62.

13. Dick R, Sauers EL, Agel J, et al. Descriptive epidemiology of collegiate men's baseball injuries: National collegiate athletic association injury surveillance system, 1988-1989 through 2003-2004. *J Athl Train*. 2007;42(2):183-193.

14. Erickson BJ, Nwachukwu BU, Rosas S, et al. Trends in medial ulnar collateral ligament reconstruction in the United States: a retrospective review of a large private-payer database from 2007 to 2011. *Am J Sports Med*. 2015;43(7):1770-1774. doi:10.1177/0363546515580304.

15. Green GA, Pollack KM, D'Angelo J, et al. Mild traumatic brain injury in major and Minor League Baseball players. *Am J Sports Med*. 2015;43(5):1118-1126. doi:10.1177/0363546514568089.

16. High School Baseball Web. Probability of playing college and professional baseball. http://www.hsbaseballweb.com/probability.htm. Accessed May 20, 2017.

17. Hodgins JL, Vitale M, Arons RR, Ahmad CS. Epidemiology of medial ulnar collateral ligament reconstruction: a 10-year study in New York state. *Am J Sports Med*. 2016;44(3):729-734. doi:10.1177/0363546515622407.

18. Hosey RG, Puffer JC. Baseball and softball sliding injuries. Incidence, and the effect of technique in collegiate baseball and softball players. *Am J Sports Med*. 2000;28(3):360-363. doi:10.1177/03635465000280031301.

19. Janda D, Maguire R, Mackesy D, Hawkins R, Fowler P, Boyd J. Sliding injuries in college and professional baseball: a prospective study com- paring standard and break-away bases. *Clin J Sports Med*. 1993;3:78-81.

20. Jobe FW, Stark H, Lombardo SJ. Reconstruction of the ulnar collateral ligament in athletes. *J Bone Jt Surg Am*. 1986;68(8):1158-1163.

21. Jones KJ, Dines JS, Rebolledo BJ, et al. Operative management of ulnar collateral ligament insufficiency in adolescent athletes. *Am J Sports Med*. 2014;42(1):117-121. doi:10.1177/0363546513507695.

22. Knowles SB, Marshall SW, Bowling JM, et al. A prospective study of injury incidence among North Carolina high school athletes. *Am J Epidemiol*. 2006;164(12):1209-1221. doi:10.1093/aje/kwj337.

23. Krajnik S, Fogarty KJ, Yard EE, Comstock RD. Shoulder injuries in US high school baseball and softball athletes, 2005-2008. *Pediatrics*. 2010;125(3):497-501. doi:10.1542/peds.2009-0961.

24. James B. *The New Bill James Historical Baseball Abstract*. Vol 2. Detroit, MI: Free Press; 2003.

25. Lewis M. *Moneyball: the Art of Winning an Unfair Game*. Vol 1. New York, NY: W. W. Norton & Company; 2004.

26. McFarland EG, Wasik M. Epidemiology of collegiate baseball injuries. *Clin J Sport Med*. 1998;8(1):10-13.

27. National Federation of State High School Associations. High school sports participation increases for 27th consecutive year. https://www.nfhs.org/articles/high-school-sports-participation-increases-for-27th-consecutive-year/. Accessed May 19, 2017.

28. Nicholls RL, Elliott BC, Miller K. Impact injuries in baseball: prevalence, aetiology and the role of equipment performance. *Sports Med*. 2004;34:17-25.

29. Petty DH, Andrews JR, Fleisig GS, Cain EL. Ulnar collateral ligament reconstruction in high school baseball players: clinical results and injury risk factors. *Am J Sports Med*. 2004;32(5):1158-1164. doi:10.1177/0363546503262166.

30. Pollack KM, D'Angelo J, Green G, et al. Developing and implementing major league Baseball's Health and injury tracking system. *Am J Epidemiol*. 2016;183(5):490-496. doi:10.1093/aje/kwv348.

31. Posner M, Cameron KL, Wolf JM, Belmont PJ, Owens BD. Epidemiology of major league baseball injuries. *Am J Sports Med*. 2011;39(8):1676-1680. doi:10.1177/0363546511411700.

32. Powell JW, Barber-Foss KD. Injury patterns in selected high school sports: a review of the 1995-1997 seasons. *J Athl Train*. 1999;34(3):277-284.

33. Powell JW, Barber-Foss KD. Sex-related injury patterns among selected high school sports. *Am J Sports Med*. 2000;28(3):385-391. doi:10.1177/03635465000280031801.

34. Rechel JA, Yard EE, Comstock RD. An epidemiologic comparison of high school sports injuries sustained in practice and competition. *J Athl Train*. 2008;43(2):197-204. doi:10.4085/1062-6050-43.2.197.

35. Rosenbaum DA, Davis SW. Injury risk due to collisions in major league baseball. *Int J Sports Med*. 2014;35(8):704-707. doi:10.1055/s-0033-1363253.

36. Shanley E, Rauh MJ, Michener LA, Ellenbecker TS. Incidence of injuries in high school softball and baseball players. *J Athl Train*. 2011;46(6):648-654.

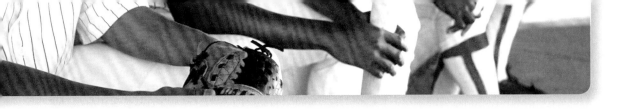

CHAPTER 2

The Biomechanics of Baseball Pitching and Throwing

Glenn S. Fleisig, PhD | Alek Z. Diffendaffer, MS | Jonathan S. Slowik, PhD

Every strike brings me closer to the next home run.

—*Babe Ruth*

INTRODUCTION

The act of throwing a baseball is a physically demanding motion that requires detailed coordination of muscles and joints and induces high loads throughout the body. Pitchers, in particular, suffer an extreme amount of throwing injuries, and their injury rate is consistently growing over time.[1] This is not surprising, as baseball pitching is among the fastest recorded human movements, resulting in ball velocities that can exceed 100 mph. This requires high velocities and accelerations in the throwing arm, and as a result the dynamic loads experienced during even a single pitch carry significant potential for injury. Pitchers may throw more than 4000 pitches per season, further increasing their injury risk. Proper throwing biomechanics are crucial to minimizing the risk of injury while simultaneously optimizing performance. While the primary focus of this chapter is on the biomechanics of pitching, the discussed concepts are valid for most overhand throwing activities.

HISTORY OF BIOMECHANICAL ANALYSIS

Technology has provided researchers, clinicians, biomechanists, and coaches with a better understanding of the joint kinematics (motions) and kinetics (forces and torques) involved in baseball pitching. Before this technology, general kinematics of baseball throwing was summarized by the naked eye.[2] As technology evolved, the use of video analysis and 3-dimensional manual digitizing helped to further investigate pitching biomechanics. Currently, the "gold standard" for studying the kinematics and kinetics of baseball pitching is using a 3D automated motion capture system,

which can be used in a laboratory setting or outdoor testing. These systems require retroreflective markers placed on the pitcher, so the camera system can track the motion of body segments. Joint kinetics is calculated using the tracked kinematics, estimated masses of body segments, and inverse dynamics equations.[3]

Future biomechanics research most likely will utilize 3D automated tracking systems that do not require markers, allowing for data capture in-game. Recent growth in computing power has shifted biomechanists toward detailed musculoskeletal modeling to simulate the throwing motion and calculate the forces and torques in specific muscles, tendons, ligaments, and bones.[4] An additional drive in technology is a growth in wearable technologies, such as inertial measurement units (IMUs) to help calculate biomechanics during pitching. IMU technology allows players and coaches to measure joint motions and stresses in real-time during a practice or game situation.[5]

THE THROWING MOTION

During the throwing motion, energy is passed up the "kinetic chain."[6] This process involves muscles and connective tissues generating, storing, and transferring energy up the body from the legs through the hips, trunk, upper arm, forearm, hand, and then finally into the ball. Proper pitching mechanics require great coordination of the entire body to enable precise sequencing and timing of segment rotations that maximize the speed of the ball without placing the thrower at high injury risk. Although the pitching kinetic chain is a continuous sequence, the motion is typically divided for easier understanding into 6 phases[3,7]: windup, stride, arm cocking, arm acceleration, arm deceleration, and follow-through (Figure 2.1).

During the windup phase (Figure 2.1A and B), the pitcher initiates his motion and generates potential energy with his lead leg. The pitcher's hands are together in front of the chest while his lead leg lifts until reaching the instant of maximum knee height (Figure 2.1B). During this phase, the forces, torques, and muscle activity in the throwing arm are low. This phase typically lasts between 0.5 and 2.0 seconds.

As the pitcher begins the stride phase (Figure 2.1B-E), the lead leg lowers while the hands simultaneously separate down and out over the lead knee (Figure 2.1C). The pitcher pushes off the back leg (Figure 2.1D) and

strides forward with the lead leg, moving his center of mass (COM) toward home plate. The instant of lead foot contact (Figure 2.1E) is a critical and coachable checkpoint where the coordinated movement of the lower body and throwing arm is evaluated. The pitcher should land with his foot placed slightly "closed" (that is, pointed inward and positioned to the right for a right-handed pitcher) with a stride length slightly less than the pitcher's height, while the lead knee should be bent to absorb the energy produced from contact. Additionally, the pitcher should begin to rotate his pelvis to face the target while the upper trunk stays closed, creating trunk

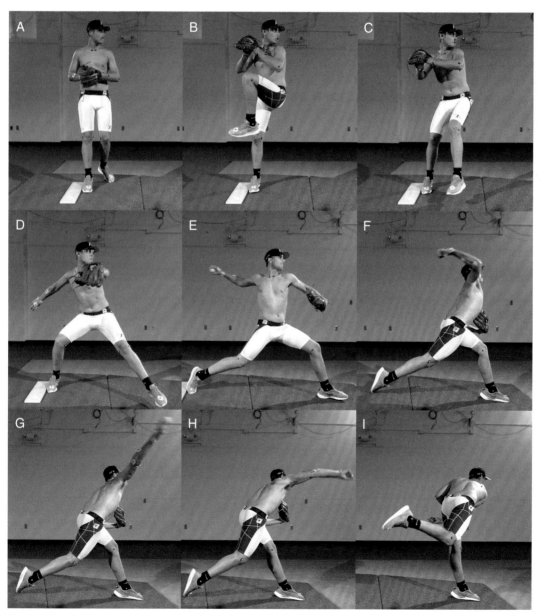

FIGURE 2.1 • Picture sequence of proper pitching biomechanics: (A) initiation, (B) maximum knee height, (C & D) mid-stride, (E) stride foot contact, (F) maximum shoulder external rotation, (G) ball release, (H) maximum shoulder internal rotation, and (I) end of pitching motion.

axial rotation and elastic energy in the trunk's musculature. At foot contact, the throwing shoulder should be abducted to 90°, horizontally abducted to 20°, and externally rotated to 50°, while the throwing elbow should be flexed to 90°. The stride phase typically lasts between 0.50 and 0.75 seconds.

During the arm cocking phase (Figure 2.1E and F), the upper body rotates to face the target while the throwing arm is externally rotated. This phase typically lasts between 0.10 and 0.15 seconds. Maximum angular velocity of pelvis and upper trunk occur during this phase. The arm cocking phase ends when the shoulder achieves its maximum external rotation (Figure 2.1F). Maximum levels of shoulder internal rotation torque and elbow varus torque occur near this instant to transition from arm cocking to arm acceleration.

The arm acceleration phase begins at the instant of external rotation (Figure 2.1F) and continues through the instant of ball release (Figure 2.1G). During this phase, the shoulder internally rotates, the elbow extends, and the wrist flexes, and as a result, all of the energy that has been generated and stored is delivered to the baseball. This phase typically lasts approximately 0.03 to 0.04 seconds. Maximum velocities of shoulder internal rotation and elbow extension occur near ball release. In fact, shoulder internal rotation during pitching (about 7500°/s) is the fastest measured human joint motion.[8] It is important to examine variables such as lead knee flexion, trunk forward tilt, trunk side tilt, shoulder abduction, and elbow flexion at the instant of ball release, to ensure that the pitcher is in the proper position.

In the arm deceleration phase (Figure 2.1G and H), eccentric forces and torques decelerate the rapidly moving arm. This phase concludes with the instant of maximum internal rotation (Figure 2.1H) and typically lasts approximately 0.03 to 0.05 seconds. Finally, the pitcher finishes the motion with the follow-through (Figure 2.1H and I) and prepares himself to field a batted ball. This phase typically lasts approximately 1 second.

To compare timing across pitches and/or pitchers, kinematic and kinetic variables are often time normalized from the instant of foot contact (0%) to the instant of ball release (100%). While this is only a small fraction of the pitch time, the critical mechanics and highest loads occur during this period. Thus this is the period with the highest risk for injury development.

It is important to optimize throwing mechanics, as poor mechanics lead to increased kinetics and an increased risk of injury from repetitive throwing.[9-12] Mechanical deficiencies can also lead to decreased velocity and performance.[9,13,14] Pitching mechanics can be improved after evaluation and instructional training; however, only about half of mechanical flaws are fixed with training, even after a comprehensive biomechanical evaluation.[15] This rate may improve in the near future, as technological advances (automated in-game digitization, IMUs) bring biomechanical measurements to more players and coaches, and younger players and coaches become more familiar with current concepts of throwing biomechanics and drills.

BIOMECHANICS OF ELBOW AND SHOULDER INJURIES

Elbow

The prevalence of ulnar collateral ligament (UCL) injuries in amateur and professional baseball continues to grow at an alarming rate.[16-18] While the general public and media have inflated confidence that "Tommy John" surgeries are always successful,[19,20] the actual percentage of pitchers returning after UCL surgery is between 67% and 83%.[21-24] Professional pitchers who successfully return after UCL reconstruction show no significant differences in pitching biomechanics or passive range of motion compared with pitchers with no history of elbow surgery.[25] However, conflicting findings have been published about whether or not professional pitchers who return exhibit diminished performance.[23,24,26]

UCL injuries occur from repetitive pitching and throwing with high elbow varus loading,[10] as tensile force in the UCL must provide nearly one-third of the total varus torque.[4] Varus torque peaks near the time of maximum shoulder external rotation (Figure 2.2), to decelerate arm cocking and initiate the forearm's forward rotation. At this point, the elbow is flexed approximately 90° and elbow varus torque in a professional pitcher is nearly 100 N m. Tension on the UCL is relatively close to the maximal tensile strength, making this ligament vulnerable to injury.[27] Compressive forces acting on the lateral radiocapitellar joint make up another 33% of the varus torque on the elbow,[10] leaving the lateral elbow susceptible to osseous injuries. From the arm-cocked position, the elbow extends and the shoulder internally rotates. During this arm acceleration, excessive shear forces in the posteromedial elbow between the olecranon and olecranon fossa may promote the development of osteophytes[28] (eg, Figure 2.3).

Shoulder

Injuries to the shoulder can manifest as pain, diminished performance (velocity and accuracy), or a decrease in strength or passive range of motion.[29] Throughout the throwing motion, the shoulder joint moves through a large range of motion in several degrees of freedom in a short duration of time. During

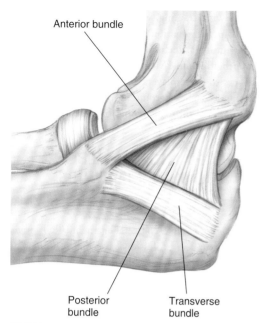

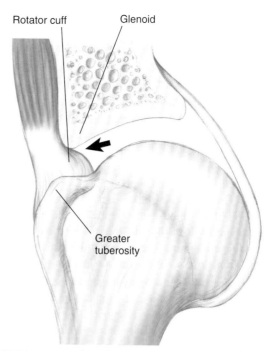

FIGURE 2.2 • Dangerously high tension occurs in the UCL—particularly in the anterior bundle—near the instant of maximum shoulder external rotation. (Illustration is adapted from Flynn JM, Skaggs DL, Waters PM. *Rockwood and Wilkins' Fractures in Children*. Philadelphia, PA: Wolters Kluwer; 2015.)

FIGURE 2.4 • When the shoulder is abducted and externally rotated, the rotator cuff can become impinged between the posterosuperior aspect of the glenoid and the greater tuberosity of the humeral head. (Illustration is adapted from Burkhart SS, Brady PC, Lo IKY. *Burkhart's View of the Shoulder: A Cowboy's Guide to Advanced Shoulder Arthroscopy*. Wolters Kluwer; 2006.)

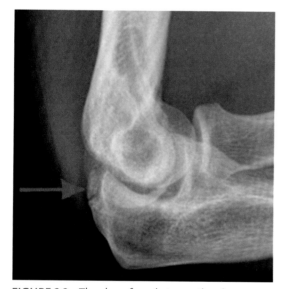

FIGURE 2.3 • The shear force between the olecranon and olecranon fossa during elbow extension can result in the development of osteophytes, such as indicated by the red arrow. (Reprinted from Fu F, ed. *Master Techniques in Orthopaedic Surgery: Sports Medicine*. 1st ed. Philadelphia, PA: Wolters Kluwer; 2010.)

the arm cocking phase, the shoulder is abducted to around 90° and maximally externally rotated (~170°). Internal impingement can occur near the instant of maximum shoulder external rotation (Figure 2.4).

As the shoulder abducts and externally rotates, the rotator cuff can become impinged between the greater tuberosity of the humeral head and the posterosuperior aspect of the glenoid.[30] A second type of impingement in overhead athletes occurs in the subacromial space. When the subacromial space becomes smaller owing to an inflamed bursae or rotator cuff muscle, this can then lead to impingement on the underside of the acromion.[31] Excessive abduction can limit the subacromial space, increasing the risk of subacromial impingement. One common labrum injury that occurs in overhead athlete is a superior labrum anterior to posterior (SLAP) lesion. Andrews and colleagues[32] were the first to report these anterosuperior labrum tears in throwers caused by the long head of the biceps pulling the labrum away from the glenoid. Biceps contraction combined with maximum external rotation results in stressful posterior shear of the biceps-labrum complex (Figure 2.5A).[33] SLAP lesions can also occur around ball release (Figure 2.5B), as the biceps contracts to resist both shoulder distraction and elbow hyperextension, creating significant stress on the anterosuperior labrum where the biceps tendon originates.[32,34] Not all SLAP tears are symptomatic, as a recent study examined asymptomatic professional pitchers, and

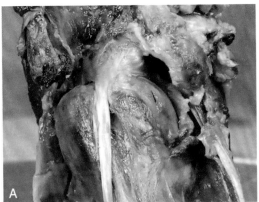
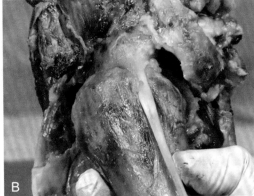

FIGURE 2.5 • Cadaveric example of the biceps tendon pulling the superior labrum: (A) shear force near the time of maximum external rotation and (B) tensile force near ball release.

TABLE 2.1 Select Biomechanical Values (Mean ± Standard Deviation) for Different Pitch Types in Professional Pitchers (n = 44)

	Pitch Type		
	Fastball	Curveball	Changeup
Arm Cocking Phase			
Maximum shoulder external rotation (°)	178 ± 10	180 ± 10	178 ± 11
Maximum varus torque (N m)	92 ± 33	88 ± 34	82 ± 30
Arm Acceleration Phase			
Maximum elbow extension velocity (°/s)	2347 ± 243	2283 ± 245	2216 ± 299
Maximum shoulder internal rotation velocity (°/s)	6904 ± 1028	6731 ± 994	6401 ± 1020
Instant of Ball Release			
Knee flexion (°)[b]	35 ± 11	38 ± 12	42 ± 11
Trunk forward tilt (°)	35 ± 8	37 ± 8	35 ± 8
Trunk side tilt (°)	25 ± 8	27 ± 8	24 ± 8
Ball velocity (m/s)[a,b,c]	37.7 ± 1.7	31.7 ± 2.3	33.8 ± 2.2

[a]Significant difference (P < .05) between fastball and curveball.

[b]Significant difference (P < .05) between fastball and changeup.

[c]Significant difference (P < .05) between curveball and changeup.

Based on data from Fleisig GS, Laughlin WA, Aune KT, Cain EL, Dugas JR, Andrews JR. Differences among fastball, curveball, and change-up pitching biomechanics across various levels of baseball. Sport Biomech. 2016;15(2):128-138.

using magnetic resonance imaging (MRI) found that 10 of 21 did in fact have SLAP tears.[35]

Although surgical repairs and rehabilitation have been implemented to treat SLAP lesions, the throwing biomechanics of these players after surgery are altered.[36] When comparing pitchers with a history of SLAP repair to a healthy-matched control group, pitchers in the SLAP repair group have less horizontal abduction at the instant of lead foot contact, less maximum shoulder external rotation, and less forward trunk tilt at the instant of ball release.

After ball release, the arm has to quickly decelerate, again placing large forces on the shoulder (Figure 2.1G and H). Rotator cuff tears can occur as the muscles attempt to resist distraction, horizontal adduction, and internal rotation during the arm deceleration phase.[37,38] If the rotator cuff and surrounding tissues are unable to stabilize the shoulder joint within the glenoid, the translation and subluxation of the humeral head in the anterior and posterior direction can cause injury to the labrum as well.

FACTORS THAT INFLUENCE THROWING BIOMECHANICS

Studies have examined a variety of pitch types (eg, fastball, curveball)[39-42] and reported only minor changes in kinematics (eg, Table 2.1). Furthermore,

TABLE 2.2 Select Kinematic Values (Mean ± Standard Deviation) for Different Levels of Baseball

	Level			
	Youth (n = 26)	High School (n = 21)	College (n = 20)	Professional (n = 44)
Instant of Lead Foot Contact				
Stride length (% of height)[b]	79 ± 7	80 ± 5	84 ± 5	82 ± 4
Lead foot oosition (cm)[a,b,c]	7 ± 14	24 ± 8	21 ± 11	25 ± 12
Shoulder external rotation (°)[b,c]	79 ± 23	60 ± 28	56 ± 26	48 ± 25
Elbow flexion (°)	83 ± 17	87 ± 17	87 ± 15	91 ± 18
Arm Cocking Phase				
Maximum pelvis angular velocity (°/s)[c]	603 ± 63	565 ± 54	562 ± 60	560 ± 74
Maximum upper trunk angular velocity (°/s)	1095 ± 78	1094 ± 88	1076 ± 92	1114 ± 81
Maximum shoulder external rotation (°)	177 ± 13	175 ± 10	177 ± 9	178 ± 10
Arm Acceleration Phase				
Maximum elbow extension velocity (°/s)	2272 ± 226	2353 ± 316	2311 ± 305	2347 ± 243
Maximum shoulder internal rotation velocity (°/s)	7077 ± 1285	7235 ± 1143	6706 ± 894	6904 ± 1028
Instant of Ball Release				
Knee flexion (°)	30 ± 10	39 ± 13	36 ± 13	35 ± 11
Trunk forward tilt (°)	34 ± 9	34 ± 7	35 ± 7	35 ± 8
Trunk side tilt (°)[b]	29 ± 9	28 ± 8	22 ± 10	25 ± 8
Ball velocity (m/s)[a,b,c,d,e,f]	26.0 ± 3.7	33.4 ± 2.4	35.6 ± 1.9	37.7 ± 1.7

[a]*Significant difference (P < .05) between youth and high school.*

[b]*Significant difference (P < .05) between youth and college.*

[c]*Significant difference (P < .05) between youth and professional.*

[d]*Significant difference (P < .05) between high school and college.*

[e]*Significant difference (P < .05) between high school and professional.*

[f]*Significant difference (P < .05) between college and professional.*

Based on data from Fleisig GS, Laughlin WA, Aune KT, Cain EL, Dugas JR, Andrews JR. Differences among fastball, curveball, and change-up pitching biomechanics across various levels of baseball. Sport Biomech. 2016;15(2):128-138.

fastballs and curveballs have been shown to generate similar kinetics, while changeups produce reduced elbow and shoulder loads.[41] These findings existed across different levels of baseball (eg, youth, high school, college, professional).[41] Studies have also specifically examined pitching changes with age and level,[41,43,44] finding remarkably similar joint angles and timing (eg, Table 2.2), but larger forces and torques at higher ages and levels.[41,45] In addition, a recent study showed that proper kinematics are developed during the first few years of pitching, while kinetic changes occur later on as the pitcher physically matures.[46] Additional studies have examined differences between pitching and training throws, finding that long-distance throws,[47] flat-ground crowhop throws,[48] and throws of balls with large differences in weights[48] may be more stressful than pitching, while flat-ground throws without a crowhop may have lower injury potential.[49] Other studies have suggested that owing to task constraints, large differences in throwing biomechanics exist between positions (eg, pitcher, catcher, infielder)[50] but that catchers in particular have similar levels of joint loading in comparison with pitchers.[51,52] Because of this, Major League Baseball and USA Baseball warn against amateur pitchers also playing as catchers.[53] Finally, differences between elite male and female pitchers have been identified, including females taking a shorter and more open (ie, positioned more to the left for a right-handed pitcher) stride and having a smaller torsional angle between the pelvis and the trunk at the instant of foot contact.[54] Female pitchers also take more time to proceed from foot contact to ball release and produce lower elbow extension angular velocity and lead knee extension during this period. This may lead to lower ball velocity and lower proximal forces at the elbow and shoulder in comparison with male pitchers.

MANAGER'S TIPS

- While the act of throwing a baseball at high velocity has inherent injury risks, the use of proper biomechanics can limit this risk while also improving performance
- It is important for sports medicine professionals to have a detailed understanding of the throwing motion and the associated potential injury mechanisms
- It is vital for sports medicine professionals who treat upper extremity injuries to understand the dynamic demands on the shoulder and elbow during throwing

REFERENCES

1. Conte SA, Requa RK, Garrick JG. Disability days in major league baseball. *Am J Sports Med.* 2001;29(4):431-436. Available at : http://www.ncbi.nlm.nih.gov/pubmed/11476381. Cited January 8, 2014.

2. Atwater AE. Biomechanics of overarm throwing movements and of throwing injuries. *Exerc Sport Sci Rev.* 1979;7(1):43-86.

3. Zheng N, Fleisig GS, Barrentine SW, Andrews JR. Biomechanics of pitching. In: Hung GK, Pallis JM, eds. *Biomedical Engineering Principles in Sports.* New York, NY: Kluwer Academic/Plenum Publishers; 2004:209-256.

4. Buffi JH, Werner K, Kepple T, Murray WM. Computing muscle, ligament, and osseous contributions to the elbow varus moment during baseball pitching. *Ann Biomed Eng.* 2014;43(2):404-415. Available at: http://link.springer.com/10.1007/s10439-014-1144-z.

5. Camp CL, Tubbs TG, Fleisig GS, et al. The relationship of throwing arm mechanics and elbow varus torque: within-subject variation for professional baseball pitchers across 82,000 throws. *Am J Sports Med.* 2017:36354651771904. Available at: http://journals.sagepub.com/doi/10.1177/0363546517719047. Cited October 3, 2017.

6. Feltner ME, Dapena J. Three-dimensional interactions in a two-segment kinetic chain. Part I: general model. *Int J Sport Biomech.* 1989;5(4):403-419. Available at: http://journals.humankinetics.com/doi/10.1123/ijsb.5.4.403. Cited May 26, 2017.

7. Fleisig GS, Barrc SW, Escamilla R, et al. Biomechanics of overhand throwing with implications for injuries. *Sport Med.* 1996;21(6):421-437.

8. Dillman CJ, Fleisig GS, Andrews JR. Biomechanics of pitching with emphasis upon shoulder kinematics. *J Orthop Sport Phys Ther.* 1993;18(2):402-408. Available at: http://www.ncbi.nlm.nih.gov/pubmed/8364594.

9. Fortenbaugh D, Fleisig GS, Andrews JR. Baseball pitching biomechanics in relation to injury risk and performance. *Sports Health.* 2009;1(4):314-320. Available at: http://www.pubmedcentral.nih.gov/articlerender.fcgi?artid=3445126&tool=pmcentrez&rendertype=abstract. Cited July 15, 2013.

10. Fleisig GS, Andrews JR, Dillman CJ, Escamilla RRFR. Kinetics of baseball pitching with implications about injury mechanisms. *Am J Sports Med.* 1995;23(2):233-239.

11. Anz AW, Bushnell BD, Griffin LP, Noonan TJ, Torry MR, Hawkins RJ. Correlation of torque and elbow injury in professional baseball pitchers. *Am J Sports Med.* 2010;38(7):1368-1374.

12. Aguinaldo AL, Chambers H. Correlation of throwing mechanics with elbow valgus load in adult baseball pitchers. *Am J Sports Med.* 2009;37(10):2043-2048. Available at: http://www.ncbi.nlm.nih.gov/pubmed/19633230. Cited February 27, 2013.

13. Urbin MA, Fleisig GS, Abebe A, Andrews JR. Associations between timing in the baseball pitch and shoulder kinetics, elbow kinetics, and ball speed. *Am J Sports Med.* 2013;41(2):336-342. Available at: http://www.ncbi.nlm.nih.gov/pubmed/23204507. Cited February 27, 2013.

14. Matsuo T, Escamilla R, Fleisig GS, Barrentine SW, Andrews JR. Comparison of kinematic and temporal parameters between different pitch velocity groups. *J Appl Biomech.* 2001;17:1-13.

15. Fleisig GS, Diffendaffer AZ, Ivey B, Aune KT. Do baseball pitchers improve mechanics after biomechanical Evaluations? *Sports Biomech.* 2018;17(3):314-321. Available at: https://www.ncbi.nlm.nih.gov/pubmed/28743205.

16. Conte SA, Fleisig GS, Aune KT, et al. Prevalence of ulnar collateral ligament surgery in professional baseball players. *Am J Sports Med.* 2015;43(7):1764-1769.

17. Hodgins JL, Vitale MA, Arons RR, Ahmad CS. Epidemiology of medial ulnar collateral ligament reconstruction: a 10-year study of New York state. *Am J Sports Med.* 2016;44(3):729-734.

18. Erickson BJ, Nwachukwu BU, Rosas S, et al. Trends in medial ulnar collateral ligament reconstruction in the United States: a retrospective review of a large private-payer database from 2007 to 2011. *Am J Sports Med.* 2015;43(7):1770-1774. Available at: http://journal.ajsm.org/cgi/doi/10.1177/0363546515580304.

19. Ahmad CS, Grantham WJ, Greiwe RM. Public perceptions of Tommy John surgery. *Phys Sportsmed.* 2012;40(2):64-72. Available at: http://www.ncbi.nlm.nih.gov/pubmed/22759607. Cited June 18, 2014.

20. Conte SA, Hodgins JL, ElAttrache NS, et al Media perceptions of Tommy John surgery. *Phys Sportsmed.* 2015;43(4):375-380.

21. Cain EL, Andrews JR, Dugas JR, et al. Outcome of ulnar collateral ligament reconstruction of the elbow in 1281 athletes: results in 743 athletes with minimum 2-year follow-up. *Am J Sports Med.* 2010;38(12): 2426-2434.

22. Osbahr DC, Cain EL, Raines BT, Fortenbaugh D, Dugas JR, Andrews JR. Long-term outcomes after ulnar collateral ligament reconstruction in competitive baseball players: minimum 10-year follow-up. *Am J Sports Med.* 2014. Available at: http://www.ncbi.nlm. nih.gov/pubmed/24705899. Cited April 9, 2014.

23. Erickson BJ, Gupta AK, Harris JD, et al. Rate of return to pitching and performance after Tommy John surgery in major league baseball pitchers. *Am J Sports Med.* 2014;42(3):536-543. Available at: http://www.ncbi.nlm.nih.gov/pubmed/24352622. Cited June 11, 2014.

24. Makhni EC, Lee RW, Morrow ZS, Gualtieri AP, Gorroochurn P, Ahmad CS. Performance, return to competition, and reinjury after Tommy John surgery in major league baseball pitchers: a review of 147 cases. *Am J Sports Med.* 2014. Available at: http:// www.ncbi.nlm.nih.gov/pubmed/24705898. Cited May 14, 2014.

25. Fleisig GS, Leddon CE, Laughlin WA, et al. Biomechanical performance of baseball pitchers with a history of ulnar collateral ligament reconstruction. *Am J Sports Med.* 2015;43(5):1045-1050. Available at: http://journal.ajsm.org/cgi/doi/10.1177/0363546515570464.

26. Jiang JJ, Leland JM. Analysis of pitching velocity in major league baseball players before and after ulnar collateral ligament reconstruction. *Am J Sports Med.* 2014;42(4):880-885. Available at: http://www.ncbi. nlm.nih.gov/pubmed/24496506. Cited June 23, 2014.

27. McGraw MA, Kremchek TE, Hooks TR, Papangelou C. Biomechanical evaluation of the docking plus ulnar collateral ligament reconstruction technique compared with the docking technique. *Am J Sports Med.* 2013;41(2):313-320.

28. Wilson FD, Andrews JR, Blackburn TA, McCluskey III GM. Valgus extension overload in the pitching elbow. *Am J Sports Med.* 1983;11(2):83-88.

29. Wilk KE, Obma P, Simpson CD, Cain EL, Dugas JR, Andrews JR. Shoulder injuries in the overhead athlete. *J Orthop Sport Phys Ther.* 2009;39(2):38-54.

30. Heyworth BE, Williams RJ. Internal impingement of the shoulder. *Am J Sports Med.* 2009;37(5):1024-1037. Available at: http://ajs.sagepub.com/lookup/doi/10.1177/0363546508324966. Cited June 14, 2017.

31. Fleisig GS, Jameson GG, Dillman CJ, Andrews JR. Biomechanics of overhead sports. In: Garrett WE, Kirkendall DT, eds. *Exercise and Sport Science.* Philadelphia: Lippincott Williams & Wilkins; 2000:563-584.

32. Andrews JR, Carson W, McLeod WD. Glenoid labrum tears related to the long head of the biceps. *Am J Sports Med.* 1985;13(5):337-341.

33. Burkhart SS, Morgan CD. The peel-back mechansim: its role in producing and extending posterior type II SLAP lesions and its effect on SLAP repair rehabilitation. *Arthroscopy.* 1998;14(6):637-640.

34. Jee WH, McCauley TR, Katz LD, Matheny JM, Ruwe PA, Daigneault JP. Superior labral anterior posterior (SLAP) lesions of the glenoid labrum: reliability and accuracy of MR arthrography for diagnosis. *Radiology.* 2001;218(1):127-132.

35. Lesniak BP, Baraga MG, Jose J, Smith MK, Cunningham S, Kaplan LD. Glenohumeral findings on magnetic resonance imaging correlate with innings pitched in asymptomatic pitchers. *Am J Sports Med.* 2013;41(9):2022-2027. Available at: http://journals. sagepub.com/doi/10.1177/0363546513491093. Cited October 3, 2017.

36. Laughlin WA, Fleisig GS, Scillia AJ, Aune KT, Cain EL, Dugas JR. Deficiencies in pitching biomechanics in baseball players with a history of superior labrum anterior-posterior repair. *Am J Sports Med.* 2014;42(12):2837-2841. Available at: http://www.ncbi.nlm.nih.gov/pubmed/25318939. Cited October 31, 2014.

37. Andrews JR, Angelo R. Shoulder arthroscopy for the throwing athlete. *Tech Orthop.* 1988;3:75-81.

38. Digiovine NM, Jobe FW, Pink M, Perry J. An electromyographic analysis of the upper extremity in pitching. *J Shoulder Elbow Surg.* 1992;1(1):15-25. Available at: http://www.ncbi.nlm.nih.gov/pubmed/22958966.

39. Escamilla R, Fleisig GS, Barrentine SW, Zheng N, Andrews JR. Kinematic comparisons of throwing different types of baseball pitches. *J Appl Biomech.* 1998;14:1-23.

40. Nissen CW, Westwell M, Ounpuu S, Patel M, Solomito MJ, Tate JP. A biomechanical comparison of the fastball and curveball in adolescent baseball pitchers. *Am J Sports Med.* 2009 Aug;37(8):1492-1498.

41. Fleisig GS, Laughlin WA, Aune KT, Cain EL, Dugas JR, Andrews JR. Differences among fastball, curveball, and change-up pitching biomechanics across various levels of baseball. *Sport Biomech.* 2016;15(2):128-138.

42. Oliver GD, Plummer H, Henning L, et al. Effects of a simulated game on upper extremity pitching mechanics and muscle activations among various pitch types in youth baseball pitchers. *J Pediatr Orthop.* 2017;1. Available at: http://insights.ovid.com/crossref?an=01241398-900000000-99084. Cited May 30, 2017.

43. Fleisig GS, Barrentine SW, Zheng N, Escamilla R, Andrews JR. Kinematic and kinetic comparison of baseball pitching among various levels of development. *J Biomech.* 1999;32(12):1371-1375.

44. Fleisig GS, Chu Y, Weber A, Andrews JR. Variability in baseball pitching biomechanics among various levels of competition. *Sport Biomech*. 2009;8(1):10-21.

45. Fleisig GS, Diffendaffer AZ, Ivey B, et al. Changes in youth baseball pitching biomechanics: a 7-year longitudinal study. *Am J Sports Med*. 2017;36354651773203. Available at: http://journals.sagepub.com/doi/10.1177/0363546517732034. Cited October 3, 2017.

46. Fleisig GS, Diffendaffer AZ, Ivey B, et al. Changes in youth baseball pitching biomechanics: a seven-year longitudinal study. *Am J Sports Med*. 2018;46(1):44-51. Available at: https://www.ncbi.nlm.nih.gov/pubmed/28968146.

47. Fleisig GS, Bolt B, Fortenbaugh D, Wilk KE, Andrews JR. Biomechanical comparison of baseball pitching and long-toss: implications for training and rehabilitation. *J Orthop Sport Phys Ther*. 2011;41(5):296-303.

48. Fleisig GS, Diffendaffer AZ, Aune KT, et al. Biomechanical analysis of weighted ball throwing exercises for baseball pitchers. *Sport Biomech*. 2017;9(3):210-215. Available at: https://www.ncbi.nlm.nih.gov/pubmed/27872403.

49. Nissen CW, Solomito MJ, Garibay EJ, Ounpuu S, Westwell M. A biomechanical comparison of pitching from a mound versus flat ground in adolescent baseball pitchers. *Sports Health*. 2013;5(6):530-536.

50. Miyanishi T, Endo S. *A Kinematic Comparison of the Delivery Motions of Catchers and Infielders in Baseball*. . Available at: https://ojs.ub.uni-konstanz.de/cpa/article/viewFile/6602/5963. Cited June 8, 2017.

51. Oliver G, Lohse K, Gascon S. Kinematics and kinetics of youth baseball catchers and pitchers. *Sports*. 2015;3(3):246-257. Available at: http://www.mdpi.com/2075-4663/3/3/246/. Cited May 30, 2017.

52. Fortenbaugh D, Fleisig G, Bolt B. *Coming down: throwing mechanics of baseball catchers*. In: *International Symposium on Biomechanics in Sports: Conference Proceedings Archive*. 2010. Available at: https://ojs.ub.uni-konstanz.de/cpa/article/view/4464. Cited June 8, 2017.

53. Major League Baseball, USA Baseball. *Pitch Smart*. 2015. Available at: www.pitchsmart.org. Cited May 13, 2015.

54. Chu Y, Fleisig GS, Simpson KJ, Andrews JR. Biomechanical comparison between elite female and male baseball pitchers. *J Appl Biomech*. 2009;25(1):22-31.

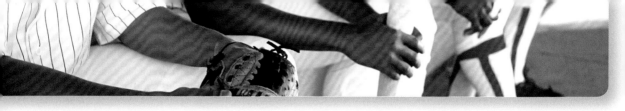

CHAPTER 3

Biomechanics of Swinging a Bat

Rafael F. Escamilla, PhD, PT, CSCS, FACSM | Brittany Dowling, MS |
Glenn S. Fleisig, PhD

A baseball swing is a very finely tuned instrument. It is repetition, and more
repetition, then a little more after that.

—*Reggie Jackson*

INTRODUCTION

Hitting a baseball is one of the most difficult skills to learn in sport.[1] Although there are several reasons why successfully hitting a baseball is so difficult, Hall of Fame pitcher Warren Spahn, who won more games than any other left-hander in Major League Baseball history, summed it up in one word, "timing," when he famously quoted "Hitting is timing. Pitching is upsetting timing." What makes the timing of hitting so challenging is the fact that both ball movement (vertical and horizontal) and ball velocity change from pitch to pitch according to the pitch type thrown. What makes it even more challenging is the fact that by the time the ball leaves a pitcher's hand, a hitter has less than one-half second to decide whether or not to swing at the pitch.

A pitcher "upsets" timing by varying ball velocity. Escamilla and colleagues[2] recently examined different pitch types in professional pitchers, which included the fastball, slider, curveball, and changeup, and reported a relatively large range of velocities among these four pitches. Using data from the Escamilla et al,[2] as well as data over the past 5 years (2012-2016),[3] it can be concluded that the fastball is the primary pitch thrown by professional baseball pitchers, thrown approximately 55% to 60% of the time with an average velocity of 92 mph. A pitcher also throws "off-speed" pitches to throw off a hitter's timing. The most common "off-speed" pitches thrown by professional baseball pitchers over the last 5 years (2012-2016) are (1) the slider, thrown approximately 15% of the time with an average velocity of 84 mph—approximately 8% slower than the fastball; (2) the changeup, thrown approximately

10% of the time with an average velocity of 83 mph—approximately 10% slower than the fastball; and (3) the curveball, thrown approximately 10% of the time with an average velocity of 78 mph—approximately 15% slower than the fastball.[3]

The different spin patterns (eg, backspin, topspin, sidespin) among different pitch types result in varying vertical and horizontal ball movements, which may also "upset" a hitter's timing, causing the batter to swing too high, low, inside, or outside relative to the ball's actual location. Using data from http://www.fangraphs.com,[3] from ball release to when the ball crosses the plate, the curveball (which has topspin) drops vertically approximately 15 inches more than a 4-seam fastball (which has backspin). Moreover, the slider drops vertically approximately 8 inches more than the fastball and the changeup drops vertically approximately 5 inches more than the fastball. Several other pitches, such as the "cutter" and "split-finger," also drop vertically more than the fastball. Compared with the fastball, these varying vertical displacements from "off-speed" pitches cause a hitter to have to adjust his swing plane, which affects a hitter's timing. Horizontal movements also vary among pitch types. The fastball and changeup both move horizontally toward the throwing arm side, whereas the slider and curveball both move horizontally toward the nonthrowing arm side. Therefore, the goal of an off-speed pitch, such as a changeup or slider, is to fool the hitter by initially looking like a fastball, therefore upsetting his timing and balance when it arrives both later and in a different location compared with the fastball.[4] How well a hitter can adjust his swing to the varying ball velocities and ball movements from each pitch determines the result of the swing, such as hitting the ball on-center resulting in a line drive, or hitting the ball off-center resulting in a pop-up or grounder.

When a hitter decides to swing at a pitch, he generates energy through the kinetic chain starting at his feet and working up through the legs, pelvis, trunk, arms, and ultimately the bat. The ultimate goal of the kinetic chain is to transfer energy from the larger, stronger, and slower moving proximal segments (hips, thighs, and trunk) to the smaller and faster moving distal segments (upper extremity and bat) to maximize bat velocity, which in turn maximizes ball exit velocity off the bat. A ball moving faster off the bat gives a fielder less time to react to and get to the batted ball, and if the ball exits off the bat both fast enough and high enough it could result in an extra base hit or a home run.

In this chapter, we will discuss the biomechanical aspects of batting. As swing biomechanics improve, a batter potentially becomes more successful as a hitter. This is important because the "success" rate (ie, getting a hit instead of an out) is relatively low, as most hitters at higher levels of baseball (college and professional) typically only succeed in hitting 25% to 35% of the time, which means they fail the majority of the time. Enhancing baseball swing biomechanics may translate to improved success in hitting.

THE FIVE PHASES OF BATTING (HITTING)

Although studies have investigated the baseball swing in various demographics, it is difficult to compare results among studies without first defining phases and key time points separating the phases. Figure 3.1 shows the five phases of the swing, which includes the stance, stride, drive, bat acceleration, and follow-through, and the key time points that define them. **Stance** is the preparatory phase of hitting before beginning the swing. The time from when the lead foot leaves the ground to when the lead foot comes back in contact with the ground is commonly referred to as the **Stride.** The transition phase from when the lead foot contacts the ground to when the hands and bat first start moving forward has also been described as the **Drive** phase. The time from when the hands and bat first start moving forward until bat-to-ball contact is the **Bat Acceleration** phase. Finally, the time from bat-to-ball contact to the end of bat and body motion is the **Follow-Through**.

Kinematic variables are presented in Table 3.1 and shown in Figure 3.2. Following the principle of

the kinetic chain, Table 3.2 illustrates that energy is transferred from the proximal larger, albeit slower segments, to the distal smaller and faster segments, and ultimately to the bat. The timing of the velocities, showing the energy progression through the kinetic chain, is shown in Table 3.3. Kinematics of the five phases of swinging are discussed in the following sections in detail.

Stance

The objective of the stance is to prepare the batter for his swing. The stance is generally self-selected and the player should be in a balanced and comfortable, athletic position. Stances vary widely among players.

When comparing batting mechanics between various competition levels, Dowling and Fleisig[5] reported professional batters had a longer stance width compared with youth batters. Similarly, when investigating batters in the same competition level, Fleisig et al[6] reported foot and trunk positioning at stance varied widely among batters. DeRenne[4] suggested that the weight should be equally distributed between the feet as this limits excessive movement during the load and stride to foot contact. However, Fortenbaugh et al[7] found professional batters shifted their weight onto their back leg during stance. It is possible that more advanced batters can load their back leg during stance and continue to control movements from load to lead foot liftoff and lead foot contact, and that youth batters might not have developed that control yet possibly resulting in longer strides and committing to the swing too early.[4]

While in the stance position, batters may move around slightly preparing for the swing. Batters can be seen swaying their hips, bending their knees, moving their hands, adjusting their weight, and even wiggling their bat as they wait for the incoming pitch. Race[8] reported the stance of a batter did not affect his batting average. Matsuo and Kasai[9] showed that even though there were differences in a batter's kinematics at stance, at ball contact there were no differences in body and bat positioning. Even though stance positions vary widely, this is a critical part of the swing. If the batter is not in his proper position, it can disrupt his timing and alter his mechanics through the entire swing.

Stride

The stride phase is identified as the time from when the batter lifts his lead foot off the ground until the time it touches back down, and according to Escamilla et al, it represents about 60% of the swing.[10,11] The height a batter lifts his foot varies considerably, both

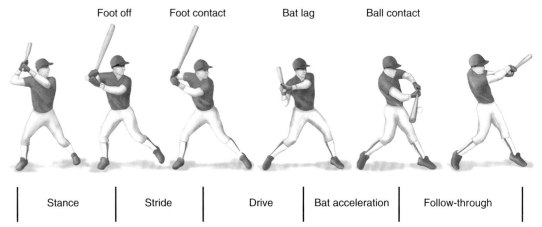

FIGURE 3.1 • Five phases of hitting a baseball: stance, stride, drive, bat acceleration, and follow-through.

among and within all levels of baseball. At higher levels of baseball (college and professional), the batter's lead foot typically lifts off the ground near the time the pitcher's lead foot contacts the ground. The batter's lead foot typically begins moving back down toward the ground at or shortly after the pitcher releases the ball. During the stride phase, the batter decides if he is going to swing at the incoming ball. When comparing youth with adult batters, Escamilla et al[10] found adult batters spent more time in the stride phase indicating adult batters took more time loading up and preparing for the swing. Conversely, Inkster et al[12] and Dowling and Fleisig[5] reported no differences in swing time between age and skill groups.

At the initial part of the stride, there is a slight rotation of the back arm and the trunk toward the catcher, combined with a shift of weight toward the rear leg. Welch[13] reported that the back leg takes on 102% of the body weight during the stride. As the batter moves forward, his hands and bat move back slightly and the pelvis slightly rotates toward the pitcher. This is considered loading, or coiling, and is illustrated by the batter moving his segments in the opposite direction of his intended movement. The stride also includes a step the batter takes toward the pitcher, generating linear momentum toward the direction of the pitch. Coaches stress the proper shift of body weight from the back leg to the lead leg during the stride, as it promotes proper timing and dynamic balance.[14] The lead foot is placed back on the ground just before the ball arrives. Professional batters have been shown to load and stride using the same mechanism for all pitches.[7] It is interesting DeRenne[4] suggests the stride length should be around 12 inches (30.5 cm) and that any longer could potentially cause a greater weight shift and cause lunging, whereas most of the reported

stride lengths in research have been between 81 and 87 cm.[10,11,13] It appears that batter's stride length is consistent between age and competition levels with a range of 39% to 48% of body height.[5,10,11] The stride causes the momentum of the batter's center of mass to shift forward toward the pitcher. In fact, the swing is initiated by ground contact of the lead foot, not the back leg as many coaches believe.[13] Lead foot contact provides a base for support and for the body to begin rotation over it, beginning with the pelvis and then energy transferred up to the upper torso.

Drive

The drive phase starts when the lead foot contacts the ground and ends at maximum bat lag. During this phase, the pelvis and upper torso rotate toward the pitcher and there is a lag between the two segments during rotation, resulting in trunk axial rotation. When the lead foot contacts the ground, it provides a base of support, stopping the body from moving forward, and begins the initiation of pelvis and trunk rotation.[13,15]

Coaches and researchers stress the importance of pelvis rotational velocity and its influence on bat velocity. Race[8] used 16 mm film to study professional batters and concluded hip (pelvis) linear velocity was of significant importance for effective hitting. More recent research has been unable to find this link. Inkster et al[12] found no difference in skilled and novice batter's pelvis linear velocity but found that skilled batters had 7% faster pelvis rotational velocity compared with the novice group. When comparing different age groups, Escamilla et al[10] found adult batters had faster pelvis rotational velocity, whereas in contrast Dowling and Fleisig[5] reported youth batters had faster pelvis rotational velocities. Dowling and Fleisig[5] suggested

TABLE 3.1 Positional Data for the Phases of the Swing

Reference	Participants	Event	Stride (cm)	Stride (% Height)	Lead Elbow Flexion	Back Elbow Flexion	Lead Knee Flexion	Back Knee Flexion	Upper Trunk Rotation	Pelvis Rotation	Twist
Welch et al[13]	7	Load	85	380% hip	70 ± 11	124 ± 10	41 ± 8	42 ± 15	29 ± 16	−4 ± 17	
		Foot contact		Width							
		Hands move forward									
		Ball contact			37 ± 8	57 ± 9	15 ± 9	45 ± 12	−66 ± 22	−83 ± 9	
Escamilla et al[11]	14 (normal grip)	Load	86 ± 9	48 ± 4	77 ± 13	126 ± 17	46 ± 12	49 ± 15	−16 ± 9	−10 ± 5	−6 ± 7
		Foot contact			57 ± 9	129 ± 8	38 ± 10	44 ± 17	−25 ± 7	−10 ± 5	−15 ± 10
		Hands move forward			66 ± 11	131 ± 19	65 ± 25	44 ± 15	−20 ± 18	−10 ± 6	−9 ± 9
		Ball contact			18 ± 7	54 ± 15	11 ± 5	64 ± 10	51 ± 8	72 ± 13	21 ± 16
	14 (choke-up)	Load	87 ± 8	48 ± 4	78 ± 14	127 ± 14	47 ± 13	49 ± 16	−13 ± 9	−9 ± 6	−4 ± 6
		Foot contact			62 ± 10	133 ± 8	39 ± 11	43 ± 15	−22 ± 8	−10 ± 6	−12 ± 9
		Hands move forward			70 ± 12	132 ± 15	64 ± 24	45 ± 16	−19 ± 7	−9 ± 6	−9 ± 8
		Ball contact			16 ± 9	54 ± 15	11 ± 5	62 ± 9	48 ± 8	65 ± 11	16 ± 14
Escamilla et al[10]	12 (youth)	Load	81 ± 7	47 ± 3	77 ± 10	140 ± 9	51 ± 12	52 ± 10	−18 ± 11	−19 ± 6	0 ± 10
		Foot contact			61 ± 11	135 ± 9	34 ± 7	44 ± 13	−25 ± 5	−12 ± 6	−13 ± 7
		Hands move forward			67 ± 10	138 ± 8	47 ± 19	43 ± 14	−27 ± 8	−16 ± 9	−11 ± 11
		Ball contact			14 ± 7	64 ± 15	15 ± 11	62 ± 6	58 ± 4	81 ± 5	22 ± 5
	12 (adult)	Load	87 ± 9	48 ± 5	77 ± 14	124 ± 18	45 ± 13	49 ± 16	−15 ± 9	−10 ± 5	−6 ± 8
		Foot contact			59 ± 10	129 ± 9	39 ± 10	46 ± 16	−24 ± 9	−10 ± 5	−14 ± 9
		Hands move forward			67 ± 14	129 ± 19	70 ± 15	47 ± 14	−17 ± 8	−12 ± 5	−6 ± 9
		Ball contact			18 ± 6	55 ± 17	11 ± 4	66 ± 10	48 ± 6	71 ± 13	23 ± 11

Study	Group	Phase							
Inkster et al[12]	10 (elite)	Load	21 ± 19% hip width						
		Foot contact							
		Hands move forward							
		Ball contact		148 ± 12	131 ± 15	136 ± 7	106 ± 4		
	10 (subelite)	Load	28 ± 14						
		Foot contact							
		Hands move forward							
		Ball contact		139 ± 14	134 ± 11	137 ± 9	100 ± 5		
Dowling and Fleisig[5]	33 (youth)	Load	41 ± 6	83 ± 13	129 ± 14	53 ± 12	56 ± 13	-10 ± 6	-20 ± 9
		Foot contact		72 ± 16	127 ± 11	46 ± 11	51 ± 10	-22 ± 10	-17 ± 11
		Hands move forward							
		Ball contact							
	69 (high school)	Load	39 ± 4	55 ± 18	89 ± 15	20 ± 8	65 ± 10	12 ± 6	92 ± 12
		Foot contact		87 ± 12	128 ± 11	60 ± 13	59 ± 12	-9 ± 6	-14 ± 8
		Hands move forward		79 ± 12	128 ± 9	51 ± 12	54 ± 11	-19 ± 8	-17 ± 9
		Ball contact							
	22 (college)	Load	41 ± 5	60 ± 16	87 ± 15	22 ± 10	56 ± 12	-9 ± 6	87 ± 12
		Foot contact		85 ± 8	128 ± 7	64 ± 11	67 ± 9	-8 ± 5	-13 ± 6
		Hands move forward		77 ± 11	128 ± 7	56 ± 11	57 ± 9	-18 ± 9	-20 ± 7
		Ball contact							
	46 (professional)	Load	41 ± 3	56 ± 13	82 ± 12	25 ± 8	61 ± 12	-10 ± 5	83 ± 10
		Foot contact		84 ± 10	125 ± 10	61 ± 12	56 ± 11	-8 ± 5	-13 ± 7
		Hands move forward		75 ± 9	123 ± 7	51 ± 10	52 ± 9	-21 ± 11	-16 ± 8
		Ball contact		55 ± 12	78 ± 12	21 ± 8	59 ± 10	-13 ± 7	81 ± 9

Twist is the difference between upper trunk rotation and pelvis rotation.

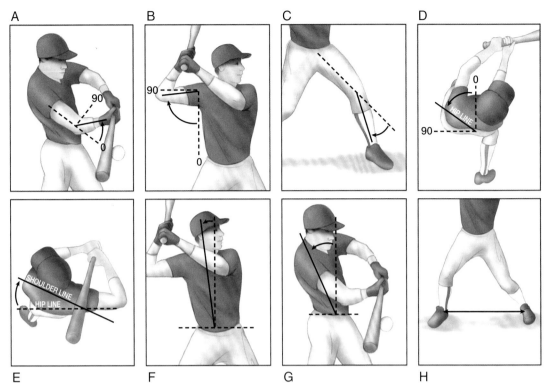

FIGURE 3.2 • Kinematic variables measured in hitting a baseball. A, Elbow flexion; B, shoulder abduction; C, knee flexion; D, pelvic rotation; E, upper trunk rotation; F, upper trunk lateral flexion; G, upper trunk flexion; H, stance width.

because youth have less mass, thus less inertia, compared with the professional group, they are able to generate faster velocities at their pelvis.

Bat Acceleration

At the end of bat lag, the hands and bat start moving and accelerating forward until bat-ball contact; this is referred to as the bat acceleration phase. The pelvis and trunk rotate toward the pitcher, initiating bat velocity.[16] Elbow extension combined with continued pelvis and trunk rotation causes the bat to increase in velocity. In fact, it has been suggested that if lead elbow extension occurs immediately after swing initiation (hands move forward), it will allow for greater bat velocity.[16] Breen suggests that poor hitters pull the bat, with a bent elbow, which inhibits the transfer of energy.[16] Inkster et al[12] investigated novice and skilled baseball players matched for height and weight and found that the skilled players had greater lead elbow extension velocity (991°/s) compared with the novice hitters (729°/s) (Table 3.2). When comparing age groups, both Escamilla et al[10] and Dowling and Fleisig[5] reported the older group had faster elbow extension velocity compared with the younger group.

However, all three studies showed no differences in the timing of when the elbow extension velocity occurred (Table 3.3).

Ideally, the bat should reach maximum velocity at the time of ball contact because it allows for optimal transfer of energy to the ball; however, there are conflicting results in the literature. Some research reports maximum bat velocity 10 to 35 ms before ball contact (Table 3.3)[13,17,18]; however, these studies processed their data differently (eg, filtering bat marker data). Conversely, Tabuchi et al[19] and Dowling and Fleisig[5] used unfiltered bat marker data and reported maximum bat velocity occurred at ball contact. Filtering data has been shown to cause a shift in peak velocity and thus causing researchers to miss true maximum velocity and acceleration curves.[20,21]

Follow-Through

The follow-through phase begins at the instant of bat-ball contact and ends when the swing is complete, generally when the lead shoulder is maximally abducted. During this phase, the batter continues to rotate his trunk and shoulders to decelerate his rapidly moving segments. Maximal trunk axial rotation has been

TABLE 3.2 Maximum Joint and Segment Angular Velocities During a Swing (°/s)

Reference	Participants	Lead Knee Extension	Back Knee Extension	Pelvis Rotation	Trunk Rotation	Lead Elbow Extension	Back Elbow Extension	Bat Velocity (m/s)
Welch[13]	7			714 ± 76	937 ± 102			31 ± 2
Escamilla et al[11]	14 (normal grip)	378 ± 65		681 ± 94	850 ± 50	722 ± 131	928 ± 120	31 ± 4
	14 (choke-up)	350 ± 60		669 ± 119	884 ± 67	732 ± 102	997 ± 110	28 ± 5
Escamilla et al[10]	12 (youth)	303 ± 76		632 ± 117	717 ± 86	598 ± 126	849 ± 151	25 ± 3
	12 (adult)	386 ± 60		678 ± 87	857 ± 53	752 ± 95	936 ± 190	30 ± 2
Inkster et al[12]	10 (elite)	386 ± 81	474 ± 183	897 ± 72		991 ± 230	1907 ± 614	37 ± 3
	10 (subelite)	474 ± 183	474 ± 368	836 ± 57		729 ± 248	1886 ± 330	34 ± 2
Dowling and Fleisig[5]	33 (youth)	367 ± 139	243 ± 83	743 ± 71	428 ± 87	225 ± 105	1174 ± 307	26 ± 3
	69 (high school)	321 ± 98	244 ± 102	686 ± 80	476 ± 121	238 ± 122	1430 ± 340	31 ± 3
	22 (college)	319 ± 79	209 ± 94	696 ± 64	530 ± 94	286 ± 117	1448 ± 281	37 ± 6
	46 (professional)	168 ± 59	168 ± 59	665 ± 63	509 ± 102	324 ± 178	1539 ± 319	38 ± 2

TABLE 3.3 Timing of Maximum Joint and Segment Angular Velocities

Reference	Participants	Lead Knee Extension	Back Knee Extension	Pelvis Rotation	Trunk Rotation	Lead Elbow Extension	Back Elbow Extension	Bat Velocity
Welch[13]**	7			−75	−65	0.5	−15	−15
Escamilla et al[11]*	14 (normal grip)	66 ± 11		60 ± 12	65 ± 7	73 ± 12	79 ± 12	
	14 (choke-up)	68 ± 10		64 ± 13	67 ± 11	77 ± 11	82 ± 11	
Escamilla et al[10]**	12 (youth)	75 ± 12		76 ± 11	77 ± 10	90 ± 13	95 ± 10	
	12 (adult)	78 ± 10		82 ± 13	88 ± 6	93 ± 12	96 ± 12	
Inkster et al[12]**	10 (elite)			−64 ± 22		−10 ± 22		
	10 (subelite)			−83 ± 21		−21 ± 33		
Dowling and Fleisig[5]**	33 (youth)	−61 ± 67	−22 ± 100	−84 ± 19	83 ± 32	−79 ± 86	25 ± 21	0 ± 0
	69 (high school)	−74 ± 90	3 ± 35	−81 ± 19	65 ± 47	−126 ± 100	31 ± 13	0 ± 0
	22 (college)	−69 ± 62	−23 ± 83	−80 ± 17	65 ± 41	−111 ± 31	25 ± 7	0 ± 0
	46 (professional)	−65 ± 55	−4 ± 94	−81 ± 14	64 ± 28	−131 ± 103	37 ± 8	0 ± 0

*, Percentage of swing; **, Time relative to ball contact (ms), 0 ms = ball contact.

shown to occur after ball contact,[6] but because of different methods of data processing between studies, it is hard to find conclusive evidence for this. However, Dowling and Fleisig[5] have reported maximum trunk angular velocity to occur after ball contact for all competition levels. The elbows extend through ball contact and finish fully extended. The only research that has reported kinematics during the follow-through phase is from Dowling and Fleisig[5] because most studies end their investigation at bat-ball contact. Dowling and Fleisig[5] report that youth batters do not extend their lead elbow as much as professional batters do

(42° flexion compared with 27°, respectively) (Table 3.1). Some batters choose to release their top hand after contact and finish the swing with one hand on the bat. Although the follow-through does not affect the path and velocity of the ball, as the ball has already left the bat, it is possible that a premature release of the top hand could lengthen the swing.[4]

PERFORMANCE

Fast bat velocity is one of the key indicators of a successful swing.[16,22] In fact it is stressed that to become a better hitter, batters should work to increase their bat velocity. Increasing bat velocity allows for batters to increase the time to decide on whether or not to swing, decrease the swing time, and increase batted-ball velocity. It takes a batter roughly 150 ms, just 2 or 3 blinks of an eye, to track the pitched ball and judge the correct response. This initial neural process of tracking the ball cannot be sped up. However, the longer the time available after the first 150 ms of the swing, the more detailed the selection process and higher probability that the best swing pattern will be chosen.

Increased Decision Time

A batter only has 400 to 500 ms to visually track a pitched ball, decide if he wants to swing at the incoming ball, and if he does want to swing, perform the swing.[23] The time the batter has to visually track the ball and decide to swing is called decision time. For high school batters the decision time is about 200 ms[24] and for major leaguers it is 260 to 350 ms.[16] The longer the batter can wait before he swings, the more time he has to recognize the type of pitch thrown, velocity and movement of the pitch, and the final location of the pitch.

Decreased Swing Time

If a hitter decides to swing, he must adjust to the incoming pitch. Swing time is defined as the time the batter initiates his swing to bat-ball contact and is inversely proportional to decision time. The shorter the swing time, the more decision time the batter has. Professional batters' swing time is 190 to 280 ms,[5,16] whereas high schoolers have a slower time of 275 to 300 ms.[5,24] It is most likely youth batters have slower swing time because they have slower bat velocities and less muscular strength.[4] If a pitcher throws a fastball at 40 m/s (90 mph), it will reach home plate in 417 ms, the batter has a decision time of 200 ms, and swing time of 200 ms. Decreased swing time allows the batter to have increased decision time and thus allow the batter to be selective to only strikes.

Increased Bat-Ball Velocity

According to Adair,[23] if a batter could swing his game bat faster or swing a heavier bat at the same velocity as his game bat, the ball would be hit harder and/or travel further. He suggests this is due to the greater momentum that is imparted on the ball by the bat. To illustrate this idea, Adair[23] demonstrated the distance a ball thrown at 38 m/s (85 mph) would travel when hit by a bat swung at four different velocities (27, 31, 36, and 30 m/s). He reported the ball would travel 99, 114, 134, and 153 m when hit with a wood bat at the center of percussion (COP), respectively. When using an aluminum bat, the ball would travel an additional 9 m further compared with the ball hit with the wood bat. Aluminum bats have been shown to have faster bat-ball velocities compared with wood bats of the same weight.[25-27] This is because aluminum bats of the same length and circumference of wood bats are lighter in weight and thus have lower moments of inertia resulting in faster bat velocities and increased bat-ball velocity.[27] Moment of inertia has shown to be more associated with bat velocity than bat weight[28-32]; in fact, bats with higher moments of inertia are swung with slower velocities.[27,28,33] Additionally, the elastic properties of the two materials are different, and aluminum bats have greater deformation during impact, resulting in less energy lost and higher batted-ball velocities compared with wood bats.[27] The composition of a bat also affects bat velocity. Fleisig et al[28] investigated the effects of bat mass properties with bat velocity. The authors reported decreased mass properties were associated with increased bat velocity; specifically, bat-ball velocity varied among the different bats and was associated with the bat's moment of inertia. Impact location has been investigated as a contributing factor to bat-ball velocity. Crisco et al[27] found a curvilinear relationship between bat-ball velocity and impact location for wood bats and identified a region on the bat that had the largest rebound effect. The location on the bat is named the "sweet spot" and produces the greatest bat-ball velocity.[27,30] In fact, for every 2.5 cm away from the sweet spot, there is an associated decrease in bat-ball velocity of 4.5 m/s.[27] However, the sweet-spot location varies between studies. Some research has identified the sweet spot as the COP, the node of the lowest vibration, whereas others have identified it as the location that minimizes the total energy lost during impact to vibration. Crisco et al[27] reported no difference in the location and size of the COP between wood and aluminum bats, whereas Bryant et al[25] reported that COP in an aluminum bat was wider than in a wood bat and last located 20.3 cm from the tip of the bat. Fleisig et al[28] identified the "sweet spot"

15 cm from the tip, and Nathan[34] reported maximum bat-ball velocity to be 13.7 cm from the tip of a wood bat.

INCREASING BAT VELOCITY

From Little League to the Major League, coaches and athletes are always looking for ways to increase bat velocity. Previous studies have reported that increasing bat velocity is important for players' long-term success.[23,35] For decades batters have tried to increase bat velocities by using weighted bats, donut rings, Power Swings, and Power Sleeves during warm-ups on deck (Table 3.4). Theoretically, it is thought that swinging a heavier bat or weighted device activates and engages more motor units and continues to function when the weighted device is removed, but it is unknown how long these effects last. Conversely, it has been suggested that the addition of weighted implements have no effect on bat velocity but instead produce a "kinesthetic after-effect" of increased bat velocity.[36,37]

The results of 6 studies showed that normal or slightly underweight bats produced the fastest bat velocities when followed by standard bats.[22,38-42] In a series of studies by DeRenne et al,[22,39,40] it was found that weighted warm-up implements between 27 and 34 oz produced the fastest bat velocities in high school[22] and college[39,40] players when swinging a standard bat (30 oz). These data imply that using slightly underweight or slightly overweight bats that were within 10% to 15% of a standard bat weight was more effective in enhancing bat velocity of a standard weight bat. In contrast, these authors reported that using a very heavy (over 42 oz) or a very light (under 27 oz) bat during warm-up actually slowed down the swing (a decrease of 2.2 m/s).[22,40] Similarly, Montoya et al[41] suggested that batters do not swing heavy bats on-deck as it produced the slowest bat velocities but that using light or standard bats produced faster bat velocities compared with the heavy bat. Researchers stress the idea of specificity training and that batters should train with the bat that is going to be used in competition, especially during preseason and in-season. Moreover, they suggest that different bat weights have different moments of inertia and cause changes in the bat path resulting in training a motor pattern not used with the standard bat. Studies have shown that the use of weighted bats during warm-up caused changes in timing and errors when using the standard game bat in competition.[33,37,38] Southard and Groomer[38] reported that heavier bats produced slower bat velocities as well as changes in the swing pattern. Similarly, Laughlin et al[33] investigated the effects of

different moments of inertia within weighted bats. They reported weighted bats with the weight added to the knob, instead of the barrel, had similar moments of inertia to a standard bat, and batters were able to replicate the swing characteristics between the standard bat and the handle-weighted bat.[33] Changing the moment of inertia from 0.24 to 0.16 kg/m² caused an increase in bat speed by 2 m/s (4.5 mph).[30] Although heavier bats (weighted bats, donut rings, sleeves, etc) used on-deck have been shown to adversely affect swing speed, heavier bats have shown to have a psychological advantage because the standard bat feels lighter.[22,37,38,42] This has led researchers to believe that using weighted implements are more of a psychological advantage rather than biomechanical. Therefore, researchers have stressed that if batters want to use warm-up devices, they should choose devices within 12% of their standard bat weight.[22,39,40,43]

Long-term effects of weighted and underweighted implements have also been shown to increase bat velocity. Focusing on the idea of specificity, 3 studies were conducted looking at the effects of weighted bat training for a period of 6 to 12 weeks. Two studies investigated the effect of swings using weighted bats 8% to 100% greater than the standard bat,[44,45] and the other studies used both underweight bats, 12% less than the standard bat, and weighted bats, as much as 100% greater weight than a standard bat.[35,44] The findings of these studies revealed that swinging underweight and overweight bats for 6 to 12 weeks increased bat velocity. DeRenne and colleagues used bat weights with 12% of the standard bat and suggested that this was more appropriate for players to use in season, whereas, Sergo and Boatwright[44] reported that any bat, overweight (62 oz) or underweight, swung 300 times a week produced greater bat velocity. However, overweight bats have been shown to change a batter's swing mechanics[35,38] and should be used with caution and only during the off-season.

Changing the grip on the bat has also been suggested by coaches as a way to increase bat velocity. Choke-up grip during batting has been suggested to increase bat velocity and bat control. Escamilla et al[11] found choke-up grip decreased the swing time compared with a normal grip swing. The decreased swing time allows the batter more time to decide if he wants to swing at the ball; however, the choke-up grip had a slower bat velocity.[11] It is possible that because the choke-up grip changes the moment of inertia of the bat, the bat-ball velocity and distance the ball traveled would decrease.

General strength has been related to bat swing velocity. Grip strength has shown to be significantly

TABLE 3.4 Effect of Bat Weight on-Deck on Bat Velocity

Reference	n	Level	Device and Weight	Results
DeRenne[39]	23	College, ex-college, and professional	Donut ring (16 3/4 oz)	The overweight and underweight bats (within 10%-15% of the weight of a standard bat) produced the fastest bat velocities.
			Power swing (32 oz)	
			Weighted bat (34 oz)	
			Light bat (23, 25, 27 oz)	
DeRenne and Branco[40]	20	College	Donut ring (16 3/4 oz)	Bats lighter than 27 oz and heavier than 34 oz produced slowest bat velocity.
			Power swing (32 oz)	
			Power sleeve (4 oz)	
			Overweight aluminum bat (32, 42, 45, 48, 51 oz)	
			Underweight aluminum bat (23, 25, 27, 29 oz)	
DeRenne et al[22]	60	High school	Donut ring (58 oz)	Slightly underweight and overweight bats (between 27 and 34 oz) produced the greatest bat velocity.
			Power swing (62 oz)	
			Power sleeve (34 oz)	
			Weighted aluminum bat (32, 42, 45, 48, 51 oz)	
			Underloaded aluminum bat (23, 25, 27, 29 oz)	
Montoya et al[41]	19	Recreational	Underweight bat (9.6 oz)	Underweight and standard bats produced fastest bat velocities.
			Standard bat (31.5 oz)	
			Overweight bat (55.2 oz)	
Southard and Groomer[38]	10	College	Standard bat (34 oz)	Swings with donut ring produced slower bat velocities. The standard bat produced the fastest bat velocities.
			Donut ring (56 oz)	
			Hallow plastic bat (12 oz)	
Reyes and Dolny[55]	19	College	Underweight bat (794 g = 28 oz)	No statistical difference between bat weights and bat velocity
			Standard bat (850 g = 30 oz)	
			Power wrap (1531 g = 54 oz)	
Szymanski et al[43]	22	College	Standard bat (30 oz)	No difference in bat velocity between all 10 different weights.
			Aluminum bat (26 oz)	
			Wood bat (34 oz)	
			Power fin (14 oz)	
			Schutt Dirx (96 oz)	
			Fungo bat (22 oz)	
			Pitcher's nightmare	
			Draz gloves (50 oz)	
			Donut ring (16 oz)	
			Power wrap (24 oz)	
Wilson et al[56]	16	College	Underweight bat (26 oz)	No difference in bat velocity between different overweight bats.
			Standard bat (30 oz)	
			Overweight bat (34 oz)	
			Overweight bat (38 oz)	
			Donut (50 oz)	

(continued)

TABLE 3.4 Effect of Bat Weight on-Deck on Bat Velocity   (continued)

Reference	n	Level	Device and Weight	Results
Otsuji et al[42]	8	College	Normal wood bat (920 g = 32.5 oz)	Swings with the overweigh bat produced slower bat speeds.
			Donut ring (800 g = 28 oz)	
Nakamoto et al[37]	8	College	Standard bat (850 g = 30 oz)	Swings with the overweight bat produced faster bat velocities.
			Overweight bat (1200 g = 42 oz)	

n, number of participants.

related to bat swing velocity in NCAA Division 1 baseball players[46] and high schoolers.[47-49] Additionally, researchers have indicated that baseball players with greater lower body strength,[49-51] upper body strength,[52] rotational power,[53,54] and lean body mass[46,50,54] have faster bat velocity. Improving bat velocity has also been shown through strength and power training. Resistance training originally was neglected and suggested by coaches to be avoided, as it could decrease baseball performance.[4] However, recently resistance training has started to play a larger role in baseball, as it is now believed that strength and power are key components to a player's performance.

REFERENCES

1. Fleisig GS, Kwon Y-H. *The Biomechanics of Batting, Swinging, and Hitting.* New York, NY: Routledge; 2014:1.

2. Escamilla RF, Fleisig GS, Groeschner D, et al. Biomechanical comparisons among fastball, slider, curveball, and changeup, pitch types and between balls and strikes in professional baseball pitchers. *Am J Sports Med.* 2017;45(14):3358-3367.

3. Levy WC, Cerqueira MD, Harp GD, et al. Effect of endurance exercise training on heart rate variability at rest in healthy young and older men. *Am J Cardiol.* 1998;82(10):1236-1241.

4. DeRenne C. *The Scientific Approach to Hitting: Research Explores the Most Difficult Skill in Sport.* 2nd ed. San Diego, CA; 2011.

5. Dowling B, Fleisig GS. Kinematic comparison of baseball batting off of a tee among various competition levels. *Sports Biomech.* 2016;15(03):255-269.

6. Fleisig GS, Hsu WK, Fortenbaugh D, et al. Trunk axial rotation in baseball pitching and batting. *Sports Biomech.* 2013;12(4):324-333.

7. Fortenbaugh D, Fleisig GS, Onar-Thomas A, et al. The effect of pitch type on ground reaction forces in the baseball swing. *Sports Biomech.* 2011;10(4):270-279.

8. Race D. A cinematographic and mechanical analysis of the external movements involved in hitting a baseball effectively. *Res Q.* 1961;32:394-404.

9. Matsuo T, Kasai T. Timing strategy of baseball-batting. *J Hum Mov Stud.* 1994;27(6):253-269.

10. Escamilla RF, Fleisig GS, DeRenne C, et al. A comparison of age level on baseball hitting kinematics. *J Appl Biomech.* 2009;25(3):210-218.

11. Escamilla RF, Fleisig GS, Derenne C, et al. Effects of bat grip on baseball hitting kinematics. *J Appl Biomech.* 2009;25:203-209.

12. Inkster B, Murphy A, Bower R, et al. Differences in the kinematics of the baseball swing between hitters of varying skill. *Med Sci Sports Exerc.* 2011;43(6):1050-1054.

13. Welch CM, Banks SA, Cook FF, et al. Hitting a baseball: a biomechanical description. *J Orthop Sports Phys Ther.* 1995;22(5):193-201.

14. Lau C, Glossbrenner A, LaRussa T, et al. *The Art of Hitting.300*. New York, NY: Penguin Group; 1992.

15. Lund RJ, Heefner D. Training the baseball hitter: what does research say? *J Phys Educ Recr Dance.* 2005;76(3):27-33.

16. Breen JL. What makes a good hitter? *J Health Phys Educ Recr.* 1967;38(4):36-39.

17. DeRenne C, Morgan CF, Escamilla RF, et al. A choke-up grip facilitates faster swing and stride times without compromising bat velocity and bat control. *Sport J.* 2010;13(2):2.

18. McIntyre DR, Pfaustch EW. A kinematic analysis of the baseball batting swings involved in opposite-field and same field hitting. *Res Q Exerc Sport.* 1982;53(3):206-213.

19. Tabuchi N, Matsuo T, Hashizume K. Bat speed, trajectory, and timing for collegiate baseball batters hitting a stationary ball. *Sports Biomech.* 2007;6(1):17-30.

20. Knudson D, Bahamonde R. Effect of endpoint conditions on position and velocity near impact in tennis. *J Sports Sci.* 2001;19(11):839-844.

21. Vint PF, Hinrichs RN. Endpoint error in smoothing and differentiating raw kinematic data: an evaluation of four popular methods. *J Biomech.* 1996;29(12):1637-1642.

22. DeRenne C, Ho KW, Hetzler RK, et al. Effects of warm up with various weighted implements on baseball bat swing velocity. *J Strength Cond Res.* 1992;6(4):214-218.

23. Adair RK. *The Physics of Baseball.* 3rd ed. New York, NY: Harper Collins; 2002:85-87.

24. Szymanski DJ, McIntyre JS, Szymanski JM, et al. Effect of wrist and forearm training on linear bat-end, center of percussion, and hand velocities and on time to ball contact of high school baseball players. *J Strength Cond Res*. 2006;20(1):231-240.

25. Bryant FO, Burkett LN, Chen SS, et al. Dynamic performance characteristics of baseball bats. *Res Q Exerc Sport*. 1979;48:505-510.

26. Greenwald RM, Penna LH, Crisco JJ. Differences in batted ball speed with wood and aluminum baseball bats: a batting cage study. *J Appl Biomech*. 2001;17(3):241-252.

27. Crisco JJ, Greenwald RM, Blume JD, et al. Batting performance of wood and metal baseball bats. *Med Sci Sports Exerc*. 2002;34(10):1675-1684.

28. Fleisig GS, Zheng N, Stodden DF, et al. Relationship between bat mass properties and bat velocity. *Sports Eng*. 2002;5(1):1-8.

29. Nicholls RL, Miller K, Elliott BC. Numerical analysis of maximal bat performance in baseball. *J Biomech*. 2006;39(6):1001-1009.

30. Crisco JJ, Rainbow MJ, Schwartz JB, et al. Batting cage performance of wood and nonwood youth baseball bats. *J Appl Biomech*. 2014;30(2):237-243.

31. Nathan AM. Characterizing the performance of baseball bats. *Am J Phys*. 2003;71(2):134-143.

32. Koenig K, Mitchell ND, Hannigan TE, et al. The influence of moment of inertia on baseball/softball bat swing speed. *Sports Eng*. 2004;7(2):105-117.

33. Laughlin WA, Fleisig GS, Aune KT, et al. The effects of baseball bat mass properties on swing mechanics, ground reaction forces, and swing timing. *Sports Biomech*. 2016;15(1):36-47.

34. Nathan AM. Dynamics of the baseball–bat collision. *Am J Phys*. 2000;68(11):979-990.

35. DeRenne C, Buxton BP, Hetzler RK, et al. Effects of weighted bat implement training on bat swing velocity. *J Strength Cond Res*. 1995;9(4):247-250.

36. Nelson RC, Nofsinger MR. effect of overload on speed of elbow flexion and the associated after effects. *Res Q*. 1965;36:174-181.

37. Nakamoto H, Ishii Y, Ikudome S, et al. Kinesthetic aftereffects induced by a weighted tool on movement correction in baseball batting. *Hum Mov Sci*. 2012;31(6):1529-1540.

38. Southard D, Groomer L. Warm-up with baseball bats of varying moments of inertia: effect on bat velocity and swing pattern. *Res Q Exerc Sport*. 2003;74(3):270-276.

39. DeRenne C. Increasing bat velocity. *Athl J*. 1982:28-31.

40. DeRenne C, Branco D. *Overloading and Under-loading in Your On-deck Preparation?* Vol 55. Scholastic Coach; 1986:32-37.

41. Montoya BS, Brown LE, Coburn JW, et al. Effect of warm-up with different weighted bats on normal baseball bat velocity. *J Strength Cond Res*. 2009;23(5):1566-1569.

42. Otsuji T, Abe M, Kinoshita H. After-effects of using a weighted bat on subsequent swing velocity and batters' perceptions of swing velocity and heaviness. *Percept Mot Skills*. 2002;94(1):119-126.

43. Szymanski DJ, Beiser EJ, Bassett KE, et al. Effect of various warm-up devices on bat velocity of intercollegiate baseball players. *J Strength Cond Res*. 2011;25(2):287-292.

44. Sergo C, Boatwright D. Training methods using various weighted bats and the *effects on bat velocity*. *J Strength Cond Res*. 1993;7(2):115-117.

45. DeRenne C, Okasaki E. Increasing bat velocity (part 2). *Athl J*. 1983;63(7):54-55.

46. Spaniol F, Bonnette R, Melrose D, et al. Physiological predictors of bat speed and batted-ball velocity in NCAA Division I baseball players. *J Strength Cond Res*. 2006;20(4):e25.

47. Spaniol F. Physiological predictors of bat speed and throwing velocity in adolescent baseball players. *J Strength Cond Res*. 2002;16(4):6.

48. Spaniol F, Bonnette R, Melrose D. The relationship between grip strength and bat speed of adolescent baseball players. *J Strength Cond Res*. 2007;20:747.

49. Szymanski DJ, Szymanski JM, Schade RL, et al. Relationship between physiological variables and linear bat swing velocity of high school baseball players. *Med Sci Sports Exerc*. 2008;40(5):S422.

50. Basile R, Otto R, Wygand J. The relationship between physical and physiological performance measures and baseball performance measures. *Med Sci Sports Exerc*. 2007;39(5):S214.

51. Szymanski J, Szymanski D, Albert J, et al. Relationship between physiological characteristics and baseball-specific variables of high school baseball players. *J Strength Cond Res*. 2008;22(6):e110.

52. Miyaguchi K, Demura S. Relationship between upper-body strength and bat swing speed in high-school baseball players. *J Strength Cond Res*. 2012;26(7):1786-1791.

53. Szymanski DJ, Szymanski JM, Schade RL, et al. The relation between anthropometric and physiological variables and bat velocity of high-school baseball players before and after 12 weeks of training. *J Strength Cond Res*. 2010;24(11):2933-2943.

54. Bonnette R, Spaniol F, Melrose D, et al. The relationship between rotational power, bat speed, and batted-ball velocity of NCAA Division I baseball players. *J Strength Cond Res*. 2008;22(6):e112.

55. Reyes GF, Dolny D. Acute effects of various weighted bat warm-up protocols on bat velocity. *J Strength Cond Res*. 2009;23(7):2114-2118.

56. Wilson JM, Miller AL, Szymanski DJ, et al. Effects of various warm-up devices and rest period lengths on batting velocity and acceleration of intercollegiate baseball players. *J Strength Cond Res*. 2012;26(9):2317-2323.

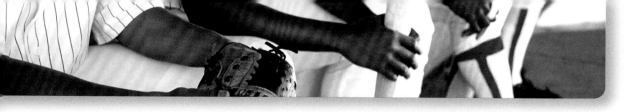

CHAPTER 4

The Biomechanics of Sliding

T. Sean Lynch, MD

If my uniform doesn't get dirty, I haven't done anything in the baseball game.
—*Rickey Henderson*

INTRODUCTION

Baseball sliding is the ability to sprint between bases and suddenly convert a vertical body to a nearly horizontal by gradually lowering the body as the player glides on top of the dirt. Sliding assists a baseball player to arrive at the base to avoid an opponent's tag or to negate a potential defensive play. There are 2 fundamental sliding techniques: head-first (HF) and feet-first (FF). The HF technique is executed with a diving motion such that the players slide on the front of their trunk and legs, arriving with the hands first at the base. Meanwhile, the FF technique is performed by sliding on the hip of a leg, which is folded underneath the other with the extended leg arriving at the base with its foot first.

SLIDING INJURIES

Sliding into a base while avoiding a tag can be an exciting play; however, proper technique is imperative to prevent injuries. For recreational athletes playing softball, sliding injuries have been found to make up approximately 70% of all injuries.[1] In college baseball, the overall rate of injury due to sliding is 9.5 per 1000 slides[2] with base runners more commonly injured than batters or position players. More than 8% of injuries occur as a result of players making contact with a base.[3]

Camp et al examined the epidemiology and the effect of sliding on professional baseball players using the MLB HITS (Health and Injury Tracking System) database.[4] Over 5 seasons (2011-2015), there were 1633 injuries that occurred as a result of sliding. The average time out from play was 14 days (range 1-173) with 8% of these injuries requiring surgery. The frequency of injury in MLB was once per every 336 slides,

and these injuries are nearly 4 times more likely to occur at second base than any other location. FF slides produced 56% of injuries, and the sliding technique utilized influences the site of injury, with HF slides most frequently producing hand, finger, and thumb injuries and FF slides most commonly causing ankle injuries.

SLIDING BIOMECHANICS

The prevalence of these injuries has shed light on injury prevention and proper technique. Additionally, MLB has made changes to rules concerning sliding into second base to reduce the number of potential collisions, particularly as players slide into second base and attempt to break up a double play. Other rule changes include that the runner is no longer allowed to slide past the base, change his pathway to the base during the approach, or utilize "roll blocks." The Centers for Disease Control and Prevention (CDC) have previously estimated that 24 million dollars could be saved annually from sliding prevention in recreational athletes and the financial implications are magnified at the professional level.[1] Although prevention is one component to decreasing injuries, it also stresses the importance of proper sliding technique to ensure the athlete places their body in the appropriate positon to execute this maneuver. Before a player can be called safe at a base, the act of sliding can be divided into 4 phases: sprinting, securing proper sliding position, airborne phase, and landing[5] (Figure 4.1).

Phase 1: Sprinting Toward the Base

In this first phase, body position and mechanical movements are identical with both sliding techniques. The success of the slide is contingent upon the athlete sprinting with a forward body angle relative to the

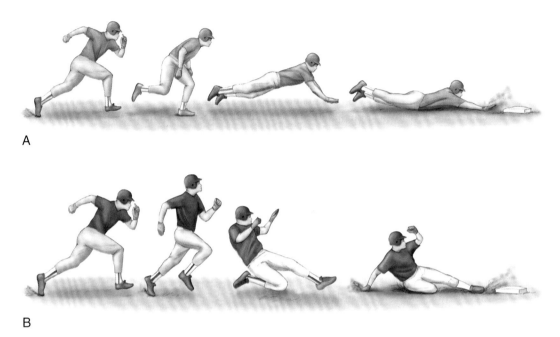

A

B

FIGURE 4.1 • Four stages of sliding; sprint → positioning → airborne → landing. A, Head-first slide, B, Feet-first slide.

ground. The runner's basic objective is to accelerate in a horizontal direction as rapidly as possible by creating significant ground reaction forces in this direction while being propelled forward by the momentum of his stride. Analysis of sliding by McCord et al revealed that the body should be approximately 70° relative to the horizontal.[6] This body lean overcomes whatever air resistance is present and also keeps the center of gravity ahead of the striding foot. If the runner inadvertently straightens his upper body, the center of gravity falls behind the foot as it contacts the ground and an abnormal decelerating force occurs.

Phase 2: Securing Sliding Position

The second phase of sliding requires the athlete to attain the appropriate sliding position. Both sliding techniques require a change in the runner's body lean. In the HF slide, the application of force against the ground continues with forward gravity always ahead of the striding foot to ensure maximum speed. With the FF slide, a relaxing phase begins about 15 feet from the base as the body transitions from a 70° lean with a counterclockwise body rotation and relaxes in preparation for a position change as the runner becomes more erect by rotating their body clockwise. As the runner's body rotation increases, the hands and arms rotate backward, the upper body shifts upward and backward, and the lower body travels downward and forward.

This clockwise rotation neutralizes the counterclockwise rotation generated from the actual sprinting movement and creates a major difference between the sliding techniques in terms of human motion.

When a runner makes the decision to slide HF, there is no relaxing phase. The runner continues to sprint while leaning slightly forward and driving hard against the ground in a forward direction. The weight remains on the balls of the feet and the center of gravity is ahead of the striding foot. The athlete lowers his body position by flexing the knees, and this crouching lowers the center of gravity to produce a more horizontal force against the ground. The runner's final push-off increases his body lean forward, and combining this with the downward force of gravity causes the runner to fall forward and slide into the base. Forward body motion continues as the runner increases body length by extending the arms and legs. The result of this angular action and reaction is that the arms and upper body move forward and downward, while the lower body moves slightly upward and backward.

Phase 3: Airborne Phase

Although a flight phase definitely exists in the FF slide, the airborne phase is not always seen in the HF slide. Regardless of the sliding technique, 2 major forces act on the runner's body during this phase: the horizontal force produced as the player leaves the ground and the vertical force of gravity once the athlete is airborne. The body's center of gravity cannot be changed or altered while airborne; however, the runner can alter the body's position around his center of gravity to accommodate flight and prepare for landing. The vertical force of gravity plays an integral role in the amount of energy encountered when landing from the airborne phase. Greater vertical displacement causes the slider to impact the ground with greater force, which can place the athlete at risk for injury from body impact with the ground. FF sliders travel further vertically than HF sliders.

In the airborne phase of the FF slide, one leg is extended forward while the other leg is flexed beneath the outstretched leg. The arms and trunk maintain a more erect position to assist the runner should they choose to abandon a slide and arriving at the base while standing. In the HF slide, there is little time for sudden movement of the body segment. Minor adjustments of the arms and legs are made in preparation for contact with the ground. The arms are forward and the remainder of the body is in a prone position with the trunk and legs extended.

Phase 4: Landing Phase

In both sliding styles, the runner's body should be completely relaxed for the landing phase. Impact with the ground should be absorbed by as much body surface area as possible. In the FF slide, initial contact with the ground is made with the extended foot and the tucked-under foot and knee. This may have some serious sports medicine implications; specifically the extended foot is at risk for catching the ground at the heel, which can cause severe plantar flexion at the ankle. This can force the foot to slap down against the ground, thus ultimately slowing the slider's progression toward the base and increasing the risk of serious trauma to the ankle and midfoot.

Meanwhile, in the HF slide, the thighs and chest provide a large surface area for initial ground contact, protecting the arms and knees. If the slide is properly executed, the force of impact should not be excessive. However, Corzatt et al evaluated real-time game footage of professional baseball players and showed that initial ground contact is made with the hands, followed quickly by the knees.[5] Significant sports medicine consequences exist owing to the small amount of body area attempting to absorb the shock of impact. These small, dangerously vulnerable body parts (hands and knees) also become subjected to high horizontal velocities as the base is impacted.

Although sliding can be a very exciting play and potentially swing a game's momentum, sliding injuries are a common cause for time out of play from recreational to professional baseball. Injury potential has been demonstrated in both sliding techniques: hands and knees of the HF slider and the ankles, knees, hips, and trailing hand of the FF slider. Better understanding of the biomechanics of this play is not only important to impart proper technique to the athletes but also to investigate areas of injury prevention. Further study into this important and impactful topic is warranted with monitoring subsequent trends in the incidence of these injuries, as rule changes take effect and better techniques are coached.

TRIP TO THE MOUND

Baseball physicians should be aware of the injury hazards of sliding into a base. Areas of particular concern include sliding into second base and HF short slides to avoid getting picked off. Thumb ulnar collateral ligament and shoulder labral tears while sliding in several high-profile baseball players have emphasized this.

MLB has looked at preventative strategies including the use of prophylactic hand bracing or taping. Another potential strategy to reduce these injuries may be the use of low-impact or breakaway bases rather than the standard bases currently used in professional baseball. Additionally, rules that prohibit defensive players from blocking second base and home plate have also been implemented to an area where sliding injuries most commonly occur.

MANAGER'S TIPS

- Two fundamental sliding techniques: head-first and feet-first
- Although sliding is an exciting play, it places baseball players at risk for injury with the average time out from play of 14 days with approximately 8% of injuries requiring surgery
- Injuries most commonly occur at second base
- Regardless of technique, the act of sliding can be divided into 4 phases: sprinting, securing proper sliding positon, airborne, and landing
- Rule changes and protective hand gear are important strategies to prevent injuries on the diamond

REFERENCES

1. Janda DH, Hankin FM, Wojtys EM. Softball injuries: cost, cause and prevention. *Am Fam Physician*. 1986;33(6):143-144.

2. Hosey RG, Puffer JC. Baseball and softball sliding injuries. Incidence, and the effect of technique in collegiate baseball and softball players. *Am J Sports Med*. 2000;28(3):360-363. doi:10.1177/03635465000280031301.

3. Dick R, Sauers EL, Agel J, et al. Descriptive epidemiology of collegiate men's baseball injuries: National Collegiate Athletic Association Injury Surveillance System, 1988-1989 through 2003-2004. *J Athl Train*. 2007;42(2):183-193.

4. Camp CL, Curriero FC, Pollack KM, et al. The epidemiology and effect of sliding injuries in Major and Minor League Baseball players. *Am J Sports Med*. 2017. doi:10.1177/0363546517704835.

5. Corzatt RD, Groppel JL, Pfautsch E, Boscardin J. The biomechanics of head-first versus feet-first sliding. *Am J Sports Med*. 1984;12(3):229-232. doi:10.1177/036354658401200312.

6. McCord J. Mechanical analysis of sliding. *Ath J*. 1971;51:66-75.

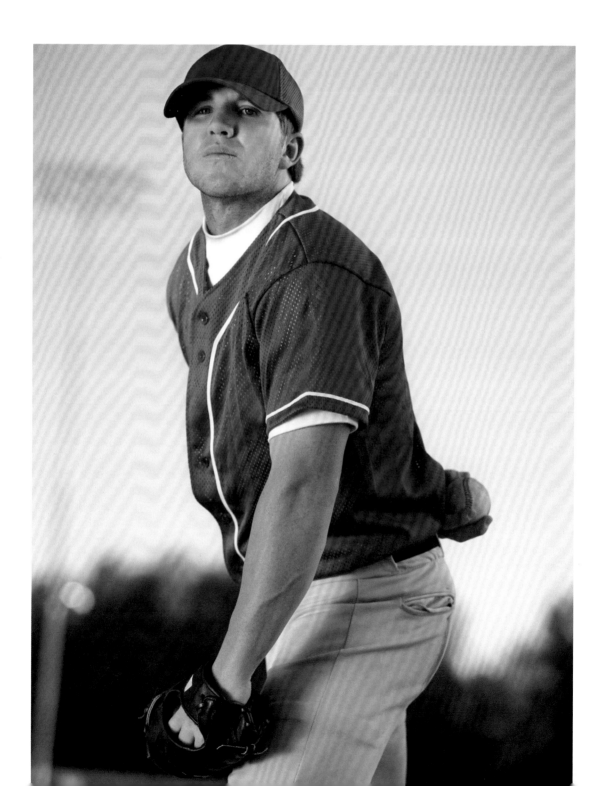

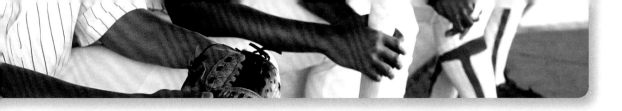

CHAPTER 5

Anatomy and Physical Examination of the Elbow

Brandon J. Erickson, MD | Peter N. Chalmers, MD

It ain't over 'til it's over.

—*Yogi Berra*

INTRODUCTION

Understanding the anatomy of the elbow and how to perform a complete and thorough physical examination of the elbow is imperative to correctly diagnose and treat the overhead throwing athlete. There are countless structures around the elbow that can be injured in the overhead athlete, and while some pathologic conditions can present with similar findings, there are often subtle differences in either the history or physical examination that can help the clinician reach the correct diagnosis. As the treatment options for varying pathology of the elbow can be different, reaching the correct diagnosis is imperative to help these athletes return to sport (RTS) in a safe, but timely, manner.

ANATOMY

The elbow joint is a complex hinge joint that is made up of 3 distinct articulations: ulnotrochlear (medially), radiocapitellar (laterally), and the proximal radioulnar joint (PRUJ) (distally), although the PRUJ does not play a role in elbow stability.[37] The elbow commonly rests in 11° to 16° of valgus to prevent the forearm and wrist from hitting the hip and leg during arm swing.[4] This is known as the valgus carrying angle (measured the angle between a line drawn down the axis of the humerus and down the axis of the forearm) and is typically higher in females than males. The restraints of the elbow can be divided into osseous and soft tissue, with each contributing 50% of elbow stability.

Medial Elbow Anatomy

Medial osseous stability of the elbow is provided by contact between the anteromedial coronoid facet and medial lip of the trochlea, as the coronoid acts as an important anterior and varus buttress to the elbow (Figure 5.1). Similarly, the congruence of the ulnotrochlear joint imparts significant stability to the elbow. The primary soft tissue restraints to valgus stress at the elbow are the flexor-pronator mass (specifically the flexor carpi ulnaris [FCU]), ulnar collateral ligament (UCL), and anterior joint capsule.[20,34] Several muscles take their origin from the medial epicondyle, including the pronator teres, flexor carpi radialis (FCR), flexor digitorum superficialis, palmaris longus, and FCU (Figure 5.2).[4]

The UCL consists of 3 separate bundles (anterior, posterior, and transverse) and is the primary restraint to valgus stress of the elbow with the elbow in flexion, with the radial head serving as a secondary stabilizer and contributing up to 30% to stability with an intact anterior band of the UCL (Figure 5.3).[14,16-18,25,37,38] The anterior bundle of the UCL, which can be broken down into 2 separate bands (anterior and posterior), provides the majority of resistance to valgus stress at the elbow.[23] The posterior bundle is a secondary valgus stabilizer, and the transverse bundle does not cross the elbow joint and therefore provides no valgus support. The anterior bundle originates at the anteroinferior aspect of the medial epicondyle of the humerus and inserts on the sublime tubercle and UCL ridge of the ulna.[23,40] The sublime tubercle is approximately 5.5 mm distal to the articular surface. This is an important landmark to understand, as the ulnar tunnel

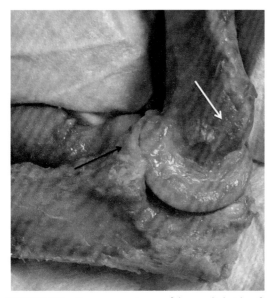

FIGURE 5.1 • Osseous anatomy of the medial side of the elbow including the coronoid (black arrow) and medial epicondyle (white arrow).

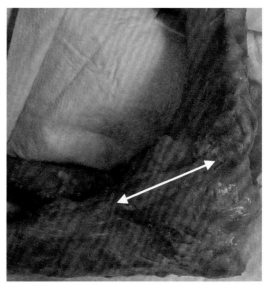

FIGURE 5.3 • Anatomic dissection of the ulnar collateral ligament (white arrow defines the course of the anterior band).

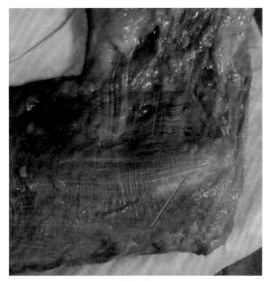

FIGURE 5.2 • Muscles of the flexor-pronator mass seen in cadaveric dissection. Blue arrow demonstrates the midpoint of the flexor-pronator, which is the typical split point for a muscle splitting approach to ulnar collateral ligament reconstruction.

should be placed in this position when performing an ulnar collateral ligament reconstruction (UCLR). Just medial to the sublime tubercle and extending distally is the UCL ridge, averaging 24.5 mm in length, onto which the UCL inserts.[11] While many initially thought the UCL inserted on one distinct location (sublime tubercle), recent evidence has shown that the

insertion of the UCL is broader and longer. The UCL originates from a 9.6-mm-wide area on the raised surface of the anteroinferior medial epicondyle, occupying 67% of the width of the epicondyle.[28] The 2 bands of the anterior bundle function are in a reciprocal fashion: the anterior band is tight in lower degrees of flexion (<90°) and the posterior band is tight in higher degrees of flexion (90°).[3,23,37] These 2 bands allow the ligament as a whole to function isometrically, potentially explaining the disagreement in prior literature as to whether the anterior band is isometric.[14,25,36]

TRIP TO THE MOUND

A 3 and 1 Count. Why Is the UCL Reconstructed With 1 Bundle When It Has 3?

The UCL is made up of 3 bundles, but the anterior bundle provides the majority of valgus restraint to the elbow. The 2 bands, anterior and posterior, of the anterior bundle function at different levels of elbow flexion to ensure the elbow remains stable to valgus stress throughout its arc of motion. Hence, when performing a UCLR, if the anatomic location of the anterior bundle is recreated, the valgus stability of the elbow is restored and the pitcher is able to compete again at a high level.

The ulnar nerve, which lies posterior to the medial intermuscular septum proximally in the arm before coursing around the medial epicondyle within the cubital tunnel, is sensitive to both micro- and macrotrauma and critical for hand function.[32] The cubital tunnel is made up of several structures: The UCL forms the floor, the arcuate (Osborne) ligament forms the roof, the medial head of the triceps forms the posterior border, the medial epicondyle forms the anterior border, and the olecranon forms the lateral border.[4] The ulnar nerve is a branch of the medial cord of the brachial plexus (C8-T1) and innervates the FCU, third and fourth lumbricals, all interossi of the hand, flexor digitorum profundus to the pinky and ring fingers, adductor pollicis, deep head of the flexor pollicis brevis, abductor digiti minimi, opponens digiti minimi, and flexor digiti minimi. It also provides sensation to the pinky and ulnar half of the ring finger. The repetitive tensile and compressive forces the ulnar nerve experiences during elbow flexion and valgus loads can lead to damage over time.[15]

Lateral Elbow Anatomy

While the medial elbow is commonly involved in pathologic conditions of the overhead throwing athlete, the anatomy of the lateral elbow must also be understood. The osseous structures of the lateral elbow consist of the radial head and capitellum. The radial head provides stability through 3 mechanisms: by acting as a buttress laterally, through the concavity-compression mechanism, and by tensioning the lateral collateral ligament complex. The lateral ligamentous complex is made up of 3 distinct bands. These include the lateral ulnar collateral ligament (LUCL), radial collateral ligament, and annular ligament. While most authors agree that the majority of stability is provided by the LUCL, there is some disagreement with the radial collateral ligament and the annular ligament also providing stability in some studies.[6,8,21,27,31,39,43] The lateral collateral ligament complex originates on the lateral condyle and inserts on the supinator crest of the ulna.[22,24]

The lateral epicondyle serves as the site of origin for several muscles of the forearm. These muscles include the extensor carpi radialis brevis (ECRB), extensor digitorum, extensor carpi ulnaris (ECU), supinator, extensor digiti minimi, and anconeus. The brachioradialis and extensor carpi radialis longus (ECRL) originate slightly proximal to the lateral epicondyle.[22]

CLINICAL EVALUATION

History

As with any evaluation, it is necessary to obtain a detailed history regarding the patient's current complaint. It is important to know the situation surrounding the injury (if there was a discrete injury), duration of symptoms, what exacerbates/alleviates the symptoms, and whether the symptoms have been getting better, staying the same, or getting worse. The pitcher should be asked about changes in velocity or accuracy or low levels of elbow pain for an extended period. When asking the overhead throwing athlete to describe when the symptoms are worse, it is important to define the phase of the pitching cycle when the symptoms flare the most. The pitching cycle can be broken down into 6 distinct phases: windup, early cocking, late cocking, acceleration, deceleration, and follow-through. Each phase imparts a different amount of stress on the elbow, with the medial elbow experiencing the most stress during the late cocking and early acceleration phases.[1,10,12,13,33] The presence of swelling should be noted, as this can often point to an intra-articular process such as an osteochondral lesion or loose body.[35] Furthermore, the patient should be asked about symptoms suggestive of ulnar neuritis, including numbness in the pinky and ulnar half of the ring finger, weakness in the hand, and clawing of the hand. Pitchers should be asked whether these symptoms occur at rest, while pitching, or following pitching to understand if these are static or dynamic in nature.

The patient should do his best to localize the symptoms to a specific area of the elbow. Whether this is the medial epicondyle, posteromedial olecranon, sublime tubercle, radial head, etc, having the patient drill down to the exact location of pain will be beneficial in making the correct diagnosis. Specific complaints including presence/absence of mechanical symptoms, snapping or subluxation of the ulnar nerve and/or triceps tendon, feelings of instability, and others should be noted. Prior treatment, including periods of rest and their duration, should be recorded. The completeness of the rest should also be recorded—for instance, many pitchers will continue bull pens and long toss while avoiding competition play and consider this a complete period of rest. Similarly, any other treatments including physical therapy, ultrasound and other modalities, and platelet-rich plasma (PRP), as well as their response to these treatments, should be recorded. Finally, if the patient has had prior surgery on the extremity in question, the details of surgery including when the surgery was performed, what the surgery was performed for, whether the patient improved after surgery, and whether they were able to RTS after surgery must be ascertained.

PHYSICAL EXAMINATION

Inspection

The physical examination of the elbow begins by completely exposing the upper extremity of the patient, maintaining modesty in females. The elbow is inspected for any previous scars, deformities, ecchymosis, and rashes. Inspection should take place through a full range of motion (ROM) of the elbow, as depending on location, focal swelling can be obscured in flexion or extension. The valgus carrying angle of the elbow should be observed. As previously mentioned, the carrying angle is typically between 11° and 16°. The carrying angles less than 11° or more than 16° could indicate prior trauma to the elbow. Subtle malunion from pediatric supracondylar humeral fracture is not uncommon and can increase medial or lateral stress.[30] In patients with a prior lateral condyle fracture, the carrying angle can be decreased or increased depending on whether the patient experienced overgrowth or undergrowth of the lateral condyle, respectively. The injured elbow should be compared with the contralateral elbow to determine if any abnormalities are symmetric (commonly congenital issues) or unilateral (indicating a prior injury or pathologic condition). The hand should be inspected for any evidence of wasting of the first dorsal interosseous muscle, and the shoulder should be inspected for any evidence of atrophy of the rotator cuff muscles or asymmetry of the shoulder girdle.

Palpation

Palpation of the elbow follows inspection and should be performed in a systematic manner to avoid overlooking any aspect of the elbow. Typically palpation should be performed before any provocative testing at the elbow to improve the examiners' ability to pinpoint pathology in a noninflamed setting. The authors typically leave the medial elbow for last and focus on the other parts of the elbow first. When palpating structures of the elbow, the examiner should be very precise with where they are pushing. Using the entire hand or several fingers to palpate is not very specific and can lead to difficulty in localizing pain to a specific structure. As such, the authors are meticulous about only using 1 or 2 fingers when palpating specific areas of the elbow in an effort to localize the patient's pain to a specific structure. Palpation begins laterally over the lateral epicondyle. The mobile wad should be palpated for any

tenderness. The ECRB should be palpated at its origin on the face of the epicondyle, as tenderness in this area can suggest lateral epicondylitis. The radial head is palpated, as the forearm is supinated and pronated. An audible or palpable click laterally can indicate the presence of a plica or chondral lesion. Palpation continues posteriorly to the posterolateral tip, posterior tip, and posteromedial tip of the olecranon. Tenderness in the region of the posteromedial olecranon can suggest valgus extension overload with a posteromedial osteophyte. The triceps tendon should be palpated along its course, ending at the triceps insertion into the olecranon. Tenderness at the level of the triceps insertion can indicate insertional triceps tendonitis. Finally, the area of the olecranon physis should be palpated in the skeletally immature individual to rule out a persistent olecranon physis.[7]

Once the lateral and posterior aspects of the elbow have been examined, the medial elbow is palpated. Palpation begins at the medial epicondyle. Tenderness over the face of the medial epicondyle can indicate a proximal tear of the UCL, medial apophysitis (also known as little leaguer's elbow) in the skeletally immature individual, medial epicondylitis, and a medial epicondyle avulsion fracture. Palpation continues along the course of the UCL down to its insertion on the sublime tubercle of the ulna. Tenderness along the path of the UCL can indicate a complete midsubstance tear or a partial thickness undersurface tear. Pain at the sublime tubercle can signal a distal tear of the UCL, which, unfortunately, portends a worse prognosis than a proximal tear.[26] The ulnar nerve should then be palpated to determine if it is sitting in the cubital tunnel or is dislocated. The nerve should be palpated through a full ROM to test for ulnar nerve instability. The medial intermuscular septum can be palpated proximally for tenderness to see if the ulnar nerve is irritated. The flexor-pronator mass is palpated to assess for a tear. The lacertus fibrosus should also be palpated, as it can be a source of localized muscular compression in select pitchers and can be surgically released.

Range of Motion

Once palpation is completed, the elbow is taken through a full ROM. This should be performed both actively and passively. Flexion and extension of the elbow assesses the ulnotrochlear joint and normally should be from approximately 0° to 140° (Figure 5.4A and B).[35] It is not uncommon for pitchers to have some loss of terminal extension secondary to an elbow contracture, loose bodies, soft tissue swelling, or a posteromedial osteophyte. If a contracture exists, the

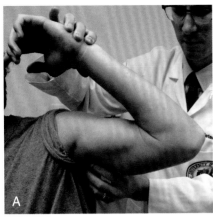
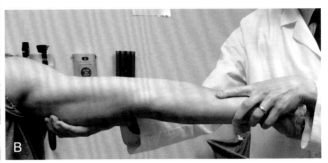

FIGURE 5.4 • Assessment of elbow flexion (A) and extension (B). Notice that the position of the examiner's left hand remains constant under the triceps to ensure the elbow remains in the same plane during range of motion testing to avoid inaccuracies.

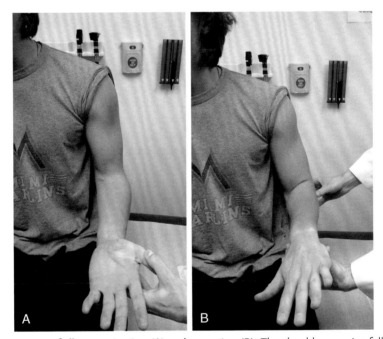

FIGURE 5.5 • Assessment of elbow supination (A) and pronation (B). The shoulder remains fully adducted and the elbow remains flexed to approximately 90° during this part of the examination.

examiner should forcefully extend the elbow to determine if this is painful for the patient. If this is painful, it may indicate a posteromedial osteophyte secondary to valgus extension overload or other intra-articular process. If it is not painful it may be adaptive, as pitchers can lose up to 20° of extension without impacting their kinematics.[2] Loss of terminal flexion can occur from osteophyte formation within the coronoid fossa. Furthermore, if the patient has pain during mid-arc ROM, this can indicate an osteochondral lesion. Any evidence of mechanical symptoms during ROM testing such as locking, catching, or crepitus should alert

the examiner to the possibility of a chondral defect or intra-articular loose body. Forearm pronation and supination, which should average 80°, should then be assessed (Figure 5.5A and B).[35] Limitation in pronation or supination can indicate problems with the radiocapitellar joint or PRUJ but can also arise owing to problems at any point along the forearm.

Special Tests

There are several tests that are specific to the UCL. These include the valgus stress test, milking maneuver, and the moving valgus stress test (Figure 5.6). The

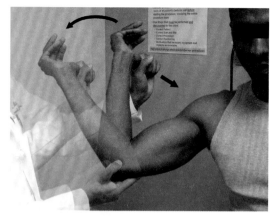

FIGURE 5.6 • Moving valgus stress test. The examiner grabs the thumb and imparts a valgus force to the elbow while flexing and extending the elbow (black arrows). Pain is reproduced at the area of the examiner's right thumb with an injury to the ulnar collateral ligament.

valgus stress test is performed in the supine or standing position. If the examiner is testing a left elbow, the right hand of the examiner should cup the humerus just proximal to the elbow while the left hand grasps the forearm just distal to the elbow. With the patient's elbow flexed to approximately 70°, a valgus stress is applied to the elbow. This test can also be performed supine on an examination table, with the edge of the table providing counterresistance on the humerus. An increase in medial gapping from side to side can be indicative of a UCL tear. However, increased medial laxity in the throwing arm of a pitcher may be adaptive, as ultrasound studies have shown that asymptomatic pitchers have almost 1 mm more of medial gapping in their throwing elbow compared with their opposite elbow.[5] Significant laxity is also uncommon among patients indicated for UCL reconstruction, calling into question the usefulness of laxity with any test as an indication for reconstruction.[19]

The milking maneuver is performed with the patient supine or standing. The shoulder is abducted and slightly externally rotated, the forearm is supinated, and the elbow is flexed to approximately 90°. This position places tension on the posterior band of the anterior bundle of the UCL. The examiner then grabs the patient's thumb and creates a valgus stress by exerting a posteriorly directed pull on the thumb. A positive test is seen with reproduction of pain indicating an injury of the UCL. The moving valgus stress test is performed with the patient standing, the shoulder abducted to 90°, and the elbow maximally flexed. If the examiner is testing a right elbow, the left hand of the examiner is placed around the back of the patient's elbow to exert

a valgus force while the examiner's right hand is placed palm to palm with the patient's right hand. The patient then flexes and extends the elbow while the examiner exerts a constant valgus force on both the elbow and palm of the patient. Reproduction of pain similar to that experienced during throwing, especially from 70° to 120° of elbow flexion, is considered a positive test (sensitivity, 100%; specificity, 75%).[29]

> ### TRIP TO THE MOUND
> #### I Thought You Only Milked a Cow?
> There are several tests that can help diagnose a UCL tear of the elbow, one of which is termed "the milking maneuver." While this test is somewhat awkward to perform, pain elicited during this test is a good indicator of an injury to the UCL.

There are several tests that should be performed to evaluate other structures about the elbow aside from the UCL. Patients who present with medial elbow pain also need to be ruled out for medial epicondylitis. Resisted wrist flexion and forearm pronation will often cause pain at the medial elbow in a patient with medial epicondylitis. Similarly, pain in the lateral elbow with resisted wrist extension and forearm supination is often indicative of lateral epicondylitis. Occasionally overhead athletes can present with instability of the medial head of the triceps tendon that can appear similar to ulnar nerve subluxation on examination. A subluxating triceps tendon can be caused by hypertrophy of the medial head of the triceps or an anatomic variation of the tendon. This can present in isolation or concomitantly with a subluxating ulnar nerve. Patients report a snapping sensation with or without pain and paresthesias shooting down the forearm during elbow flexion in both cases.

Ulnar Nerve

Once the focused examination of the elbow is complete, the ulnar nerve should be evaluated for irritability and subluxation. It is important to perform a detailed ulnar nerve examination, as patients with ulnar nerve symptoms who are going to undergo a surgical procedure to address some other form of elbow pathology will often necessitate an ulnar nerve transposition at the time of their surgery. Two-point discrimination (normal is ≤5 mm) should be tested on the ring and small fingers. A Tinel test should be performed at the elbow where the examiner taps along the course of the ulnar nerve in an attempt to elicit shooting pain

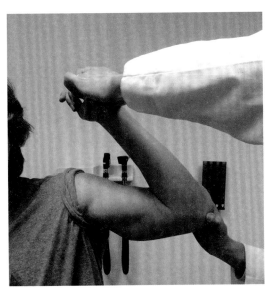

FIGURE 5.7 • Ulnar nerve compression test. The patient's elbow is maximally flexed and the examiner exerts direct pressure over the ulnar nerve at the level of the cubital tunnel. Progressive numbness in the pinky and ulnar half of the erring fingers indicates a positive test.

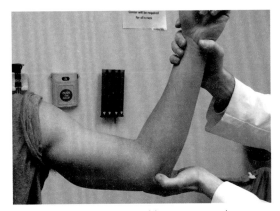

FIGURE 5.8 • Ulnar nerve subluxation test. The examiner holds a finger over the medial epicondyle as he brings the patient's elbow repeatedly from flexion into extension. If the ulnar nerve subluxates out of the cubital tunnel in flexion and reduces in extension, this is considered a positive test.

down the forearm and into the pinky and ring fingers. If the patient complains of pain that radiates into the radial side of the hand during the Tinel test, this is not considered a positive examination. An ulnar nerve compression test can also be performed by maximally flexing the patient's elbow and exerting a constant pressure over the ulnar nerve with the examiner's thumb at the level of the cubital tunnel or slightly distal to this (Figure 5.7). Progressive numbness in the ring and small fingers indicates a positive test. The stability of the ulnar nerve can be assessed with the ulnar nerve subluxation test. To perform this test, the patient can be supine or standing and the examiner places his or her index and long fingers over the cubital tunnel. As the patient flexes and extends his elbow, the examiner feels for nerve subluxation in and out of the cubital tunnel (Figure 5.8).

The strength of the patient's first dorsal interossei should be tested by abducting the index finger and having the patient resist while the examiner attempts to adduct the finger. Weakness with this maneuver can indicate compression of the ulnar nerve. Two different signs can indicate ulnar neuropathy: the Wartenberg sign and Froment sign. A Wartenberg sign is seen when the patient adducts the pinky finger but experiences inadvertent abduction and extension of the pinky finger secondary to ulnar overpull of the extensor digiti minimi and weakness in the palmar interosseous muscle. A Froment sign is seen with compensatory thumb interphalangeal flexion (from the flexor pollicis longus [FPL]) due to loss of function of the adductor pollicis upon attempted pinch.[15,32]

> ### TRIP TO THE MOUND
>
> #### Just a Little High and Inside: Why Do We Care So Much About the Ulnar Nerve?
>
> The ulnar nerve is a vital structure to all patients, but specifically the overhead athlete, as it contributes a significant amount of function to the hand. Dynamic compression or static constant irritation and decreased blood flow to the ulnar nerve can cause wasting of the intrinsic muscles of the hand. If a patient has symptoms of ulnar neuropathy, these should be addressed at the same time as their concomitant elbow pathology to prevent bigger issues down the line. Indeed, the first UCL reconstruction to be performed, on Tommy John himself, had to be revised for persistent ulnar neuritis.

Other Pertinent Physical Examinations

Any overhead throwing athlete who presents with elbow pain should have a complete examination of their cervical spine, core, shoulder, and wrist. It is important to assess the shoulder for scapulothoracic dyskinesis, glenohumeral internal rotation deficit, loss of total arc of motion of the glenohumeral joint, and posterior capsular tightness. Studies have found that a decrease in total arc of motion of the throwing shoulder compared with the nonthrowing shoulder increases a player's risk of elbow, as well as shoulder, injuries.[41,42] If the athlete is suffering from posterior capsular tightness, starting them on a sleeper stretching program will often help with shoulder and elbow pain. Spurling test, which is performed with passive extension and lateral rotation of the cervical spine, can also reveal otherwise occult radicular pain. Recent evidence has suggested that core weakness can have an effect on the pitching motion and possibly increase a player's risk of injury.[9] Assessing these athletes for core muscle strength and intervening with a core strengthening program in those who demonstrate weakness may help prevent elbow injuries, especially as pitchers begin to fatigue. A wide variety of tests have been developed to test core strength, including the plank and side plank tests, the Trendelenburg test, and the single-leg squat test.

MANAGER'S TIPS

- Elbow pain in the throwing athlete is often secondary to repetitive overuse, although this can occur from a one time, traumatic injury
- The UCL is made up of 3 distinct bundles, with the anterior bundle contributing the majority of stability to the medial elbow
- A thorough history should precede the physical examination
- The physical examination should be performed in a systematic manner to avoid overlooking any potential sources of pathology
- The ulnar nerve should be critically evaluated both with history and physical examination to uncover pathology if any exists
- All overhead athletes who present with elbow pain should undergo a complete cervical spine, shoulder, and wrist examination to confirm that these other areas are not the source of the problem or contributing to the problem

REFERENCES

1. Aguinaldo AL, Chambers H. Correlation of throwing mechanics with elbow valgus load in adult baseball pitchers. *Am J Sports Med.* 2009;37(10):2043-2048.
2. Cain EL Jr, Dugas JR, Wolf RS, Andrews JR. Elbow injuries in throwing athletes: a current concepts review. *Am J Sports Med.* 2003;31(4):621-635.
3. Callaway GH, Field LD, Deng XH, et al. Biomechanical evaluation of the medial collateral ligament of the elbow. *J Bone Joint Surg Am.* 1997;79(8):1223-1231.
4. Chen FS, Rokito AS, Jobe FW. Medial elbow problems in the overhead-throwing athlete. *J Am Acad Orthop Surg.* 2001;9(2):99-113.
5. Ciccotti MG, Atanda A Jr, Nazarian LN, Dodson CC, Holmes L, Cohen SB. Stress sonography of the ulnar collateral ligament of the elbow in professional baseball pitchers: a 10-year study. *Am J Sports Med.* 2014;42(3):544-551.
6. Cohen MS. Lateral collateral ligament instability of the elbow. *Hand Clin.* 2008;24(1):69-77.
7. Crowther M. Elbow pain in pediatrics. *Curr Rev Musculoskelet Med.* 2009;2(2):83-87.
8. Dunning CE, Zarzour ZD, Patterson SD, Johnson JA, King GJ. Ligamentous stabilizers against posterolateral rotatory instability of the elbow. *J Bone Joint Surg Am.* 2001;83-A(12):1823-1828.
9. Erickson BJ, Sgori T, Chalmers PN, et al. The impact of fatigue on baseball pitching mechanics in adolescent male pitchers. *Arthroscopy.* 2016;32(5):762-771.
10. Escamilla RF, Barrentine SW, Fleisig GS, et al. Pitching biomechanics as a pitcher approaches muscular fatigue during a simulated baseball game. *Am J Sports Med.* 2007;35(1):23-33.
11. Farrow LD, Mahoney AJ, Stefancin JJ, Taljanovic MS, Sheppard JE, Schickendantz MS. Quantitative analysis of the medial ulnar collateral ligament ulnar footprint and its relationship to the ulnar sublime tubercle. *Am J Sports Med.* 2011;39(9):1936-1941.
12. Fleisig GS, Andrews JR, Dillman CJ, Escamilla RF. Kinetics of baseball pitching with implications about injury mechanisms. *Am J Sports Med.* 1995;23(2):233-239.
13. Fleisig GS, Kingsley DS, Loftice JW, et al. Kinetic comparison among the fastball, curveball, change-up, and slider in collegiate baseball pitchers. *Am J Sports Med.* 2006;34(3):423-430.
14. Fuss FK. The ulnar collateral ligament of the human elbow joint. Anatomy, function and biomechanics. *J Anat.* 1991;175:203-212.
15. Harris JD, Lintner DM. Nerve injuries about the elbow in the athlete. *Sports Med Arthrosc.* 2014;22(3):e7-e15.
16. Hotchkiss RN, Weiland AJ. Valgus stability of the elbow. *J Orthop Res.* 1987;5(3):372-377.
17. Josefsson PO, Gentz CF, Johnell O, Wendeberg B. Surgical versus non-surgical treatment of ligamentous injuries following dislocation of the elbow joint. A prospective randomized study. *J Bone Joint Surg Am.* 1987;69(4):605-608.
18. Josefsson PO, Johnell O, Wendeberg B. Ligamentous injuries in dislocations of the elbow joint. *Clin Orthop Relat Res.* 1987(221):221-225.
19. Joyner PW, Bruce J, Hess R, Mates A, Mills FB, Andrews JR. Magnetic resonance imaging-based classification for ulnar collateral ligament injuries of the elbow. *J Shoulder Elbow Surg.* 2016;25(10):1710-1716.

20. Loftice J, Fleisig GS, Zheng N, Andrews JR. Biomechanics of the elbow in sports. *Clin Sports Med.* 2004;23(4):519-530 [vii-viii].

21. McAdams TR, Masters GW, Srivastava S. The effect of arthroscopic sectioning of the lateral ligament complex of the elbow on posterolateral rotatory stability. *J Shoulder Elbow Surg.* 2005;14(3):298-301.

22. Morrey BF. Applied anatomy and biomechanics of the elbow joint. *Instr Course Lect.* 1986;35:59-68.

23. Morrey BF, An KN. Articular and ligamentous contributions to the stability of the elbow joint. *Am J Sports Med.* 1983;11(5):315-319.

24. Morrey BF, An KN. Functional anatomy of the ligaments of the elbow. *Clin Orthop Relat Res.* 1985(201):84-90.

25. Morrey BF, Tanaka S, An KN. Valgus stability of the elbow. A definition of primary and secondary constraints. *Clin Orthop Relat Res.* 1991(265):187-195.

26. Nassab PF, Schickendantz MS. Evaluation and treatment of medial ulnar collateral ligament injuries in the throwing athlete. *Sports Med Arthrosc.* 2006;14(4):221-231.

27. O'Driscoll SW, Bell DF, Morrey BF. Posterolateral rotatory instability of the elbow. *J Bone Joint Surg Am.* 1991;73(3):440-446.

28. O'Driscoll SW, Jaloszynski R, Morrey BF, An KN. Origin of the medial ulnar collateral ligament. *J Hand Surg Am.* 1992;17(1):164-168.

29. O'Driscoll SW, Lawton RL, Smith AM. The "moving valgus stress test" for medial collateral ligament tears of the elbow. *Am J Sports Med.* 2005;33(2):231-239.

30. O'Driscoll SW, Spinner RJ, McKee MD, et al. Tardy posterolateral rotatory instability of the elbow due to cubitus varus. *J Bone Joint Surg Am.* 2001;83-A(9):1358-1369.

31. Olsen BS, Henriksen MG, Sojbjerg JO, Helmig P, Sneppen O. Elbow joint instability: a kinematic model. *J Shoulder Elbow Surg.* 1994;3(3):143-150.

32. Palmer BA, Hughes TB. Cubital tunnel syndrome. *J Hand Surg Am.* 2010;35(1):153-163.

33. Pappas AM, Zawacki RM, Sullivan TJ. Biomechanics of baseball pitching. A preliminary report. *Am J Sports Med.* 1985;13(4):216-222.

34. Park MC, Ahmad CS. Dynamic contributions of the flexor-pronator mass to elbow valgus stability. *J Bone Joint Surg Am.* 2004;86-A(10):2268-2274.

35. Redler LH, Watling JP, Ahmad CS. Physical examination of the throwing athlete's elbow. *Am J Orthop (Belle Mead NJ).* 2015;44(1):13-18.

36. Regan WD, Korinek SL, Morrey BF, An KN. Biomechanical study of ligaments around the elbow joint. *Clin Orthop Relat Res.* 1991(271):170-179.

37. Schwab GH, Bennett JB, Woods GW, Tullos HS. Biomechanics of elbow instability: the role of the medial collateral ligament. *Clin Orthop Relat Res.* 1980(146):42-52.

38. Sojbjerg JO, Ovesen J, Nielsen S. Experimental elbow instability after transection of the medial collateral ligament. *Clin Orthop Relat Res.* 1987(218):186-190.

39. Tashjian RZ, Katarincic JA. Complex elbow instability. *J Am Acad Orthop Surg.* 2006;14(5):278-286.

40. Timmerman LA, Andrews JR. Histology and arthroscopic anatomy of the ulnar collateral ligament of the elbow. *Am J Sports Med.* 1994;22(5):667-673.

41. Wilk KE, Macrina LC, Fleisig GS, et al. Deficits in glenohumeral passive range of motion increase risk of elbow injury in professional baseball pitchers: a prospective study. *Am J Sports Med.* 2014;42(9):2075-2081.

42. Wilk KE, Macrina LC, Fleisig GS, et al. Deficits in glenohumeral passive range of motion increase risk of shoulder injury in professional baseball pitchers: a prospective study. *Am J Sports Med.* 2015;43(10):2379-2385.

43. Wyrick JD, Dailey SK, Gunzenhaeuser JM, Casstevens EC. Management of complex elbow dislocations: a mechanistic approach. *J Am Acad Orthop Surg.* 2015;23(5):297-306.

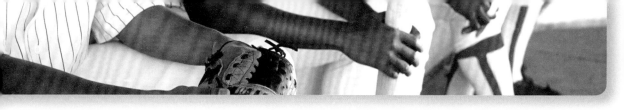

CHAPTER 6

MRI and Ultrasound Imaging of the Throwing Athlete's Elbow

Michael C. Ciccotti, MD | Meghan Bishop, MD | Michael G. Ciccotti, MD

Competing at the highest level is not about winning. It's about preparation, courage, understanding and nurturing your people, and heart. Winning is the result.

—Joe Torre

INTRODUCTION

Overhead-throwing places a significant amount of stress on the elbow, particularly to the medial structures that are subjected to repetitive valgus and extension loads.[1,2] The forces generated during throwing are distributed throughout the soft tissues and osseous structures of the elbow, often leading to a predictable series of chronic changes.[2] The combination of high valgus force with rapid extension of the elbow during the late cocking and early acceleration phases of throwing places significant tensile forces on the medial elbow structures, including the medial ulnar collateral ligament (UCL), flexor-pronator mass, ulnar nerve, and medial epicondyle apophysis.[1,2] Concurrently, the elbow posterior compartment, which includes the posteromedial tip of the olecranon and olecranon fossa, is subjected to large shear forces, while the radial head and capitellum in the lateral compartment withstand large compressive forces.[1,2] Also known as "valgus extension overload syndrome," the combination of medial tensile, posterior shear, and lateral compressive forces contribute to the pathophysiology of the commonly seen injuries in the thrower's elbow.[3] These include flexor-pronator strain, peri-elbow soft tissue contracture, UCL injury with medial laxity, ulnar nerve irritation, olecranon or medial epicondyle stress fracture/apophysitis, posterior medial impingement with olecranon osteophytes, radiocapitellar osteochondral injury, and loose bodies/free osteochondral fragments.[1] The general population, however, is not routinely exposed to this cascade of pathophysiologic changes that are often seen in the thrower's elbow.

A number of epidemiologic studies suggest that with the increase in youth sports participation and popularization of "Tommy John" surgery, the number of UCL injuries and those undergoing reconstruction is increasing.[4-7] This is particularly notable for pitchers, who are at the greatest risk of sustaining injury to the medial structures of the elbow.[8] Our recently published review of elbow injuries in the professional baseball player utilizing the Major League Baseball Injury Surveillance System noted that elbow injuries account for the highest number of days missed of all musculoskeletal injuries in this sport.[8] The most common elbow injuries are ligamentous; the most common ligament injuries involve the UCL; and the most commonly performed elbow surgery in this throwing population is UCL reconstruction.[8]

A combination of history, physical examination, and imaging is essential to diagnosing injuries of the throwing athlete's elbow. Throwers often complain of progressive medial elbow pain during the late cocking or early acceleration phases of throwing with associated decreased throwing velocity.[9] Alternatively, throwers may describe an acute pop from a single episode of throwing. Pain is often centralized to the medial or posteromedial aspect of the elbow and may be exacerbated by valgus stress testing, specifically

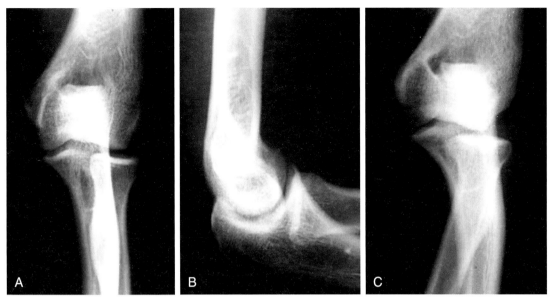

FIGURE 6.1 • Plain X-ray views of normal elbow: (A) AP (45°), (B) lateral, (C) oblique.

through the milking maneuver or moving valgus stress test.[10,11] While history and physical examination provide essential information concerning the athlete's injury, imaging is most often beneficial in assessing the elbow pathology and directing appropriate treatment modalities.

A variety of imaging studies have been used to assess elbow injuries in the throwing athlete with specific indications for each study based on anatomic location of the pathology. Elbow pathology to be assessed on imaging include bony changes (medial UCL ossification, radiocapitellar flattening/osteochondral defects [OCDs], olecranon/coronoid spurring), musculotendinous changes (flexor-pronator and extensor tendon degeneration/fraying/tearing), ligamentous changes (UCL degeneration/fraying/tearing), and nerve changes (ulnar nerve edema/scarring/subluxation).[12-16] This chapter will further explore the appropriate imaging modalities to best evaluate these changes radiographically in the throwing elbow.

IMAGING TECHNIQUES

Plain Radiographs

Radiographic evaluation should begin with standard plain radiographs of the elbow, including anteroposterior (AP) (45°), lateral, oblique, and axial views (Figure 6.1A-C). These radiographs can be used to assess for loss of joint space, osteophyte formation, loose bodies,

calcifications, OCD lesions, cystic changes, and fractures.[1,2,17-19] A radiograph of the contralateral elbow should always be utilized for comparison. Common standard radiographic findings unique to the thrower's elbow include medial calcifications, radiocapitellar chondrosis, and posteromedial spurring from chronic changes of valgus extension overload (Figure 6.2A-C).[15,20] In younger patients, widening of the growth plate of the medial epicondyle or the olecranon with or without fragmentation of the ossification center may be seen as a chronic stress response to the repetitive throwing motion.[21] It is important to recognize that asymptomatic abnormalities may be present on radiographs owing to the repetitive chronic nature associated with the throwing mechanism, but often more advanced imaging modalities are necessary to further define the extent of injury, particularly for soft tissue and intra-articular pathologies.[15]

If an injury to the UCL is suspected, dynamic stress AP radiographs can be performed either manually or using a calibrated stress device (Telos, Weiterstadt, Germany) to determine the presence of ulnohumeral medial joint gapping.[1,22,23] Forces up to 15 dN of valgus stress are applied to the injured elbow at 25° to 30° of flexion and compared with the contralateral side for evaluation of medial gapping with increasing valgus stress.[1,22] Rijke et al showed in a cadaveric study using stress radiography that medial joint gapping more than 0.5 mm compared with the contralateral elbow was indicative of complete and large partial UCL tears.[22] Bruce et al later

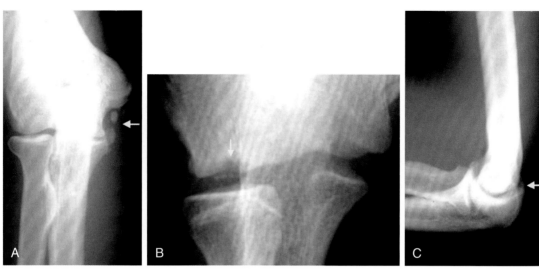

FIGURE 6.2 ● Plain X-ray examples of common elbow pathology seen in the thrower indicated by arrows: (A) medial calcifications, (B) radiocapitellar chondrosis, (C) posteromedial spurring.

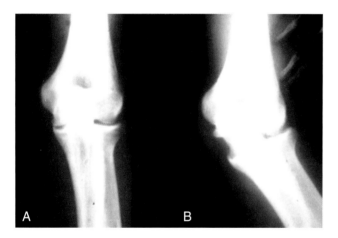

FIGURE 6.3 ● Stress radiography of UCL injured elbow: (A) stressed, (B) unstressed.

showed using stress radiography that the thrower's elbow with a UCL injury opened 0.4 mm more than the uninjured side and those with complete tears (diagnosed by MRI) gapped an average of 0.6 mm, which was significantly more than 0.1 mm for partial tears.[23] However, stress radiography evaluations of elbows of elite level pitchers have found increased medial joint gapping in asymptomatic uninjured elbows compared with the nondominant arm, suggesting that baseline-increased medial joint laxity may be present in the thrower's elbow.[24] This emphasizes the importance of interpreting stress radiographic findings within the context of the history and physical examination (Figure 6.3A and B). While still a useful diagnostic modality, the difficulty in measuring such small distances with accuracy on plain stress radiographs has led to other advanced imaging modalities such as MRI/MRA to be a more accurate and widely used diagnostic test for elbow injuries in the thrower.

Magnetic Resonance Imaging/ Arthrography

Magnetic resonance imaging (MRI) of the elbow, with or without intra-articular gadolinium arthrography, has been considered an optimal way to diagnose elbow pathology in the athlete, in particular injury to the UCL.[18,19,25-28] MR utilizes a magnetic field to align the spin of protons within the nuclei of various tissues and measures the wave emitted by the decay of these protons to their resting state. T1- and T2-weighted

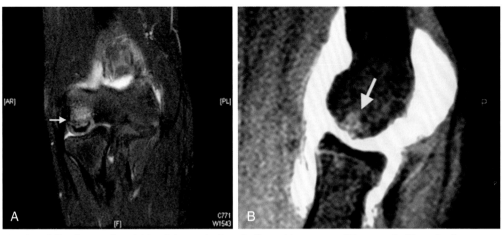

FIGURE 6.4 • MR of osteochondritis of the capitellum indicated by arrows: (A) coronal, (B) sagittal.

images are generated by altering repetition time (TR) and echo time (TE), respectively, and provide the clinician with complimentary information regarding injured tissue. Fat-enhancing T1-weighted images are typically used to assess anatomy, whereas water-content-enhancing T2-weighted images are useful for detecting edema/inflammation associated with injury/pathology. As with CT, images are typically produced in the sagittal, coronal, and axial/transverse planes. As with the interpretation of any imaging study, the clinician should systematically evaluate all visualized structures as a potential source of pathology, including bone, cartilage, ligament, tendon, muscle, and neurovascular structures.

MRI allows the evaluation of multiple osseous and cartilaginous pathologies common in overhead throwers. MR is excellent for evaluating osteochondritis of the capitellum, with the ability to demonstrate disruption of the capitellar cartilage, the extent of underlying bony edema, the stability of the chondral lesion, and the presence of any loose bodies[29,30] (Figure 6.4A and B). However, it is important to note that the so-called pseudodefect, a groove at the junction and overhanging lateral edges of the capitellum, should not be mistaken for an OCD lesion.[31] Posteromedial impingement or valgus extension overload can be assessed on MR with edema manifesting as increased signal of the posterior medial articular surface on T2-weighted images. Cohen et al described the characteristic findings for posteromedial impingement as articular pathology of the posterior trochlea, insertional tendinosis of the medial border of the triceps, and synovitis in the posteromedial recess[13] (Figure 6.5A and B). MR is similarly valuable for evaluating olecranon stress reaction, characterized by bony edema or high signal intensity

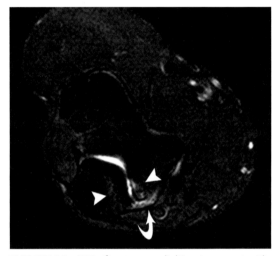

FIGURE 6.5 • MR of posteromedial impingement with impingement site indicated by arrows. (Reprinted with permission from Cohen SB, Valko C, Zoga A, Dodson CC, Ciccotti MG. Posteromedial elbow impingement: magnetic resonance imaging findings in overhead throwing athletes and results of arthroscopic treatment. *Arthroscopy*. 2011;27(10):1364-1370. Copyright © 2011 Arthroscopy Association of North America.)

on T2-weighted images, and distinguishing it from olecranon stress fracture in which a fracture line can be visualized[32] (Figure 6.6).

The UCL is typically visualized on MR as a linear structure of low signal intensity on T1-weighted or proton density–weighted images that runs perpendicular to the medial joint line[33-36] (Figure 6.7A). Injuries are best appreciated on T2-weighted images as intraligamentous hyperintensity, discontinuity of fibers, and possible retraction[36,37] (Figure 6.7B). The "T sign" is commonly seen as an undersurface partial tear at the insertion of the UCL[12,38]

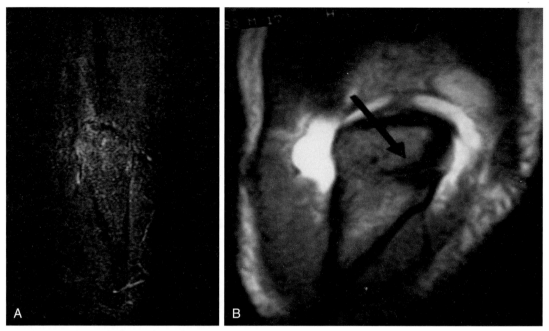

FIGURE 6.6 ⬥ MR of olecranon: (A) sagittal view of stress reaction as diffuse increased signal, (B) sagittal view of stress fracture indicated by black arrow.

(Figure 6.7C). Chronic injury can be appreciated as thickening, intrasubstance hyperintensity, and redundancy[27,36] (Figure 6.7D).

Although conventional MRI provides excellent visualization of acute, complete ruptures of the UCL, it may be less accurate for the diagnosis of partial tears.[25-28,39] As a result, MR arthrography (MRA) has been proposed as an optimal way to evaluate UCL injury with accuracy, specificity, and sensitively all above 95%.[26-28,40] Joyner et al have recently proposed the first MR classification system for UCL injury based on the severity and location of injury (Table 6.1). Type 1 injuries are low-grade partial tears of the UCL, with only edema visualized within the UCL substance.[12] Type 2 injuries are high-grade partial tears with no extravasation of intra-articular contrast. Type 3 injuries are complete, full-thickness UCL tears in which contrast extravasates from the joint, through the UCL, and into the surrounding superficial tissue. Finally, type 4 injuries represent injuries in multiple locations along the ligament, ie, at both the ulnar and humeral attachments. All types of injuries can be further subclassified by the location of injury: U (ulna), M (midsubstance), and H (humerus). In this review of 240 patients with UCL injury, Joyner et al defined the incidence of each type as follows: type 1 (9.2%); type 2 (58%); type 3 (27.5%); and type 4 (5.4%). Furthermore, 44.6% of injures were humeral, 37.5% were ulnar, 12.5% were midsubstance, and 5.4% were multiple locations. This suggests that approximately two-thirds of injuries seen clinically are partial injuries (67.2%) and that they occur in a broad distribution of anatomic locations along the ligament. The precise significance of this remains to be seen and is the focus of ongoing research. Despite the tremendous value of MRA for diagnoses of these injuries, it is not without shortcomings, as it remains expensive, time-consuming, and invasive, with many athletes reluctant to have dye injected into the elbow of their throwing arm. Furthermore, it remains a static study that is unable to functionally evaluate structures under an applied stress.

Common musculotendinous pathology at the elbow can also be evaluated on MR. Medial epicondylitis has been characterized by common flexor tendon thickening on T1-weighted imaging and/or tendon edema on T2-weighted imaging.[41,42] Younger athletes with acute injuries have been reported to show a spectrum of injury ranging from edema in the surrounding tissues in the absence of common flexor tendon inflammation to tendon fiber disruption[42] (Figure 6.8A and B). Similar findings can be seen with injury to the common extensor tendons. Furthermore, both distal biceps and triceps tendon pathology can be well assessed with MR. Injury ranging from partial- to full-thickness tears can be visualized (Figure 6.9A and B).

Ulnar neuritis can also be evaluated on MR with sensitivity and specificity of 83% and 88%,

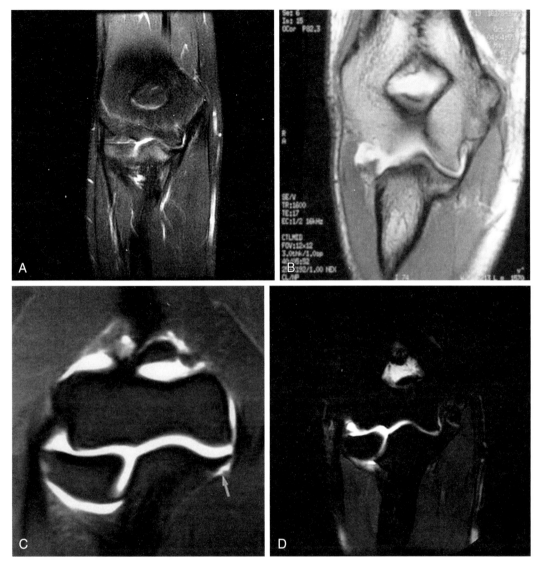

FIGURE 6.7 • MR of UCL: (A) normal coronal view, (B) abnormal coronal view with tear, (C) abnormal coronal view with T sign indicated by white arrow, (D) abnormal coronal view with chronic changes.

TABLE 6.1 Joyner Ulnar Collateral Ligament Injury Classification on Magnetic Resonance Imaging (MRI)

Classification	Qualitative Description	Reported Prevalence by Joyner et al
Type I	Low-grade partial tear—involves only edema within UCL	9.2%
Type II	High-grade partial tear—partial tear of UCL without extravasation of fluid on arthrogram	58.0%
Type III	Complete/full-thickness tear—extravasation of fluid through torn UCL on arthrogram	27.5%
Type IV	Tear/pathology in more than 1 anatomic location within the UCL (ie, ulna and humerus)	5.4%

Humerus, ulna, and midsubstance are used to further identify anatomic location of injury.

UCL, ulnar collateral ligament.

Joyner et al have proposed the above classification system for UCL injury based on MRI appearance. Injuries are classified by type and then further identified based on anatomic location. Prevalence as reported by Joyner et al is also provided.

Adapted from Joyner PW, Bruce J, Hess R, Mates A, Mills FB IV, Andrews JR, Magnetic resonance imaging-based classification for ulnar collateral ligament injuries of the elbow. J Shoulder Elbow Surg. 2016;25:1710-1716. Copyright © 2016 Elsevier. With permission.

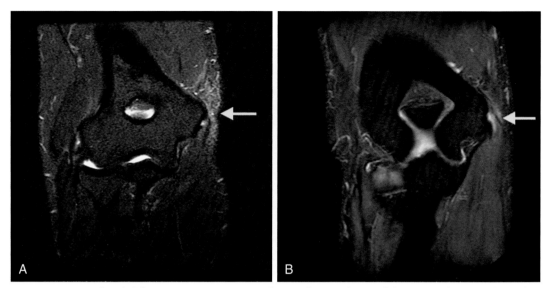

FIGURE 6.8 • MR of medial flexor-pronator injury: (A) abnormal coronal view of chronic tendinosis indicated by arrow, (B) abnormal coronal view of acute tear indicated by arrow.

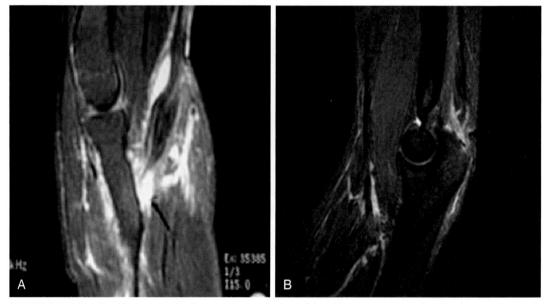

FIGURE 6.9 • MR of tendon tears: (A) abnormal sagittal view of distal biceps tear, (B) abnormal sagittal view of distal triceps tear.

respectively, and is best evaluated on axial imaging, the so-called cubital/ulnar tunnel view.[37,43,44] Irritation and inflammation are commonly indicated by thickening as well as increased signal intensity, which may be accompanied by fascicular distortion or "mottling" and perineural edema[42,45] (Figure 6.10). Chronic ulnar neuropathy can also be evaluated by its effect on distally innervated muscles, which may show fatty infiltration, increased signal, and atrophy from denervation.[45,46]

Ultrasound

Musculoskeletal ultrasonography (US) utilizes reflected pulses of high frequency sound waves to visualize tendons, ligaments, muscles, nerves, vessels, joints, cartilage, bone surfaces, soft tissue masses, and fluid-containing structures. The intensity of the reflected sound wave is depicted using a gray scale, and the time it takes to return to the transducer determines the depth of the structure on the image. Linear array transducers, as opposed to curved transducers, are typically used

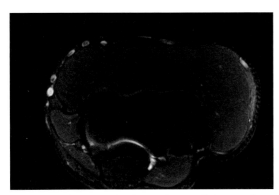

FIGURE 6.10 • MR cubital tunnel view of abnormal ulnar nerve.

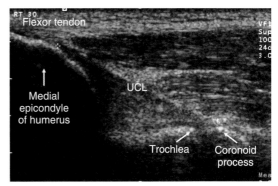

FIGURE 6.11 • Longitudinal ultrasound view of medial elbow showing the flexor-pronator tendon, medial epicondyle of the humerus, the sublime tubercle of the coronoid process of the ulna, and the UCL.

in musculoskeletal US. High-frequency transducers sacrifice depth of tissue penetration to yield improved axial resolution ranging from 0.15 mm at 10 MHz to 0.04 mm at 20 MHz. At the elbow, the need for significant tissue penetration is limited; thus 13 MHz transducers are commonly used, yielding the image resolution necessary for detailed evaluation of musculoskeletal tissues. The orientation of the transducer can quickly provide views analogous to the axial, coronal, and sagittal views seen using other advanced imaging.

A number of common imaging artifacts may be encountered with the use of musculoskeletal ultrasound. Anisotropy is commonly seen in tendons (to a lesser degree in muscles, nerves, and ligaments), in which the beam is reflected into another plane and only partially reflected to the transducer, yielding an uncharacteristic hypoechogenic image. Acoustic shadowing is the inability to visualize behind structures that completely reflect sound waves, such as intact bone or dense calcification. In contrast, acoustic enhancement causes structures deep to areas that do not absorb much of the beam (such as cysts and other fluid-filled structures) to appear brighter than similar adjacent tissues. Metal objects such as needles, implants, and prostheses cause reverberation, in which multiple echoes are seen.

The characteristic ultrasound appearance of musculoskeletal tissues has been well described. Bone is typically hyperechoic (white/bright) and, as described above, exhibits acoustic shadowing. In contrast, articular cartilage is often anechoic (black) with a smooth surface. Degenerative cartilage is characterized by increased echogenicity and surface irregularities. Synovium demonstrates intermediate echogenicity; joint capsule can be identified as the boundary between hypoechoic synovium and anechoic synovial fluid, which can be displaced by pressure from the transducer. Tendons typically possess a fine, organized internal fibrillar pattern; are slightly hyperechoic; and

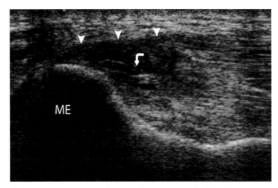

FIGURE 6.12 • Longitudinal ultrasound view of flexor-pronator tear demonstrated the medial epicondyle (ME), flexor-pronator tendon (arrowheads), and disruption of the undersurface of the tendon (arrow).

may exhibit anisotropy. Nerves possess a similar echogenicity to tendon, but the internal fascicular pattern is less tightly packed than the fibrillary pattern of tendon. Muscle is largely hypoechoic, although interspersed with hyperechoic lines representing the peri- and epimysium, and surrounded by hyperechoic lines indicating septae and investing fascia. Finally, ligaments, such as the UCL, demonstrate similar echogenicity to tendon but contain multiple layers of fibrillary patterns running in different directions (Figure 6.11).

Abnormal ultrasound findings are common in the overhead-throwing athlete and may be symptomatic or asymptomatic. Common findings for musculotendinous pathology include flexor-pronator and extensor tendinosis and tearing (Figure 6.12). The distal biceps and triceps tendons can also be assessed for rupture with measurement of retraction (Figure 6.13A and B). Finally, neurovascular structures such as the ulnar nerve can be evaluated for edema, scarring, and dynamic subluxation (Figure 6.14A and B). Ultrasound is also valuable for evaluating the UCL.

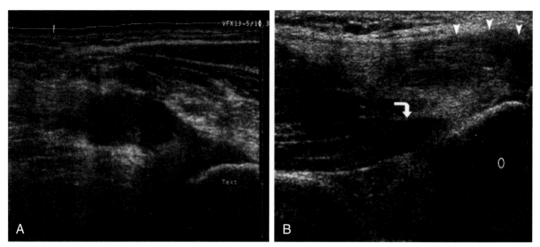

FIGURE 6.13 • Sagittal ultrasound view of tendon tears: (A) distal biceps, (B) triceps tears demonstrating the olecranon (O), the triceps tendon (arrowheads), and disruption of the triceps tendon at its insertion (arrow).

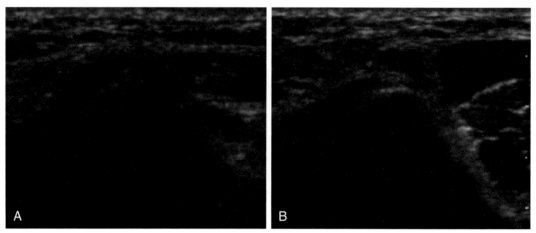

FIGURE 6.14 • Axial ultrasound view of ulnar nerve: (A) in the cubital tunnel with surrounding edema, (B) subluxated ulnar nerve.

Asymptomatic UCL changes include thickening of the anterior band in the dominant arm compared with the nondominant arm, calcifications, and hypoechoic foci (Figure 6.15A and B). Tears of the UCL can be visualized as disruption of the substance of the UCL with loss of tension within the fibers and anechoic fluid within the tear (Figure 6.15C).

Musculoskeletal ultrasound of the symptomatic athlete's elbow should systematically evaluate all potential sources of pathology. A careful inspection should be performed of the UCL, flexor-pronator tendons and musculature, extensor tendons and musculature, ulnar nerve, olecranon, and radiocapitellar joint. In addition to the aforementioned superior spatial resolution of US, this modality benefits from the ability to dynamically assess the function of these structures. As with stress radiographs, a valgus stress can be applied to the elbow with a standardized device. Thereby, the

functional integrity of the UCL can be assessed by comparing the amount of ulnohumeral joint gapping with and without valgus stress. At the authors' institution, a Telos device (Weiterstadt, Germany) is utilized to apply a standardized valgus stress of 15 daN during stress ultrasound evaluation. Stress is applied to the injured elbow at 30° of flexion and compared with the contralateral side for evaluation of the increase in ulnohumeral gapping from the rest state to the stressed state (Figure 6.16A and B).

Over the last decade, numerous studies have investigated stress US for the diagnosis of UCL injury in the throwing athlete. In 2003, at our institution, Nazarian et al was the first to describe the aforementioned stress ultrasound technique in 26 asymptomatic Major League Baseball (MLB) pitchers.[40] Stress ultrasound demonstrated that the anterior band of the UCL is thicker in the pitching arm, more likely to have

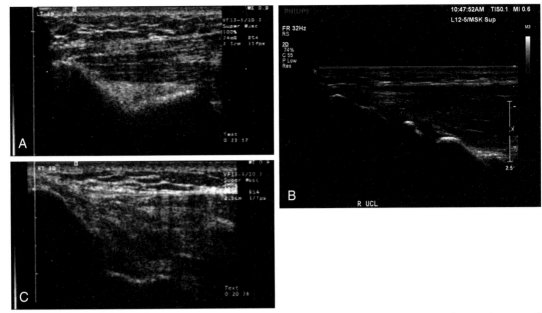

FIGURE 6.15 • Longitudinal ultrasound views of the UCL: (A) normal, (B) chronic changes of hypoechoic signal and calcifications, (C) acute tear.

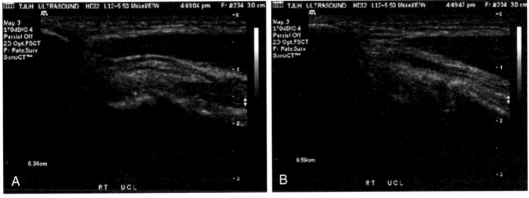

FIGURE 6.16 • Longitudinal ultrasound of UCL demonstrating: (A) the width of the ulnohumeral joint at rest and (B) the width of the ulnohumeral joint with applied valgus stress.

hypoechoic foci and calcifications, and demonstrates greater ulnohumeral joint gapping with stress with applied valgus stress. In 2014, Ciccotti et al followed up this initial study with a 10-year, prospective evaluation of this technique in 368 asymptomatic MLB pitchers, corroborating the findings of Nazarian et al.[47] Furthermore, in this longitudinal study, ulnohumeral joint gapping was seen to increase with time among pitchers who were examined in multiple years. A concurrent cadaveric study by Ciccotti et al utilized the stress ultrasound technique in anatomic elbow specimens to evaluate the contribution to ulnohumeral joint stability of the various medial elbow structures.[14] Sequential sectioning confirmed the greatest increase in gapping occurred with sectioning of the anterior

band of the UCL. These findings, in conjunction with the 2 clinical studies mentioned earlier, allowed the authors to establish a threshold of approximately 1.5 mm of increased ulnohumeral joint gapping from rest to stress compared with the contralateral arm as suggestive of clinically significant UCL injury.

Stress US has also been studied in youth and adolescent pitchers. In 2015, Atanda et al performed SUS on asymptomatic professional pitchers aged 17 to 21 years and divided them into groups by age and experience, finding that UCL thickness significantly increased with the number of years of professional pitching.[48] This suggests that a thickening ligament may be the first adaptive or pathologic change to occur. Furthermore, in 2016, Atanda et al reported on 102 youth and adolescent pitchers divided into 2 groups based on age (12-14 and 15-18 years).[49] In this study, a thicker UCL was correlated with more time pitching, with more pitches per appearance, and with more than 5.5 years of pitching, adding greater nuance to our understanding of the sequence of pathologic/adaptive change in the UCL as a result of repeated valgus stress.

TRIP TO THE MOUND

In currently unpublished work, Ciccotti et al utilized stress US to more thoroughly evaluate the functional consequences of partial tears of the UCL in a cadaveric model. The authors simulated clinically noted patterns of partial tears at different anatomic locations within the anterior band of UCL, comparing the resultant ulnohumeral joint gapping with stress to the intact and completely torn states. They noted different amounts of gapping at different locations of partial tears within the UCL, suggesting that some partial tears may be more stable than others and therefore more amenable to nonoperative treatment, whereas others may be indicated for early reconstruction. Although further research is necessary to define the in vivo behavior of different partial tears, it appears more important than ever to define both the location and degree of UCL injury to inform optimal management.

CURRENT RECOMMENDATIONS IN THE THROWING ATHLETE

The current approach advocated by the authors is a combined approach using both MRA and stress US to improve diagnostic accuracy. In 2016, at our institution, Roedl et al reported the results of such a combined approach in 144 baseball players at all levels of competition who had obtained both MRA and US/SUS preoperatively.[50] Imaging findings individually and in combination were correlated with surgical findings as the gold standard for diagnosis. MRA alone yielded sensitivity, specificity, and accuracy for UCL tears of 81%, 91%, and 88%. SUS alone yielded sensitivity, specificity, and accuracy of 96%, 81%, and 87% for UCL tears. The combination of MRA and US/SUS increased sensitivity, specificity, and accuracy for UCL tears to 96%, 99%, and 98%. For ulnar

neuritis, MRA yielded sensitivity, specificity, and accuracy of 74%, 92%, and 88%. In comparison, US yielded sensitivity, specificity, and accuracy of 94%, 74%, and 79%. Combined MRA and US improved sensitivity, specificity and accuracy for the diagnosis of ulnar neuritis to 90%, 100%, and 98%. However, combination of MR and US did not provide similar improvement for diagnosis of myotendinous injury or posteromedial impingement. Statistically significant increased diagnostic value was noted with the combined use of ultrasound and MRA for medial elbow pain, especially the UCL. This significant amount of research on imaging of the elbow in the throwing athlete has allowed the authors to establish a clinical algorithm for the diagnosis and management of medial elbow injury in this population (Table 6.2).

MANAGER'S TIPS

- Any evaluation of the throwing athlete's elbow requires a thorough history and physical examination to provide context for subsequent imaging studies
- It is important to recognize that asymptomatic changes exist with all imaging, particularly in overhead throwers
- As in the majority of musculoskeletal complaints, plain radiographs should be obtained initially
- If the athlete's symptoms and examination suggest structural injury, it is appropriate to progress to advanced imaging. MRA is typically the imaging study of choice
- Recent research suggests that a combined approach with stress US may increase diagnostic accuracy, particularly in the setting of UCL injury, from partial to full and recurrent
- Regardless of the imaging obtained, it is critical to never consider the imaging studies in isolation, but always interpret those findings with respect to the athlete's history and physical examination findings to provide optimal care

ACKNOWLEDGMENTS

We would like to take this opportunity to acknowledge the gracious contribution of our colleagues in the Division of Musculoskeletal Radiology in the Department of Radiology at Thomas Jefferson University Hospital, Philadelphia, Pennsylvania. Drs Levon Nazarian and Adam Zoga were invaluable in identifying and sharing many of the images displayed in this chapter.

TABLE 6.2 Clinical Algorithm for the Diagnosis and Treatment of Ulnar Collateral Ligament (UCL) Injury Including the Use of Stress Ultrasound, Magnetic Resonance Imaging, and Magnetic Resonance Arthrography

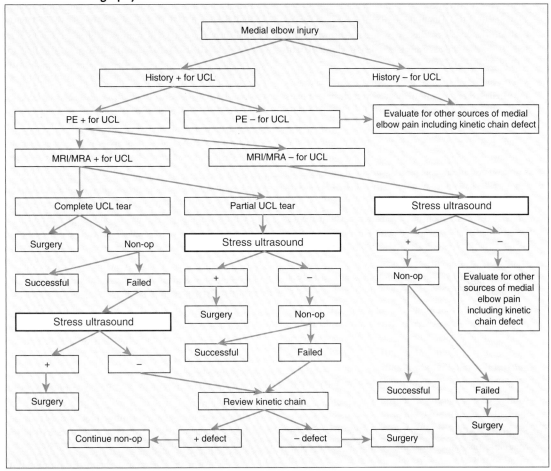

Reprinted with permission from Ciccotti MC, Nazarian LN, Ciccotti MG. Ultrasound imaging of ulnar collateral ligament injury. In: Dines JS, Altchek DW, eds. Elbow Ulnar Collateral Ligament Injury: A Guide to Diagnosis and Treatment. US, New York, NY: Springer; 2015:79-91. Copyright © 2015 Springer Science+Business Media New York.

REFERENCES

1. Cain EL, Dugas JR, Wolf RS, Andrews JR. Elbow injuries in throwing athletes: a current concepts review. *Am J Sports Med*. 2003;31(4):621-635. doi:10.1177/03635 465030310042601.

2. Patel RM, Lynch TS, Amin NH, Calabrese G, Gryzlo SM, Schickendantz MS. The thrower's elbow. *Orthop Clin North Am*. 2014;45(3):355-376. doi:10.1016/j. ocl.2014.03.007.

3. Wilson FD, Andrews JR, Blackburn TA, Mccluskey G. Valgus extension overload in the pitching elbow. *Am J Sports Med*. 1983;11(2):83-88. doi:10.1177/036354658301100206.

4. DeFroda SF, Kriz PK, Hall AM, Zurakowski D, Fadale PD. Risk stratification for ulnar collateral ligament injury in major league baseball players. *Orthop J Sports Med*. 2016;4(2). doi:10.1177/2325967 115627126.

5. Hodgins JL, Vitale M, Arons RR, Ahmad CS. Epidemiology of medial ulnar collateral ligament reconstruction. *Am J Sports Med*. 2016;44(3):729-734. doi:10.1177/0363546515622407.

6. Mahure SA, Mollon B, Shamah SD, Kwon YW, Rokito AS. Disproportionate trends in ulnar collateral ligament reconstruction: projections through 2025 and a literature review. *J Shoulder Elbow Surg*. 2016;25(6):1005-1012. doi:10.1016/j.jse.2016.02.036.

7. Erickson BJ, Nwachukwu BU, Rosas S, et al. Trends in medial ulnar collateral ligament reconstruction in the United States. *Am J Sports Med*. 2015;43(7):1770-1774. doi:10.1177/0363546515580304.

8. Ciccotti MG, Pollack KM, Ciccotti MC, et al. Elbow injuries in professional baseball: epidemiological findings from the major league baseball injury surveillance system. *Am J Sports Med*. 2017;45(10):2319-2328. doi:10.1177/0363546517706964.

9. Hariri S, Safran MR. Ulnar collateral ligament injury in the overhead athlete. *Athletes Elb*. 2010;29(4):619-644. doi:10.1016/j.csm.2010.06.007.

10. Veltri DM, O'Brien SJ, Field LD, Deutsch A, Altchek DW, Potter HG. The milking manuever-a new test to evaluate the MCL of the elbow in the throwing athlete. *J Shoulder Elbow Surg*.1995; 4:S10. doi:10.1016/S1058-2746(95)80048-4.

11. O'Driscoll SWM, Lawton RL, Smith AM. The "moving valgus stress test" for medial collateral ligament tears of the elbow. *Am J Sports Med*. 2005;33(2):231-239. doi:10.1177/0363546504267804.

12. Joyner PW, Bruce J, Hess R, Mates A, Mills FB IV, Andrews JR. Magnetic resonance imaging-based classification for ulnar collateral ligament injuries of the elbow. *J Shoulder Elbow Surg*. 2016;25(10):1710-1716. doi:10.1016/j.jse.2016.05.006.

13. Cohen SB, Valko C, Zoga A, Dodson CC, Ciccotti MG. Posteromedial elbow impingement: magnetic resonance imaging findings in overhead throwing athletes and results of arthroscopic treatment. *Arthrosc J Arthrosc Relat Surg*. 2011;27(10):1364-1370. doi:10.1016/j.arthro.2011.06.012.

14. Ciccotti MC, Hammoud S, Dodson CC, Cohen SB, Nazarian LN, Ciccotti MG. Stress ultrasound evaluation of medial elbow instability in a cadaveric model. *Am J Sports Med*. 2014;42(10):2463-2469. doi:10.1177/0363546514542805.

15. Gustas CN, Lee KS. Multimodality imaging of the painful elbow. *Imaging Athlete*. 2016;54(5):817-839. doi:10.1016/j.rcl.2016.04.005.

16. Sampath SC, Sampath SC, Bredella MA. Magnetic resonance imaging of the elbow: a structured approach. *Sports Health*. 2013;5(1):34-49. doi:10.1177/1941738112467941.

17. Bowerman JW, McDonnell EJ. Radiology of athletic injuries: baseball. *Radiology*. 1975;116(3):611-615. doi:10.1148/116.3.611.

18. Mulligan SA, Schwartz ML, Broussard MF, Andrews JR. Heterotopic calcification and tears of the ulnar collateral ligament. *Am J Roentgenol*. 2000;175(4):1099-1102. doi:10.2214/ajr.175.4.1751099.

19. Popovic N, Ferrara MA, Daenen B, Georis P, Lemaire R. Imaging overuse injury of the elbow in professional team handball players: a bilateral comparison using plain films, stress radiography, ultrasound, and magnetic resonance imaging. *Int J Sports Med*. 2002;22(1):60-67. doi:10.1055/s-2001-11333.

20. Dugas JR. Valgus extension overload: diagnosis and treatment. *Athletes Elb*. 2010;29(4):645-654. doi:10.1016/j.csm.2010.07.001.

21. Saltzman BM, Chalmers PN, Mascarenhas R, Cole BJ, Romeo AA. Upper extremity physeal injury in young baseball pitchers. *Phys Sportsmed*. 2014;42(3):100-111. doi:10.3810/psm.2014.09.2081.

22. Rijke AM, Goitz HT, McCue FC, Andrews JR, Berr SS. Stress radiography of the medial elbow ligaments. *Radiology*. 1994;191(1):213-216. doi:10.1148/radiology.191.1.8134574.

23. Bruce JR, Hess R, Joyner P, Andrews JR. How much valgus instability can be expected with ulnar collateral ligament (UCL) injuries? A review of 273 baseball players with UCL injuries. *J Shoulder Elbow Surg*. 2014;23(10):1521-1526. doi:10.1016/j.jse.2014.05.015.

24. Ellenbecker TS, Mattalino AJ, Elam EA, Caplinger RA. Medial elbow joint laxity in professional baseball pitchers. *Am J Sports Med*. 1998;26(3):420-424. doi:10.1177/03635465980260031301.

25. Brunton LM, Anderson MW, Pannunzio ME, Khanna AJ, Chhabra AB. Magnetic resonance imaging of the elbow: update on current techniques and indications. *J Hand Surg*. 2006;31(6):1001-1011. doi:10.1016/j.jhsa.2006.04.006.

26. Cotten A, Jacobson J, Brossmann J, et al. Collateral ligaments of the elbow: conventional MR imaging and MR arthrography with coronal oblique plane and elbow flexion. *Radiology*. 1997;204(3):806-812. doi:10.1148/radiology.204.3.9280264.

27. Kaplan LJ, Potter HG. MR imaging of ligament injuries to the elbow. *Imaging Up Extrem*. 2006;44(4):583-594. doi:10.1016/j.rcl.2006.04.007.

28. Schwartz ML, al-Zahrani S, Morwessel RM, Andrews JR. Ulnar collateral ligament injury in the throwing athlete: evaluation with saline-enhanced MR arthrography. *Radiology*. 1995;197(1):297-299. doi:10.1148/radiology.197.1.7568841.

29. Mesgarzadeh M, Sapega AA, Bonakdarpour A, et al. Osteochondritis dissecans: analysis of mechanical stability with radiography, scintigraphy, and MR imaging. *Radiology*. 1987;165(3):775-780. doi:10.1148/radiology.165.3.3685359.

30. Peiss J, Adam G, Casser R, Urhahn R, Günther RW. Gadopentetate-dimeglumine-enhanced MR imaging of osteonecrosis and osteochondritis dissecans of the elbow: initial experience. *Skeletal Radiol*. 1995;24(1):17. doi:10.1007/BF02425939.

31. Rosenberg ZS, Beltran J, Cheung YY. Pseudodefect of the capitellum: potential MR imaging pitfall. *Radiology*. 1994;191(3):821-823. doi:10.1148/radiology.191.3.8184072.

32. Furushima K, Itoh Y, Iwabu S, Yamamoto Y, Koga R, Shimizu M. Classification of olecranon stress fractures in baseball players. *Am J Sports Med*. 2014;42(6):1343-1351. doi:10.1177/0363546514528099.

33. Regan WD. Biomechanical study of ligaments around the elbow joint. *Clin Orthop*. 1991(271):170-179.

34. Dewan A, Chhabra A, Khanna AJ, Anderson M, Brunton L. MRI of the elbow: techniques and spectrum of disease: AAOS exhibit selection. *J Bone Joint Surg Am*. 2013;95(14):e99 1-e99 13.

35. Hill NB Jr, Bucchieri JS, Shon F, Miller TT, Rosenwasser MP. Magnetic resonance imaging of injury to the medial collateral ligament of the elbow: a cadaver model. *J Shoulder Elbow Surg*. 2000;9(5):418-422. doi:10.1067/mse.2000.107392.

36. Mirowitz SA, London SL. Ulnar collateral ligament injury in baseball pitchers: MR imaging evaluation. *Radiology.* 1992;185(2):573-576. doi:10.1148/radiology.185.2.1410375.

37. Ouellette H, Kassarjian A, Tretreault P, Palmer W. Imaging of the overhead throwing athlete. *Semin Musculoskelet Radiol.* 2005;9(4):316-333. doi:10.1055/s-2005-923377.

38. Timmerman LA, Schwartz ML, Andrews JR. Preoperative evaluation of the ulnar collateral ligament by magnetic resonance imaging and computed tomography arthrography. *Am J Sports Med.* 1994;22(1):26-32. doi:10.1177/036354659402200105.

39. Fritz RC. MR imaging of the elbow. An update. *Radiol Clin North Am.* 1997;35(1):117-144.

40. Nazarian LN, McShane JM, Ciccotti MG, O'Kane PL, Harwood MI. Dynamic US of the anterior band of the ulnar collateral ligament of the elbow in asymptomatic major league baseball pitchers. *Radiology.* 2003;227(1):149-154. doi:10.1148/radiol.2271020288.

41. Stevens KJ, McNally EG. Magnetic resonance imaging of the elbow in athletes. *Clin Sports Med.* 2010;29(4):521-553. doi:10.1016/j.csm.2010.06.004.

42. Kijowski R, Tuite M, Sanford M. Magnetic resonance imaging of the elbow. Part II: Abnormalities of the ligaments, tendons, and nerves. *Skeletal Radiol.* 2005;34(1):1-18. doi:10.1007/s00256-004-0854-y.

43. Ouellette H, Bredella M, Labis J, Palmer WE, Torriani M. MR imaging of the elbow in baseball pitchers. *Skeletal Radiol.* 2008;37(2):115-121. doi:10.1007/s00256-007-0364-9.

44. Bäumer P, Dombert T, Staub F, et al. Ulnar neuropathy at the elbow: MR neurography—nerve T2 signal increase and caliber. *Radiology.* 2011;260(1):199-206. doi:10.1148/radiol.11102357.

45. Kijowski R, Tuite M, Sanford M. Magnetic resonance imaging of the elbow. Part I: Normal anatomy, imaging technique, and osseous abnormalities. *Skeletal Radiol.* 2004;33(12):685-697. doi:10.1007/s00256-004-0853-z.

46. Bordalo-Rodrigues M, Rosenberg ZS. MR imaging of entrapment neuropathies at the elbow. *Magn Reson Imaging Clin N Am.* 2004;12(2):247-263. doi:10.1016/j.mric.2004.02.002.

47. Ciccotti MG, Atanda A, Nazarian LN, Dodson CC, Holmes L, Cohen SB. Stress sonography of the ulnar collateral ligament of the elbow in professional baseball pitchers. *Am J Sports Med.* 2014;42(3):544-551. doi:10.1177/0363546513516592.

48. Atanda A, Buckley PS, Hammoud S, Cohen SB, Nazarian LN, Ciccotti MG. Early anatomic changes of the ulnar collateral ligament identified by stress ultrasound of the elbow in young professional baseball pitchers. *Am J Sports Med.* 2015;43(12):2943-2949. doi:10.1177/0363546515605042.

49. Atanda A, Averill LW, Wallace M, Niiler TA, Nazarian LN, Ciccotti MG. Factors related to increased ulnar collateral ligament thickness on stress sonography of the elbow in asymptomatic youth and adolescent baseball pitchers. *Am J Sports Med.* 2016;44(12):3179-3187. doi:10.1177/0363546516661010.

50. Roedl JB, Gonzalez FM, Zoga AC, et al. Potential utility of a combined approach with US and MR arthrography to image medial elbow pain in baseball players. *Radiology.* 2016;279(3):827-837. doi:10.1148/radiol.2015151256.

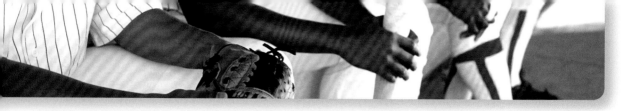

CHAPTER 7

Epicondylitis and Baseball Players

Djuro Petkovic, MD | Brian Shiu, MD | Christopher S. Ahmad, MD

My philosophy has always been simple: Believe in yourself.

—*Tommy John*

LATERAL EPICONDYLITIS— INTRODUCTION

Lateral epicondylitis is characterized by pathologic changes to the musculotendinous origin of the extension-supination musculature at the lateral elbow. Although overhead athletes more commonly develop medial elbow symptoms because of the valgus forces placed on the medial side of the elbow, they frequently experience symptoms from lateral aspect of the elbow as well. Specifically, the repetitive throwing cycle with intense gripping of the baseball may contribute to lateral epicondylitis. Forceful grasping of the bat can also cause or exacerbate symptoms. In many cases, the strength and conditioning routines of baseball players also contribute to the disease process, and exercises that require stressful gripping such as using kettle bells are most concerning.

In the general population, the incidence of lateral epicondylitis is up to 3%, with the age of onset between 40 and 50 years and affects occupations that involve high-repetition forceful activities.[1,2] Although most patients who develop lateral epicondylitis do not play tennis, almost half of tennis players develop the condition.[3] Baseball players are at increased risk based on their repetitive forceful activities coupled with their extensive workouts.

Despite the name epicondylitis, histological analysis of lateral epicondylitis shows no significant inflammation and can be classified as a tendinosis. After repeated muscular contraction, microtears develop in the tendon followed by an ineffective healing process that leads to a chronic degeneration classically termed angiofibroblastic hyperplasia.[4] Lateral epicondylitis most commonly affects the extensor carpi radialis brevis (ECRB) but can also involve the entire extensor tendon.[5]

TRIP TO THE MOUND

In baseball players, throwing activities contribute less than hitting and exercises performed in the weight room to the development of lateral epicondylitis. As players grip and lift weights away from the center of the body, stress is placed on the extensor origin on the lateral aspect of the elbow, which can start the cascade leading to lateral epicondylitis. Kettle bell lifts, for example, can be a major culprit. Early treatment of players who develop this condition can be as simple as avoiding these weight room exercises.

CLINICAL EVALUATION

History

The pain develops insidiously and may radiate distally from the lateral epicondyle. The pain is worse with gripping activity where the wrist and elbow are extended. The player may also complain of discomfort with holding objects such as a gallon of milk in the pronated position. Many players aggressively work on strengthening their grip in effort to improve hitting despite research demonstrating no improvement in bat velocity with increased grip strength.[6,7] Throwing speed has been found to be related to wrist extension strength.[8] Thus, if the player's grip strength is compromised because of lateral epicondylitis, it can potentially decrease his throwing velocity.

Physical Examination

Lateral epicondylitis classically demonstrates tenderness slightly distal to the lateral epicondyle. Pain can be elicited with resisted wrist and finger extension. Tenderness located more distal than 1 cm from the epicondyle or associated with severe weakness may suggest a posterior interosseous nerve compression syndrome. A radial neck stress fracture or intra-articular processes such as radiocapitellar arthritis, posterior plica, or osteochondritis dissecans of the capitellum can similarly mimic lateral epicondylitis and should be evaluated with radiographic and/or advanced imaging. A cervical spine examination should also be performed to rule out any radicular component of pain.

Imaging and Other Studies

Although radiographic imaging is not required to diagnose lateral epicondylitis, standard radiographs should be obtained to rule out bony pathology. Radiographs can often be normal or calcifications may be present, although the significance of these findings have yet to be determined.[9] Calcifications may also develop secondary to repeated corticosteroid injections.[10] If a compression neuropathy is suspected, electromyography (EMG) and nerve conduction studies (NCSs) should be performed.

Evaluation of the soft tissue structures can be performed with ultrasound or magnetic resonance imaging (MRI). Ultrasound is noninvasive and can reliably detect calcifications, tendon thickening, and heterogeneity of lateral soft tissue structures.[11] However, even with an experienced ultrasound radiologist or practitioner, the specificity and implications of these findings has still yet to be determined.

MRI detects tendon tears or signal changes related to tendinopathy. However, asymptomatic individuals can have signal changes within the ECRB, so interpretation of imaging must be assessed in the context of clinical findings. In elite baseball players, MRI is often used to evaluate the degree of epicondylitis and potential intra-articular pathology that may coexist (Figure 7.1).

TRIP TO THE MOUND

An MRI of the elbow often shows pathologic processes in elite baseball players. In addition, radiology reports often note the presence of lateral tendon tears. The original imaging should be interpreted by an experienced physician to determine the true magnitude of the pathology because in reality many "tears" are merely areas of increased signal related to the pathologic process of lateral epicondylitis. On evaluation of an MRI, the treating practitioner should carefully examine for other intra-articular pathology that could be a cause of the player's symptoms. Such confounding conditions that can mimic lateral epicondylitis include radiocapitellar arthrosis, a synovial plica, capitellar osteochondritis dissecans, an inflamed radial bursa, and loose bodies. Certainly, if the player had a baseline MRI obtained at the time of the player's draft or trade, the clinician should compare any processes in the new MRI with baseline imaging.

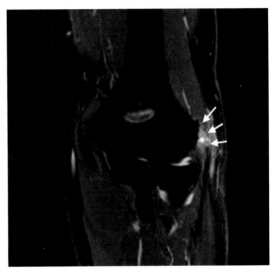

FIGURE 7.1 • A T2 coronal MRI of the throwing elbow of a professional outfielder showing the white bright signal change in the extensor tendon origin at the lateral epicondyle. The white arrows point to this high signal area suggesting lateral epicondylitis. (Courtesy Christopher S. Ahmad, MD.)

TREATMENT

Nonoperative

Nonsurgical management of lateral epicondylitis is the cornerstone of treatment. The majority of these patients will have symptomatic relief from conservative management with some series reporting as high as 95% of patients obtaining significant relief.[12] The most important initial step is to eliminate the activities producing the tendinopathy such as overhand or pronated lifts in the weight room and hitting. Initial treatment also includes NSAIDs and a rehabilitation protocol that includes modalities that decrease inflammation such as icing and gentle compression wrapping.

Other nonoperative treatments including night-time and periodic extension wrist splinting may be attempted. Counterforce bracing during the day may further assist athletes during their daily activities. Directed physiotherapy with additional modalities and eccentric strengthening are important components of conservative treatment. Injection treatment can be performed consisting of a corticosteroid, autologous blood, or platelet-rich plasma (PRP), the results of which will be reviewed later in this chapter. PRP in particular has an important role in the treatment of recalcitrant lateral epicondylitis based on various studies.[13-17] Various other modalities include ultrasound, acupuncture, laser therapy, acupuncture, and extracorporeal shock-wave therapy, although few high-quality trials exist for these treatments.[18-21]

The progression of rehabilitation begins once the thrower sufficiently rests his elbow to the point where it is no longer painful, at which point he can begin to increase range of motion followed by strengthening. Isometric exercises should be performed followed by integration of eccentric and then concentric exercises. Gradual resistance is added until the strength reaches or surpasses preinjury levels. Return to sport should begin with a gradual increase in throwing intensity, hitting, strength, and conditioning. Exercises should be continued under the supervision of a physician or physical therapist to maintain strength and motion during the season.

Operative

Indications

A minority of patients will fail a conservative management period of 6 to 12 months and will be indicated for surgery. In professional athletes, a shortened timeline may be appropriate depending where in the season the injury occurs. No absolute contraindications exist to surgery besides comorbidities that would make surgical treatment an unacceptable risk for a particular patient.

Surgical Options

The goal of operative management is to debride the painful, diseased tendon. The two primary techniques for treatment of lateral epicondylitis include open debridement with or without tendon repair and arthroscopic debridement. Open treatment is currently the gold standard for effective debridement of the extensor origin. Alternatively, arthroscopic debridement allows the surgeon to evaluate for intra-articular pathology such as loose bodies, chondral wear, or synovitis.[10] Although elbow arthroscopy

has a significant learning curve, arthroscopic debridement has recently gained popularity because of ability for faster return to work.[22-24] Recent anatomic work has designated a safe zone during elbow arthroscopy to limit injury to the lateral ulnar collateral ligament (LUCL), significantly improving the safety profile of the procedure.[25] Consistently favorable results have been achieved with both treatment methods, leaving the decision at the surgeon's discretion.

Authors' Preferred Surgical Technique

Preoperative Planning

Preoperative X-rays are evaluated for any bony pathology that can be responsible for the patient's symptoms. As noted earlier, a preoperative MRI can also be examined for intra-articular pathology as well as any tear of the extensor origin off the lateral epicondyle. If there is no suspicion of intra-articular pathology, or in the setting of a clear case of chronic lateral epicondylitis, an open debridement is the gold standard and is preferred with the patient positioned in the supine position with the arm internally rotated across his chest. However, in the event of suspicion or confirmation of intra-articular pathology based on preoperative imaging, a diagnostic arthroscopy is performed to treat any intra-articular pathology as well as treatment of the lateral epicondylitis from inside the joint. Arthroscopic management can then be converted to a mini-open debridement and repair of the extensor origin. This is done from the lateral position with the arm suspended on an arm holder.

Equipment Needed

If doing isolated open approach:

- Standard operating room table
- Hand table extension
- Hand tray including a small rongeur and curettes
- 2.0 preloaded suture anchor
- Free Mayo needle
- Pneumatic or cordless drill
- Size 0 nonabsorbable braided suture

If including arthroscopy, the following additional instruments are needed:

- Lateral arm holder
- Bean bag (for lateral position)
- 4.0 mm 30° arthroscope
- 2.7 mm arthroscope as needed
- 3.5 and 4.5 mechanical shaver
- Electrocautery device
- Switching stick(s)

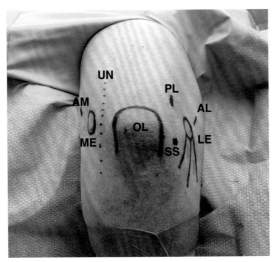

FIGURE 7.2 • Before surgery, all bony prominences and potential portal sites are marked. The anteromedial (AM) portal, medial epicondyle (ME), ulnar nerve (UN), olecranon (OL), posterolateral (PL) portal, "soft spot" (SS) portal, lateral epicondyle (LE), and anterolateral (AL) portal are shown. (Courtesy Christopher S. Ahmad, MD.)

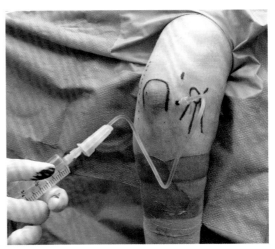

FIGURE 7.3 • An 18-gauge needle connected to flexible tubing is inserted into the "soft spot" portal and once through the elbow joint capsule, saline is injected to insufflate the joint. (Courtesy Christopher S. Ahmad, MD.)

- Fully threaded and partially threaded graspers
- Blunt tipped elevator
- Osteotomes (1/4 inch both straight and curved)
- Articulating retractor
- 60 cc syringe with normal saline and 18G needle
- 10 cc syringe with Lidocaine

Step by Step Surgical Technique (Arthroscopy)

- The patient is positioned in the lateral decubitus position with the arm on a lateral arm positioner. The major anatomical landmarks are marked out as well as the intended portal sites (Figure 7.2). These will include the following:
  - Olecranon
  - Lateral epicondyle
  - Radial head
  - Medial epicondyle
  - Path of the ulnar nerve
  - Anteromedial (AM) portal, which is 2 cm proximal to the medial epicondyle and 1 cm anterior to intermuscular septum. This can be 1 to 13 mm from the medial antebrachial cutaneous nerve[26]
  - Anterolateral (AL) portal: 1 cm anterior and proximal to the lateral epicondyle
  - Posterolateral (PL) portal: located in a vertical line anywhere on the lateral border of the triceps

tendon usually about 1 cm proximal to the olecranon tip (to minimize neurovascular risk)
  - Soft spot (SS) portal: Also known as the direct lateral portal, placed in the recess formed between the olecranon tip, radial head, and lateral epicondyle
  - Accessory posterolateral portals can be made about 2 cm proximal to the PL portal along the lateral border of the triceps for retractor insertion (not shown in this image)
  - Direct posterior portal: located 2 to 3 cm proximal to the tip of the olecranon in the midline of the triceps (not shown in this image)

Anterior Elbow Arthroscopy

- An 18-gauge needle is placed through the SS portal and capsule percutaneously and connected to a 60 mL syringe filled with sterile saline via flexible tubing (Figure 7.3)
- By injecting 20 to 30 mL into the joint, the bone to nerve distance is increased by distending the capsule[27]
- The skin is incised at the proximal AM portal and spread through the subcutaneous tissues with a hemostat clamp (Figure 7.4)
- The arthroscope is then inserted into the joint through the AM portal using a blunt trocar followed by insertion of the camera (Figure 7.5)
- A diagnostic arthroscopy is performed in the anterior joint and the diseased, tendinotic tissue of the ECRB is identified as well as any tears (Figure 7.6)

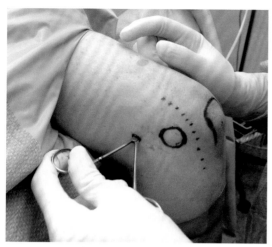

FIGURE 7.4 • A hemostat clamp is used to spread and create a path through the soft tissues through the AM (anteromedial) portal and used to pierce the anterior capsule. (Courtesy Christopher S. Ahmad, MD.)

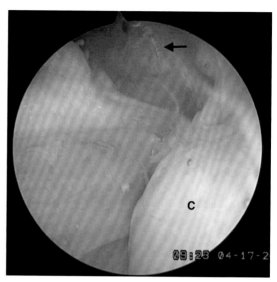

FIGURE 7.6 • View from the AM (anteromedial) portal in the anterior elbow joint showing a rent in the ECRB (extensor carpi radialis brevis) (arrow). C, capitellum. (Courtesy Christopher S. Ahmad, MD.)

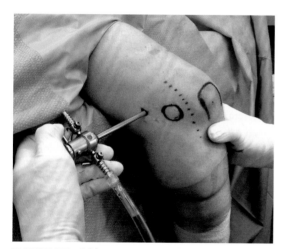

FIGURE 7.5 • A blunt trocar is used to advance the cannula through the AM (anteromedial) portal. (Courtesy Christopher S. Ahmad, MD.)

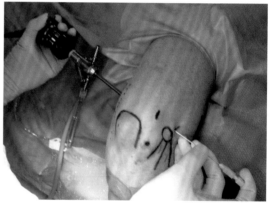

FIGURE 7.7 • The anterolateral (AL) portal is created under needle localization. (Courtesy Christopher S. Ahmad, MD.)

- The AL portal is created under needle localization (Figure 7.7), followed by scalpel incision through the skin. A hemostat clamp is again used to spread through the soft tissues and capsule (Figure 7.8)
- One can insert a switching stick or articulating retractor through the AL portal or through an accessory proximal AL portal as necessary to retract anterior soft tissues (including the posterior interosseous nerve and anterior capsule) during the case (Figure 7.9)
- A mechanical shaver is inserted through the AL portal, and the ECRB tendon is debrided. The fibers of the extensor carpi radialis longus (ECRL) are visualized more superficial and

anterior once the ECRB tendon is adequately debrided (Figure 7.10)
- More posteriorly, one may find the fibers of the extensor digitorum communis
- One has to be mindful not to debride more posterior than the equator of the radial head, or risk compromising the LUCL
- Continue debridement of the ECRB tendon until the entire tendon is excised and the four corners of the window into the more superficial fibers of the ECRL are visualized (Figure 7.11)
- Other pathology in the elbow joint can be addressed as needed (Figure 7.12)

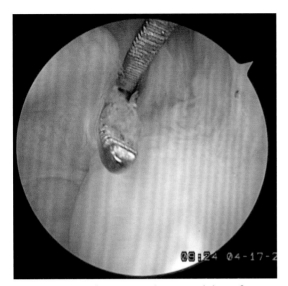

FIGURE 7.8 • A clamp is used to spread the soft tissues through the capsule from the AL (anterolateral) portal. (Courtesy Christopher S. Ahmad, MD.)

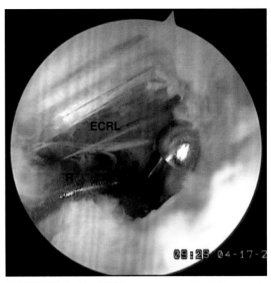

FIGURE 7.10 • The ECRB (extensor carpi radialis brevis) is being debrided, exposing the horizontal fibers of the more superficial ECRL (extensor carpi radialis longus). R, retractor. (Courtesy Christopher S. Ahmad, MD.)

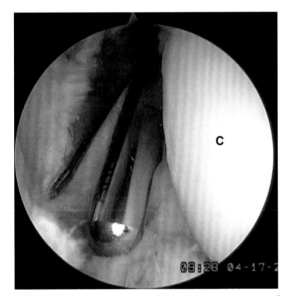

FIGURE 7.9 • A switching stick is used as a retractor of the anterior soft tissues through the same portal (AL [anterolateral] portal) as the shaver, which is debriding the ECRB (extensor carpi radialis brevis). R, retractor; C, capitellum. (Courtesy Christopher S. Ahmad, MD.)

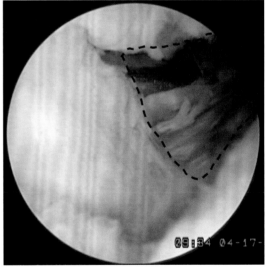

FIGURE 7.11 • A window is now visible, outlined by the dashed line, where the previous ECRB (extensor carpi radialis brevis) fibers used to be, exposing the more superficial ECRL (extensor carpi radialis longus) fibers. (Courtesy Christopher S. Ahmad, MD.)

Open Debridement and Repair of Extensor Origin

- An open approach to the lateral elbow can be employed to obtain a more thorough debridement and repair of the extensor tendon origin
- The arm is held in internal rotation and a longitudinal incision is made over the extensor origin and across the radiocapitellar joint just anterior to the lateral epicondyle (Figure 7.13)
- Metzenbaum scissors are used to dissect off the soft tissues down to the fascia overlying the extensor origin (Figure 7.14)
- The muscle is elevated off the underlying fascia with an elevator (Figure 7.15). The diseased tendon is now clearly visible (Figure 7.16)

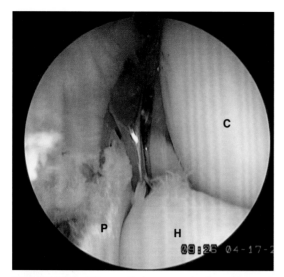

FIGURE 7.12 • Other pathology can also be addressed with an arthroscope. In this case, the patient had a symptomatic radiocapitellar plica (P), which is being excised with an arthroscopic biter. C, capitellum, H, radial head. (Courtesy Christopher S. Ahmad, MD.)

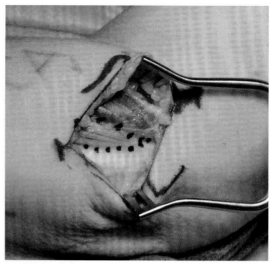

FIGURE 7.14 • After incision, the subcutaneous tissues are dissected down to the fascia overlying the extensor origin. The EDC (extensor digitorum communis) tendon is outlined. ECRB (extensor carpi radialis brevis) is deep to it. (Courtesy Christopher S. Ahmad, MD.)

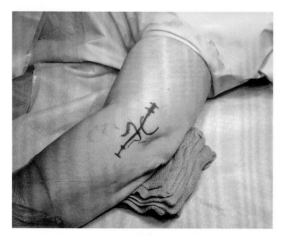

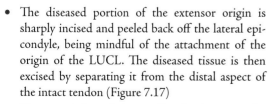

FIGURE 7.13 • A patient's left arm is shown prepped and draped with the planned incision drawn over the lateral aspect of the radiocapitellar joint. The wrist is to the bottom left and the shoulder is toward the upper right part of the picture. (Courtesy Christopher S. Ahmad, MD.)

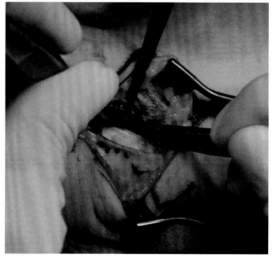

FIGURE 7.15 • : The EDC (extensor digitorum communis) fascia is incised and muscle is elevated, exposing the ECRB (extensor carpi radialis brevis). (Courtesy Christopher S. Ahmad, MD.)

- The diseased portion of the extensor origin is sharply incised and peeled back off the lateral epicondyle, being mindful of the attachment of the origin of the LUCL. The diseased tissue is then excised by separating it from the distal aspect of the intact tendon (Figure 7.17)
- The remainder of the tendinotic tissue on the underside of the extensor origin is excised and the lateral epicondyle is then debrided using a rongeur, curette, or other instrumentation down to a healthy bleeding surface to optimize healing potential (Figure 7.18)
- The extensor origin is now repaired
  - A 2.0 or 2.4 anchor single-loaded with high-strength #2 suture is inserted into the lateral epicondyle (Figure 7.19)

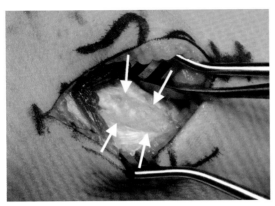

FIGURE 7.16 • The ECRB (extensor carpi radialis brevis) tendon origin is exposed and the diseased tissue is clearly delineated by the change in color and tendon quality, as indicated with the arrows. (Courtesy Christopher S. Ahmad, MD.)

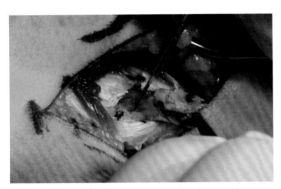

FIGURE 7.17 • The distal extent of the diseased tissue is separated from the surrounding healthy tendon and excised. (Courtesy Christopher S. Ahmad, MD.)

• Because the size of the sutures is too large for the repair, the sutures in the anchor are changed out for a size 0 braided suture
  ◆ This can be done by piercing a size 0 suture through one of the limbs of the #2 suture, then pulling the 0 suture halfway through its length
  ◆ This size 0 suture is then shuttled across the eyelet of the suture anchor and cut at its midpoint, leaving 4 limbs of sutures coming out of the suture anchor (Figure 7.20)
• Using free needles, each size 0 suture limb is passed through opposite sides of the extensor origin and tied to its opposite limb to pull the extensor aponeurosis down to the suture anchor and to the lateral epicondyle (Figure 7.21)
• A 3-0 braided suture is used to close the remainder of the aponeurosis (Figure 7.22)
• The skin is closed in a layered fashion with 3-0 braided suture in the deep dermal layer and a 4-0 monofilament used to close the skin in a subcuticular fashion

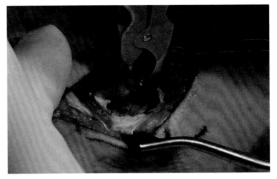

FIGURE 7.18 • The remainder of the tissue overlying the lateral epicondyle is debrided of soft tissue until a healthy bleeding bony bed is visualized. (Courtesy Christopher S. Ahmad, MD.)

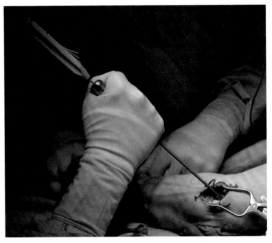

FIGURE 7.19 • A suture anchor preloaded with #2 braided suture is advanced into the lateral epicondyle. (Courtesy Christopher S. Ahmad, MD.)

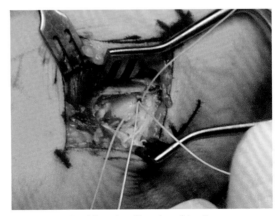

FIGURE 7.20 • After shuttling the white 0 suture across the eyelet of the suture anchor, the looped end of the suture will be cut, and the blue #2 suture will be pulled from the anchor, resulting in 4 white suture limbs coming out of the anchor. (Courtesy Christopher S. Ahmad, MD.)

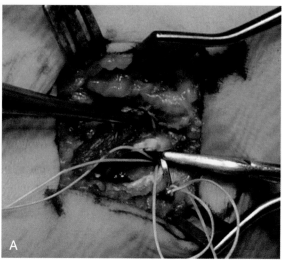
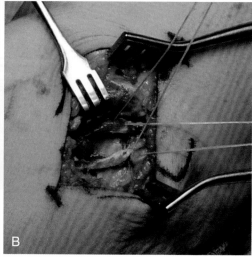

FIGURE 7.21 • A, Sutures from the suture anchor are passed across the anterior leaflet of the remaining extensor origin. B, All 4 limbs of suture are passed across the anterior and posterior leaflets of the extensor origin. (Courtesy Christopher S. Ahmad, MD.)

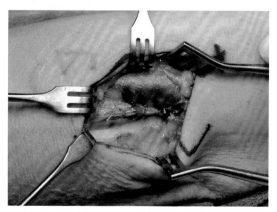

FIGURE 7.22 • The completed repair of the aponeurosis is shown. (Courtesy Christopher S. Ahmad, MD.)

POSTSURGICAL REHABILITATION

All patients are placed in a sling for comfort postoperatively until the effects of the perioperative nerve block wear off. Patients are also placed in a wrist extension brace to take pressure off the lateral elbow extensor origin. They continue this brace until the first postoperative visit. The patient can begin gentle elbow range of motion immediately. After about 4 weeks they can begin gentle wrist and elbow flexion exercises with some resistance, but avoid active wrist extension or passive flexion exercises. At 6 weeks postoperatively, the patient can begin light resistance exercises for wrist extension, progressing as tolerated. At 3 months postoperatively, if pain-free, the throwing athlete can begin a return to a throwing program and progress to full play as per protocol. Full return to play should be expected in the throwing athlete by 4 to 6 months.

RESULTS

Overall the treatment of lateral epicondylitis has been found to be very amenable to both operative and nonoperative treatment. The lack of consensus may be related to the fact that the condition is self-limited, the incomplete evidence on mechanism, or poor methodology.[28] Classically, it has been determined that 90% to 95% of patients will recover from lateral epicondylitis with conservative treatment alone.[12,29] Simple observation can be as effective a treatment as any; one study found that successful treatment at 52 weeks was 69% for injections, 91% for physiotherapy, and 83% for a "wait-and-see" type of treatment.[30]

Despite the fact that this is not an inflammatory condition, the use of NSAIDs alone has had mixed results; one study has shown oral NSAIDs to have a beneficial effect.[31] However, there have been randomized control trials comparing NSAIDs with placebo for treatment of lateral epicondylitis and found no significant difference.[32,33] Topical NSAIDs have also shown promise as a potential treatment.[34]

Physical therapy has also received mixed results in the literature. A systematic review on physical therapy modalities could only give Grade A recommendations for short-term interventions including pulsed ultrasound, friction massage, strengthening, stretching, and exercise, but after 6 months they could not recommend therapy as an effective modality beyond a "wait-and-see" approach.[35] Female gender and nerve-related symptoms are poor prognostic factors regarding early results with physical therapy.[36]

Bracing has also been extensively examined over time. EMG activity has been examined using various braces and it was found that the lateral elbow counter-force brace led to decreased activity in the extensor origin muscles.[37] One study found significant decrease in pain with a brace at 2 weeks, but this decrease did not persist at 6 weeks of follow-up.[38] A Cochrane review could not find any differences in the literature for different types of bracing for lateral epicondylitis, including no differences between wrist and elbow bracing.[39] However, a recent randomized trial did find greater improvement with a wrist extension brace compared with a forearm brace.[40]

Injections have been used in various forms, ranging from corticosteroid to PRP injections. One study randomized patients with lateral epicondylitis to corticosteroid or placebo injections ± physiotherapy. They found that patients who had a steroid injection, while enjoying more improvement at 4 weeks, had worse results at 1 year with lower complete recovery (83% vs 96%) and greater 1 year recurrence (54% vs 12%).[41] Others have found short-term improvement with corticosteroid injection that was not maintained after the first month.[15] Botulinum toxin has been noted to provide marginal benefit but with the risk of temporary paralysis of finger extension.[42] Other biologic treatments have also been extensively studied with mixed results. Well-designed randomized studies have found no significant differences between injection with placebo, autologous blood, or corticosteroid,[43] whereas a systematic review has found autologous blood as well as PRP to be effective.[42] PRP injection is a promising treatment with randomized studies showing improvement maintained at over 2 years compared with corticosteroid[16,17] and also superior results compared with autologous whole blood.[14] However, even here there is disagreement as other randomized studies have found no improvement with PRP compared with placebo.[15]

Open surgical techniques have consistently good long-term outcomes, with as high as 97% improvement.[44] Improvements after arthroscopic management have also been found to continue long term with 87% being satisfied, 97% reporting feeling "better" or "much better," and 93% saying they would have the surgery again.[45] A retrospective series of open and arthroscopic treatment found similar results at 3 to 6 years of follow-up, with a slightly higher rate of excellent results in the arthroscopic group (78%) compared with the open group (67%).[46] Another systematic review found approximately 80% good results with either technique, with a slightly faster return to work with the arthroscopic group.[47] A promising new method is a percutaneous tenotomy of the common extensor tendon, which is a minimally invasive technique done under ultrasound guidance with 80% good to excellent results.[48] Further study will help delineate the ideal treatment protocol with optimal results.

COMPLICATIONS

There are a number of potential complications with treatment of lateral epicondylitis, including poor function, elbow instability from damage to the LUCL, persistent muscle weakness, potential iatrogenic damage to the posterior interosseous nerve, and painful neuroma of the posterior cutaneous nerve.[49] However, actual reports of these complications in the literature are extremely rare. Repeated injection of corticosteroid into the lateral epicondyle can also lead to problems with fat atrophy and changes in skin pigmentation, although actual reports of these complications are also uncommon.[13]

MANAGER'S TIPS

- Most athletes will sustain lateral epicondylitis from the weight room, not from throwing
- Nonoperative treatment will be effective for a large majority of cases
- Strengthening should focus on the wrist flexion, ulnar deviation and pronation; avoid strengthening the extensor muscle mass in the early stages of rehab to avoid irritation of the condition
- Later stages of rehabilitation from lateral epicondylitis should include eccentric exercises, which have demonstrated excellent results[50]

MEDIAL EPICONDYLITIS— INTRODUCTION

Medial epicondylitis or "golfer's elbow" represents pathologic changes to the musculotendinous origin of the flexor-pronator musculature at the elbow. In overhead athletes, the repetitive valgus loads coupled with muscular contractions contribute to the development of this condition. In addition to overhead throwers, medial epicondylitis has also been reported in other athletes who require repeated wrist flexion such as javelin throwers, weightlifters, golfers, and bowlers.[9,51-53] However, because of the valgus stress placed on the medial aspect of the elbow with throwing, medial epicondylitis can be a significant burden on baseball players. It also presents a diagnostic challenge to the professional taking care of baseball players as they attempt to differentiate this condition from other medial elbow pathology.

The incidence of medial epicondylitis is 5 to 20 times less common than lateral epicondylitis in the general population.[9,51] In the working population, approximately 4% to 5% of individuals have this condition with nearly 80% having relief of symptoms at 3 years.[54] Given their requirement of a predictable return to play timetable, such recovery time is not acceptable in overhead athletes, and so more aggressive diagnosis and treatment is warranted in this population. Other confounding conditions such as ulnar collateral ligament (UCL) injury, flexor strains, flexor tendon avulsions, or valgus extension overload can either mimic or be present in addition to medial epicondylitis, so the treating practitioner must have a high index of suspicion for these related conditions.

Despite the name, histological analysis of medial epicondylitis demonstrates no significant inflammation and can be classified as a tendinosis. Although most literature has focused on lateral epicondylitis, it is generally accepted that the underlying cause is similar in both processes. After repeated muscle contraction, microtears develop in the tendon and are followed by a chronic ineffective healing process that leads to a degeneration of the tendinous origin.[4] Based on EMG activity, during the acceleration phase of throwing, the flexor carpi radialis has the highest muscle activity, whereas the pronator teres has the lowest.[55] The flexor-pronator musculature microtears not only occur primarily in the interface between these 2 muscles but can also affect the remainder of the flexor-pronator muscles.[55-59] Understanding the pathology, diagnosis and treatment will be important to optimize their return to play.

CLINICAL EVALUATION

History

The diagnosis of medial epicondylitis in the throwing athlete centers around activity-related pain about the medial elbow. The pain may radiate distally from the medial epicondyle. The patient may also complain of pain with grasping or pulling heavy loads. Ulnar neuritis and UCL instability are differential diagnoses and must be excluded. The pain of medial epicondylitis will be of gradual onset and worse during the acceleration phases of the throwing motion. Symptoms will often improve significantly with NSAIDs and rest. If the patient complains of paresthesias, this can suggest ulnar nerve pathology, which can be confirmed with physical examination.

Physical Examination

Inspection and range-of motion testing should occur before eliciting maneuvers that could generate discomfort. The elbow will likely have no significant swelling or excessive warmth although this has occasionally been reported.[57] Asymptomatic flexion contractures can be expected in throwers and can be relatively common especially in professional baseball players.[60]

Tenderness at the origin of the flexor-pronator mass will likely be present within 1 cm of the epicondyle. The pain will be worse with active pronation as well as flexion at the forearm and wrist. Grip strength can be reduced in severe cases when compared with the contralateral side and can be tested with a dynamometer.

Ulnar nerve pathology can easily be elicited with a positive Tinel sign. The elbow flexion test is assessed with the elbow in hyperflexion and the wrist in extension for approximately 60 seconds causing the patient paresthesias or pain radiating to their ulnar digits. The course of the ulnar nerve should be examined for subluxation over the medial epicondyle as the elbow is brought through a range of motion.

UCL insufficiency is best determined with pain or subtle opening on the moving valgus stress test. The moving valgus stress test involves elicitation of pain and instability with application of a valgus force applied through a 70° to 120° range of motion, compared with the milking maneuver that places the valgus stress at 90°. Pain or apprehension during these maneuvers signifies a positive test. In general, pain with UCL injury is often over the ligament itself rather than the origin of the flexor musculature.

TRIP TO THE MOUND
Determining the specific cause of medial elbow pathology can be challenging, but a few tips on physical examination can be helpful. When checking for UCL injury, palpate along the path of the UCL from the inferior aspect of the medial epicondyle to sublime tubercle of the ulna. Medial epicondylitis tenderness will be present anterior to the UCL, again within 1 cm of the epicondyle itself. The moving valgus stress test is the most sensitive and specific test for UCL pathology. It is best to perform this test with the patient supine and

the shoulder in abduction and external rotation to not only stabilize the shoulder but also have the patient maximally relaxed. To check for ulnar nerve pathology, the Tinel sign, ulnar nerve compression test, and elbow flexion test can all be performed. Hypermobility can be assessed by actively flexing the elbow and placing the examiner's finger on the medial epicondyle to check if there is entrapment of the ulnar nerve anterior to the epicondyle as the patient actively extends the elbow.[61] If the nerve is overly mobile, this may be an indication for an ulnar nerve transposition if surgical treatment is pursued.

Imaging

Standard radiographs can provide information to rule out bony pathology. Radiographs can often be normal. Medial epicondyle calcifications and ulnar traction spurs can also be present, although the significance of these findings is to be determined.[9] Posteromedial olecranon bone spurs and loose bodies are commonly identified on axillary views of the elbow joint in pitchers.[62] The significance of these findings should be assessed in light of the clinical history and physical examination, as this can be a normal finding in many throwers.

If ulnar nerve pathology is suspected, EMG and NCSs can be performed. Transient sensory disturbances found on NCS can be observed, but evidence of muscle wasting or motor weakness should be investigated with an EMG. (*See chapter 12*)

Evaluation of the soft tissue structures can be performed with ultrasound or MRI. If an experienced ultrasound radiologist or practitioner is available, a dynamic, stress ultrasound is an accurate and noninvasive modality to evaluate medial elbow structures including the UCL.[63] MRI imaging, with or without contrast, is the gold standard for evaluation of the UCL complex and can evaluate for inflammation of the flexor-pronator muscle and tendon, intra-articular pathology, and other potential traumatic etiologies (Figure 7.23).

TREATMENT

Nonoperative

The foundation of medial epicondylitis management is nonsurgical. The most important initial step is to remove the painful activities from an athlete's daily routine. The majority of these patients will have symptom

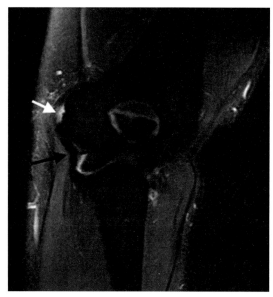

FIGURE 7.23 • A coronal T2 MRI of an elbow showing inflammation signified by increased signal at the origin of the flexor musculature on the medial epicondyle (white arrow). The ulnar collateral ligament is intact (long black arrow). (Courtesy Christopher S. Ahmad, MD.)

relief from conservative management, although nearly a quarter of patients will have recurrence.[64]

After discontinuing the painful and often repetitive upper extremity activities, such as throwing, patients will initiate a rehabilitation protocol that includes modalities that decrease inflammation. This protocol may incorporate icing, gentle compression wrapping, and nonsteroidal anti-inflammatory medications. It is important during this rest period to continue daily activities and ensure no elbow or wrist range of motion is lost. Although the etiology of medial epicondylitis is not histologically inflammatory, anti-inflammatory treatments often improve the short-term symptoms of patients, likely because of calming other concomitant pathology such as synovitis, tendonitis, and muscle strains. There are some reports that PRP injections can be effective for medial epicondylitis, but further study is warranted to definitively support this as an effective option.[65,66]

After a 2 to 6 weeks trial of nonoperative modalities, nighttime wrist splinting may be attempted. Counterforce bracing during the day may further assist athletes during their daily activities. Throwers may also be candidates for medial epicondyle injections consisting of a corticosteroid or autologous whole blood. A range of other treatments includes ultrasound, acupuncture, and shock-wave therapy, although they have not been well studied.

The progression of rehabilitation begins once the thrower sufficiently rests his elbow and develops a pain-free motion from which he can begin to increase activity followed by strengthening. Isometric exercises should be performed followed by integration of eccentric and then concentric exercises. Gradual resistance is added until strength is equal to or greater than preinjury level. Return to sport should begin with a gradual increase in throwing intensity. Progressive strengthening exercises should be advanced under the supervision of a physician or physical therapist to maintain strength and motion during the season.

Operative

Indications

A minority of patients will fail a conservative management period of 6 months and will be indicated for surgery. In professional athletes, a shortened timeline may be appropriate depending on seasonal timing of the injury. Furthermore, if the detection of full-thickness tendon tear is found, a poorer conservative therapy prognosis can be expected and surgery can be pursued sooner.[52]

Surgical Options

The current standard of care for operative treatment of medial epicondylitis is open debridement with repair of the tendon. Although arthroscopic debridement has gained in popularity for the treatment of lateral epicondylitis, the proximity of the ulnar nerve to the medial epicondyle has limited its potential use for medial epicondylitis.

Author's Preferred Surgical Technique

Preoperative Planning

As with every patient, a history and physical examination will guide preoperative workup. Differentiating between medial epicondylitis and confounding conditions such as ulnar neuropathy and UCL injury is paramount to executing a successful surgical plan. If there is a suspicion of neurologic deficit or symptoms, an EMG can help determine if there are objective findings of compression. In a throwing athlete, an MRI can be especially helpful to define if there is an associated UCL tear or traumatic tear of the flexor-pronator origin. By understanding the pathology with this workup, the operative treatment will be guided accordingly.

Equipment Needed

- Standard operating room table
- Hand table extension
- Hand tray including a small rongeur and curettes

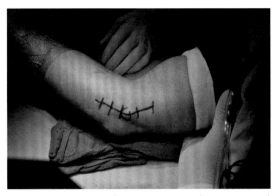

FIGURE 7.24 • A curvilinear incision is drawn centered over the medial epicondyle. In this series of photos, the wrist is to the left (where the iodoform dressing is visible) and the shoulder is to the right (toward the tourniquet). (Courtesy Christopher S. Ahmad, MD.)

- 0.062 K wire
- 2-0 drill
- Nonabsorbable braided sutures
- Free needle for suture passage
- Pneumatic or cordless drill

Positioning

- The patient is positioned supine on a regular table with the operative arm abducted onto an arm table
- A tourniquet is applied to the upper arm for adequate hemostasis
- The operative arm is prepped and draped in a standard sterile fashion and then is externally rotated to expose the medial aspect of the elbow
- The relevant anatomy is marked, particularly the medial epicondyle and the ulnar nerve path usually running posterior to the medial epicondyle
- A curvilinear incision is drawn centered over the medial epicondyle following the medial intermuscular septum proximally and the center of the flexor-pronator mass distally (Figure 7.24)

Exposure and Dissection

- An Esmarch is used to exsanguinate the arm and the tourniquet is inflated
- The incision is made through the skin and Metzenbaum scissors are used to dissect down to the flexor-pronator fascia (Figure 7.25)
- The ulnar nerve can be decompressed and transposed as needed
- The flexor origin tendon is palpated for where there is a difference in quality between normal and abnormal tissue. A U-shaped flap corresponding to this change in quality is marked in the fascia based distally (Figure 7.26)

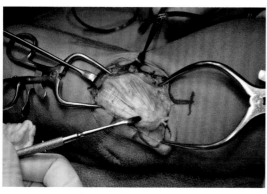

FIGURE 7.25 • The superficial aspect of the flexor-pronator fascia is fully exposed. (Courtesy Christopher S. Ahmad, MD.)

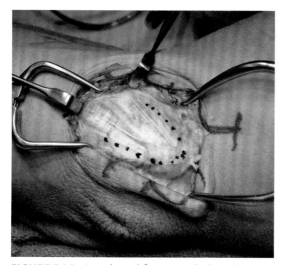

FIGURE 7.26 • A U-shaped flap is marked out based on palpation of the junction of normal and abnormal tendon. (Courtesy Christopher S. Ahmad, MD.)

- The flap of fascia is elevated off the medial epicondyle along with the diseased underside of the flexor-pronator fascia (Figure 7.27A and B)
- One must take care not to include the UCL in the tissue flap
- The diseased tissue is identified then peeled off the underside of the flexor origin with a sharp knife (Figure 7.28)
- The completed debridement of the tendon is inspected and the fascia is mobilized back to its origin

Repair of Fascia

- Next the fascia is repaired back to the medial epicondyle through transosseous drill holes
- An 0.062 K wire is used to create proximal to distal drill holes: one at the far anterior aspect and one at the far posterior aspect of the footprint on the

medial epicondyle (Figure 7.29), protecting the ulnar nerve with either one's finger or a retractor

- A 2-0 drill bit is used to create multiple drill holes in the footprint to produce a bleeding bony bed and stimulate a healing response (Figure 7.30)
- There are now a total of 2 drill paths each with a drill hole on either end of the medial epicondyle
- Two high-tensile strength, nonabsorbable size 0 sutures are passed through each of the drill holes from proximal to distal (Figure 7.31) and one suture is passed proximally through one drill path and then distally through the other drill path, such that both ends of the suture emerge distally (Figure 7.32)
- The tendon flap is then brought proximally to its origin and the repair is initiated
- Two sutures are passed distally through the tendon and tied, compressing the tendon down to the distal aspect of its origin (Figure 7.33)
- The other distal sutures are passed through the tendon and pulled over the tendon proximally in a cross and box pattern. These are then tied to their proximal counterparts, compressing the tendon down to its origin
- The longitudinal splits in the tendon are repaired with a 2-0 braided absorbable suture (Figure 7.34)
- The skin is then repaired in layers until closed with a subcuticular monofilament suture

POSTSURGICAL REHABILITATION

The patient is placed in a posterior slab splint postoperatively for protection of the wound. The patient will remove the splint on his or her own within 1 week and begin gentle active and passive range of motion as tolerated, with avoidance of passive wrist extension or active wrist flexion. The patient then begins gentle isometric exercises after a month, progressing to more intensive exercises with resistance at the 6 weeks postoperative period. At this 6-week postoperative mark, the patient can begin resistance strengthening of wrist flexors as well and progress as tolerated. He or she continues to progressively strengthen until about 3 months, at which time he or she can begin a return to throwing program if he or she is pain-free and eventually advances to full participation as he or she goes through the protocol.

RESULTS

Similar to lateral epicondylitis, nonoperative treatment is the mainstay of treatment and has been very successful. Therapy includes a program of

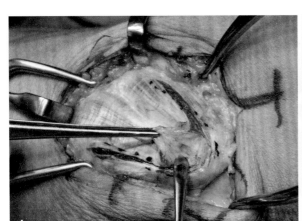
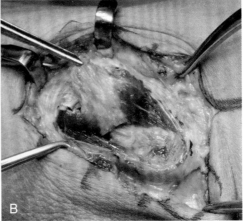

FIGURE 7.27 • A, The U-shaped flap is elevated off the medial epicondyle. B, The underside of the flexor-pronator origin is fully exposed showing the diseased tissue indicative of medial epicondylitis. (Courtesy Christopher S. Ahmad, MD.)

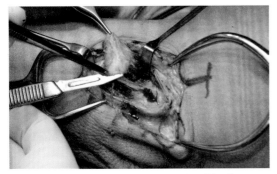

FIGURE 7.28 • The diseased underside of the flexor-pronator origin is debrided sharply with a scalpel. (Courtesy Christopher S. Ahmad, MD.)

flexor-pronator stretching as well as progressive exercises. Although classically it has been reported that there are 85% to 90% success rates, recurrence of symptoms may be underreported with over 40% complaining of prolonged minor discomfort.[64] Furthermore, in throwing athletes the rate of failure of nonoperative treatment is higher as the thrower begins to resume throwing, especially in cases of valgus instability.[59]

Injections have been found to be beneficial to this condition, at least in the short term. In a randomized double blind study, injection of the patients with corticosteroid below the muscle origin at the medial epicondyle resulted in significant pain relief compared with controls at 6 weeks, although this effect did not last past 3 months.[54] Biologic injections have been attempted on the medial aspect of the elbow as well. One study found significant improvements in pain and symptoms even 10 months after a single treatment of dry needling and autologous blood injection under ultrasound guidance.[67]

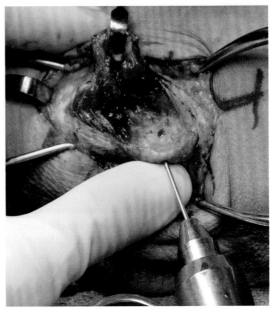

FIGURE 7.29 • A K wire is used to create an anterior drill hole from proximal to distal to allow passage of sutures. The ulnar nerve is protected using the thumb during drilling. (Courtesy Christopher S. Ahmad, MD.)

When surgical treatment has been necessary, the results have been excellent. As many as 97% of patients can have good or excellent results, with 95% returning to their previous level of sport, and 86% having full use of their elbow.[52] These results have been reflected in other similar investigations as well.[52,58,68] Percutaneous techniques have also been used with success in 83% of patients in another small study.[68] However, those with preoperative ulnar nerve symptoms had inferior outcomes, so these patients should be counseled accordingly.[52,69]

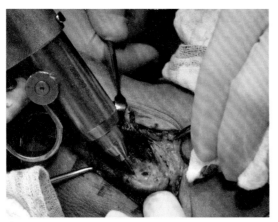

FIGURE 7.30 • A 2-0 drill bit is used to place multiple shallow drill holes in the medial epicondyle to optimize the potential healing surface at the flexor origin. (Courtesy Christopher S. Ahmad, MD.)

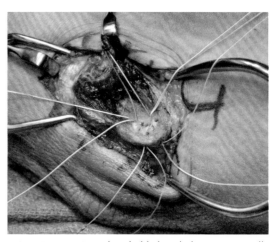

FIGURE 7.32 • Nonabsorbable braided sutures are all passed through the drill holes in the medial epicondyle before passage through the flexor-pronator tendon origin. Note the perforations in the bone to enhance biologic healing. (Courtesy Christopher S. Ahmad, MD.)

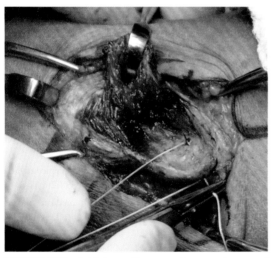

FIGURE 7.31 • A high-tensile strength suture is passed from proximal to distal through the anterior drill hole followed by a second suture through the same drill hole. This will be repeated with the posterior drill hole. (Courtesy Christopher S. Ahmad, MD.)

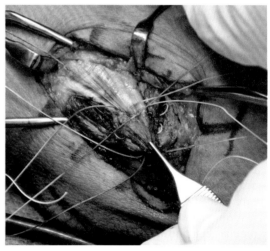

FIGURE 7.33 • The origin of the flexor-pronator tendon is reduced. Sutures from the drill holes are passed distally through the tendon and tied, compressing the tendon down to the origin. (Courtesy Christopher S. Ahmad, MD.)

Complications

Reports of complications after medial epicondylitis surgery are rare. Vangsness and Jobe reported one patient with a postoperative hematoma requiring aspiration and 2 patients out of 35 who had postoperative ulnar nerve symptoms.[52] Performing an arthroscopic debridement of the medial epicondyle could potentially risk injury to the ulnar nerve if not properly protected.

MANAGER'S TIPS

• One must differentiate medial epicondylitis from UCL tears; epicondylitis will be found more anterior and proximal

• Most cases of medial epicondylitis can be effectively treated nonoperatively

• An MRI report may describe both UCL tears and medial epicondylitis. It is essential that the clinician use physical examination to determine the true pathology that correlates with imaging

• Strengthening exercises during rehabilitation should focus on wrist extension, radial deviation, and supination; avoid strengthening the flexor muscle mass early in rehab to avoid irritation of the condition

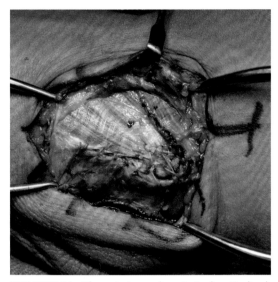

FIGURE 7.34 • The anterior and posterior longitudinal splits in the flexor origin are repaired with side-to-side interrupted absorbable sutures. (Courtesy Christopher S. Ahmad, MD.)

TRIP TO THE MOUND

Flexor-Pronator Ruptures

Another confounding condition on the medial side of the elbow is a traumatic injury to the flexor-pronator tendon. The flexor-pronator origin is helpful for maintaining dynamic stability to the elbow with valgus loads and thus can take pressure off the UCL.[59] However, throwing beyond the limit of muscle fatigue can lead to complete rupture of the flexor-pronator origin.[70] On examination, these patients will present much like medial epicondylitis with tenderness just distal to the medial epicondyle and pain with resisted wrist flexion. Also similar to medial epicondylitis, the pain will be found more anterior and proximal to that of the UCL. With these injuries, MRI will help delineate the ultimate cause. Small partial tears will be treated successfully with rest and NSAIDs, whereas complete ruptures may require operative treatment. Return to play after operative treatment of flexor-pronator tears in the absence of UCL pathology can be as low as 4 to 6 months. In the setting of concomitant UCL and flexor-pronator rupture, reconstruction in these throwing athletes is associated with a worse outcome than UCL reconstruction alone, with return to previous play as low as 12.5% and as high as 78%.[71,72]

REFERENCES

1. Calfee RP, Patel A, DaSilva MF, Akelman E. Management of lateral epicondylitis: current concepts. *J Am Acad Orthop Surg.* 2008;16(1):19-29.

2. Shiri R, Viikari-Juntura E. Lateral and medial epicondylitis: role of occupational factors. *Best Pract Res Clin Rheumatol.* 2011;25(1):43-57.

3. Priest JD, Braden V, Gerberich SG. The elbow and tennis, Part 1: An analysis of players with and without pain. *Phys Sportsmed.* 1980;8(4):80-91.

4. Regan W, Wold LE, Coonrad R, Morrey BF. Microscopic histopathology of chronic refractory lateral epicondylitis. *Am J Sports Med.* 1992;20(6):746-749.

5. Nirschl RP. Elbow tendinosis/tennis elbow. *Clin Sports Med.* 1992;11(4):851-870.

6. Hughes SS, Lyons BC, Mayo JJ. Effect of grip strength and grip strengthening exercises on instantaneous bat velocity of collegiate baseball players. *J Strength Condit Res.* 2004;18(2):298-301.

7. Szymanski DJ, McIntyre JS, Szymanski JM, Molloy JM, Madsen NH, Pascoe DD. Effect of wrist and forearm training on linear bat-end, center of percussion, and hand velocities and on time to ball contact of high school baseball players. *J Strength Condit Res.* 2006;20(1):231-240.

8. Pedegana LR, Elsner RC, Roberts D, Lang J, Farewell V. The relationship of upper extremity strength to throwing speed. *Am J Sports Med.* 1982;10(6): 352-354.

9. Jobe FW, Ciccotti MG. Lateral and medial epicondylitis of the elbow. *J Am Acad Orthop Surg.* 1994;2(1):1-8.

10. Dlabach JA, Baker CL. Lateral and medical epicondylitis in the overhead athlete. *Operat Tech Orthop.* 2001;11(1):46-54.

11. Levin D, Nazarian LN, Miller TT, et al. Lateral epicondylitis of the elbow: US findings. *Radiology.* 2005;237(1):230-234.

12. Coonrad RW, Hooper WR. Tennis elbow: its course, natural history, conservative and surgical management. *J Bone Joint Surg.* 1973;55(6):1177-1182.

13. Murray D, Javed S, Jain N, Kemp S, Watts A. Platelet—rich—plasma injections in treating lateral epicondylosis: a review of the recent evidence. *J Hand Microsurg.* 2015;7(2):320-325.

14. Thanasas C, Papadimitriou G, Charalambidis C, Paraskevopoulos I, Papanikolaou A. Platelet-rich plasma versus autologous whole blood for the treatment of chronic lateral elbow epicondylitis a randomized controlled clinical trial. *Am J Sports Med.* 2011;39(10):2130-2134.

15. Krogh TP, Fredberg U, Stengaard-Pedersen K, Christensen R, Jensen P, Ellingsen T. Treatment of lateral epicondylitis with platelet-rich plasma, glucocorticoid, or saline: a randomized, double-blind, placebo-controlled trial. *Am J Sports Med.* 2013;41(3):625-635.

16. Peerbooms JC, Sluimer J, Bruijn DJ, Gosens T. Positive effect of an autologous platelet concentrate in lateral epicondylitis in a double-blind randomized controlled trial platelet-rich plasma versus corticosteroid injection with a 1-year follow-up. *Am J Sports Med.* 2010;38(2):255-262.

17. Gosens T, Peerbooms JC, van Laar W, den Oudsten BL. Ongoing positive effect of platelet-rich plasma versus corticosteroid injection in lateral epicondylitis: a double-blind randomized controlled trial with 2-year follow-up. *Am J Sports Med.* 2011;39(6):1200-1208.

18. De Smedt T, de Jong A, Van Leemput W, Lieven D, Van Glabbeek F. Lateral epicondylitis in tennis: update on aetiology, biomechanics and treatment. *Br J Sports Med.* 2007;41(11):816-819.

19. Buchbinder R, Green S, Youd JM, Assendelft WJ, Barnsley L, Smidt N. Shock wave therapy for lateral elbow pain. *Cochrane Libr.* 2005;(4):CD003524.

20. Bisset L, Paungmali A, Vicenzino B, Beller E. A systematic review and meta-analysis of clinical trials on physical interventions for lateral epicondylalgia. *Br J Sports Med.* 2005;39(7):411-422.

21. Maher S. Is low-level laser therapy effective in the management of lateral epicondylitis? *Phys Ther.* 2006;86(8):1161-1167.

22. Kwon BC, Kim JY, Park K-T. The Nirschl procedure versus arthroscopic extensor carpi radialis brevis débridement for lateral epicondylitis. *J Shoulder Elbow Surg.* 2017;26(1):118-124.

23. Peart RE, Strickler SS, Schweitzer K Jr. Lateral epicondylitis: a comparative study of open and arthroscopic lateral release. *Am J Orthoped.* 2004;33(11):565-567.

24. Baker CL, Murphy KP, Gottlob CA, Curd DT. Arthroscopic classification and treatment of lateral epicondylitis: two-year clinical results. *J Shoulder Elbow Surg.* 2000;9(6):475-482.

25. Lattermann C, Romeo AA, Anbari A, et al. Arthroscopic debridement of the extensor carpi radialis brevis for recalcitrant lateral epicondylitis. *J Shoulder Elbow Surg.* 2010;19(5):651-656.

26. Unlu MC, Kesmezacar H, Akgun I, Ogut T, Uzun I. Anatomic relationship between elbow arthroscopy portals and neurovascular structures in different elbow and forearm positions. *J Shoulder Elbow Surg.* 2006;15(4):457-462.

27. Miller CD, Jobe CM, Wright MH. Neuroanatomy in elbow arthroscopy. *J Shoulder Elbow Surg.* 1995;4(3):168-174.

28. Hong QN, Durand M-J, Loisel P. Treatment of lateral epicondylitis: where is the evidence? *Joint Bone Spine.* 2004;71(5):369-373.

29. Nirschl RP, Pettrone F. Tennis elbow. The surgical treatment of lateral epicondylitis. *J Bone Joint Surg Am.* 1979;61(6):832-839.

30. Smidt N, Van Der Windt DA, Assendelft WJ, Devillé WL, Korthals-de Bos IB, Bouter LM. Corticosteroid injections, physiotherapy, or a wait-and-see policy for lateral epicondylitis: a randomised controlled trial. *Lancet.* 2002;359(9307):657-662.

31. Nirschl RP, Ashman ES. Elbow tendinopathy: tennis elbow. *Clin Sports Med.* 2003;22(4):813-836.

32. Labelle H, Guibert R. Efficacy of diclofenac in lateral epicondylitis of the elbow also treated with immobilization. The University of Montreal Orthopaedic Research Group. *Arch Fam Med.* 1996;6(3):257-262.

33. Hay EM, Paterson SM, Lewis M, Hosie G, Croft P. Pragmatic randomised controlled trial of local corticosteroid injection and naproxen for treatment of lateral epicondylitis of elbow in primary care. *BMJ.* 1999;319(7215):964-968.

34. Burnham R, Gregg R, Healy P, Steadward R. The effectiveness of topical diclofenac for lateral epicondylitis. *Clin J Sport Med.* 1998;8(2):78-81.

35. Kohia M, Brackle J, Byrd K, Jennings A, Murray W, Wilfong E. Effectiveness of physical therapy treatments on lateral epicondylitis. *J Sport Rehabil.* 2008;17(2):119-136.

36. Waugh EJ, Jaglal SB, Davis AM, Tomlinson G, Verrier MC. Factors associated with prognosis of lateral epicondylitis after 8 weeks of physical therapy. *Arch Phys Med Rehabil.* 2004;85(2):308-318.

37. Groppel JL, Nirschl RP. A mechanical and electromyographical analysis of the effects of various joint counterforce braces on the tennis player. *Am J Sports Med.* 1986;14(3):195-200.

38. Öken Ö, Kahraman Y, Ayhan F, Canpolat S, Yorgancioglu ZR, Öken ÖF. The short-term efficacy of laser, brace, and ultrasound treatment in lateral epicondylitis: a prospective, randomized, controlled trial. *J Hand Ther.* 2008;21(1):63-68.

39. Struijs PA, Smidt N, Arola H, Van Dijk C, Buchbinder R, Assendelft WJ. Orthotic devices for the treatment of tennis elbow. *Cochrane Libr.* 2002;(1):CD001821.

40. Garg R, Adamson GJ, Dawson PA, Shankwiler JA, Pink MM. A prospective randomized study comparing a forearm strap brace versus a wrist splint for the treatment of lateral epicondylitis. *J Shoulder Elbow Surg.* 2010;19(4):508-512.

41. Coombes BK, Bisset L, Brooks P, Khan A, Vicenzino B. Effect of corticosteroid injection, physiotherapy, or both on clinical outcomes in patients with unilateral lateral epicondylalgia: a randomized controlled trial. *JAMA.* 2013;309(5):461-469.

42. Krogh TP, Bartels EM, Ellingsen T, et al. Comparative effectiveness of injection therapies in lateral epicondylitis: a systematic review and network meta-analysis of randomized controlled trials. *Am J Sports Med.* 2013;41(6):1435-1446.

43. Wolf JM, Ozer K, Scott F, Gordon MJ, Williams AE. Comparison of autologous blood, corticosteroid, and saline injection in the treatment of lateral epicondylitis: a prospective, randomized, controlled multicenter study. *J Hand Surg.* 2011;36(8):1269-1272.

44. Dunn JH, Kim JJ, Davis L, Nirschl RP. Ten-to 14-year follow-up of the Nirschl surgical technique for lateral epicondylitis. *Am J Sports Med.* 2008;36(2):261-266.

45. Baker CL. Long-term follow-up of arthroscopic treatment of lateral epicondylitis. *Am J Sports Med.* 2008;36(2):254-260.

46. Solheim E, Hegna J, Øyen J. Arthroscopic versus open tennis elbow release: 3-to 6-year results of a case-control series of 305 elbows. *Arthrosc J Arthrosc Relat Surg.* 2013;29(5):854-859.

47. Lo MY, Safran MR. Surgical treatment of lateral epicondylitis: a systematic review. *Clin Orthop Relat Res.* 2007;463:98-106.

48. McShane JM, Nazarian LN, Harwood MI. Sonographically guided percutaneous needle tenotomy for treatment of common extensor tendinosis in the elbow. *J Ultrasound Med.* 2006;25(10):1281-1289.

49. Meknas K, Odden-Miland Å, Mercer JB, Castillejo M, Johansen O. Radiofrequency microtenotomy a promising method for treatment of recalcitrant lateral epicondylitis. *Am J Sports Med.* 2008;36(10):1960-1965.

50. Cullinane FL, Boocock MG, Trevelyan FC. Is eccentric exercise an effective treatment for lateral epicondylitis? A systematic review. *Clin Rehabil.* 2014;28(1):3-19.

51. Leach RE, Miller JK. Lateral and medial epicondylitis of the elbow. *Clin Sports Med.* 1987;6(2):259-272.

52. Vangsness C, Jobe F. Surgical treatment of medial epicondylitis. Results in 35 elbows. *Bone Joint J.* 1991;73(3):409-411.

53. Miller J. Javelin thrower's elbow. *Bone Joint J.* 1960;42(4):788-792.

54. Stahl S, Kaufman T. The efficacy of an injection of steroids for medial epicondylitis. A prospective study of sixty elbows. *J Bone Joint Surg Am.* 1997;79(11):1648-1652.

55. Hamilton CD, Glousman RE, Jobe FW, Brault J, Pink M, Perry J. Dynamic stability of the elbow: electromyographic analysis of the flexor pronator group and the extensor group in pitchers with valgus instability. *J Shoulder Elbow Surg.* 1996;5(5):347-354.

56. Davidson PA, Pink M, Perry J, Jobe FW. Functional anatomy of the flexor pronator muscle group in relation to the medial collateral ligament of the elbow. *Am J Sports Med.* 1995;23(2):245-250.

57. Bennett JB. Lateral and medial epicondylitis. *Hand Clin.* 1994;10(1):157-163.

58. Gabel GT, Morrey BF. Operative treatment of medial epicondylitis. Influence of concomitant ulnar neuropathy at the elbow. *J Bone Joint Surg Am.* 1995;77(7):1065-1069.

59. Chen FS, Rokito AS, Jobe FW. Medial elbow problems in the overhead-throwing athlete. *J Am Acad Orthop Surg.* 2001;9(2):99-113.

60. King JW, Brelsford HJ, Tullos HS. Analysis of the pitching arm of the professional baseball pitcher. *Clin Orthop Relat Res.* 1969;67:116-123.

61. Calfee RP, Manske PR, Gelberman RH, Van Steyn MO, Steffen J, Goldfarb CA. Clinical assessment of the ulnar nerve at the elbow: reliability of instability testing and the association of hypermobility with clinical symptoms. *J Bone Joint Surg.* 2010;92(17):2801-2808.

62. ElAttrache NS, Ahmad CS. Valgus extension overload syndrome and olecranon stress fractures. *Sports Med Arthrosc Rev.* 2003;11(1):25-29.

63. Ciccotti MG, Atanda A Jr, Nazarian LN, Dodson CC, Holmes L, Cohen SB. Stress sonography of the ulnar collateral ligament of the elbow in professional baseball pitchers: a 10-year study. *Am J Sports Med.* 2014;42(3):544-551.

64. Ciccotti MC, Schwartz MA, Ciccotti MG. Diagnosis and treatment of medial epicondylitis of the elbow. *Clin Sports Med.* 2004;23(4):693-705.

65. Hechtman KS, Uribe JW, Botto-vanDemden A, Kiebzak GM. Platelet-rich plasma injection reduces pain in patients with recalcitrant epicondylitis. *Orthopedics.* 2011;34(2):92.

66. Mishra A, Pavelko T. Treatment of chronic elbow tendinosis with buffered platelet-rich plasma. *Am J Sports Med.* 2006;34(11):1774-1778.

67. Suresh S, Ali KE, Jones H, Connell D. Medial epicondylitis: is ultrasound guided autologous blood injection an effective treatment? *Br J Sports Med.* 2006;40(11):935-939.

68. Baumgard SH, Schwartz DR. Percutaneous release of the epicondylar muscles for humeral epicondylitis. *Am J Sports Med.* 1982;10(4):233-236.

69. Ciccotti MG, Ramani MN. Medial epicondylitis. *Tech Hand Up Extrem Surg.* 2003;7(4):190-196.

70. Norwood LA, Shook JA, Andrews JR. Acute medial elbow ruptures. *Am J Sports Med.* 1981;9(1):16-19.

71. Osbahr DC, Swaminathan SS, Allen AA, Dines JS, Coleman SH, Altchek DW. Combined flexor-pronator mass and ulnar collateral ligament injuries in the elbows of older baseball players. *Am J Sports Med.* 2010;38(4):733-739.

72. Conway J, Jobe FW, Glousman R, Pink M. Medial instability of the elbow in throwing athletes. Treatment by repair or reconstruction of the ulnar collateral ligament. *J Bone Joint Surg Am.* 1992;74(1):67-83.

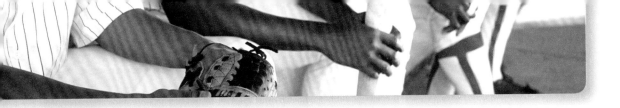

CHAPTER 8

Valgus Extension Overload

Justin L. Hodgins, MD | Christopher S. Ahmad, MD | Anthony A. Romeo, MD

Every day that goes by and we don't win a ballgame, that's a missed opportunity for us to battle back.

—*Brett Gardner*

INTRODUCTION

The mechanics of high-velocity throwing generates distinctive forces in the elbow, which are resisted by articular, ligamentous, and muscular constraints. In the posterior compartment, as the elbow reaches terminal extension, the combined valgus and angular moments are dissipated, as the posteromedial olecranon contacts the trochlea and the olecranon fossa. The resultant shear and compressive forces can be amplified by poor dynamic muscular control and, in some cases, chronic attenuation of the medial ulnar collateral ligament (UCL) (Figure 8.1). The repetitive traumatic abutment during extension induces reactive bone formation, resulting in osteophyte formation at the tip of the posteromedial olecranon. Corresponding "kissing lesions" of chondromalacia may exist within the olecranon fossa and posteromedial trochlea, combined with symptomatic loose bodies. This constellation of pathology is referred to as *valgus extension overload (VEO) syndrome*, which is unique to the overhead throwing athlete.[1]

The relationship between the abnormal contact of the posteromedial olecranon and valgus instability of the elbow has been the focus of several clinical and biomechanical investigations.[2-5] Olecranon tip exostosis has been identified in up to 24% of lateral radiographs of asymptomatic professional pitchers.[3] However, for those players with exostosis formation, 34% had relative valgus laxity of 1.0 mm or greater on stress radiographs compared with only 16% without exostosis, supporting a plausible relationship between posteromedial impingement and valgus laxity.[3] Similarly, a biomechanical study investigated the effect of partial- and full-thickness UCL injuries on the contact forces

of the posterior elbow.[2] UCL insufficiency was found to alter the contact area and pressure forces between the posteromedial trochlea and olecranon, helping to explain the development of posteromedial osteophyte formation.

CLINICAL EVALUATION

History

Patients are most often athletes with a history of throwing or repetitive overhead activity.

In pitchers, symptoms may be preceded by a decrease in pitch velocity, control, and early fatiguability. With isolated VEO, elbow pain is localized to the posteromedial aspect of the olecranon immediately after ball release in the deceleration phase of throwing. Players may report limited elbow extension, which results from impinging posterior osteophytes, or mechanical symptoms of locking and catching from loose bodies or chondral injury. Symptoms of UCL insufficiency may be overshadowed in these patients, and a history of UCL or flexor-pronator injury should be noted. Ulnar neuritis or subluxation may manifest as paresthesia in the fourth and fifth digits when throwing.

Physical Examination

Physical examination may demonstrate tenderness and/or crepitus over the posteromedial olecranon with an associated loss of extension and a firm endpoint. The *extension impingement test* elicits pain within the posterior compartment when the elbow is snapped into terminal extension. During the *arm bar test*, the patient's shoulder is positioned at 90°

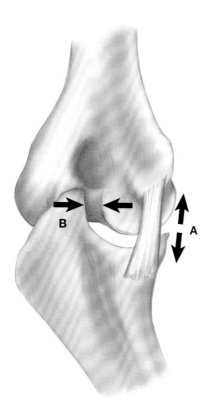

FIGURE 8.1 • In the posterior compartment, the olecranon experiences medial shearing forces with valgus stress, which may be heightened by increased valgus laxity. A, Ligament tension. B, Posterior medial contact and shear.

of forward flexion and full internal rotation and the patient's hand is placed on the examiner's shoulder.[6] The reproduction of posterior pain when the examiner pulls down on the olecranon to simulate forced extension is considered a positive test. Possible UCL insufficiency should be evaluated with valgus stress testing, the milking maneuver, and the moving valgus stress test. The presence of ulnar neuritis and a subluxing ulnar nerve should be noted, particularly if planning the use of medial portals with arthroscopic treatment.

Imaging

Standard anteroposterior (AP), lateral, oblique, and axillary radiographs of the elbow may reveal posteromedial olecranon osteophytes and/or loose bodies (Figure 8.2). A modified AP radiograph with 140° of external rotation may best elicit osteophytes on the posteromedial olecranon.[3] A computed tomography (CT) scan with 2-dimensional sagittal and coronal images and 3-dimensional surface rendering can best demonstrate morphologic abnormalities, loose

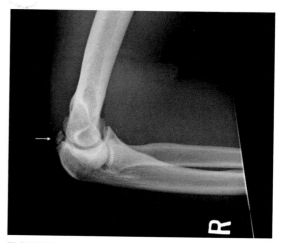

FIGURE 8.2 • Lateral elbow radiograph demonstrating large posterior olecranon osteophyte (arrow).

bodies, and osteophyte formation and help plan for future osteophyte removal[16] (Figure 8.3). Additional abnormalities including bony hypertrophy, ligament ossification, and osteophyte fracture may be observed, especially in the symptomatic elbow. Magnetic resonance imaging (MRI) can further assess soft tissue and chondral injury, including UCL insufficiency, synovial plicae, bone edema, and stress fractures of the olecranon.

TREATMENT

Nonoperative

Nonoperative treatment options include the use of oral anti-inflammatory medications (such as NSAIDs and acetaminophen), activity modification, and possible intra-articular corticosteroid injection of the elbow. Posterior elbow symptoms may be exacerbated by heavy throwing volumes, and players often benefit from a resting period combined with the abovementioned modalities. A global assessment of pitching mechanics should be performed to correct errors in technique and identify muscular imbalances. Strengthening of the dynamic musculature surrounding the elbow and forearm, particularly the flexor-pronator mass, can help control the valgus stresses experienced in the elbow during arm deceleration and ultimately reduce symptoms and help prevent further injury. After the resting period, a supervised throwing program is initiated under the direction of an experienced therapist and trainer and later patients return to play after its completion.

The clinical results of nonoperative treatment in throwers are limited. Satisfactory outcomes have been

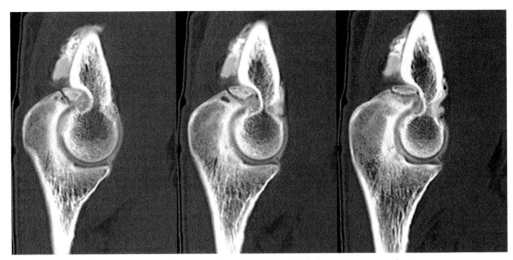

FIGURE 8.3 • Sagittal CT sequences demonstrating posteromedial olecranon osteophyte.

described in professional javelin throwers, although the patients were identified to have olecranon osteophytes retrospectively.[17]

Operative

Surgical decompression is indicated for patients with persistent symptoms of posteromedial impingement despite nonoperative treatment and for those who wish to return to the same level of performance. Posteromedial decompression is not indicated in patients with negative provocative testing on physical examination even in the setting of olecranon abnormalities on radiographs or advanced imaging. Such finding, including olecranon osteophytes and loose bodies, may be routinely found in asymptomatic professional baseball players.[3,7] A relative contraindication to performing isolated olecranon resection is the presence of UCL insufficiency, which may become symptomatic after posteromedial decompression, and excessive resection of osteophytes should be avoided because olecranon debridement alone is unlikely to benefit these patients.[9] Therefore, careful history, physical examination, and advanced imaging are necessary to avoid missed UCL injuries when considering posteromedial decompression.

Surgical Options

Surgical options include arthroscopic or limited incision arthrotomy to decompress the posterior compartment. Arthroscopic debridement offers the advantages of reduced soft tissue morbidity and allows a complete intra-articular assessment of the elbow. Open decompression is indicated in patients with significant heterotopic ossification and prior ulnar nerve transposition and when concomitant UCL reconstruction and ulnar nerve release is anticipated.

Authors' Preferred Surgical Technique

Preoperative Planning

For isolated posteromedial decompression, sagittal and coronal CT reconstructions and 3-dimensional surface images should be reviewed for planned removal of pathologic osteophytes and/or loose bodies. Anesthesia and patient positioning are carried out according to surgeon preference and anticipated surgical procedures. The patient may be positioned supine, prone, or lateral decubitus. If concomitant UCL reconstruction is planned, the supine position may be preferred to avoid repositioning the patient after arthroscopy. As an alternative method, arthroscopy may be performed in the lateral position, followed by repositioning and draping for UCL reconstruction.

Equipment Needed

- Esmarch to exsanguinate the limb and a nonsterile tourniquet preset to 250 mm Hg
- 4.0-mm 30° arthroscope, 3.5- and 4-mm mechanical shavers and burrs, and grasping instruments
- Osteotomes, 1/8 inch straight and curved, freer elevators, and switching sticks
- Curved 3.2-mm articulating retractor (Figure 8.4)
- 60-mL syringe with normal saline and 18-G needle with flexible tubing
- Mini C-arm to obtain optional intraoperative fluoroscopy of the elbow after resection

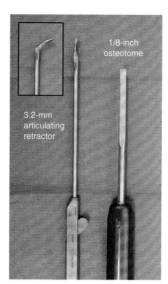

FIGURE 8.4 • Curved 3.2-mm articulating retractor used to protect the ulnar nerve and tension soft tissues and 1/8-inch osteotome used for olecranon resection.

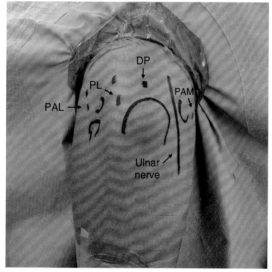

FIGURE 8.5 • External skin markings for portal placement. PAM, proximal anteromedial; PAL, proximal anterolateral; PL, posterolateral; DP, direct posterior.

Technique, Step by Step

- The authors' preferred method is the lateral decubitus position and to start with anterior compartment diagnostic arthroscopy followed by posterior compartment decompression and debridement
- Anatomic landmarks and portals are appropriately marked including the location of the ulnar nerve (Figure 8.5)
- The elbow joint is distended using normal saline via the lateral soft spot portal to increase the working distance from neurovascular structures and ease the introduction of the scope trochar

- Diagnostic anterior arthroscopy is performed from the proximal anteromedial (PAM) portal. The joint is systematically evaluated for the presence of loose bodies, chondromalacia of the anterior radiocapitellar joint, and osteophytes of the coronoid tip and fossa. A proximal anterolateral (PAL) working portal of the anterior compartment may be established using an inside-out technique to facilitate loose body removal and debridement as well as alternative viewing vectors

---

TRIP TO THE MOUND
Dynamic Valgus Stress Examination and UCL Insufficiency

With the arthroscope in the PAL portal, a valgus stress is manually applied to the elbow in 70° of flexion. UCL insufficiency is indicated with gapping of 3 mm or more between the coronoid process and the medial trochlea.[8] The utility of this test to diagnose UCL insufficiency is controversial. It is often difficult to objectively measure joint space opening within 1 mm without using specifically sized probes, and there is no absolute degree of valgus laxity that mandates surgery. Almost exclusively, the decision to perform UCL surgery (repair or reconstruction) is made before the initial skin incision to treat gross ligament insufficiency rather than valgus laxity.

- For posterior compartment arthroscopy, a posterolateral (PL) viewing portal is established and then a direct posterior (DP) working portal through the triceps tendon. Under direct visualization, a motorized shaver and/or ablation device is used to remove synovitis and create a working space to improve visualization. The posterior compartment is evaluated for loose bodies, osteophytes on the posteromedial olecranon, and chondromalacia (Figure 8.6). The posterior radiocapitellar joint should be inspected for loose bodies and may require an accessory midlateral portal through the soft spot to facilitate removal
- The ulnar nerve is located superficial to the capsule in the posteromedial gutter and may be injured when working with motorized instruments or ablation devices. The suction normally attached to the shaver and ablation device should be removed when working in this area to avoid inadvertent suction of the nerve. A curved articulating retractor can also be placed through an accessory PL portal to assist in protecting the ulnar nerve and displace the soft tissues to improve visualization (Figure 8.7)

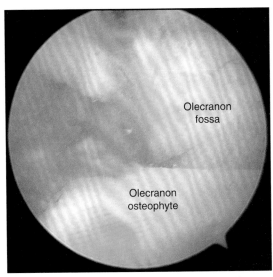

FIGURE 8.6 • Posterior diagnostic arthroscopy demonstrating posteromedial olecranon osteophyte.

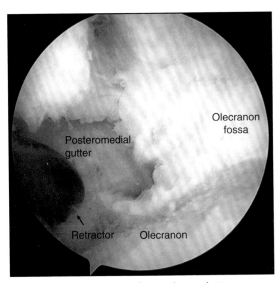

FIGURE 8.7 • Placement of curved articulating retractor in posteromedial gutter to assist in protecting the ulnar nerve and displace the soft tissues to improve visualization.

- Olecranon osteophytes can be removed using a 1/8-inch osteotome inserted through the DP portal at the margin of osteophyte and normal olecranon. A motorized shaver and/or burr can be introduced through either the posterior portal or the PL portal to contour the olecranon tip (Figure 8.8). An intraoperative lateral radiograph can be obtained to confirm sufficient bone removal and to ensure that no bone debris remains within the soft tissues of the elbow

TRIP TO THE MOUND
Olecranon Osteophyte Resection and UCL Insufficiency

The posteromedial olecranon shares an intricate relationship with the UCL acting as a stabilizing buttress to medial tensile forces. Biomechanical analysis has demonstrated that sequential partial resection of the posteromedial olecranon results in a stepwise increase in elbow valgus angulation.[4] Similarly, cadaver model testing has identified that posteromedial resection of the olecranon beyond 3 mm significantly increases the strain experienced in the anterior bundle of the UCL.[5] The role of the olecranon in resisting valgus instability has also been observed clinically. In a large case series, 25% of professional baseball players who underwent olecranon debridement eventually required UCL reconstruction.[9] Therefore, only pathologic osteophytes should be removed during olecranon resection. Effort should be made to preserve normal olecranon which is an important restraint to valgus loading and UCL strain.

- Osteophytes within the olecranon fossa and debridement of kissing lesions on the posteromedial trochlea are then addressed. When a significant chondral injury is present, cartilage flaps are contoured using curettes and shavers to create a "well-shouldered" or stable rim. Microfracture is then performed via anterograde drilling of the lesion with perforations separated by 2 to 3 mm to stimulate the marrow elements and facilitate fibrocartilage development

- On completion of arthroscopy, the fluid is evacuated from the posterior cannulas, and the portals are closed with simple interrupted 3.0 nylon sutures

Postsurgical Rehabilitation

For isolated posteromedial decompression, early active elbow flexion and extension exercises can be initiated in the immediate postoperative period. Emphasis is placed on restoring the dynamic muscular constraints around the elbow, particularly the flexor-pronator mass. At 6 weeks, a progressive throwing program can be initiated combined with plyometric, neuromuscular, and endurance exercises. Return to competition is typically achieved 3 to 4 months after surgery, once preoperative motion and strength have been restored and no pain is exhibited during stress testing or palpation of the olecranon.

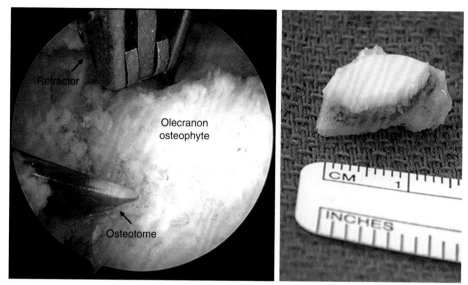

FIGURE 8.8 ● Removal of posteromedial olecranon osteophyte with 1/8-inch osteotome and removed osteophyte en bloc after resection.

TABLE 8.1 Clinical Outcomes of Posteromedial Decompression for Valgus Extension Overload

References	No. of Elbows	Surgical Technique	Mean Patient Age (Years)	Mean Follow-up (Months)	Results
Park et al[13,*]	13	Arthroscopic	15.4	39	85% return to sport, 62% excellent result
Reddy et al[12,*]	96	Arthroscopic	30	42	85% good or excellent, 85% return to the same level of competition
Helper et al[11]	28	Arthroscopic	29	54	95% satisfactory results, no reported complications
Andrews and Timmerman[9]	34	Arthroscopic	24.2	42	68% return to play, 41% reoperation rate
Rosenwasser and Steinmann[10]	9	Arthroscopic	30.2	26	83% return to sport at 6 mo post-op
Wilson et al[1]	5	Open	24	12	All patients returned to throwing for 1 season

*Reported results include multiple diagnoses and/or procedures that were not isolated to posteromedial decompression for valgus extension overload.

RESULTS

Early case series reported high patient satisfaction and return to competition with both open and arthroscopic posteromedial decompression (Table 8.1).[1,9-11] However, in a large study of professional baseball players, the reoperation rate was 41%, and 25% of players developed valgus instability requiring subsequent UCL reconstruction.[9] On later review, the authors have since suggested that the incidence of UCL injury was underestimated in the study population and that treating the secondary effects of UCL insufficiency without the underlying UCL pathology will lead to unsatisfactory results.

More recently, good to excellent outcomes have been reported in 87% of patients after arthroscopic posteromedial decompression.[12] In this series of 187 elbow procedures, 85% of baseball players were able to return to the same level of competition. Similarly, an overall return to play of 85% was demonstrated in adolescent baseball players with VEO.[13] Patients who underwent isolated arthroscopic decompression reported less pain and achieved higher outcome scores compared with those who had concomitant UCL insufficiency.

COMPLICATIONS

The most common complications are those inherent to elbow arthroscopy. Minor complications including ulnar neuritis and superficial wound infections have been reported to occur in 7% to 11% of cases, and major complications such as permanent ulnar nerve injury or deep infection, in only 0.5% to 0.8% of procedures.[12,14,15] A high level of clinical suspicion before the decision to operate and conservative olecranon resection during debridement may help mitigate the incidence of UCL insufficiency after posteromedial decompression.

MANAGER'S TIPS

- Careful patient selection is required to surgically treat only those patients with persistent symptomatic VEO and corresponding radiographic pathology
- A thorough history, physical examination, and advanced imaging are required to avoid missing UCL injury in the patient presenting with VEO symptoms
- The ulnar nerve should be protected during posteromedial decompression with precise portal placement, the removal of suction from mechanical or ablation devices, and the use of intra-articular retractors
- Only pathologic osteophyte should be removed from the posteromedial olecranon during debridement, as the anatomic articulation provides an important restraint to valgus loading and UCL strain

REFERENCES

1. Wilson FD, Andrews JR, Blackburn TA, McCluskey G. Valgus extension overload in the pitching elbow. *Am J Sports Med.* 1983;11:83-88.
2. Ahmad CS, Park MC, Elattrache NS. Elbow medial ulnar collateral ligament insufficiency alters posteromedial olecranon contact. *Am J Sports Med.* 2004;32:1607-1612.
3. Conway J. *Elbow Arthroscopy: Beginners to Advanced.* Las Vegas, NV: American Academy of Orthopaedic Surgeons; 2009.
4. Kamineni S, ElAttrache NS, O'Driscoll SW, et al. Medial collateral ligament strain with partial posteromedial olecranon resection. A biomechanical study. *J Bone Joint Surg Am.* 2004;86-A:2424-2430.
5. Kamineni S, Hirahara H, Pomianowski S, et al. Partial posteromedial olecranon resection: a kinematic study. *J Bone Joint Surg Am.* 2003;85-A:1005-1011.
6. O'Driscoll SW, Morrey BF. Arthroscopy of the elbow. Diagnostic and therapeutic benefits and hazards. *J Bone Joint Surg Am.* 1992;74:84-94.
7. Kooima CL, Anderson K, Craig JV, Teeter DM, van Holsbeeck M. Evidence of subclinical medial collateral ligament injury and posteromedial impingement in professional baseball players. *Am J Sports Med.* 2004;32(7):1602-1606.
8. Field LD, Altchek DW. Evaluation of the arthroscopic valgus instability test of the elbow. *Am J Sports Med.* 1996;24:177-181.
9. Andrews JR, Timmerman LA. Outcome of elbow surgery in professional baseball players. *Am J Sports Med.* 1995;23:407.
10. Rosenwasser MP, Steinmann S. *Elbow Arthroscopy in the Treatment of Posterior Olecranon Impingement.* San Diego: AANA Annual Meeting; 1991.
11. Helper MD, Steinman S, Rosenwasser M. Elbow arthroscopy in the treatment of posterior olecranon impingement. *Arthroscopy.* 1998;14:430.
12. Reddy AS, Kvitne RE, Yocum LA, Elattrache NS, Glousman RE, Jobe FW. Arthroscopy of the elbow: a long-term clinical review. *Arthroscopy.* 2000;16:588-594.
13. Park JY, Yoo HY, Chung SW, et al. Valgus extension overload syndrome in adolescent baseball players: clinical characteristics and surgical outcomes. *J Shoulder Elbow Surg.* 2016;25(12):2048-2056.
14. Kelly EW, Morrey BF, O'Driscoll SW. Complications of elbow arthroscopy. *J Bone Joint Surg Am.* 2001;83-A(1):25-34.
15. Elfeddali R, Schreuder MH, Eygendaal D. Arthroscopic elbow surgery, is it safe? *J Shoulder Elbow Surg.* 2013;22(5):647-652.
16. Hodgins JL, Ahmad CS, Conway JE. The thrower's elbow. In: *Morrey's the Elbow and its Disorders.* 5th ed. Philadelphia: Elsevier; 2015:630-636.
17. Waris W. Elbow injuries of javelin throwers. *Acta Chir Scand.* 1946;93:563-575.

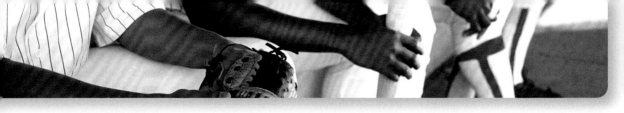

CHAPTER 9

Elbow Stress Reactions and Fractures

Lee D. Kaplan, MD | Paul M. Rothenberg, MD | Philip N. Collis, MD

You just can't beat the person who never gives up.

—*Babe Ruth*

INTRODUCTION

Bone is a dynamic connective tissue whose shape and internal structure are influenced by the mechanical loads associated with normal function.[1] In accordance to Wolf's law, bone adapts to increased stress by changing its form to meet this new demand. This process is called bone remodeling and involves cycles of bone resorption by osteoclasts and formation by osteoblasts. Stress injury occurs when repetitive stresses overwhelm normal bone remodeling and recovery.[2] The injury unfolds over a continuum time, starting with stress injury and eventually progressing to stress fracture.[3] In athletes, this is typically due to abnormal stress on normal bone; however, one must also consider normal stress on deficient bone.[4]

Stress fractures in athletes are rare, representing 0.8% of all injuries among high school athletes. Of those stress fractures, only 3% involve the upper extremity.[5] Stress fractures of the lower extremity are secondary to repetitive weight-bearing forces, whereas stress fractures of the upper extremity are predominantly caused by muscle forces on bone.[4]

In baseball, the most common site of stress fracture is the olecranon.[6] Stress fractures, or stress reactions, of the olecranon have seldom been reported in the literature. However, it has gained more attention recently and we, as clinicians, are now starting to better identify this clinical entity. There are 3 types of olecranon stress fractures described: transverse, oblique, and those of the olecranon tip (Figure 9.1). It is thought that transverse stress fractures are more likely to result from repetitive triceps strain, oblique fractures from valgus overload, and olecranon tip fracture from posterior impingement.[7]

CLINICAL EVALUATION

History

The throwing athlete will complain of a gradual, vague, and progressive elbow pain. The pain is usually posteromedial or posterolateral but may also be difficult to localize. The pain typically presents during and shortly after throwing and is worse during the follow-through phase of throwing. This can be associated with decreased range of motion and weakness of the elbow. Pain is usually absent when at rest.

Physical Examination

Physical examination begins with inspection of the elbow joint. This may reveal localized swelling of the olecranon. Range of motion is usually decreased with lack of full terminal extension. Palpation reveals tenderness over the posteromedial elbow. This tenderness must be differentiated from pain over the ulnar collateral ligament or flexor-pronator mass, as patients may have concomitant injuries.[8] The pain associated with this injury may only be present during the dynamic phases of throwing; therefore, special tests mimicking these movements can be critical in making the diagnosis. Special tests specific for olecranon stress injuries include the snapping extension test and the arm bar test.[7]

In the snapping extension test, the examiner quickly and forcefully extends the athletes elbow from 20° to 30° of flexion, into full terminal extension (Figure 9.2). This maneuver causes the olecranon to drive into the fossa, with positive test eliciting pain at the olecranon.[7]

In the arm bar test, the examiner positions the patient's arm into internal rotation and forward elevation to 90°. The patient then rests his arm on the

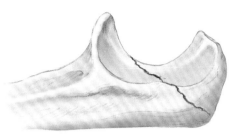

Oblique mid–olecranon stress fracture

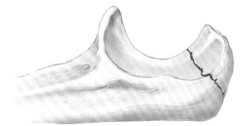

Proximal transverse olecranon stress fracture

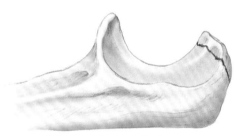

Olecranon tip stress fracture

FIGURE 9.1 • Olecranon stress fractures.

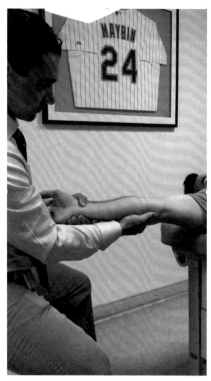

FIGURE 9.2 • Snapping extension test.

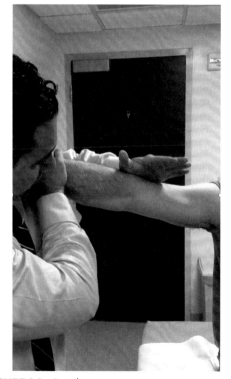

FIGURE 9.3 • Arm bar test.

examiner's shoulder, as the examiner places a downward pressure on the olecranon (Figure 9.3). A positive test will elicit pain.[7]

Imaging

Initial workup should consist of standard anteroposterior (AP), lateral, and axial radiographs. Radiographic findings of stress fractures are usually apparent 2 to 8 weeks after the onset of symptoms.[9] The most common early sign in stress fractures is a subtle area of focal periosteal bone formation.[9] Over time, as the fracture progresses, a discrete lucent fracture line will be seen, often with associated sclerosis. However, X-rays are not very sensitive for the detection of stress fractures.[9] Therefore, additional imaging is necessary in patients with high clinical suspicion for stress fracture.

Radionuclide scanning is the most sensitive imaging method for bone stress injuries. Triphasic bone scans will be positive as early as 2 to 8 days after the onset of symptoms.[10] The 3 phases of the bone scan are blood flow, blood pool, and delayed phases. The blood flow and pool phases demonstrate the perfusion and inflammation of an affected area, respectively. The delayed phase is an indicator of bone turnover. In an acute stress fracture, there will be increased uptake in all 3 phases, compared with soft tissue injuries, which

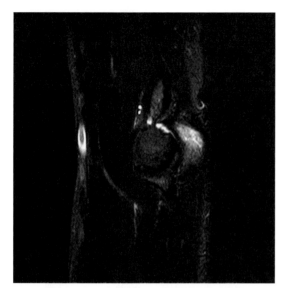

FIGURE 9.4 • Olecranon stress reaction on fluid-sensitive MRI sequence. This image demonstrates enhanced olecranon signal without discrete fracture line.

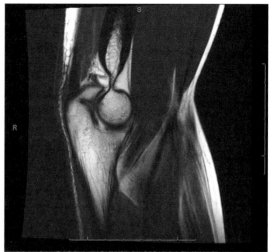

FIGURE 9.5 • Proximal transverse olecranon stress fracture on T1 MRI sequence.

will only demonstrate increased uptake in the first 2 phases.[9] Although very sensitive for acute injuries, bone scans are not very specific and can lead to false positives.[9] Furthermore, false negatives are possible in injuries that are subacute.[8] In addition, the study is very inconvenient for the patient.

Magnetic resonance imaging (MRI) for stress injuries has been shown to be just as sensitive and more specific than bone scans, with a positive and negative predictive value of 93% and up to 100%, respectively.[11] In the setting of stress reaction, fluid-sensitive MR images demonstrate high signal in the olecranon bone marrow (Figure 9.4). If stress reaction has progressed to stress fracture, MRI will also show an irregular T1 hypointense line surrounded by abnormal marrow signal (Figures 9.5 and 9.6).[12]

Computed tomography (CT) scans may play a role for determining fracture orientation for preoperative planning. However, owing to its low sensitivity and inability to evaluate soft tissues for concomitant injuries, it is not first-line diagnostic test.

TREATMENT

Treatment for stress injuries without fracture and early stress fractures should start with a trial of nonoperative management. This consists of a period of rest, in which no throwing or valgus stress for at least 6 weeks. Sports specific rehabilitation can begin at 6 weeks with a throwing program at 8 weeks.[14] Return to play can be considered once the patient has returned to preinjury range

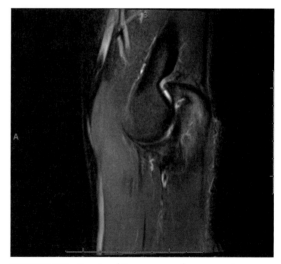

FIGURE 9.6 • Proximal transverse olecranon stress fracture on T2 MRI sequence.

of motion, has no pain on the arm bar test or snapping extension test, and is radiographically healed.[7,13,14] It is important to address throwing mechanics during this period of rehabilitation, to detect any technical issues that may be contributing to the injury. Stress fractures heal slower than regular fracture healing, and restriction from sports for up to 3 to 6 months may be necessary.[13]

Surgical intervention is reserved for those who have failed nonoperative management. Although, some recommend surgical fixation for any patient with visible fracture lines on conventional radiographs.[8] The most common procedure for oblique and transverse stress fractures is internal fixation with a single cannulated screw directed perpendicular to the fracture line (Figure 9.7).[8,15-19] However, some surgeons prefer to treat oblique fractures

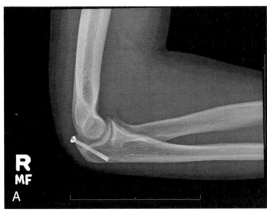
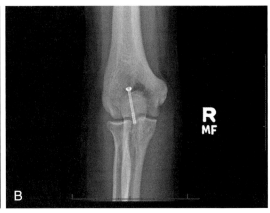

FIGURE 9.7 • A, AP and B, lateral radiographs of an olecranon stress fracture treated with cannulated screw fixation.

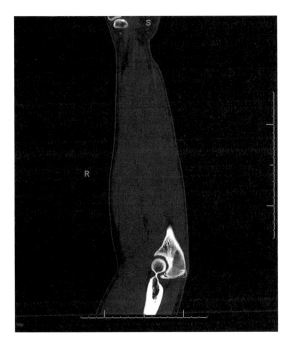

FIGURE 9.8 • CT scan demonstrating a stress fracture of the olecranon tip.

with a single screw directed down the ulnar canal and not perpendicular to the fracture line.[16]

Olecranon tip stress fractures (Figure 9.8) follow a similar treatment plan. An initial trial of nonoperative management is followed by surgical treatment for refractory cases. The mainstay of surgical treatment is arthroscopic olecranon tip excision.[8]

AUTHORS' PREFERRED SURGICAL TECHNIQUE

Before surgery, all radiographs should be reviewed to determine exact orientation of the fracture. If an MRI or CT scan was used during the workup, those can

also be used to assess the fracture orientation. The diameter of the proximal ulnar canal can be measured to help select the appropriate-size cannulated screw.

The equipment needed for the procedure include the following:

1. Fluoroscopy
2. Hand table
3. Partially threaded cannulated screw set with appropriate drill and guidewire (appropriate size varies depending on fracture)
4. Reduction clamp
5. Curettes

Technique

1. Patient is placed supine with a hand table
2. Sterile tourniquet is placed high on the operative arm to avoid surgical field
3. Using fluoroscopy and the guidewire, the starting point is determined. The starting point should avoid the tip of the olecranon, as this may cause hardware to be prominent and likely to require removal at a later date. The trajectory should be perpendicular to the fracture. A stab incision, large enough to accommodate the screw, is then made at the starting point
4. In cases of nonunion, a separate incision should be made longitudinally over the fracture site. The nonunion site should be debrided using bone curettes before guidewire insertion. Alternatively, the stab incision over the starting point can be extended to the fracture site
5. If the fracture is displaced, pointed reduction clamps placed from the tip of the olecranon and toward the mid-ulna can be used for reduction and compression

6. The guidewire is then inserted under fluoroscopic guidance perpendicular to the fracture. The guide-wire is then advanced passing through the fracture site. The guidewire should be advanced to a depth that will allow all threads of the partially threaded screw to lie beyond the fracture

7. Screw length is then measured over the wire using a cannulated depth gauge

8. Proximal cortex is then drilled over the guidewire with a cannulated drill bit

9. A partially threaded cannulated screw is advanced by hand over the wire using fluoroscopic guidance, confirming that adequate compression is achieved. All threads of the partially threaded screw must lie beyond the fracture site to achieve compression

POSTSURGICAL REHABILITATION

After surgery, the patient is placed in a posterior splint with the elbow at 90° of flexion for a period of 7 to 10 days. While immobilized, the patient can perform wrist, hand, and shoulder range of motion. Progressive, unlimited passive range of motion can begin once splint is removed. Active range of motion can also begin once splint is removed, except for active flexion past 90°, which is avoided until 6 weeks postoperatively. Full range of motion at the elbow should be achieved by 6 weeks. Weeks 6 to 12 focus on strengthening of elbow flexion and extension, and forearm pronation and supination. At 12 weeks, an interval throwing program can begin.

RESULTS

Schickendantz et al reported on the successful nonoperative treatment of 7 professional baseball players with stress reactions but no fracture.[14] All athletes returned to play. Paci et al reported on the largest case series of surgically treated olecranon stress fractures. In their report, 25 elite level baseball players underwent cannulated screw fixation, with 18 available for follow-up. Evidence of bony union occurred at an average of 10.9 weeks. Of the 18 players, 17 returned to play at their previous level. Of those 17, the average time to return to throwing was 29 weeks, and they played, on average, an additional 3.1 years of baseball after surgery.[16]

COMPLICATIONS

The biggest complication of nonoperative management is the development of a nonunion. In this instance, surgical fixation is indicated. The most common complication reported after surgical management is symptomatic hardware requiring removal. In a study, 22% of their patients required hardware removal for reasons other than infection.[16]

TRIP TO THE MOUND

Two techniques predominate for surgical fixation of oblique olecranon stress fractures. Either a single cannulated screw through the olecranon down the center of the ulna shaft or 1 or 2 screws directed perpendicular to the fracture site. There are very limited data to support one versus the other. I recommend a case-by-case approach depending on the obliquity of the fracture. For minimally oblique fractures, the trajectory of a screw placed perpendicular to the fractures should be within a safe zone confined to the bony olecranon devoid of any elbow stabilizers. As obliquity increases, the trajectory of the screw starts to shift more lateral and potentially compromise the elbow's lateral collateral ligament. For these fractures, I recommend a single cannulated screw directed down the ulnar shaft.

MANAGER'S TIPS

- Suspect olecranon injury in the throwing athlete who presents with vague, progressive elbow pain that is worse while throwing with tenderness to palpation over olecranon

- Initial X-rays are often negative, so the clinician should have a low threshold for ordering an MRI for further investigation

- Initial treatment is nonoperative; however, in the high-level athlete with discrete fracture line, immediate surgical treatment can be considered

- Throwing mechanics should be addressed during nonoperative management or after surgical intervention

REFERENCES

1. Morgan EF, Barnes GL, Einhorn TA. Chapter 1: The bone organ system: form and function. In: *Fundamentals of Osteoporosis*. Elsevier; 2010.

2. Miller TL. *Stress Fractures in Athletes: Diagnosis and Management*. New York, NY: Springer; 2015.

3. Bope ET, Kellerman RD. Rheumatology and the musculoskeletal system. In: *Conn's Current Therapy*. Elsevier; 2017.

4. Boden BP, Osbahr DC, Jimenez C. Low-risk stress fractures. *Am J Sports Med*. 2001;29(1):100-111.

5. Changstrom BG, Brou L, Khodaee M, et al. Epidemiology of stress fracture injuries among US high school athletes, 2005-2006 through 2012-2013. *Am J Sports Med.* 2015;43(1):26-33.

6. Iwamoto J, Sato Y, Takeda T, et al. Analysis of stress fractures in athletes based on our clinical experience. *World J Orthop.* 2011;2(1):7-12.

7. Makhni EC, Jegede KA, Ahmad CS. Pediatric elbow injuries in athletes. *Sports Med Arthrosc.* 2014;22(3):e16-e24.

8. Osbahr DC, Bedi A, Conway JE. Chapter 23: Olecranon stress fractures. In: Brown B, ed. *Sports Medicine of Baseball.* Philadelphia, PA: Lippincott Williams & Wilkins; 2012.

9. Fredericson M, Jennings F, Beaulieu C, et al. Stress fractures in athletes. *Top Magn Reson Imaging.* 2006;17(5):309-325.

10. Roub LW, Gumerman LW, Hanley EN Jr, et al. Bone stress: a radionuclide imaging perspective. *Radiology.* 1979;132(2):431-438.

11. Kiuru MJ, Pihlajamaki HK, Hietanen HJ, et al. MR imaging, bone scintigraphy, and radiography in bone stress injuries of the pelvis and the lower extremity. *Acta Radiol.* 2002;43(2):207-212.

12. Wenzke DR. MR imaging of the elbow in the injured athlete. *Radiol Clin North Am.* 2013;51(2):195-213.

13. Ahmad CS, ElAttrache NS. Valgus extension overload syndrome and stress injury of the olecranon. *Clin Sports Med.* 2004;23(4):665-676 [x].

14. Schickendantz MS, Ho CP, Koh J. Stress injury of the proximal ulna in professional baseball players. *Am J Sports Med.* 2002;30(5):737-741.

15. Fujioka H, Tsunemi K, Takagi Y, et al. Treatment of stress fracture of the olecranon in throwing athletes with internal fixation through a small incision. *Sports Med Arthrosc Rehabil Ther Technol.* 2012;4(1):49.

16. Paci JM, Dugas JR, Guy JA, et al. Cannulated screw fixation of refractory olecranon stress fractures with and without associated injuries allows a return to baseball. *Am J Sports Med.* 2013;41(2):306-312.

17. Stephenson DR, Love S, Garcia GG, et al. Recurrence of an olecranon stress fracture in an elite pitcher after percutaneous internal fixation: a case report. *Am J Sports Med.* 2012;40(1):218-221.

18. Rettig AC, Wurth TR, Mieling P. Nonunion of olecranon stress fractures in adolescent baseball pitchers: a case series of 5 athletes. *Am J Sports Med.* 2006;34(4):653-656.

19. Nakaji N, Fujioka H, Tanaka J, et al. Stress fracture of the olecranon in an adult baseball player. *Knee Surg Sports Traumatol Arthrosc.* 2006;14(4):390-393.

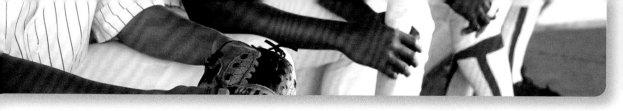

CHAPTER 10

Ulnar Collateral Ligament Injuries

Christopher S. Ahmad, MD | Brandon J. Erickson, MD | Anthony A. Romeo, MD

When they operated, I told them to put in a Koufax fastball. They did-but it was Mrs. Koufax's.

—*Tommy John*

INTRODUCTION

The ulnar collateral ligament (UCL), commonly referred to as the "Tommy John" ligament, is one of the most important structures of the elbow for a baseball pitcher. With each pitch, a pitcher generates a tremendous amount of stress across the medial elbow that pushes the UCL toward failure. In fact, without the supporting structures about the elbow including the flexor-pronator mass, joint capsule, and osseous restraints to help diffuse this stress, the stress on the UCL exceeds the force necessary to tear the ligament. Hence, for a pitcher to throw successfully and efficiently, the UCL must be functioning properly.

Over the past 10 years, there has been an increasing interest in UCL injuries, as the number of UCL tears has risen dramatically in pitchers of all levels of competition.[1-3] In fact, as much as 25% of Major League Baseball (MLB) professional pitchers have had UCL reconstructive surgery.[4] Several studies have tried to determine why the number of UCL tears has increased and what modifiable risk factors exist to decrease the rate of injury. While the reason some pitchers sustain UCL tears whereas others do not has not completely been elucidated, studies have shown many risk factors that contribute to these tears. These risk factors include that high pitch counts, pitching >100 innings per year, pitching for multiple teams, pitching while fatigued, pitching with higher velocity, pitching on consecutive days, geography (pitching while growing up in warmer climates), and pitching with a glenohumeral internal rotation deficit or a loss of total arc of shoulder motion increase the risk of elbow injuries.[5-12]

CLINICAL EVALUATION

History

When a pitcher presents with medial elbow pain, it is important to obtain a thorough history including the exact location of the pain (medial, posteromedial, etc), onset of symptoms, phase of the pitching cycle when the symptoms arise, whether the patient has pain at rest, and what prior treatments the player has had.[13] This will help the clinician focus on the patient's physical examination and ensure the proper diagnosis is reached. Players who sustain a UCL injury will often complain of vague elbow pain that has been bothering them on and off for some time, as well as a change in their velocity and accuracy.[14] Occasionally, pitchers present following an acute, traumatic event in which they experience a "pop" in their elbow after a specific pitch without having had significant symptoms before the injury.[15] The clinician should also inquire about ulnar nerve symptoms such as numbness and tingling in the pinky and ulnar half of the ring finger. It is important to note if these ulnar nerve symptoms are static (present at rest) or dynamic (only happen during pitching), as this can have treatment implications.

Physical Examination

The examination begins with general inspection of the neck, scapula, shoulder, elbow, and hand. Areas of ecchymosis, swelling, prior scars, muscle atrophy, or bony deformities should be noted. Palpation of the elbow is then conducted with special attention paid to tenderness over the medial epicondyle, sublime tubercle, and olecranon.[16] The throwing and nonthrowing elbows are then taken through passive and active range of motion (ROM), with special attention paid to loss of extension or pain with forced extension of the throwing elbow that could indicate posteromedial impingement. Stability and irritability of the ulnar nerve should be assessed during elbow ROM. Subluxation of the ulnar should be noted, as this may affect treatment options. Hypermobility alone is not pathologic, as up to one-third of ulnar nerves are hypermobile in the general population.[17] ROM of the shoulder is then conducted to look for scapular dyskinesis, loss of glenohumeral internal rotation, and loss of total shoulder rotation of the throwing arm, as these findings have been correlated with increased risk of elbow injuries.[6] A complete physical examination should also include a global musculoskeletal assessment, as problems within the kinetic chain are intimately related to the shoulder, elbow, and core in high-level performance athletes.

The examiner then performs resisted forearm pronation and forced elbow extension maneuvers to rule out other sources of medial elbow pain such as medial epicondylitis, tears of the flexor-pronator mass, and valgus extension overload. Several special tests to evaluate the UCL are then performed, including the valgus stress test, moving valgus stress test, and milking maneuver. To perform the milking maneuver, the patient's elbow is flexed to approximately 90°, the forearm is supinated, and the shoulder is abducted and slightly externally rotated, thereby placing tension on the posterior band of the anterior bundle of the UCL. The examiner holds the patient's thumb and creates a valgus stress on the elbow by exerting a posteriorly directed pull. A positive test, which indicates an injury to the UCL, is confirmed by reproduction of the pain the athlete experiences when throwing during the test. The moving valgus stress test is preferred, as studies have found a sensitivity of 100% and specificity of 75% in diagnosing tears of the UCL if the patient complains of pain during valgus load of the elbow while also flexing and extending the elbow between 70° and 120° of flexion.[18] Finally, one should check for presence of a palmaris longus in both forearms by having the patient touch his thumb and pinky finger together while slightly flexing his wrist. If the palmaris longus is not present in either arm, the hamstring tendon becomes the graft of choice.

Imaging

Every player presenting with elbow pain should have a high-quality 3-view series of the elbow (anteroposterior [AP], lateral, and oblique) to evaluate for the integrity of the UCL, calcifications within the ligament, posteromedial osteophytes, degenerative changes within the ulnohumeral and radiocapitellar joints, capitellar osteochondral defects, loose bodies, and persistent physes, or stress fracture. Enthesophytes on the sublime tubercle and prior avulsion injury to the medial epicondyle should also be assessed. Stress radiographs to look for medial widening are not commonly performed, although a difference of 1 to 3 mm between elbows can indicate a UCL injury (Figure 10.1A and B).[19] Stress ultrasound of the elbow may be valuable in the hands of expert technicians but has yet to become a standard part of the elbow evaluation.[19]

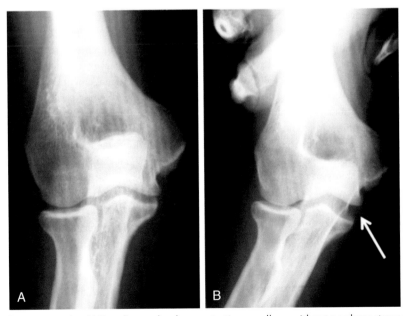

FIGURE 10.1 • Anteroposterior (AP) radiographs demonstrating an elbow without a valgus stress (A) and with a valgus stress (B) demonstrating medial gapping (white arrow).

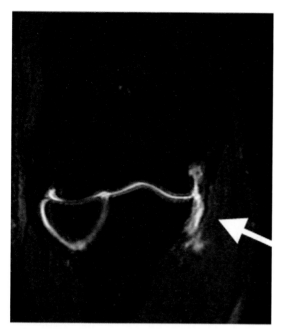

FIGURE 10.2 • Magnetic resonance imaging scan with a white arrow indicating full-thickness ulnar collateral ligament (UCL) tear from its attachment to the sublime tubercle.

While X-rays are useful to rule out bony pathology, magnetic resonance imaging (MRI) (Figure 10.2) and magnetic resonance arthrography (MRA) are the best imaging modalities to evaluate both full- and partial-thickness UCL tears, as well as concomitant elbow injuries. MRA has been shown to outperform MRI for the diagnosis of UCL tears (sensitivity and specificity, 92% and 100%, respectively, compared with 57% and 100%, respectively).[20] The normal, intact UCL has a low signal on T1-weighted images while a tear of the UCL, often seen at the level of the humeral attachment of the UCL on the medial epicondyle, will be bright on T2-weighted images secondary to edema within the ligament.[21-23] Conventional MRI studies are capable of identifying thickening within the ligament from chronic injury and large full-thickness tears. MRA, enhanced with intra-articular gadolinium contrast, improves the diagnostic ability of partial undersurface tears. Therefore, when plain MRI is inconclusive, the preferred imaging technique is MRA using a high-field closed magnet with narrow slice images. Contrast can often be seen migrating proximally and distally forming a T in some UCL lesions. MRI can also identify concomitant edema and injury in the flexor-pronator origin and posteromedial ulnohumeral chondromalacia.[24]

A computed tomography (CT) scan is often unnecessary in the setting of a primary UCL tear unless there is concern for a concomitant posteromedial osteophyte, olecranon stress fracture, and large enthesophytes on the sublime tubercle, which needs to be better classified, or to clearly define the 3-dimensional nature of the bone prominence if surgical excision of osteophytes is planned. However, in a patient with a previous ulnar collateral ligament reconstruction (UCLR), a CT scan can be useful to evaluate the placement of the ulnar and humeral tunnels and sockets to aid in preoperative planning for the revision UCLR. The CT can also help quantify bone loss in the revision setting (discussed in Chapter 11) and, again, clearly define the 3-dimensional anatomy of osteophytes. A 3D CT reconstruction, especially with either the ulna and radius or humerus subtracted away, can give the surgeon a better idea of where the bone loss is and where the tunnels were placed.

TREATMENT

Nonoperative

There are many factors that must be considered when counseling a patient on nonoperative versus operative management of UCL injuries. Above all, the patient's expectations must be considered.

While the UCL is critical to and must be functioning properly in pitchers, gymnasts, and javelin throwers who wish to continue to compete at a high level, a near-normal UCL is not typically necessary for patients who do not wish to compete in these sports.[25-27] Patients who desire to perform activities of daily living or play other sports than the ones previously listed, such as football, can often function well with an incompetent UCL and therefore can avoid surgery.[28] Furthermore, the length of rehabilitation after surgery is significantly longer than that of nonoperative management. Hence, some older pitchers at the end of their career may elect to undergo nonoperative management and attempt to return to sport (RTS) sooner so that they can finish their career without having surgery. Regardless of the UCL injury and associated pathology, the goals and expectations of the patient should be clearly identified, and the treatment plan should be tailored to meet these goals.

Nonoperative treatment for UCL injuries involves rest, rehabilitation, and a progressive return to throwing program over the course of several months (listed in the rehabilitation section at the end of this chapter).[29,30] The rehabilitation process must focus on maximizing shoulder ROM, increasing core strength, posterior capsular stretching, and proper scapulothoracic motion, as deficits in some of these parameters have been shown to be risk factors for elbow injuries.[6] Previous results following nonoperative treatment of UCL injuries with rest and rehabilitation alone have yielded less than 50% ability of pitchers to successfully RTS.[29] However, newer studies have found more encouraging RTS rates in specific subsets of patients with the addition of certain rehabilitation modalities, including electrical stimulation, soft tissue mobilization, massage, scraping, ultrasound, and laser therapy.[31] The subset of patients in this study had incomplete UCL tears diagnosed by MRI and had a >80% RTS rate following nonoperative management. Patients in this study with complete UCL tears underwent UCLR. This indicates that there may be certain tear patterns that are more amenable to successful nonoperative treatment than others, although a classification of partial UCL tears based on MRI findings and expected outcomes of nonsurgical management has yet to be validated. Clearly, certain tear patterns, such as avulsion of the distal ligament attachment on the ulna, have a poor prognosis and earlier surgical intervention may be warranted.[32]

While nonoperative treatment of UCL injuries classically involved rest and rehabilitation, newer biologic treatment modalities, such as platelet-rich plasma (PRP) and most recently pluripotent mesenchymal cells (stem cells), have been implemented with encouraging, but limited, results. Two recent studies have reported greater than 70% RTS rates after PRP injections coupled with rehabilitation in players with UCL tears.[21,33] While these results are promising, further work must be carried out in this area to identify which patients are most likely to benefit from the addition of some form of biologic augmentation to their nonoperative treatment regimen. When counseling patients regarding the success of treatment, high-grade partial tears, complete tears, and tears in a distal location have a worse prognosis than proximal and low-level partial tears.[34]

Operative Indications

Patients who desire to continue with competitive throwing, have failed nonoperative treatment, have an accurate diagnosis of UCL injury, and are willing to participate in the postsurgical rehabilitation are indicated for surgical reconstruction. In addition, seasonal timing may influence the decision for early surgical intervention in select situations. Contraindications to UCL reconstruction include athletes with asymptomatic tears that may be common in sports with little

valgus demands on the elbow. Patients with coexisting ulnohumeral or radiocapitellar arthritis considering UCL reconstruction should be informed of the possibility of continued or worsening pain after reconstruction.

Surgical Options

Operative treatment for UCL injures can be divided into UCL repair and UCLR. While previous reports on UCL repair have shown inferior results to UCLR, more recent studies have shown encouraging results after UCL repair with RTS rates above 90%.[15,35,36] Furthermore, a modification of the repair was recently introduced in which the UCL repair is augmented by a synthetic tape fixed with bone anchors at each end (InternalBrace, Arthrex, Naples) to act as a checkrein, prevent excessive stress on the repaired ligament, and possibly permanently reinforce the ligament when it is integrated into the native tissue.[37,38] The goal of this treatment modification is to allow a less invasive surgery with a faster rehabilitation and earlier RTS rate. Outcome studies on this technique are necessary to determine its efficacy compared with UCLR, which is the current gold standard treatment option for a high-level athlete with a UCL tear who wishes to RTS at a high level. Repair, with or without an InternalBrace construct, appears to be more readily used in younger athletes where the majority of the UCL appears normal on MRI with an avulsion or stretch injury at the humeral or ulnar attachment that remains symptomatic after nonoperative treatment.

Since its initial description in the literature in 1986 by Dr Jobe (Figure 10.3), the UCLR surgical technique has undergone several modifications in an attempt to reduce complications and improve outcomes (Figure 10.4).[24,27,39-42] These modifications have included the introduction of a muscle-splitting approach, modifications in graft choice, and different methods of fixation of the graft on the ulna and humerus. While the initial UCLR description called for a release and repair of the flexor-pronator mass, modifications in the technique have moved toward a muscle split to preserve flexor carpi ulnaris (FCU) attachments to the medial epicondyle and potentially decrease the rate of postoperative ulnar neuropathy. Based on several reviews of the literature, this modification has worked, as the rates of ulnar neuropathy for the docking and double-docking techniques are significantly lower than that of the original Jobe technique.[43,44] However, another commonly used technique, especially in MLB

hamstring autograft (gracilis or semitendinosus), hamstring allograft, and others.[25,27,47] No studies to date have found one graft to be superior to others, either biomechanically or clinically.[48-50] Similarly, no one surgical technique or method of fixation has proven superior to any others. Surgeons should use the technique with which they are most familiar and comfortable and can achieve reliable and reproducible outcomes.

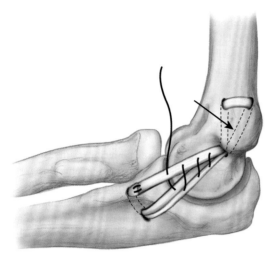

FIGURE 10.3 • Classic Jobe ulnar collateral ligament (UCL) reconstruction. Notice the graft has been looped through the tunnels on the medial epicondyle (black arrow) and sutured back onto itself to make it thicker.

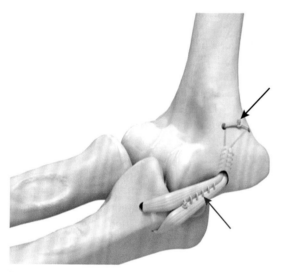

FIGURE 10.4 • Docking ulnar collateral ligament (UCL) reconstruction. Notice the graft is docked into the medial epicondyle and then tied over a bone bridge (black arrow). The graft is sutured to itself to increase stability (red arrow).

pitchers, is to partially elevate the FCU attachment from posterior to the anterior edge of the UCL after releasing the ulnar nerve in anticipation of including a subcutaneous ulnar nerve transposition with the UCLR.[45,46]

There are now several acceptable graft choices for UCLR, including ipsilateral/contralateral palmaris longus autograft, ipsilateral/contralateral

---

TRIP TO THE MOUND
A "Walk" Out to the Mound

There are countless options for graft choice when performing a UCLR. Currently, no study has shown one graft choice to be superior to another in RTS, clinical outcomes scores, or revision rates. There are certain surgical techniques that necessitate a slightly smaller diameter graft (palmaris in the docking technique) or a larger diameter graft (semitendinosus or gracilis in the double-docking technique). Each graft choice has risks and benefits that should be discussed with the patient (knee pain/weakness with hamstring autograft; wrist pain with palmaris autograft; disease transmission with allograft). If the technique allows, the patient and surgeon should make a shared decision on what graft they think is the best option for the athlete.

There is limited evidence on the value or necessity of concomitant ulnar nerve transposition and/or elbow arthroscopy in patients undergoing UCLR. Some surgical techniques necessitate ulnar nerve transposition, whereas others do not. It is currently not well defined whether players undergoing UCLR should undergo an obligatory ulnar nerve transposition, although many authors will only transpose the nerve if it is clinically symptomatic (symptoms with subluxation or symptoms of numbness) preoperatively.[43,44] Likewise, the value of concomitant elbow arthroscopy is not well defined when there are no intra-articular symptoms. No evidence exists to promote or refute concomitant elbow arthroscopy at the time of UCLR. In practice, most surgeons only use concomitant arthroscopy if there is additional intra-articular pathology that must be addressed at the time of UCLR.

TRIP TO THE MOUND
To Scope or Not to Scope? That Is the Question

When performing a UCLR, the surgeon has the option to perform a concomitant elbow arthroscopy to evaluate intra-articular structures for concomitant pathology that may not have been seen on the MRI/MRA. No studies to date have compared obligatory concomitant elbow arthroscopy with selective elbow arthroscopy when performing a UCLR. Whether or not to perform an elbow arthroscopy should be based on the individual surgeon's preference, preoperative physical examination, diagnostic imaging studies, and evidence of intra-articular pathology that the surgeon can successfully treat with his or her elbow arthroscopy skills. The authors prefer to perform elbow arthroscopy to treat concomitant symptomatic valgus extension overload.

TRIP TO THE MOUND
What's the Deal With the Ulnar Nerve?

How to address the ulnar nerve during UCLR reconstruction remains a controversial topic without evidence-based objective criteria to guide the surgeon. While certain techniques require an obligatory ulnar nerve transposition, most do not. Hence, the decision of whether to transpose the ulnar nerve is based on the surgeon's experience and expertise, often persuaded by his or her educational mentors. Most surgeons agree that patients with consistent preoperative ulnar nerve symptoms (numbness/tingling in the pinky and ulnar half of the ring finger, wasting of the first dorsal interosseous) or symptomatic ulnar nerve instability (subluxation of the nerve upon flexion/extension of the elbow) should undergo a concomitant subcutaneous ulnar nerve transposition. However, in patients without consistent preoperative symptoms, most surgeons who routinely perform the flexor-pronator muscle split exposure do not move the ulnar nerve. The risks and benefits of the ulnar nerve transposition should be discussed with the patient, and a shared decision should be reached with the patient.

Authors' Preferred Surgical Technique

The authors preferred surgical technique when performing a UCLR is via the modified docking technique.

Preoperative Planning

- Before surgery, the surgical technique and graft choice should be discussed with the patient, as well as whether the ulnar nerve will be transposed and whether concomitant elbow arthroscopy will be performed. Risks and benefits of each type of autograft, as well as allograft, should be explained in detail to allow for a shared decision with the patient
- Equipment needed:
  - Hand table
  - Sterile tourniquet
  - Two #1 or #2 high-strength nonabsorbable sutures
  - 2.0-mm drill
  - 3.5-mm drill
  - 4.5-mm drill
  - Two high-tensile passing sutures
  - Malleable wire suture passers
  - One high-tensile suture used to close the capsule and native UCL, again, either #1 or #2
  - Chamfer for the tunnel openings
  - Curette, preferably angled
  - Mineral oil (optional—assist with graft passage through bone tunnels)

Patient Setup

- Regional anesthesia, commonly a supraclavicular block, is performed with the addition of light sedation. Local anesthetic is injected at the site of incision before the tourniquet is inflated. General anesthesia and local anesthetic to the graft harvest site can be added if the preoperative plan involves harvesting a hamstring autograft
- Patients are placed supine on the operating table with the bed rotated 90° to the standard position with the operating room, and the operative extremity is placed on a hand table that is facing out toward the center of the room
- A nonsterile tourniquet is placed on the upper arm
- Preoperative antibiotics are given, the patient is prepped and draped, and a sterile tourniquet is applied
- The authors prefer to use the ipsilateral palmaris longus or contralateral gracilis/semitendinosus as their autograft for the modified docking technique. Allograft hamstring tendon, either gracilis or semitendinosus, is also a viable option

Step-by-Step Procedure

- Concomitant elbow arthroscopy is only performed if intra-articular pathology has been identified by pre-operative history/physical examination or imaging
- Palmaris longus harvest
  - A transverse incision is made at the wrist flexion crease over the palpable tendon. The tendon is dissected free, and small hemostat clamp is placed deep to it. Care is taken to avoid neuro-vascular structures, especially the median nerve
  - A second incision is made 5 cm proximal
  - A third incision is made and the tendon is identified. Muscle should be attaching onto the tendon at this location. The tendon is then divided at the wrist crease and delivered out the most proximal incision
  - To prepare the graft, a #1 or #2 high-tensile strength nonabsorbable is used. Five passes are performed over a distance of 2 cm. The graft is freed from the muscle attachments. Size the graft at this point. Note that the tunnel in the ulna is 3.5 mm, so grafts much larger than this will have a difficult time passing. Use a sharp pair of tenotomy scissors to trim the graft if necessary, but take care not to delaminate the graft. The second end of the graft is not prepared until the proper length is determined at the docking point of the medial epicondyle of the humerus
  - If a hamstring autograft is being used, a 4-cm incision is made along the medial border of the tibia, slightly distal to the tibial tubercle extending distally. The sartorius is elevated, and the gracilis and semitendinosus are exposed. A tendon stripper is used to harvest the hamstring graft of choice
- The medial epicondyle, olecranon, medial intermuscular septum, and path of the ulnar nerve are marked out. The incision is either directly over the ulnar nerve if this is being transposed or anterior to this if it is not being transposed. The incision should not be placed directly over the medial epicondyle (Figure 10.5)
- A 10 or 15 blade is used to incise the skin. A bipolar or standard electrocautery is used to cauterize the skin bleeders
- Dissection with tenotomy scissors is taken down to the fascia of the FCU. Care is taken to dissect and protect the branches of the medial antebrachial cutaneous nerve (Figure 10.6). Failure to protect these will result in numbness in the forearm and potentially a symptomatic neuroma

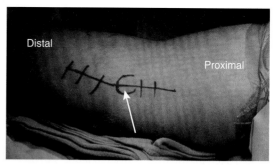

FIGURE 10.5 • Patient position and incision outlined. The white arrow is pointing to the medial epicondyle.

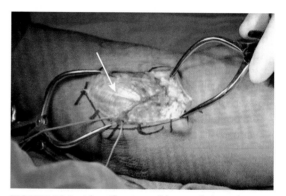

FIGURE 10.6 • Identification of the medial antebrachial cutaneous nerve (blue vessel loop is on the nerve) superficial to the flexor-pronator fascia (white arrow).

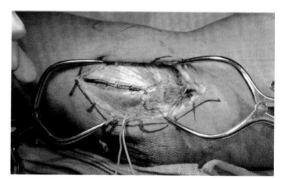

FIGURE 10.7 • Flexor carpi ulnaris (FCU) fascia incision marked with a pen.

- A muscle-splitting approach to the FCU is used when there are no preoperative ulnar nerve symptoms. The fascia is split and dissection is bluntly taken down to the joint capsule and UCL (Figure 10.7)
- A pen is used to mark the sublime tubercle and the path of the UCL on the joint capsule. The UCL is incised and medial gapping of the ulnohumeral joint is observed (Figures 10.8 and 10.9)

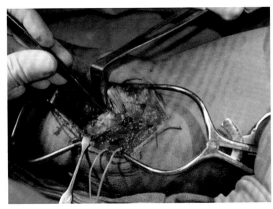

FIGURE 10.8 • Muscle-splitting approach with retractors in place and forceps pointing to the ulnar collateral ligament (UCL) which is well visualized.

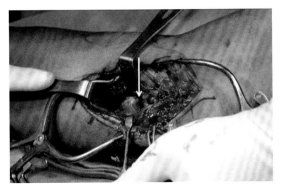

FIGURE 10.9 • Ulnar collateral ligament incised demonstrating ulnohumeral gapping of the ulnohumeral joint (white arrow).

- Tunnel creation
  - ◆ Ulnar tunnels are created with constant vigilance to the location of the ulnar nerve (Figure 10.10A and B)
  - ◆ Converging 3.2- or 3.5-mm drill holes, depending on the selected graft size, are made with a drill sleeve in the ulna anterior and posterior to the sublime tubercle with a minimum 5-mm bone bridge (essentially straddling the ridge of the sublime tubercle)
  - ◆ The drill holes should be 2 to 4 mm from the joint line and are connected through the ulnar medullary canal. An angled curette and chamfer are then used to ensure the tunnel is connected and patent, allowing the graft to slide through it without significant resistance
  - ◆ A looped suture is placed through the tunnels for subsequent graft shuttling
- Humeral tunnels
  - ◆ A 4.5-mm drill hole is made at the site of the anatomic origin of the anterior bundle of UCL

on the medial epicondyle, taking care not to penetrate the posterior cortex (Figure 10.11)

- ◆ The socket should be approximately 15 mm deep. A chamfer is used to smooth the opening of the socket
- ◆ The upper border of the epicondyle is exposed by incising the overlying fascia. Two sequential 2-mm tunnels are drilled from superior to inferior to communicate with the larger tunnel at its apex. Extreme caution must be used when creating the posterior drill hole to avoid the ulnar nerve if it remains in its normal location, or the surgeon can choose to put 2 anterior drill holes separated by 1 cm or more
- ◆ A bone bridge of 5 to 10 mm separates these tunnels, which are created to allow suture passage from the ends of the graft that are stationed in the primary humeral tunnel (Figure 10.12)
- ◆ Suture loops are then placed from the primary humeral tunnel through the exit tunnels to facilitate graft passing
- Graft passing and native UCL repair
  - ◆ With the elbow in forearm supination and mild varus stress, the horizontal incision in the native UCL is repaired with a 0 nonabsorbable suture. The free end of this running suture is left free for later passage into the central distal tunnel after graft docking
  - ◆ The graft is then passed through the ulnar tunnel from anterior to posterior. The posterior limb of the graft is passed into the humeral tunnel and is tensioned on the far humeral cortex using its associated suture
  - ◆ The final length of the anterior limb of the graft is determined by laying it superficial to the epicondyle and visually estimating the required length to tension within the humeral tunnel
  - ◆ The estimation of graft length should be performed with the elbow flexed to 60° while applying a varus stress to reduce medial laxity. The graft is marked at the 1 cm point so that 1 cm of graft will enter the socket. Leaving too much graft will cause the graft to bottom out in the socket before it is completely tensioned and cause a big problem
  - ◆ A No. 1 braided nonabsorbable suture is placed into the anterior graft limb in a running locking fashion. The excess graft is excised, and the anterior graft limb is passed into the humeral tunnel with the sutures exiting the anterior 2-mm tunnel. Alternatively, if the graft diameter is small, a 3- or even 4-strand graft can be created by not excising the graft

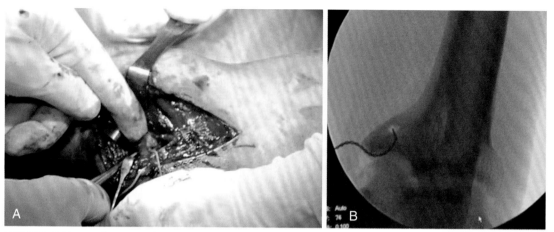

FIGURE 10.10 • A, Ulnar tunnels created anterior and posterior to the sublime tubercle. The surgeon's index finger marks the anterior tunnels and the forceps mark the posterior tunnel. B, Anteroposterior radiograph demonstrating the ulnar tunnel with a radiopacity through the tunnel.

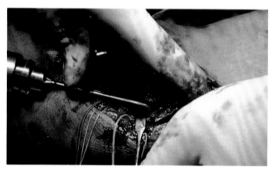

FIGURE 10.11 • Inferior humeral tunnel created using the drill at anatomic ulnar collateral ligament origin.

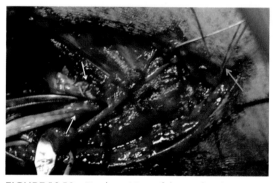

FIGURE 10.13 • Final position of the graft (white arrows) with tensioning of sutures (blue arrow). This is before the graft is looped back onto itself.

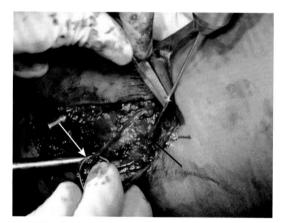

FIGURE 10.12 • Exit holes created on superior aspect of epicondyle. The drill is creating 1 of the 2 exit holes (black arrow). A curette is placed into the socket of the medial epicondyle to help with the trajectory of the drill, thereby ensuring the tunnels converge (white arrow).

- Final graft tensioning is performed by holding tension on the graft and ranging the elbow through repeated flexion-extension to remove creep and confirm graft isometry. The sutures are then tied over the bony bridge on the humeral epicondyle with the elbow in 45° of flexion, supination, and varus stress (Figure 10.13)

- The anterior and posterior limbs of the graft may be sutured together to add further graft tension

- If extra limbs of graft passing are desired, the free end of the graft is sutured with 0 nonabsorbable suture and passed back through the ulnar posterior tunnel and out the anterior portion of the tunnel. The graft sutures can then be passed through the native ligament and tied for a 3-strand graft or passed through the anterior epicondyle tunnel for a 4-strand graft (Figures 10.14 and 10.15)

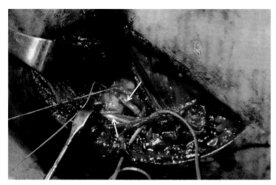

FIGURE 10.14 • Three-strand graft indicated by the white arrows.

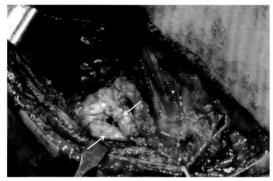

FIGURE 10.15 • Four-strand graft indicated by the white arrows.

- The sutures from the folded end of the graft are passed though the posterior tunnel in the medial epicondyle. This limb of the graft is now docked into the socket. Tension is pulled on the sutures from both ends of the graft to ensure the graft is completely seated within the socket

- The remaining sutures are tied to the sutures that were previously tied down. This helps make the knot lower profile

- Closure
  - The incision is closed in layers. #1 Vicryl is used to securely close the FCU fascia, 2-0 Monocryl is used to close the subcutaneous tissue, and a 3-0 running Monocryl is used for skin along with Steri-Strips
  - A hinged elbow brace fixed at 75° of flexion is used postoperatively to protect the reconstruction in the immediate postoperative time frame

POSTSURGICAL REHABILITATION

Much of the research surrounding UCL tears has focused on prevention and modifications to surgical techniques to achieve better outcomes. Relatively little work has been done on the rehabilitation process. Current opinion is to avoid accelerated rehabilitation, as studies have shown this to be a risk factor for reinjury to the reconstructed UCL.[51] Many rehabilitation protocols follow the same general guidelines. Even at the highest level of performance, there remains significant variability in the rehabilitation protocols provided to MLB players. The rehabilitation process can be divided into 4 phases and is further detailed in chapter 12.[52,53]

Phase I (weeks 0-3): The goals of phase I are to healing, prevention of stiffness, and protecting the reconstruction. After 1 week of immobilization, gentle ROM of the elbow in a hinged elbow brace is started from 30° to 100° for 1 week and progressed to 15° to 110° for the third week. The brace is removed at 4 weeks and ROM is progress toward full ROM of extension and flexion.

Phase II (weeks 4-8): The goals of phase II are to increase strength. ROM continues toward full ROM if any limitation persists, and the athlete begins working with very light weight and gradually progressed in resistance. Scapular stabilization exercise, shoulder ROM, as well as shoulder strengthening exercises are performed.

Phase III (weeks 9-13): This phase focuses on flexibility, restoring upper extremity neuromuscular control, and progressing toward sports-related activities. It is imperative that the athlete establishes proper throwing mechanics during this phase as well. Proprioception and dynamic stabilization exercises as well as manual resistance and isotonic exercises are performed. Toward the end of this phase, a sports-specific plyometrics program is initiated.

Phase IV (weeks 14-26): This phase involves a throwing progression program. The athlete begins with short toss (45 feet), progresses to lofted long toss (120 feet), and then long toss on a line. Once the athlete has progressed through the early return to thrown program, they can throw from the mound, then in a simulated game, and finally return to game competition. Competitive throwing is commonly permitted in controlled situations at approximately 7 to 9 months. However, it typically takes 10 to 18 months before pitchers are fully game ready, which means the ability to throw more than 3 innings and a minimum of 50 pitches at high-level competition.

RESULTS

Several studies in the last 10 years have reported the outcomes after UCLR in athletes of varying levels (Table 10.1).[1,13,24,25,27,47,49,54-60] The largest series to date by Cain et al evaluated 942 patients at a minimum

TABLE 10.1 Clinical Outcomes After Ulnar Collateral Ligament Reconstruction (UCLR) in the Literature

Author	# UCLR	# UCL Repair	Dates	Mean Age in Years (Range)	Number of Males	Sport	Surgical Technique
Erickson et al	188	0	2004-2014	19.6 (14-32)	173/188 92%	Baseball: 165 Football: 6 Gymnast: 4 Softball: 4 Volleyball: 2 97 college, 68 HS 1 MS, 7 pro	Docking Double docking
O'Brien et al	3	0	2004-2009	20.3 (16-33)	31/33 94%	Baseball: 30 Javelin: 3	Modified Jobe Docking
Merolla et al	15	0	2006-2012	38	12/15 80%	N/A	Docking Modified Jobe
Jones et al	55	0	2008-2010	17.6 (15-18)	51/55 92.7%	Baseball: 47 Gymnast: 3 Javelin: 5 All HS	Docking
Bowers et al	21	0	2005-2007	20 (16-27)	21/21 100%	Baseball: 21 5 pro, 11 college, 5 HS	Modified docking
Dines et al	10	0	2006-2009	18.5 (18-21)	N/A	Javelin: 10 5 college, 5 HS	Docking
Cain et al	1266	15	1988-2006	21.5 (14-59)	1253/1281 98%	Baseball: 1213 Javelin: 15 Football: 13 Softball: 9 Tennis: 7	Modified Jobe
Dines et al	22	0	N/A	20.1 (16-24)	N/A	Baseball: 20 1 pro, 16 college, 3 HS Hockey: 1 Football: 1	DANE TJ
Savoie et al	116	0	2005-2009	20.4 (14-32)	N/A	Baseball, softball, javelin 23 pro, 28 college, 45 HS	Docking
Hechtman et al	34	0	1997-2002	18.7 (15-23)	34/34 100%	Baseball: 34 20 college, 14 HS	Hybrid

DASH, disability of the arm, shoulder, and hand score; HS, high school; KJOC, Karla-Jobe Orthopaedic Clinic Shoulder and Outcome Score; MEPS, Mayo Elbow Performance Score; MS, middle school; N/A: not applicable; OCD, osteochondritis dissecans; OES, Oxford Elbow Score; PM, posteromedial.

Graft Choice	Concomitant Procedures	Arthroscopy Performed?	Average Follow-up	Outcomes	Mean Time to RTS	Complications
Palmaris auto: 113 Hamstring auto: 48 Allograft: 26 Triceps auto: 2	None listed	4/188 2.12%	60 mo	94.1% returned to previous level KJOC: 90.4 Andrews-Timmerman: 92.5	N/A	Subsequent surgery: 10
Palmaris auto: 24 Hamstring auto: 5 Achilles auto: 4	3 flexor-pronator tendon repairs, 2 loose body removals, 1 excision of olecranon spur, 1 ulnar nerve neurolysis without transposition	No	3.7 y	KJOC: 76 Returned to previous level of competition: 82%	Baseball: 10.4 mo Javelin: 9.5 mo	Subsequent surgery: 3
Palmaris auto: 5 Hamstring allo: 10	None listed	No	3 y	MEPS: 93.8 ± 6.1 OES: 45.8 ± 2.8 DASH: 1.81 ± 0.98	N/A	None
Palmaris auto: 45 Gracilis auto: 10	Transhumeral drilling for capitellar OCD: 2 PM olecranon osteophyte debridement: 2	4/55 7.3%	31 mo	KJOC: 88 ± 6 Andrews-Timmerman: 83.6 ± 7.2	Average: 11.5 mo Range: 9-14 mo	Ulnar neuritis: 4
Not specified	None listed	N/A	28 mo	Conway: 90% excellent results	N/A	None
Palmaris auto: 9 Gracilis auto: 1	None listed	N/A	28.9 mo	Conway: 90% excellent results Andrews-Timmerman: 97	Average 15 mo	None
Palmaris auto: 935 Gracilis auto: 294 Plantaris auto: 30	Done in 437 patients; primarily excision of PM olecranon osteophytes	N/A	38.4 mo	Returned to previous level of competition or higher: 83%	Average: 11.6 mo Range: 3-72 mo	Ulnar neuropraxia: 121 Failure: 9
Palmaris auto: 12 Gracilis auto: 10	PM olecranon osteophyte debridement: 3 Synovectomy and chondroplasty: 1	3/22 13.6%	35.9 mo	Conway: 86% excellent results	N/A	Ulnar neuritis: 2 Revision for lysis of adhesions: 2
Hamstring allo: 123	None listed	"Most"	39 mo	Conway: 80% excellent results	Average: 9.5 mo Range: 4.5-18 mo	Ulnar neuropathy: 3 Wound problems: 2 Medial humeral epicondyle fracture: 1 FP muscle and tendon tear: 1
Palmaris auto: 29 Plantaris auto: 3 Achilles auto: 2	Olecranon osteophyte and loose body removal: 1	N/A	6.9 y	Returned to previous level of competition or higher: 85%	Average: 10 mo Range: 7-13 mo	Ulnar neuropathy: 1

2-year follow-up and found 83% were able to RTS at the same or higher level of competition.[25] Many other studies have found similar RTS rates, with higher levels of RTS often seen in adolescents compared with professional athletes.[27,47] However, despite the common perception that pitchers increase their velocity after UCLR, studies have found this to be inaccurate. Pitchers are often able to reestablish their preinjury velocity or lose only a small amount of velocity upon RTS but typically do not exceed their average preinjury velocity.[61,62] Furthermore, while specific inning limits set on pitchers for a season have not been found effective in preventing revision UCLR based on an in-depth analysis of MLB pitchers over the past 20 years who have had UCLR, recent evidence implies that limiting pitchers' postoperative workload based on their preoperative workload may decrease their risk of requiring a revision UCLR.[51,63]

Although most studies cite the >80% RTS rate after UCLR, there are several confounding factors that, when present, can dramatically decrease the success of the UCLR procedure. A concomitant tear of the flexor-pronator mass, while uncommon (reported in only 4% of patients with UCLR tears), results in a poor outcomes in 62.5% of patients.[64] Similarly, concomitant ulnohumeral chondromalacia, also uncommon (cited at 18%), portends a poor prognosis for patients after UCLR. Whether this chondromalacia is treated with observation, debridement, or microfracture at the time of UCLR, the rate of RTS at the same or higher level is 76%, suggesting a slightly less predictable RTS result when compared with patients without concomitant posteromedial chondromalacia.[65] Finally, significant calcification in the native UCL is associated with inferior results after UCLR, possibly due to the extended area of ligament pathology, as well as the risk of removing capsule and ligament tissue with the excision of the calcification. Patients who had significant calcifications within the UCL and were treated with excision of the bone fragments and UCLR using contralateral gracilis autograft had a RTS rate of 81% compared with 91% in patients with no calcifications within the native UCL.[66] Understanding the confounding variables that can affect the results after UCLR provides the opportunity for surgeons to better manage patient expectations accordingly before they undergo their surgical procedure.

While the results after primary UCLR have been consistent, the results after revision UCLR are much less predictable. As the number of primary UCLR continues to increase, especially in adolescent patients, the number of revision UCLR will increase as well.[2,3,55,56] Unfortunately, the RTS rates after revision UCLR in the hands of expert surgeons have been cited at 65.5%.[55] Patients are counseled preoperatively so they understand the challenges they will face postoperatively in terms of rehabilitation and RTS. The rehabilitation process is typically slowed in the revision setting to allow the best environment for healing of the reconstruction and biologic incorporation of the graft, providing the pitchers the best opportunity to succeed upon RTS.

COMPLICATIONS

With meticulous attention to detail, complication rates after UCLR are relatively low. Studies have reported the complication rate after UCLR between 3% and 40%, with the rate significantly higher in revision cases.[45,67] The most common complication after UCLR is transient ulnar neuropathy, which, depending on the surgical technique used, can range from 3% with the docking technique to 26% with the original Jobe technique.[15,43,44] Less frequent complications include stiffness, synovitis, graft harvest site problems, stiffness, heterotopic ossification, and failure of the UCLR leading to revision.[45,56,67,68]

Intraoperative complications include ulnar tunnel fracture (if the bone bridge is too small or if it is too close to the joint line) and graft length issues for docking (too little graft in humeral tunnel or too long of a graft that bottoms out and does not tension properly). Early postoperative complications include hematoma and stiffness. Late postoperative complications include sublime tubercle stress reaction, catastrophic fracture of the medial epicondyle, flexor tendinitis, graft ossification or failure, and flexor-pronator tears.

MANAGER'S TIPS

- The number of UCL injuries is increasing
- Pitchers with a decrease in velocity and loss of accuracy in the setting of medial elbow pain should be evaluated, as this can be a sentinel finding for UCL deficiency or tear
- MRI or MRA are the imaging modalities of choice to diagnose UCL tears, with dynamic ultrasound imaging providing a new clinical imaging study that has the potential to provide a rapid assessment in the training room and during postoperative rehabilitation
- Nonoperative treatment can be successful in athletes with partial-thickness UCL tears, although distal UCL injury has a poorer prognosis for successful RTS

- Modern techniques used to perform a primary UCLR afford patients >80% RTS rates
- There is no single surgical technique or graft choice for UCLR that has clearly outperformed all others, but most surgeons use a technique that minimizes iatrogenic injury to the flexor-pronator muscle group, preserves and repairs the native UCL, and incorporates a tendon graft into the UCL after reliable fixation to the anatomic footprint region of the ulna and humerus
- The rehabilitation process after UCLR is long, tedious for the athlete, and strenuous. Patients should be prepared to participate in the rehabilitation process for more than 1 year before realizing their ability to fully compete at their preinjury level of competition

REFERENCES

1. Erickson BJ, Gupta AK, Harris JD, et al. Rate of return to pitching and performance after Tommy John surgery in major league baseball pitchers. *Am J Sports Med*. 2014;42(3):536-543.
2. Erickson BJ, Nwachukwu BU, Rosas S, et al. Trends in medial ulnar collateral ligament reconstruction in the United States: a retrospective review of a large private-payer database from 2007 to 2011. *Am J Sports Med*. 2015;43(7):1770-1774.
3. Hodgins JL, Vitale M, Arons RR, Ahmad CS. Epidemiology of medial ulnar collateral ligament reconstruction: a 10-year study of New York state. *Am J Sports Med*. 2016;44(3):729-734.
4. Conte SA, Fleisig GS, Dines JS, et al. Prevalence of ulnar collateral ligament surgery in professional baseball players. *Am J Sports Med*. 2015;43(7):1764-1769.
5. Erickson BJ, Harris JD, Tetreault M, Bush-Joseph C, Cohen M, Romeo AA. Is Tommy John surgery performed more frequently in major league baseball pitchers from warm weather areas? *Orthop J Sports Med*. 2014;2(10):2325967114553916.
6. Wilk KE, Macrina LC, Fleisig GS, et al. Deficits in glenohumeral passive range of motion increase risk of elbow injury in professional baseball pitchers: a prospective study. *Am J Sports Med*. 2014;42(9):2075-2081.
7. Bushnell BD, Anz AW, Noonan TJ, Torry MR, Hawkins RJ. Association of maximum pitch velocity and elbow injury in professional baseball pitchers. *Am J Sports Med*. 2010;38(4):728-732.
8. Chalmers PN, Erickson BJ, Ball B, Romeo AA, Verma NN. Fastball pitch velocity helps predict ulnar collateral ligament reconstruction in major league baseball pitchers. *Am J Sports Med*. 2016;44(8):2130-2135.
9. Fleisig GS, Andrews JR, Cutter GR, et al. Risk of serious injury for young baseball pitchers: a 10-year prospective study. *Am J Sports Med*. 2011;39(2):253-257.
10. Erickson BJ, Chalmers PN, Bush-Joseph CA, Romeo AA. Predicting and preventing injury in major league baseball. *Am J Orthop*. 2016;45(3):152-156.
11. Erickson BJ, Sgori T, Chalmers PN, et al. The impact of fatigue on baseball pitching mechanics in adolescent male pitchers. *Arthroscopy*. 2016;32(5):762-771.
12. Byram IR, Bushnell BD, Dugger K, Charron K, Harrell FE Jr, Noonan TJ. Preseason shoulder strength measurements in professional baseball pitchers: identifying players at risk for injury. *Am J Sports Med*. 2010;38(7):1375-1382.
13. Erickson BJ, Romeo AA. The ulnar collateral ligament injury: evaluation and treatment. *J Bone Joint Surg Am*. 2017;99(1):76-86.
14. Makhni EC, Morrow ZS, Luchetti TJ, et al. Arm pain in youth baseball players: a survey of healthy players. *Am J Sports Med*. 2015;43(1):41-46.
15. Conway JE, Jobe FW, Glousman RE, Pink M. Medial instability of the elbow in throwing athletes. Treatment by repair or reconstruction of the ulnar collateral ligament. *J Bone Joint Surg Am*. 1992;74(1):67-83.
16. Redler LH, Watling JP, Ahmad CS. Physical examination of the throwing athlete's elbow. *Am J Orthop*. 2015;44(1):13-18.
17. Calfee RP, Manske PR, Gelberman RH, Van Steyn MO, Steffen J, Goldfarb CA. Clinical assessment of the ulnar nerve at the elbow: reliability of instability testing and the association of hypermobility with clinical symptoms. *J Bone Joint Surg Am*. 2010;92(17):2801-2808.
18. O'Driscoll SW, Lawton RL, Smith AM. The "moving valgus stress test" for medial collateral ligament tears of the elbow. *Am J Sports Med*. 2005;33(2):231-239.
19. Ciccotti MG, Atanda A Jr, Nazarian LN, Dodson CC, Holmes L, Cohen SB. Stress sonography of the ulnar collateral ligament of the elbow in professional baseball pitchers: a 10-year study. *Am J Sports Med*. 2014;42(3):544-551.
20. Magee T. Accuracy of 3-T MR arthrography versus conventional 3-T MRI of elbow tendons and ligaments compared with surgery. *AJR Am J Roentgenol*. 2015;204(1):W70-W75.
21. Podesta L, Crow SA, Volkmer D, Bert T, Yocum LA. Treatment of partial ulnar collateral ligament tears in the elbow with platelet-rich plasma. *Am J Sports Med*. 2013;41(7):1689-1694.
22. Kim NR, Moon SG, Ko SM, Moon WJ, Choi JW, Park JY. MR imaging of ulnar collateral ligament injury in baseball players: value for predicting rehabilitation outcome. *Eur J Radiol*. 2011;80(3):e422-e426.
23. Wear SA, Thornton DD, Schwartz ML, Weissmann RC III, Cain EL, Andrews JR. MRI of the reconstructed ulnar collateral ligament. *AJR Am J Roentgenol*. 2011;197(5):1198-1204.
24. Dines JS, ElAttrache NS, Conway JE, Smith W, Ahmad CS. Clinical outcomes of the DANE TJ technique to treat ulnar collateral ligament insufficiency of the elbow. *Am J Sports Med*. 2007;35(12):2039-2044.

25. Cain EL Jr, Andrews JR, Dugas JR, et al. Outcome of ulnar collateral ligament reconstruction of the elbow in 1281 athletes: results in 743 athletes with minimum 2-year follow-up. *Am J Sports Med.* 2010;38(12):2426-2434.

26. Dines JS, Jones KJ, Kahlenberg C, Rosenbaum A, Osbahr DC, Altchek DW. Elbow ulnar collateral ligament reconstruction in javelin throwers at a minimum 2-year follow-up. *Am J Sports Med.* 2012;40(1):148-151.

27. Erickson BJ, Bach BR Jr, Cohen MS, et al. Ulnar collateral ligament reconstruction: the Rush experience. *Orthop J Sports Med.* 2016;4(1):2325967115626876.

28. Kenter K, Behr CT, Warren RF, O'Brien SJ, Barnes R. Acute elbow injuries in the National Football League. *J Shoulder Elbow Surg/American Shoulder and Elbow Surgeons [et al].* 2000;9(1):1-5.

29. Rettig AC, Sherrill C, Snead DS, Mendler JC, Mieling P. Nonoperative treatment of ulnar collateral ligament injuries in throwing athletes. *Am J Sports Med.* 2001;29(1):15-17.

30. Wilk KE, Arrigo CA, Hooks TR, Andrews JR. Rehabilitation of the overhead throwing athlete: there is more to it than just external rotation/internal rotation strengthening. *PM R.* 2016;8(3 suppl):S78-S90.

31. Ford GM, Genuario J, Kinkartz J, Githens T, Noonan T. Return-to-Play outcomes in professional baseball players after medial ulnar collateral ligament injuries: comparison of operative versus nonoperative treatment based on magnetic resonance imaging findings. *Am J Sports Med.* 2016;44(3):723-728.

32. Frangiamore SJ, Lynch TS, Vaughn MD, et al. Magnetic resonance imaging predictors of failure in the nonoperative management of ulnar collateral ligament injuries in professional baseball pitchers. *Am J Sports Med.* 2017:363546517699832.

33. Dines JS, Williams PN, ElAttrache N, et al. Platelet-rich plasma can Be used to successfully treat elbow ulnar collateral ligament insufficiency in high-level throwers. *Am J Orthop.* 2016;45(5):296-300.

34. Nassab PF, Schickendantz MS. Evaluation and treatment of medial ulnar collateral ligament injuries in the throwing athlete. *Sports Med Arthrosc Rev.* 2006;14(4):221-231.

35. Savoie FH III, Trenhaile SW, Roberts J, Field LD, Ramsey JR. Primary repair of ulnar collateral ligament injuries of the elbow in young athletes: a case series of injuries to the proximal and distal ends of the ligament. *Am J Sports Med.* 2008;36(6):1066-1072.

36. Erickson BJ, Bach BR Jr, Verma NN, Bush-Joseph CA, Romeo AA. Treatment of ulnar collateral ligament tears of the elbow: is repair a viable option? *Orthop J Sports Med.* 2017;5(1):2325967116682211.

37. Dugas JR, Walters BL, Beason DP, Fleisig GS, Chronister JE. Biomechanical comparison of ulnar collateral ligament repair with internal bracing versus modified jobe reconstruction. *Am J Sports Med.* 2016;44(3):735-741.

38. Dugas JR. Ulnar collateral ligament repair: an old idea with a new wrinkle. *Am J Orthop.* 2016;45(3):124-127.

39. Jobe FW, Stark H, Lombardo SJ. Reconstruction of the ulnar collateral ligament in athletes. *J Bone Joint Surg Am.* 1986;68(8):1158-1163.

40. Rohrbough JT, Altchek DW, Hyman J, Williams RJ III, Botts JD. Medial collateral ligament reconstruction of the elbow using the docking technique. *Am J Sports Med.* 2002;30(4):541-548.

41. Andrews JR, Timmerman LA. Outcome of elbow surgery in professional baseball players. *Am J Sports Med.* 1995;23(4):407-413.

42. Morgan RJ, Starman JS, Habet NA, et al. A biomechanical evaluation of ulnar collateral ligament reconstruction using a novel technique for ulnar-sided fixation. *Am J Sports Med.* 2010;38(7):1448-1455.

43. Vitale MA, Ahmad CS. The outcome of elbow ulnar collateral ligament reconstruction in overhead athletes: a systematic review. *Am J Sports Med.* 2008;36(6):1193-1205.

44. Erickson BJ, Chalmers PN, Bush-Joseph CA, Verma NN, Romeo AA. Ulnar collateral ligament reconstruction of the elbow: a systematic review of the literature. *Orthop J Sports Med.* 2015;3(12):2325967115618914.

45. Azar FM, Andrews JR, Wilk KE, Groh D. Operative treatment of ulnar collateral ligament injuries of the elbow in athletes. *Am J Sports Med.* 2000;28(1):16-23.

46. Andrews JR, Jost PW, Cain EL. The ulnar collateral ligament procedure revisited: the procedure we use. *Sports Health.* 2012;4(5):438-441.

47. Savoie FH III, Morgan C, Yaste J, Hurt J, Field L. Medial ulnar collateral ligament reconstruction using hamstring allograft in overhead throwing athletes. *J Bone Joint Surg Am.* 2013;95(12):1062-1066.

48. Saltzman BM, Erickson BJ, Frank JM, et al. Biomechanical testing of the reconstructed ulnar collateral ligament: a systematic review of the literature. *Musculoskelet Surg.* 2016;100(3):157-163.

49. Erickson BJ, Cvetanovich GL, Frank RM, et al. Do clinical results and return-to-sport rates after ulnar collateral ligament reconstruction differ based on graft choice and surgical technique? *Orthop J Sports Med.* 2016;4(11):2325967116670142.

50. Dargel J, Kupper F, Wegmann K, Oppermann J, Eysel P, Muller LP. Graft diameter does not influence primary stability of ulnar collateral ligament reconstruction of the elbow. *J Orthop Sci.* 2015;20(2):307-313.

51. Keller RA, Mehran N, Khalil LS, Ahmad CS, ElAttrache N. Relative individual workload changes may be a risk factor for rerupture of ulnar collateral ligament reconstruction. *J Shoulder Elbow Surg/American Shoulder and Elbow Surgeons [et al].* 2017;26(3):369-375.

52. Seto JL, Brewster CE, Randall CC, Jobe FW. Rehabilitation following ulnar collateral ligament reconstruction of athletes. *J Orthop Sports Phys Ther.* 1991;14(3):100-105.

53. Bernas GA, Ruberte Thiele RA, Kinnaman KA, Hughes RE, Miller BS, Carpenter JE. Defining safe rehabilitation for ulnar collateral ligament reconstruction of the elbow: a biomechanical study. *Am J Sports Med.* 2009;37(12):2392-2400.

54. O'Brien DF, O'Hagan T, Stewart R, et al. Outcomes for ulnar collateral ligament reconstruction: a retrospective review using the KJOC assessment score with two-year follow-up in an overhead throwing population. *J Shoulder Elbow Surg/American Shoulder and Elbow Surgeons [et al].* 2015;24(6):934-940.

55. Marshall NE, Keller RA, Lynch JR, Bey MJ, Moutzouros V. Pitching performance and longevity after revision ulnar collateral ligament reconstruction in Major League Baseball pitchers. *Am J Sports Med.* 2015;43(5):1051-1056.

56. Wilson AT, Pidgeon TS, Morrell NT, DaSilva MF. Trends in revision elbow ulnar collateral ligament reconstruction in professional baseball pitchers. *J Hand Surg.* 2015;40(11):2249-2254.

57. Bowers AL, Dines JS, Dines DM, Altchek DW. Elbow medial ulnar collateral ligament reconstruction: clinical relevance and the docking technique. *J Shoulder Elbow Surg/American Shoulder and Elbow Surgeons [et al].* 2010;19(2 suppl):110-117.

58. Jones KJ, Dines JS, Rebolledo BJ, et al. Operative management of ulnar collateral ligament insufficiency in adolescent athletes. *Am J Sports Med.* 2014;42(1):117-121.

59. Merolla G, Del Sordo S, Paladini P, Porcellini G. Elbow ulnar collateral ligament reconstruction: clinical, radiographic, and ultrasound outcomes at a mean 3-year follow-up. *Musculoskelet Surg.* 2014(98 suppl 1):87-93.

60. Hechtman KS, Zvijac JE, Wells ME, Botto-van Bemden A. Long-term results of ulnar collateral ligament reconstruction in throwing athletes based on a hybrid technique. *Am J Sports Med.* 2011;39(2):342-347.

61. Ahmad CS, Grantham WJ, Greiwe RM. Public perceptions of Tommy John surgery. *Phys Sportsmed.* 2012;40(2):64-72.

62. Jiang JJ, Leland JM. Analysis of pitching velocity in major league baseball players before and after ulnar collateral ligament reconstruction. *Am J Sports Med.* 2014;42(4):880-885.

63. Erickson BJ, Cvetanovich GL, Bach BR Jr, Bush-Joseph CA, Verma NN, Romeo AA. Should we limit innings pitched after ulnar collateral ligament reconstruction in major league baseball pitchers? *Am J Sports Med.* 2016;44(9):2210-2213.

64. Osbahr DC, Swaminathan SS, Allen AA, Dines JS, Coleman SH, Altchek DW. Combined flexor-pronator mass and ulnar collateral ligament injuries in the elbows of older baseball players. *Am J Sports Med.* 2010;38(4):733-739.

65. Osbahr DC, Dines JS, Rosenbaum AJ, Nguyen JT, Altchek DW. Does posteromedial chondromalacia reduce rate of return to play after ulnar collateral ligament reconstruction? *Clin Orthop Relat Res.* 2012;470(6):1558-1564.

66. Dugas JR, Bilotta J, Watts CD, et al. Ulnar collateral ligament reconstruction with gracilis tendon in athletes with intraligamentous bony excision: technique and results. *Am J Sports Med.* 2012;40(7):1578-1582.

67. Dines JS, Yocum LA, Frank JB, ElAttrache NS, Gambardella RA, Jobe FW. Revision surgery for failed elbow medial collateral ligament reconstruction. *Am J Sports Med.* 2008;36(6):1061-1065.

68. Andrachuk JS, Scillia AJ, Aune KT, Andrews JR, Dugas JR, Cain EL. Symptomatic heterotopic ossification after ulnar collateral ligament reconstruction: clinical significance and treatment outcome. *Am J Sports Med.* 2016;44(5):1324-1328.

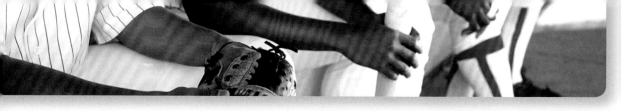

CHAPTER 11

Revision Ulnar Collateral Ligament Reconstruction

Anthony A. Romeo, MD | Brandon J. Erickson, MD | Christopher S. Ahmad, MD

Baseball is the only field of endeavor where a man can succeed three times out of ten and be considered a good performer.

—Ted Williams

INTRODUCTION

The number of ulnar collateral ligament (UCL) injuries in pitchers of all levels has been increasing over the last 10 years.[12,14,17] The current gold standard of treatment for pitchers with a symptomatic, deficient UCL who have failed conservative treatment and wish to return to sport (RTS) at a high level is an ulnar collateral ligament reconstruction (UCLR).[1,13,15,29] This can be performed through a variety of techniques, using a variety of different grafts (see chapter 10).[4,6,11] The success rates after UCLR have been encouraging, with greater than 80% of patients commonly able to RTS at a high level.[4,6,9,24] Unfortunately, as the number of primary UCLR continues to rise, the number of revision UCLR will continue to rise as well.[23,32] Studies have cited the revision rate for UCLR between 3.9% and 15%.[12,32] In fact, the rate of recent increasing UCLRs in MLB is related, in part, to the dramatic number of revisions.[5,21] There were more revision UCLRs in the 3 years from 2012 to 2014 than in the prior 12 years combined. The time between the index UCLR and revision UCLR is variable, with studies reporting an average of anywhere from 3 to 5.3 years.[8,32] Our experience is that failure of the graft can occur anytime from the postoperative throwing program to after 7 years of effective postoperative pitching.

Revision surgery is also extremely concerning because the results are inferior to primary UCLR. This will be discussed later in this chapter on the Results section. Reasons for the increase in revision UCLR may be related to the number of increasing UCLRs being performed, especially in younger patients. It is also believed that many patients who, in the past, would have discontinued baseball with a failed UCLR are now more incentivized to keep playing and undergo a revision. Studies have attempted to identify modifiable risk factors in an effort to decrease the number of revision UCLR.[10,19] A shorter time from the index UCLR to RTS has been linked to an increase risk of revision UCLR (13.7 months in those requiring a revision UCLR vs 15.2 months for those who did not require a revision).[19] Initially, some thought the number of innings pitchers threw in the seasons after their index UCLR was a risk factor for sustaining a re-tear and needing a revision UCLR. However, recent evidence has shown that no significant difference exists in the likelihood of necessitating a revision UCLR between starters who pitched more than 180 innings in their first full season after UCLR and those who pitched fewer than 180.[10] Furthermore, no difference existed in revision rates between pitchers who pitched more than 150 innings in the first full season after UCLR and those who pitched fewer than 150.[10]

What has been shown to be a risk factor for necessitating a revision UCLR is an increase in pitching workload after UCLR compared with that before the injury.[19] Studies have found that pitchers requiring a revision UCLR pitched 14.1% more games (4.3 games) after compared with before their primary UCLR, whereas those who did not require a revision UCLR pitched an average of 13.6% fewer games (5.1 games) after their primary UCLR relative to their pre–primary UCLR workload.[19] Similarly, pitchers requiring revision UCLR had a reduction in total inning workload by only 9.8% after surgery versus before surgery compared with pitchers who did not require a revision UCLR who had a significantly greater reduction in average number of innings after reconstruction by 26% versus before surgery.[19] Unfortunately, younger age at the time of index UCLR (22.9 for those requiring revision UCLR vs 27.3 for those not requiring revision UCLR) has been shown to be a risk factor for requiring a revision UCLR.[19] Management of players who sustain a re-tear of their UCL after UCLR presents a variety of problems for both the player and the treating surgeon.

TRIP TO THE MOUND

What's the Deal With Inning Limits After UCLR?

Studies have shown that pitching more than an arbitrary cutoff of innings (180 and 150 innings) and pitch counts in the seasons after primary UCLR does not increase a players' risk for revision UCLR. However, what has been shown to increase their risk of UCLR is an increase in their workload (games played and innings pitched) compared with their preinjury workload. That is to say, if a pitcher was throwing 150 innings per year before their injury, having them throw 200 innings per year after surgery will increase their risk of needing a revision UCLR.

CLINICAL EVALUATION

History

Similar to patients who sustain a tear of their native UCL, pitchers who re-tear their UCL after UCLR often complain of pain at the medial elbow as well as loss of accuracy and velocity. The pain is often nagging and continues to worsen over time. Alternatively, some patients complain of a single, distinct injury when they felt a "pop" in their elbow following a specific pitch, although this can happen, especially if the patient sustained a fracture through their one of their bone tunnels. When evaluating a player with a history of a UCLR, it is imperative to obtain the operative report of the initial surgery if it was performed by another surgeon. The graft choice, surgical technique (including surgical approach: muscle split vs elevation), management of the ulnar nerve, and any concomitant elbow pathology should be noted. Furthermore, the age of

the patient at the time of the index UCLR should be recorded. This may help the surgeon understand the etiology of the failure. If a player was unable to RTS at all after his index UCLR because of persistent pain and instability of the elbow, the cause of failure could have been from an error in surgical technique. However, if the patient was able to successfully RTS at a high level and compete for some period without issue, then the cause of failure is less likely from technique and more likely from failure of the reconstructed ligament over time. We therefore categorize failures as early or late failures.

TRIP TO THE MOUND

Who Cares What the Details of Their First Surgery Are?

It is extremely important to understand what the player had done at his index UCLR, so one can properly plan for the revision UCLR. Knowing the graft choice, surgical technique (including the method of tunnel creation), position of the ulnar nerve, and other details will help the revision surgery go much smoother.

Physical Examination

Physical examination of the patient with a presumed UCL tear is discussed in chapter 10.[26] The same examination that was described in chapter 10 should be performed in the re-tear setting with some additions. The location of the previous scar should be critically evaluated. The ulnar nerve should be thoroughly assessed. If the nerve was not previously transposed, stability of the nerve should be assessed by bringing the elbow from flexion into extension while holding a finger over the medial epicondyle to feel if the ulnar nerve subluxates. If the nerve was previously transposed, the new location of the nerve should be palpated. Stability should still be assessed even if the nerve underwent prior transposition. A Tinel test, as well as an ulnar nerve compression test, should be performed at the elbow to assess the irritability of the ulnar nerve. If an autograft was used in the index UCLR, the prior harvest site incision should be evaluated. Furthermore, it is imperative to evaluate for sources of a graft should the patient and surgeon desire to use an autograft. The presence/absence of the palmaris longus tendon in both forearms should be noted, as well as prior incisions along the medial tibia indicating a hamstring harvest from the index UCLR or a prior anterior cruciate ligament reconstruction (ACLR).

Kinetic chain issues such as spine or core injuries as well as improper throwing mechanics should be ascertained. These are modifiable factors that can lead to increased stress on the graft and as such should be corrected in the revision setting.

Imaging

While the initial radiographs for patients presenting with medial elbow pain and no history of UCLR are often normal and only useful to rule out concomitant pathology, the radiographs of patients with a history of a UCLR can be much more useful. A standard 3-view series of the elbow (anteroposterior [AP], lateral, oblique) is required (Figure 11.1). A supplemental cubital tunnel view can sometimes be useful to look for posteromedial osteophytes. The radiographs should be carefully scrutinized to ensure there is no fracture through the prior tunnels and to determine the position of the prior tunnels. The surgeon should also look for any heterotopic ossification within or around the reconstructed UCL, capitellar osteochondral defects, evidence of elbow instability, and any loose bodies.[2]

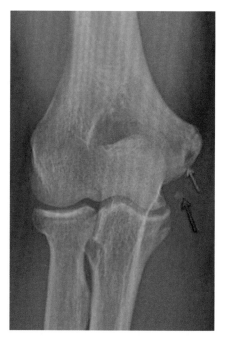

FIGURE 11.1 • Preoperative anteroposterior (AP) X-ray on a patient with a failed ulnar collateral ligament reconstruction (UCLR). The original humeral tunnel is marked by the green arrow. The original tunnel is very superficial and short, which does not allow adequate graft length to be placed into the humeral tunnel. Notice the calcification within the ligament (red arrow).

As mentioned in chapter 10, magnetic resonance imaging (MRI) and MR angiography (MRA) are very useful in evaluating the previously reconstructed UCL as well as any concomitant elbow pathology including cartilage injuries, flexor pronator injuries, and osseous stress injuries.[20,22,30] Unfortunately, evaluation of the reconstructed UCL can be difficult, and assistance by a well-trained musculoskeletal radiologist can be invaluable in determining the status of the ligament. Studies have shown that the healthy reconstructed UCL looks homogeneously low on both T1- and T2-weighted images in almost 75% of patients but can occasionally have intermediate signal on T1-weighted or intermediate to high signal on T2-weighted images. The reconstructed graft should appear thickened (compared with a native UCL) and taut. If the graft appears wavy, this indicates a tear in, or functional incompetence of the graft. Similarly, if there is diffuse intermediate signal within the graft on T1 images or hyperintensity with the graft on T2 images, this indicates damage to the reconstructed UCL (Figures 11.2 and 11.3). A fluid signal within the graft is also seen when the graft is torn.[30]

While computed tomography (CT) images are helpful in the primary setting to evaluate for posteromedial osteophytes, they are not particularly useful in

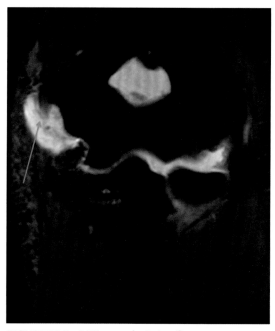

FIGURE 11.2 • MRI scan depicting flexor-pronator injury and graft failure from the medial epicondyle (blue arrow).

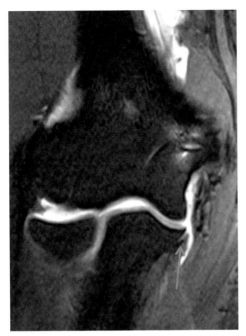

FIGURE 11.3 • MRI scan depicting graft failure from the sublime tubercle (blue arrow).

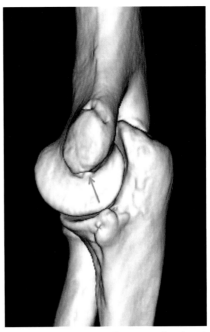

FIGURE 11.4 • CT scan revealing superficial and posterior position of the humeral tunnel (blue arrow). The inferior aspect of the humeral tunnel should be at the 7- to 8-o'clock position. The tunnel in this case is at approximately the 5-o'clock position. If the tunnel is too posterior, the graft will be tight in flexion and lose in extension, which led to failure in this case.

evaluating the native UCL. However, in the setting of a previously reconstructed UCL, a CT scan can add a significant amount of information. The CT scan can provide the exact location of the prior ulnar and humeral tunnels as well as the bone quality of these tunnels (Figure 11.4). The tunnels can be assessed for widening, fracture, and malposition.[3,28]

The status of these tunnels can have significant implications on the surgical technique used for the revision UCLR. The tunnels on the ulnar side should ideally be located 2 to 4 mm distal to the joint line and equidistant on both sides of the sublime tubercle. Sublime tubercle morphology can change owing to enthesophyte formation and often is more hypertrophic posteriorly. The medial ulnar ridge can serve as a guide to the proper location of the sublime tubercle (Figure 11.5). The inferior position of the humeral tunnel should start at least 5 mm anterior to the 6-o'clock position of the medial epicondyle. In the coronal view, the tunnel should start lateral to the midline of the medial epicondyle. Malpositioned tunnels result in a nonisometric graft. For example, if the tunnels are placed too far posterior, which is a common error, this will result in a tight graft in flexion. As a result, either elbow flexion will be limited or, if flexion is obtained, the graft subsequently becomes loose. A graft that is placed too superficial on the epicondyle will result in a small length of the epicondyle and will be less isometric.

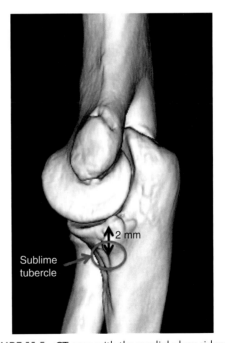

FIGURE 11.5 • CT scan with the medial ulnar ridge outlined and the proper position of the sublime tubercle indicated. Notice the hypertrophic bone posteriorly, which needs to be taken into consideration when planning the ulnar tunnel.

TREATMENT

Nonoperative

As with a tear of the native UCL, an injury to the reconstructed UCL can be managed initially in a nonoperative manner. Nonoperative treatment includes rest, rehabilitation, electrical stimulation, ultrasound, and other modalities used by therapists. Use of biologics such as platelet-rich plasma (PRP) has shown positive results in the setting of primary UCL tears, but there is no evidence on the efficacy of PRP injections for treatment of UCL re-tears.[7,25] While limited data exist on the success of nonoperative management of primary UCL tears, there are currently no studies that have looked at the effectiveness of nonoperative management in the setting of a tear of the reconstructed UCL.[16,27]

Operative

Operative management of a failed UCLR presents an extremely difficult task for the treating orthopedic surgeon that should not be taken lightly. The surgeon must determine the cause of failure of the index UCLR to correct this issue (if it is correctable) during the second surgery. The causes of failure after primary UCLR can be broken down into technical errors, patient factors, rehabilitation problems, or failure of the graft. Surgical technique errors include poor tunnel placement, improper tensioning of the graft, and poor graft fixation. If the medial epicondyle socket is not placed at the isometric point, it will cause the graft to load unevenly and can lead to increased stress seen by the graft and ultimate failure. Similarly, if the ulnar tunnel is not parallel to the joint surface, or is too proximal or too distal, it may lead to failure of the graft. If less than a 1-cm bone bridge is left for the ulnar tunnel, or if the medial epicondyle socket is too far medial, these bone bridges can break and cause catastrophic failure. Depending on the surgical technique used, if the graft is not properly secured, it runs the risk of loosening over time. There are patient factors that can lead to failure of graft incorporation and ultimately failure of the primary UCLR such as steroid use, smoking, and failure to comply with rehabilitation protocols. Likewise, if the patient does not participate in therapy, or if the therapy being given is not tailored to the specific patient, the pitcher may never optimize his throwing mechanics and can continue to improperly stress his UCL. Failure to achieve full shoulder and elbow range of motion (ROM) can put the pitcher at increased risk for a recurrent UCL tear.[31] Finally,

there is the chance that the ligament will degenerate and wear out over time. Studies have shown that pitchers who have their index UCLR at earlier ages are more likely to require a revision UCLR.[19] This is likely because the number of pitches the reconstructed UCL sees in a younger patient is higher than that in a pitcher at the end of his career.

Once the cause of the failure is determined, the surgical variables for the revision UCLR need to be determined. These variables include graft choice, management of the ulnar nerve, contaminant elbow arthroscopy, and surgical technique. As in primary UCLR, there are several graft choices available in the revision setting. If the index procedure was performed with an ipsilateral palmaris longus autograft, the surgeon may choose to use the contralateral palmaris (if the patient has one), hamstring autograft, or allograft. No studies to date have compared the results of graft choice in the revision setting and so one graft cannot definitively be recommended over another. If the patient has preoperative ulnar nerve symptoms as previously discussed, the ulnar nerve should be subcutaneously transposed. However, if the patient had a previous ulnar nerve transposition, the nerve should be identified intraoperatively, isolated, protected, and retransposed at the end of the procedure. Great care should be taken when isolating the nerve, as this is often encased in scar tissue and can be easily injured. The decision of whether to perform a concomitant elbow arthroscopy was discussed in chapter 10. Briefly, if the patient has concomitant intra-articular elbow pathology that should be addressed at the time of the revision UCLR, an elbow arthroscopy should be performed. Otherwise, the decision of whether to perform a concomitant elbow arthroscopy can be at the discretion of the treating surgeon.

One of the most difficult decisions in preoperatively planning for a revision UCLR is to decide on the proper surgical technique. While every described surgical technique can be used in the primary UCLR setting, revision UCLR is much more complicated. If the patient had a fracture through their ulnar tunnel, or has significant widening on the ulnar or humeral tunnel, the standard docking technique may not be effective. Modifications to the technique may need to be made to properly secure the graft. One option is to perform the double docking technique in which the graft is docked on both the humerus and ulna.[9] This technique avoids the need for an ulnar tunnel in the setting of tunnel widening or fracture through the tunnel by docking the graft into a socket on the ulna and tying the sutures over a bone bridge.

Authors' Preferred Surgical Technique

Late Failure

If the patient had a well-functioning UCLR (late failure) and physical examination and imaging studies indicate simple attenuation and failure of the graft without technical surgical error, UCLR is carried out similar to a primary UCLR. The previously existing tunnels are re-created and the graft choice is most often a gracilis tendon autograft.

Early Failure

Sources of early failure include failure of graft incorporation, overaccelerated rehabilitation, and surgical technical error. If the patient has a collagen disorder, the examiner may elect an allograft for his UCLR. If the tunnels are malpositioned, then the tunnels should be modified to a more accurate position. This usually involves either ignoring a previously used malpositioned tunnel if it is far from the normal position or creating the tunnel at a more precise location with partial overlap with the previous tunnel if it is close to its normal position. A large gracilis tendon graft is commonly used.

Preoperative Planning

- Physical examination, X-rays, MRI, and CT are evaluated specifically for location of the ulnar nerve, status of the flexor pronator mass, and tunnel position
- If the tunnels are malpositioned, then tunnels should be accurately planned relative to the prior tunnels

Equipment Needed

- Standard UCLR equipment (see chapter 10)
- Cortical buttons
- Gracilis tendon graft harvest equipment (including tendon stripper)
- Intraoperative fluoroscopy

Step-by-Step Surgical Technique

- Patient set up is the same as for primary UCL reconstruction
- The prior incision should be used. This may be extended proximally and distally
- If the ulnar nerve has been previously transposed, a meticulous dissection of the ulnar nerve is carried out. Often the ulnar nerve is best identified proximally where there is less scar tissue (Figure 11.6)
- A split in the flexor carpi ulnaris (FCU) fascia is created, and the prior ligament graft is identified. The graft often has to be debulked (Figure 11.7)

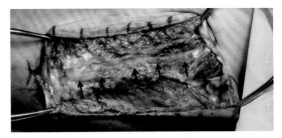

FIGURE 11.6 • Image of a previous ulnar nerve transposition. The black arrows indicate the course of the ulnar nerve.

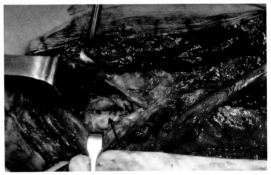

FIGURE 11.7 • Intraoperative photo of graft failure. The black arrow indicates the failed graft.

- Ulnar tunnels
- The medial ulnar ridge on the ulna is used to help identify the proper location of the sublime tubercle. Small curettes are used to identify the prior tunnel on the ulna, both anterior and posterior to the sublime tubercle. If the tunnel position and bone quality allow for an adequate bone bridge (approximately 5-10 mm) and distance from the joint line (approximately 2-4 mm), a 3.5-mm drill is used to re-create converging bone tunnels. These are connected with curettes and are chamfered similar to a primary UCLR
- If the prior tunnels do not allow for traditional converging bone tunnels, a single point of fixation is chosen. A pin is placed at the sublime tubercle to allow for at least a 4-mm or up to a 5.5-mm reamer to create a unicortical socket to accommodate the size of the graft. There should be adequate bone bridge from the joint line of at least 2 mm and depth of 15 mm. The far cortex of the ulna is penetrated with small pin to allow cortical button to pass and flip (see Figures 11.8A-C and 11.9). Fluoroscopy is used to make sure proximal radioulnar joint is not violated
- Humeral tunnel creation

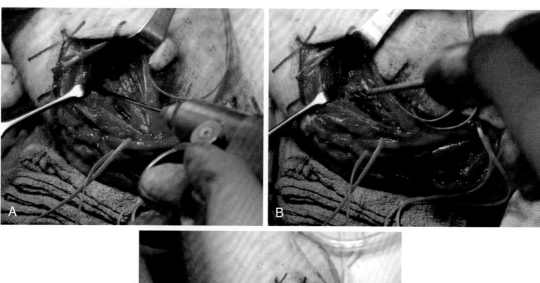

FIGURE 11.8 • A-C, Single ulnar tunnel socket creation. A pin is used to drill into the ulna at the level of the sublime tubercle (A). The pin is overdrilled using a reamer (B). A pin to shuttle the cortical button is then placed though the previously drilled socket (C).

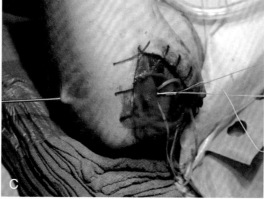

FIGURE 11.9 • Graft prepared with cortical button for ulnar fixation.

- If the humeral socket and smaller drill tunnels are an appropriate size and in an anatomic location, the humeral socket and small tunnels are re-created similar to those in a primary reconstruction
- If the humeral tunnel at its inferior location is slightly incorrect, a guide pain is placed at the ideal anatomic location of the humeral tunnel. The pin will most likely pass through the old tunnel but will not be in the center of this tunnel. The guide pin is then overreamed with a 4.5-mm reamer

- Superior exit tunnels to allow for docking of the graft are then created as in a primary UCLR
- If the humeral tunnel is located at a poor position such as too medial or posterior, a new tunnel can be created completely independent of the previous tunnel. A 4.5-mm drill creates a more isometric and anatomic anterior and lateral starting point. In this setting, a single, superior exit tunnel is created using a 2-mm drill to avoid further compromise to the structural integrity to the epicondyle that could result in fracture. Fixation in this situation will be achieved with a cortical button

Graft Passing

- The graft is passed as in primary UCLR if a traditional ulnar tunnel has been created. If a single-point fixation with cortical button is chosen, the cortical button is passed through the far ulnar cortex, and fluoroscopy is used to visualize whether the cortical button has flipped and is in good position. The graft is tensioned into the ulnar tunnel

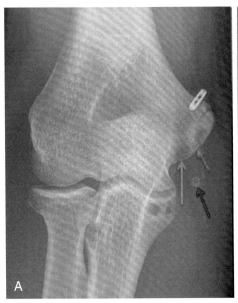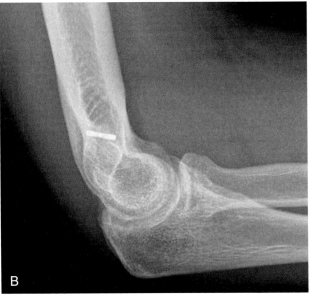

FIGURE 11.10 • A and B, Anteroposterior (A) and lateral (B) X-rays depicting cortical button fixation on the medial epicondyle. The new humeral tunnel is shown with the blue arrow. The prior humeral tunnel is seen with the green arrow. Notice the new tunnel is significantly longer than the original tunnel. The preoperative calcification within the ligament is still seen (red arrow), as the removal of this calcification would have necessitated.

- The graft length is then estimated for humeral tunnel fixation. If standard humeral exit tunnels were created, then the graft is managed as for a primary UCLR docking technique (see chapter 10)
- If humeral cortical button fixation is required, the graft limb lengths are estimated and sutured with number 1 nonabsorbable suture. The sutures are passed through the single superior epicondyle tunnel. The sutures are then passed through a cortical button and tied over the cortical button with elbow flexion, forearm supination, and a varus stress
- Elbow motion is ascertained, as well as graft isometry
- The prior graft can be sutured into the new reconstruction with simple 0 nonabsorbable sutures
- The fascia is closed with 2-0 absorbable suture
- The ulnar nerve is transposed subcutaneously if necessary
- A soft dressing is applied followed by a posterior mold splint that extends past the wrist to ensure complete immobilization. Alternatively, a soft dressing and hinged elbow brace can be applied
- Postoperative radiographs are obtained at the first office visit (Figure 11.10A and B)

Postsurgical Rehabilitation

Rehabilitation after revision UCLR is similar to that after primary UCLR (described in chapter 10),

although the phases are typically extended by 4 to 6 weeks depending on how the athlete is progressing. Timing of RTS after revision UCLR is typically longer than that after primary UCLR and can often be as long as 12 to 20 months, with some patients taking even longer to reach their preoperative level of competition. Recent studies have found the average time from revision UCLR to RTS in Major League Baseball (MLB) pitchers to be 20.76 months.[21] To an even bigger extent than after a primary UCLR, special attention must be paid to teaching the pitcher proper pitching mechanics to prevent excess stress on the graft. Similarly, ensuring the pitcher regains strength of both the upper extremities and core is paramount, as is avoiding pitching while the pitcher is fatigued. A slower throwing progression program is also advocated. Further details about rehabilitation can be found in chapter 12.

RESULTS

Unfortunately, the results after revision UCLR are inferior to those after primary UCLR. Studies have found that between 33% and 78% of pitchers after revision UCLR were able to RTS at their previous level within 2 years of their revision surgery but that an even lower percentage (29%) were able to continue to pitch more than 2 seasons after they returned.[8,18,21,23] Furthermore, pitchers who are able to RTS at the same level often cannot handle the same workload as before the revision UCLR.[18] Some studies have found that relief pitchers were able to resume only 50% of their preinjury workload whereas starting pitchers only achieved 35% of their preinjury workload.[18] In pitchers who are able to RTS, studies have found mixed results regarding their performance on RTS. Studies have reported a decline in the number of innings pitched and wins after revision UCLR, but there is no significant decline in performance in regard to earned run average (ERA) or WHIP ([walks + hits]/innings pitched).[23]

TRIP TO THE MOUND

Bottom of the Ninth

Results after revision UCLR are inferior to those of primary UCLR. There is a lower rate of RTS and a decreased chance the pitcher will be able to compete at the same level for several seasons. Furthermore, certain performance variables may decline after revision UCLR.

One confounding factor when discussing results after revision UCLR is the number of concomitant surgeries these patients have. While most primary UCLRs are performed in isolation, revision UCLRs can have several other procedures performed on the elbow at the same time, thereby complicating the rehabilitation process and affecting the results. Some studies have found that more than 45% of pitchers undergoing revision UCLR had concomitant procedures including revision ulnar nerve transposition, flexor pronator repair, posteromedial osteophyte excision, and medial antebrachial cutaneous nerve transposition.[8]

COMPLICATIONS

Just as the clinical results after revision UCLRs are inferior to primary UCLRs, the complication rates after revision UCLR are higher than that after primary UCLR.[6,8] Some studies have reported the complication rate as high as 40%.[8] These complications include re-tear, postoperative stiffness (sometimes requiring surgical release), reactive synovitis, graft harvest site problems, medial epicondylitis, and transient ulnar neuritis.[8]

MANAGER'S TIPS

- As the number of primary UCLR continues to increase, the number of revision UCLR will increase as well
- While a CT scan in the primary setting is oftentimes not necessary, a CT scan in the revision setting is crucial to assess tunnel placement, fracture, widening, etc
- Unlike a primary UCLR where many surgical techniques are at the surgeon's disposal, the surgical technique used in the revision setting may be dictated by prior tunnel placement, status of the ulnar nerve, etc
- The results after revision UCLR are inferior to those after primary UCLR
- The complication rates after revision UCLR are higher than those after primary UCLR

REFERENCES

1. Anakwenze OA, Iyengar JJ, Ahmad CS. Treatment of medial collateral ligament injuries of the elbow with use of the "Tommy John" operation: indications and results. *JBJS Rev.* 2014;2(6).

2. Andrachuk JS, Scillia AJ, Aune KT, Andrews JR, Dugas JR, Cain EL. Symptomatic heterotopic ossification after ulnar collateral ligament reconstruction: clinical significance and treatment outcome. *Am J Sports Med.* 2016;44(5):1324-1328.

3. Byram IR, Khanna K, Gardner TR, Ahmad CS. Characterizing bone tunnel placement in medial ulnar collateral ligament reconstruction using patient-specific 3-dimensional computed tomography modeling. *Am J Sports Med.* 2013;41(4):894-902.

4. Cain EL Jr, Andrews JR, Dugas JR, et al. Outcome of ulnar collateral ligament reconstruction of the elbow in 1281 athletes: results in 743 athletes with minimum 2-year follow-up. *Am J Sports Med.* 2010;38(12):2426-2434.

5. Conte SA, Fleisig GS, Dines JS, et al. Prevalence of ulnar collateral ligament surgery in professional baseball players. *Am J Sports Med.* 2015;43(7):1764-1769.

6. Dines JS, ElAttrache NS, Conway JE, Smith W, Ahmad CS. Clinical outcomes of the DANE TJ technique to treat ulnar collateral ligament insufficiency of the elbow. *Am J Sports Med.* 2007;35(12):2039-2044.

7. Dines JS, Williams PN, ElAttrache N, et al. Platelet-rich plasma can be used to successfully treat elbow ulnar collateral ligament insufficiency in high-level throwers. *Am J Orthop (Belle Mead NJ).* 2016;45(5):296-300.

8. Dines JS, Yocum LA, Frank JB, ElAttrache NS, Gambardella RA, Jobe FW. Revision surgery for failed elbow medial collateral ligament reconstruction. *Am J Sports Med.* 2008;36(6):1061-1065.

9. Erickson BJ, Bach BR Jr, Cohen MS, et al. Ulnar collateral ligament reconstruction: the rush experience. *Orthop J Sports Med.* 2016;4(1):2325967115626876.

10. Erickson BJ, Cvetanovich GL, Bach BR Jr, Bush-Joseph CA, Verma NN, Romeo AA. Should we limit innings pitched after ulnar collateral ligament reconstruction in major league baseball pitchers? *Am J Sports Med.* 2016;44(9):2210-2213.

11. Erickson BJ, Cvetanovich GL, Frank RM, et al. Do clinical results and return-to-sport rates after ulnar collateral ligament reconstruction differ based on graft choice and surgical technique? *Orthop J Sports Med.* 2016;4(11):2325967116670142.

12. Erickson BJ, Gupta AK, Harris JD, et al. Rate of return to pitching and performance after Tommy John surgery in Major League Baseball pitchers. *Am J Sports Med.* 2014;42(3):536-543.

13. Erickson BJ, Harris JD, Chalmers PN, et al. Ulnar collateral ligament reconstruction: anatomy, indications, techniques, and outcomes. *Sports Health.* 2015;7(6):511-517.

14. Erickson BJ, Nwachukwu BU, Rosas S, et al. Trends in medial ulnar collateral ligament reconstruction in the United States: a retrospective review of a large private-payer database from 2007 to 2011. *Am J Sports Med.* 2015;43(7):1770-1774.

15. Erickson BJ, Romeo AA. The ulnar collateral ligament injury: evaluation and treatment. *J Bone Joint Surg Am.* 2017;99(1):76-86.

16. Ford GM, Genuario J, Kinkartz J, Githens T, Noonan T. Return-to-play outcomes in professional baseball players after medial ulnar collateral ligament injuries: comparison of operative versus nonoperative treatment based on magnetic resonance imaging findings. *Am J Sports Med.* 2016;44(3):723-728.

17. Hodgins JL, Vitale M, Arons RR, Ahmad CS. Epidemiology of medial ulnar collateral ligament reconstruction: a 10-year study of New York state. *Am J Sports Med.* 2016;44(3):729-734.

18. Jones KJ, Conte S, Patterson N, ElAttrache NS, Dines JS. Functional outcomes following revision ulnar collateral ligament reconstruction in major league baseball pitchers. *J Shoulder Elbow Surg.* 2013;22(5):642-646.

19. Keller RA, Mehran N, Khalil LS, Ahmad CS, ElAttrache N. Relative individual workload changes may be a risk factor for rerupture of ulnar collateral ligament reconstruction. *J Shoulder Elbow Surg.* 2017;26(3):369-375.

20. Kim NR, Moon SG, Ko SM, Moon WJ, Choi JW, Park JY. MR imaging of ulnar collateral ligament injury in baseball players: value for predicting rehabilitation outcome. *Eur J Radiol.* 2011;80(3):e422-e426.

21. Liu JN, Garcia GH, Conte S, ElAttrache N, Altchek DW, Dines JS. Outcomes in revision Tommy John surgery in major league baseball pitchers. *J Shoulder Elbow Surg.* 2016;25(1):90-97.

22. Magee T. Accuracy of 3-T MR arthrography versus conventional 3-T MRI of elbow tendons and ligaments compared with surgery. *AJR Am J Roentgenol.* 2015;204(1):W70-W75.

23. Marshall NE, Keller RA, Lynch JR, Bey MJ, Moutzouros V. Pitching performance and longevity after revision ulnar collateral ligament reconstruction in major league baseball pitchers. *Am J Sports Med.* 2015;43(5):1051-1056.

24. O'Brien DF, O'Hagan T, Stewart R, et al. Outcomes for ulnar collateral ligament reconstruction: a retrospective review using the KJOC assessment score with two-year follow-up in an overhead throwing population. *J Shoulder Elbow Surg.* 2015;24(6):934-940.

25. Podesta L, Crow SA, Volkmer D, Bert T, Yocum LA. Treatment of partial ulnar collateral ligament tears in the elbow with platelet-rich plasma. *Am J Sports Med.* 2013;41(7):1689-1694.

26. Redler LH, Watling JP, Ahmad CS. Physical examination of the throwing athlete's elbow. *Am J Orthop (Belle Mead NJ).* 2015;44(1):13-18.

27. Rettig AC, Sherrill C, Snead DS, Mendler JC, Mieling P. Nonoperative treatment of ulnar collateral ligament injuries in throwing athletes. *Am J Sports Med.* 2001;29(1):15-17.

28. Timmerman LA, Schwartz ML, Andrews JR. Preoperative evaluation of the ulnar collateral ligament by magnetic resonance imaging and computed tomography arthrography. Evaluation in 25 baseball players with surgical confirmation. *Am J Sports Med.* 1994;22(1):26-31 [discussion 32].

29. Vitale MA, Ahmad CS. The outcome of elbow ulnar collateral ligament reconstruction in overhead athletes: a systematic review. *Am J Sports Med.* 2008;36(6):1193-1205.

30. Wear SA, Thornton DD, Schwartz ML, Weissmann RC III, Cain EL, Andrews JR. MRI of the reconstructed ulnar collateral ligament. *AJR Am J Roentgenol.* 2011;197(5):1198-1204.

31. Wilk KE, Macrina LC, Fleisig GS, et al. Deficits in glenohumeral passive range of motion increase risk of elbow injury in professional baseball pitchers: a prospective study. *Am J Sports Med.* 2014;42(9):2075-2081.

32. Wilson AT, Pidgeon TS, Morrell NT, DaSilva MF. Trends in revision elbow ulnar collateral ligament reconstruction in professional baseball pitchers. *J Hand Surg Am.* 2015;40(11):2249-2254.

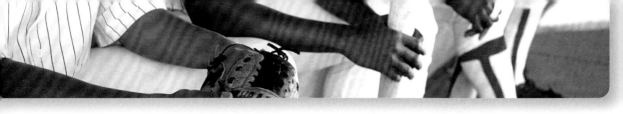

CHAPTER **12**

Neurovascular Compression Injuries in Baseball Players

Samuel E. Galle, MD | David P. Trofa, MD | Christopher S. Ahmad, MD | Melvin P. Rosenwasser, MD

It's like deja-vu, all over again.

—*Yogi Berra*

INTRODUCTION

Throwing athletes experience significant biomechanical stresses on the bone and soft tissues of the elbow. These repetitive stresses place throwers at risk for elbow peripheral nerve injuries.[1] Nerve injury typically follows a course of local edema, progressive ischemia, and eventually neural conduction changes. Of the 3 major nerves traversing the elbow joint, the ulnar nerve is most commonly injured given its medial position where tension is greatest during the throwing motion; however, median and radial nerve pathology have been reported as well. In general, initial treatment consists of nonoperative treatment, and if nonoperative treatment fails, surgery may be necessary. In this chapter, we will review the pathoanatomy, clinical manifestations, and management of ulnar neuropathy in throwers in detail and also briefly review radial and median neuropathies.

ULNAR NERVE

Pathoanatomy

In treating patients and athletes with ulnar neuritis, a sound understanding of the nerve's function and its anatomic course through the upper extremity is necessary. Functionally, the ulnar nerve provides motor innervation to the flexor digitorum profundus (FDP) of the ring and small finger, the hypothenar musculature, the ulnar 2 lumbricals, and the adductor pollicis. It also provides sensation to the ulnar forearm, palm, small finger, and ulnar half of the ring finger.

The ulnar nerve is a terminal branch of the medial cord of the brachial plexus and receives contributions from the C8 and T1 spine roots. It is helpful to divide the ulnar nerve's course through the arm and into the forearm into 3 zones (Figure 12.1).[2] Zone 1 includes the course of the nerve on entering the anterior compartment of the arm through the medial intermuscular septum. From there, it travels through the arcade of Struthers approximately 8 cm above the medial epicondyle. The arcade of Struthers is comprised of the medial intermuscular septum, the interbrachial ligament attachment, the deep investing fascia of the distal arm, and the superficial fibers of the medial head of the triceps. In Zone 2 the nerve rests posterior to the medial epicondyle and consistently gives off a sensory branch to the joint capsule of the elbow. This area is termed the cubital tunnel and is bounded by the medial trochlea, the medial epicondylar groove, the posterior portion of the ulnar collateral ligament (UCL), and Osborne ligament that connects the medial epicondyle to the medial border of the olecranon. After exiting the cubital tunnel, the ulnar nerve enters Zone 3 where it passes between the humeral and ulnar heads of the flexor carpi ulnaris (FCU).

Neuropathy of the ulnar nerve is the most common nerve injury about the elbow in the general population and in throwers.[3,4] The mechanism of irritation may be a result of compression, traction, friction, or any combination of the 3 about the medial elbow. Regarding compressive etiologies, various points of constriction along the course of the ulnar nerve have been identified. In Zone 1 these include the medial intermuscular septum, the arcade of Struthers, and the interbrachial ligament. In Zone 2 these include the anatomic boundaries of the cubital tunnel such as Osborne ligament and the UCL. And finally, in Zone 3 these include

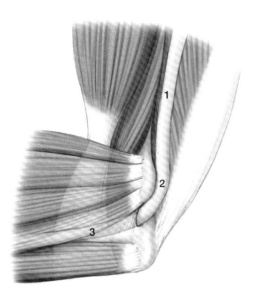

FIGURE 12.1 • The boundaries of the 3 anatomic zones of the ulnar nerve.

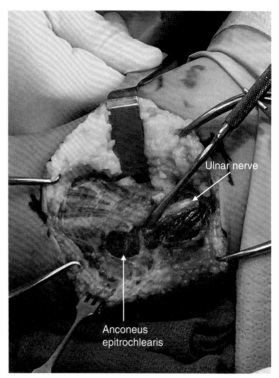

FIGURE 12.2 • The ulnar nerve, as it curves under the medial epicondyle, is compressed by an overlying muscle belly of the anconeus epitrochlearis.

the aponeurosis of the FCU as well as the deep flexor pronator retinaculum. Throwers may have additional points of compression, however, owing to hypertrophied muscles of the medial head of the triceps (Zone 1) or the FCU (Zone 3) that may also cause pathology. Finally, anatomic variants may also be culprits of compression. For instance, the anconeus epitrochlearis is a congenital accessory muscle that covers the posterior aspect of the cubital tunnel between the medial epicondyle and the olecranon that can also cause ulnar compression in Zone 2 and possibly Zone 1 if large enough (Figures 12.2 and 12.3).[5-7] These potential sites of compression, if present, may seriously compromise the ulnar nerve in throwers because, as with all nerves, free gliding is necessary for normal function.[8] However, this is even more significant in overhead athletes, as the ulnar nerve elongates an average of 4.7 mm during normal elbow range of motion and up to 12.4 mm during the windup phase of throwing.[10,11] This amount of gliding and elongation is not possible without pathology if the nerve is constricted.

In addition to compression, the ulnar nerve can also be compromised by traction-related injury. The late cocking and early acceleration phases of throwing impart significant valgus stresses of up to 60 to 65 Nm on all of the medial structures of the elbow including the ulnar nerve and UCL.[12,13] Not only may throwers develop ulnar neuritis from the repetitive microtrauma of the tension sustained during throwing, but also UCL insufficiency with valgus laxity can further increase the tensile forces on the nerve with throwing.

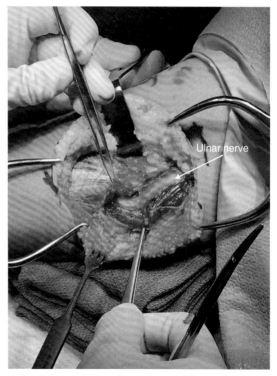

FIGURE 12.3 • A complete release of the anconeus epitrochlearis reveals the decompressed ulnar nerve.

Similarly, ulnar nerve symptoms are associated with other pathologies frequently seen in throwers, such as subluxation of the ulnar nerve.[14,15] Ulnar neuritis has also been identified in 40% of players with valgus extension overload syndrome and in 60% of those with medial epicondylitis.[16,17] Baseball players are also prone to adhesions, calcium deposits, synovitis, and osteophytes all of which may result in friction or compression injury to the nerve.[4,6]

Clinical Evaluation

History

It is imperative to perform an in-depth history for any thrower with ulnar neuropathy. As throwing athletes may have a history of prior surgery, it is important to know the exact details of any prior intervention, particularly if an ulnar nerve transposition was performed. Clinical complaints of athletes with ulnar neuritis may include pain along the medial joint line that is provoked or exacerbated by overhead activities.[4] Associated paresthesias are found in the ulnar 2 digits with activity at first and may progress to include periods of rest. In the setting of a subluxating ulnar nerve, athletes may complain of a painful "snapping" or "popping" sensation during elbow flexion and extension. Clumsiness due to motor weakness of the hand intrinsics and extrinsic forearm musculature are late findings and generally not common in the initial presentation.[1]

Physical Examination

A comprehensive elbow examination is necessary for any athlete presenting with ulnar nerve symptoms.[18] This includes examination for any cervical radiculopathy, brachial plexopathy, or other neurologic pathology. Clinical evaluation may also reveal muscle hypertrophy, elbow flexion contracture, and/or valgus instability. A number of special tests have been described to assess for ulnar nerve symptoms. For example, testing for nerve irritation may reveal tenderness to palpation of the nerve about the cubital tunnel as well as a positive Tinel sign when the nerve is tapped along the cubital tunnel. The elbow flexion test can be performed by holding the elbow in maximum flexion for 1 minute and is considered positive if paresthesias are elicited in the ulnar 2 digits. Ulnar nerve subluxation should also be assessed, as hypermobility has been identified in 37% of elbows.[19] Hypermobility may be assessed by having the patient actively flex the elbow with the forearm in supination. While the examiner places a finger on the posteromedial aspect of the medial epicondyle, the patient actively extends the elbow. A nerve dislocation is noted when the nerve is trapped anterior to the examiner's finger as the elbow is moved from flexion to extension.[19] Late

symptoms resulting from chronic ulnar neuropathy include resting numbness in the ulnar digits, clawing of the ulnar digits, Wartenberg sign (inability to adduct the small finger), Froment sign (using the flexor pollicis longus to supplement weakness in the thumb adductor during pinch), and intrinsic muscle atrophy.

Imaging and Nerve Conduction Studies

Standard anteroposterior (AP), lateral, and cubital tunnel radiographs are obtained to evaluate for bony and static ligamentous pathology. Bony pathology includes osteophytes, loose bodies, malunions, and fractures. Instability of the UCL complex may present on plain radiographs as 3 mm of medial ulno-humeral joint line widening with or without applied valgus stress.[20] The cubital tunnel view may reveal bony encroachment in the form of osteophytes. In the setting of nerve injury, magnetic resonance imaging (MRI) presents an opportunity to evaluate the internal/external nerve architecture and the presence of denervated musculature.[21] It can further delineate the exact etiology of the patient's symptoms by ruling out common associated pathologies presenting as medial elbow pain, for example, UCL tears. However, advanced imaging is not always necessary.

Electromyography (EMG) and nerve conduction studies (NCS) are considered standard for neurologic evaluation of the upper extremity; however, they are not a prerequisite for the diagnosis of ulnar neuritis.[4] Generally they are helpful to identify sites of compression when cervical pathology is also suspected. Unfortunately, EMG has not been found to be predictive of nerve recovery potential, but nerve conduction tests can monitor nerve recovery when compared with preoperative values.[22,23] There is some basis for EMG being able to delineate healthy pitchers from injured ones; however, it was unable to demonstrate a difference between injured pitchers and healthy nonpitchers, confounding its usefulness and role as a diagnostic examination.[24] Abnormal results include a nerve conduction velocity across the elbow of less than 49 m/second or greater than 10 m/second difference from the contralateral extremity.[25]

Treatment

Nonoperative

Conservative management options include rest, cryotherapy, activity modification, oral nonsteroidal anti-inflammatory drugs (NSAIDS), and a guided rehabilitation program focused on optimizing throwing mechanics.[3,26] Night splinting in slight flexion has been shown in conjunction with activity modification to have a positive effect on ulnar neuritis symptoms.[27] The athlete is allowed to return to sport with symptom resolution and rehabilitation program completion. It should be noted that in the setting of valgus instability, athletes are often found to have recurrence of ulnar neuritis symptoms with resumption of throwing if treatment does not address the underlying instability.

Operative

Surgical intervention is considered in the setting of failed conservative management, persistent or worsening symptoms, nerve subluxation, and persistent ongoing abnormalities as demonstrated on EMG. Decompression of the ulnar nerve at the cubital tunnel has been described via a medial epicondylectomy, in situ decompression, and subcutaneous/submuscular/adipose flap transposition. It is the opinion of the authors that medial epicondylectomy is contraindicated in throwers, given the potential to damage the origin of the UCL and cause weakness of the flexor muscles.[28] With regard to in situ decompression, the technique has been shown to be less effective than ulnar nerve transposition and may be associated with nerve instability (see Trip to the Mound #1).[29] The author's preferred technique involves anterior transposition of the ulnar nerve using a locally derived adipofascial flap, which is described in detail below. Of note, valgus instability must be thoroughly evaluated, as surgical techniques to address ulnar nerve pathology will not preserve nerve function nor restore athletic performance without appropriate intervention to address the underlying instability.[30] Furthermore, as ulnar neuritis is a known complication of UCL reconstruction, the appropriate management of the ulnar nerve in the setting of UCL instability continues to be a debated topic (see Trip to the Mound #2).

TRIP TO THE MOUND

In Situ Decompression Versus Transposition

Ulnar neuropathy literature remains controversial regarding the optimal surgical technique in the general patient population. Some authors recommend simple decompression of the ulnar nerve, as this preserves the vascular supply and avoids any iatrogenic traction injury to the nerve itself.[31] Additionally, 1 large meta-analysis failed to find a statistical difference between the 2 techniques with regard to relief of symptoms.[32] In contrast, however, this has not been the experience of the senior author with the professional baseball player population. Experience has shown that an in situ ulnar nerve decompression does not address the significant tractional forces from repetitive throwing that are sustained on the medial aspect of the elbow in the professional athlete. In addition, the violent repetitive force places throwing athletes at risk for ulnar nerve instability following decompression. The adipofascial sling with anterior ulnar nerve transposition is the author's preferred surgical technique, as it protects the nerve with local adipose tissue, avoids complications related to mobilization of the flexor origin, and prevents posterior subluxation while minimizing recurrence risks.[33] Contraindications to surgery are limited to those athletes with insufficient subcutaneous adipose tissue.

TRIP TO THE MOUND

Ulnar Nerve Management in the Setting of UCL Instability

Management of the ulnar nerve in the setting of a UCL instability has been a significant discussion point with surgeons ever since Dr Frank Jobe described his original UCL reconstructive technique involving detachment of the flexor pronator mass and an obligatory submuscular transposition.[34-36] However, many authors now recommend against obligatory transposition of the asymptomatic ulnar nerve during UCL reconstruction to avoid postoperative neuritis. In a recent systematic review, Vitale et al found a 12.0% prevalence of postoperative ulnar neuropathy following UCL reconstruction.[37] The authors found that detachment of the flexor pronator mass was the surgical approach associated with the highest risk of postoperative ulnar neuropathy (21.9%). Alternatively, a muscle-splitting approach resulted in a significantly smaller, 3.9%, incidence of ulnar neuropathy. In any case, 3 prior systematic reviews independently concluded that ulnar neuropathy is the most common complication associated with UCL reconstruction.[35,38,39] As such, ulnar nerve decompression and anterior transposition is recommended only for athletes with ulnar nerve symptoms before UCL reconstruction.

Authors' Preferred Surgical Technique

Preoperative Planning

Anterior transposition of the ulnar nerve with an adipofascial sling is indicated in the athlete with ulnar neuritis without significant ligamentous instability. In the setting of UCL deficiency, however, this procedure can be performed in tandem with a UCL reconstruction or repair in the appropriate clinical setting. Regional or general anesthesia is used per surgeon preference, per patient requirement, or based on required commiserate procedures. The patient may be placed supine with a hand table using a sterile tourniquet to allow for adequate proximal dissection to the arcade of Struthers.

Equipment Needed

- Hand table
- Esmarch to exsanguinate the upper extremity and sterile tourniquet preset to 250 mm Hg
- 15-blade scalpels
- Metzenbaum dissecting scissors
- Vessel loops
- Self-retaining retractors
- 3-0 monocryl and 4-0 or 5-0 nylon suture

Technique, Step by Step

- A posteromedial incision is created sharply in-line with the intermuscular septum 10 cm proximal to the medial epicondyle to 4 cm distal. Care is used to prevent injury to branches of the medial antebrachial cutaneous nerve

- Blunt dissection begins proximally to identify the ulnar nerve about the level of the arcade of Struthers just posterior to the intermuscular septum
- Dissection proceeds distally along the anterograde path of the nerve taking care to prevent iatrogenic injury. Every effort should be used to preserve the epineurial vascular mesentery
- Osborne ligament is sharply divided in-line with the ulnar nerve, and dissection proceeds to the aponeurosis of the FCU
- The ulnar nerve motor branches to the FCU are carefully preserved
- The medial intermuscular septum is excised to prevent secondary compression after ulnar nerve transposition. This usually occurs approximately 4 cm proximal to the medial epicondyle, but intraoperative evaluation is crucial to identify possible compression points and adequate resection. Examples illustrating the full exposure of the ulnar nerve can be seen in Figure 12.4A and B
- An adipose flap is sharply elevated from the anterior skin flap while preserving the underlying vascular pedicle and ensuring adequate anterior subcutaneous tissue remains (Figure 12.5)
- With the ulnar nerve anteriorly transposed, the adipofascial flap is placed deep to the ulnar nerve (Figure 12.6) and wrapped around it to create an adipose "tunnel." The flap is loosely sutured together using a 3-0 monocryl suture (Figure 12.7). Alternatively, if the patient is thin and does not have enough adipose tissue to create a complete tunnel, a smaller flap may be created and sutured to the medial epicondyle

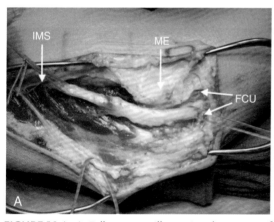
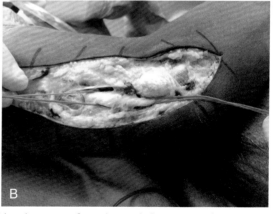

FIGURE 12.4 ● A, Full exposure illustrating the course of the ulnar nerve from the medial intermuscular septum (IMS) to the aponeurosis of the 2 heads of the flexor carpi ulnaris (FCU). The ulnar nerve is controlled with vessel loops and has not yet been transposed over the medial epicondyle (ME). B, A second demonstration of the course of the ulnar nerve. In this case, the patient was hit by a pitch and developed an ulnar nerve neuroma that required decompression and transposition.

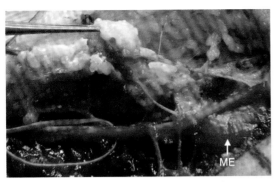

FIGURE 12.5 • An axially based adipofascial flap is raised sharply from the anterior skin flap as identified by the forceps. The ulnar nerve has been transposed over the medial epicondyle (ME).

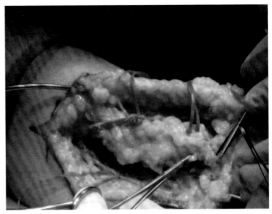

FIGURE 12.7 • The adipofascial flap is loosely sutured to itself to envelope the ulnar nerve. The ulnar nerve should be able to slide freely within the flap. This protects the nerve from further traction-related injuries.

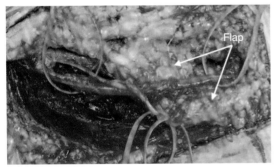

FIGURE 12.6 • The adipofascial flap is adequately released to allow circumferential enveloping of the ulnar nerve. The ulnar nerve has been anteriorly transposed and is placed superficial to the flap in preparation for final suturing of the flap about the nerve.

- Intraoperative evaluation of elbow flexion and extension should reveal gliding of the nerve within the adipofascial tunnel without evidence of kinking
- The tourniquet is released to evaluate and address appropriate hemostasis
- Closure is obtained with 4-0 or 5-0 nylon sutures in a simple, interrupted fashion. A soft dressing is applied, and the patient is placed in a sling for comfort

Postsurgical Rehabilitation

Postoperative rehabilitation must be baseball specific and can be accelerated in patients with a stable UCL complex. Elbow range of motion is initiated in the immediate postoperative setting within the confines of the soft dressing. Dressings and sutures are removed at 2 weeks postoperatively, and full, active range of motion is started. This is followed by a gradual strengthening program over the subsequent 4 weeks. At 3 months postoperatively the patient begins light throwing with the expectation of returning to full athletic activity. After an additional 3 to 4 months, the program increases both speed and endurance.

Results

Ulnar neuropathy is a common source of elbow disability in baseball players and accounts for 15% of all elbow operations among these athletes in a single surgeon series over 5 years.[16] In throwers, this is a pathology that is best treated operatively, as only 60% of patients treated conservatively have been found to return to play.[40] The author's current preferred technique has reported a 94% patient satisfaction rate among the general population.[33] In throwing athletes specifically, ulnar nerve decompression and transposition results in good functional outcomes and return to play rates.[4,41-44] For instance, results have shown that 95% of throwers are asymptomatic at an average of 19 months postoperatively and that anywhere from 83% to 100% of throwers are able to return to play.[16,40,44,45]

Complications

Complications from surgery related to ulnar nerve transposition with an adipofascial flap are similar to other documented ulnar nerve transpositions.[46] The most common is hematoma, which can be avoided with adequate hemostasis throughout the case. Iatrogenic damage to the medial brachial and antebrachial cutaneous nerves is possible, as they cross directly through the incision in many cases; however, this can be avoided by careful surgical technique.

MANAGER'S TIPS

- Ulnar nerve decompression must include release of the entire course of the ulnar nerve from the arcade of Struthers to the decussation of the 2 heads of the FCU
- The medial intermuscular septum should be excised with bipolar cautery
- Careful dissection should be exercised to avoid injury to the medial antebrachial cutaneous nerve, the ulnar nerve extrinsic vascular supply, and the adipofascial vascular pedicle
- The adipofascial tunnel should not kink the ulnar nerve and should not prevent nerve gliding during elbow flexion and extension
- In the setting of a previously transposed ulnar nerve, any future reconstruction of the ulnar collateral ligament complex should begin with proximal identification of the nerve to prevent iatrogenic injury

OTHER NEUROPATHIES

Compression of the median and radial nerve may also occur in throwers but is much less frequent than pathology of the ulnar nerve.[9] In fact, there is a paucity of literature detailing median and radial nerve injuries in baseball athletes.[47] Nevertheless, below we briefly describe the pathology, clinical presentations, pertinent examination findings, and treatment of median and radial nerve pathology, including pronator syndrome, anterior interosseous nerve (AIN) syndrome, radial tunnel syndrome, and posterior interosseous nerve (PIN) syndrome. Despite not being commonly described in the literature regarding throwing athletes, it is imperative to accurately recognize and diagnose these compression neuropathies, as they can present concomitantly with more commonly encountered pathologies such as lateral epicondylitis, extensor muscle strains, and insertional biceps tendinopathy.

Median Nerve

The median nerve is formed by the confluence of the medial and lateral cords of the brachial plexus. At the antecubital fossa, the nerve lies medial to the brachial artery and passes under the lacertus fibrosus where it enters the forearm between the 2 heads of the pronator teres. It continues into the forearm between the flexor digitorum superficialis (FDS) and the FDP. The median nerve proper provides motor innervation to the pronator teres, FDS, flexor carpi radialis (FCR), and palmaris longus. It also gives off 2 main branches

before traversing the wrist at the carpal tunnel. The first is the AIN, which normally branches off at the level of the radiohumeral joint line and is a purely motor nerve traveling in the deep volar compartment of the forearm. The AIN innervates the pronator quadratus, flexor pollicis longus (FPL), and FDP tendons to the index and middle finger. The second branch is the palmar cutaneous nerve, which provides sensory innervation to the thenar aspect of the palm.[48]

Potential compression sites of the median nerve about the elbow include the bicipital aponeurosis (aka lacertus fibrosus), the 2 heads of the pronator teres, and the FDS aponeurotic arch. Furthermore, aberrant anatomy may cause compression of the median nerve including a supracondylar process with an associated ligament of Struthers or an accessory FPL muscle belly (also known as Gantzer muscle).[9,49] In throwers specifically, the median nerve is particularly at risk for compression under the ligament of Struthers and/or a supracondylar process during the late cocking and early acceleration phases when the elbow is flexed between 90° and 120° with forearm pronation approaching 90°.[1] The nerve can also be compressed by the lacertus fibrosus during early acceleration owing to strong contractions of the biceps muscle.[50] Finally, the nerve can be subjected to compression from muscle hypertrophy in the dominant arm of throwers.

Compression of the median nerve can occur along any of the sites noted above and clinically presents as either pronator syndrome or AIN syndrome. A recent review on pronator syndrome stated that it is a rare diagnosis in the general population, which makes its incidence among throwing athletes even more difficult to discern.[48] In fact, there are no specific case reports in the literature regarding median nerve compression in throwers despite the fact that the lead author has treated a number of throwing athletes with this pathology.

Pronator syndrome usually encompasses both sensory and motor abnormalities. Patients typically complain of vague proximal volar forearm and antecubital fossa pain associated with numbness or paresthesias of the radial 3 digits and thenar eminence. The thenar eminence is supplied by the palmar cutaneous branch of the median nerve, which helps to differentiate this pathology from carpal tunnel syndrome.[49] On examination, provocative maneuvers can be performed to confirm the diagnosis and identify the anatomic location of compression. Compression under the lacertus fibrosus is assessed via resisted elbow flexion with the forearm supinated, whereas compression by the pronator teres is assessed by resisted forearm pronation with the elbow in extension. Finally, compression

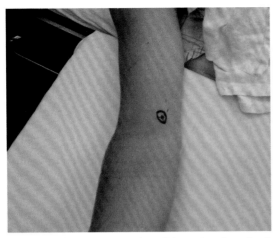

FIGURE 12.8 • Demonstration of the point of maximal tenderness, as indicated by the circle, about the antecubital fossa in a thrower who presented with pronator syndrome requiring surgical decompression.

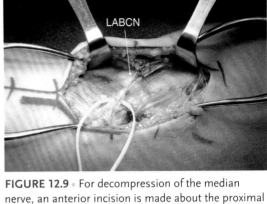

FIGURE 12.9 • For decompression of the median nerve, an anterior incision is made about the proximal aspect of the forearm. Branches of the lateral antebrachial cutaneous nerves (LABCN) are identified and protected with a vessel loop.

under the FDS aponeurotic arch can be assessed by resisted long finger proximal interphalangeal joint flexion.[49] A positive Tinel sign may reproduce a patient's symptomatology and can also localize the site of compression. Figure 12.8 provides an example of the point of maximal tenderness about the antecubital fossa in a thrower who presented with pronator syndrome requiring surgical decompression.

AIN syndrome presents with similar proximal vague forearm pain but primarily causes motor weakness of the deep volar compartment without any sensory deficits.[50] Patients will have weakness of grip and pinch and will be unable to make an "OK sign" owing to weakness of both the FPL and FDP to the index finger.

The diagnostic workup for compression of the median nerve is similar to what has been previously described for ulnar neuropathy. Generally, a thorough history and physical examination is sufficient to diagnose a nerve injury in a thrower. Nonetheless, elbow radiographs should be obtained, as a supracondylar process may be seen and suggest the presence of a ligament of Struthers.[49] Advanced imaging is generally not necessary, but MRI may show an accessory FPL muscle belly. Finally, nerve conduction studies and electromyography may be helpful for the diagnosis of AIN syndrome but is often nondiagnostic in pronator syndrome.[48,50]

There are no set treatment guidelines for pronator or AIN syndrome in throwers, specifically. In general, nonsurgical management is recommended for at least 3 months, which may take the form of rest and throwing cessation, possibly a brief period of immobilization,

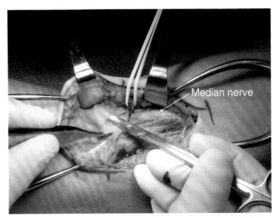

FIGURE 12.10 • The lacerates fibrosis, as identified by the metzenbaum scissor, is visualized overlying the median nerve for subsequent release.

forearm flexor muscle stretching, nerve-gliding exercises, and NSAIDS.[49,50] A supervised rehabilitation process through an interval throwing program should then be initiated. If symptoms persist beyond this time period and a thrower is unable to rehabilitate, the nerve can be explored surgically and decompressed; however, this decision should not be taken lightly by the athlete or surgeon. Decompression requires a full open exposure to release the entire nerve, which can threaten a thrower's career.[50] This is performed through a standard anterior antecubital approach that permits access to the median nerve. Focus should be placed on the surgical release of the lacertus fibrosus, fibrous bands of the pronator teres, and the aponeurosis of the FDS (Figures 12.9-12.11). In this approach, the lateral antebrachial cutaneous nerve should be identified and preserved.

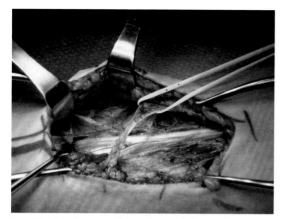

FIGURE 12.11 • Complete release of the median nerve.

Radial Nerve

Radial nerve compression occurs even less frequently than both ulnar and median nerves. The radial nerve originates from the C6, C7, and C8 nerve roots and is 1 of the 2 terminal branches of the posterior cord. This nerve courses on the posterior wall of the axilla and travels to the posterior compartment of the arm by traversing through the triangular interval with the deep brachial artery. Next, it courses around the humerus in the spiral grooves to pass from the posterior to the anterior compartment through the lateral intermuscular septum. The nerve then runs between the brachialis and brachioradialis passing the elbow anterior to lateral epicondyle. At the level of the radiohumeral joint line, the radial nerve divides into the PIN and the superficial sensory branch. The PIN provides motor innervation to the supinator and extensor muscles of the wrist and digits while the superficial sensory nerve provides sensory innervation to the dorsoradial hand.[49]

Compression of the radial nerve may occur at any of the following locations: fascial bands at the radial head, the recurrent leash of Henry, the extensor carpi radialis brevis (ECRB) edge, the arcade of Frohse (the proximal edge of the supinator), and the distal edge of the supinator muscle. Among these, compression at the arcade of Frohse is most common, especially in the setting of muscular hypertrophy.[9] In throwers specifically, injury to the radial nerve during throwing likely occurs during the deceleration and follow-through stages where there is eccentric loading at the distal elbow and forearm as well as repetitive forceful pronation-supination motions.[47,50] The muscles undergoing eccentric contractions that can contribute to radial nerve compression includes the triceps, brachialis, and lateral extensors. Furthermore, near ball release, the forearm pronates resulting in eccentric supinator

muscle contraction that may compress the PIN.[50] This is in contrast to both ulnar and medial nerve compression during throwing, both of which occur in late cocking and early acceleration.

Clinically, patients with PIN syndrome experience lateral elbow, dorsal forearm, and wrist pain associated with motor weakness of wrist, finger, and thumb extension.[50] Given these associated motor deficits, it is important to rule out extensor tendon injuries with a passive tenodesis test of the wrist. In contrast to PIN syndrome, radial tunnel syndrome is a pure pain syndrome without any associated paresthesias or motor weakness. Pain from both etiologies is most commonly over the patient's lateral forearm approximately 3 to 5 cm distal to the elbow over the supinator muscle. Palpation of the lateral forearm in supination should reproduce the patient's pain, which should remit on pronation of the forearm.[49,51] Finally, provocative maneuvers for both radial tunnel syndrome and PIN syndrome include resisted middle finger extension and forearm supination. Similar to ulnar and median nerve compression in throwers, the typical workup depends on clinician impression but may include plain radiographs, MRI, and electrodiagnostic studies. Electrodiagnostic studies often lack specific findings for radial tunnel syndrome but may help in the diagnosis of PIN syndrome.[49,50]

There is only 1 case report in the literature describing PIN compression in a baseball pitcher. Robb et al presented a case report of a 21-year-old male elite thrower who presented with acute pain, fatigue, and altered sensation of his right posterior forearm.[47] His pain was worse during the follow-through phase of throwing and was associated with altered sensation over the dorsum of the thumb and index finger. On examination, the patient exhibited pain with resisted wrist extension with the elbow extended, similar to a lateral epicondylitis examination, and pain with palpation of the supinator muscle. Despite this symptomatology, a nerve conduction analysis was within normal limits. The patient initiated nonoperative management in the form of pitching cessation, soft tissue therapy, augmented soft tissue mobilization technique, low-level laser therapy, and neural gliding. The patient returned to pitching after 3 weeks with minimal symptoms and pain-free pitching within 38 days. Unfortunately, given the paucity of other case reports, the success rate of nonoperative treatment is unknown. However, the failure of nonoperative treatment in a thrower with radial nerve compression requires a serious discussion on the risks and benefits of a decompression owing to the possible surgical morbidity associated with an extensive lateral decompression.[50]

REFERENCES

1. Cummins CA, Schneider DS. Peripheral nerve injuries in baseball players. *Phys Med Rehabil Clin N Am.* 2009;20(1):175-193.

2. Conway J. *Ulnar nerve issues in throwers.* In: *1st Annual Baseball Sports Medicine: Game-Changing Concepts.* 2016.

3. Keefe DT, Lintner DM. Nerve injuries in the throwing elbow. *Clin Sports Med.* 2004;23(4):723-742 [xi].

4. Glousman RE. Ulnar nerve problems in the athlete's elbow. *Clin Sports Med.* 1990;9(2):365-377.

5. Dahners LE, Wood FM. Anconeus epitrochlearis, a rare cause of cubital tunnel syndrome: a case report. *J Hand Surg Am.* 1984;9(4):579-580.

6. Li X, Dines JS, Gorman M, et al. Anconeus epitrochlearis as a source of medial elbow pain in baseball pitchers. *Orthopedics.* 2012;35(7):e1129-e1132.

7. Struthers J. On some points in the abnormal anatomy of the arm. *Foreign Med Chir Rev.* 1854;14:170-179.

8. Andrews JR, Whiteside JA. Common elbow problems in the athlete. *J Orthop Sports Phys Ther.* 1993;17(6):289-295.

9. Kim RY, Wolfe VM, Rosenwasser MP. Orthopaedic sports medicine principle and practice. In: DeLee JC, Drez D Jr, Miller MD, eds. *Entrapment Neuropathies Around the Elbow.* 3rd ed. Saunders, Elsevier; 2010:1311-1318.

10. Buehler MJ, Thayer DT. The elbow flexion test. A clinical test for the cubital tunnel syndrome. *Clin Orthop Relat Res.* 1988;(233):213-216.

11. Aoki M, Takasaki H, Muraki T, et al. Strain on the ulnar nerve at the elbow and wrist during throwing motion. *J Bone Joint Surg Am.* 2005;87(11):2508-2514.

12. Fleisig GS, Andrews JR, Dillman CJ, et al. Kinetics of baseball pitching with implications about injury mechanisms. *Am J Sports Med.* 1995;23(2):233-239.

13. Werner SL, Fleisig GS, Dillman CJ, et al. Biomechanics of the elbow during baseball pitching. *J Orthop Sports Phys Ther.* 1993;17(6):274-278.

14. Childress HM. Recurrent ulnar-nerve dislocation at the elbow. *Clin Orthop Relat Res.* 1975;108:168-173.

15. Behr CT, Altchek DW. The elbow. *Clin Sports Med.* 1997;16(4):681-704.

16. Andrews JR, Timmerman LA. Outcome of elbow surgery in professional baseball players. *Am J Sports Med.* 1995;23(4):407-413.

17. Bennett GE. Shoulder and elbow lesions of the professional baseball pitcher. *J Am Med Assoc.* 1941;117(7):510-514.

18. Redler L, Watling J, Ahmad CS. 5 points on physical examination of the throwing athlete's elbow. *Am J Ophthalmol.* 2012;33136(8):380-382.

19. Calfee RP, Manske PR, Gelberman RH, et al. Clinical assessment of the ulnar nerve at the elbow: reliability of instability testing and the association of hypermobility with clinical symptoms. *J Bone Joint Surg Am.* 2010;92(17):2801-2808.

20. Schwab GH, Bennett JB, Woods GW, et al. Biomechanics of elbow instability: the role of the medial collateral ligament. *Clin Orthop Relat Res.* 1980:42-52.

21. Mitchell CH, Brushart TM, Ahlawat S, et al. MRI of sports-related peripheral nerve injuries. *Am J Roentgenol.* 2014;203(5):1075-1084.

22. Friedman RJ, Cochran TP. A clinical and electrophysiological investigation of anterior transposition for ulnar neuropathy at the elbow. *Arch Orthop Trauma Surg.* 1987;106(6):375-380.

23. Glousman RE, Barron J, Jobe FW, et al. An electromyographic analysis of the elbow in normal and injured pitchers with medial collateral ligament insufficiency. *Am J Sports Med.* 1992;20(3):311-317.

24. Wei S-H, Jong Y-J, Chang Y-J. Ulnar nerve conduction velocity in injured baseball pitchers. *Arch Phys Med Rehabil.* 2005;86(1):21-25.

25. Eisen A. Early diagnosis of ulnar nerve palsy. An electrophysiologic study. *Neurology.* 1974;24(3):236.

26. Thomas DR, Plancher KD, Hawkins RJ. Prevention and rehabilitation of overuse injuries of the elbow. *Clin Sports Med.* 1995;14:459-477.

27. Shah CM, Calfee RP, Gelberman RH, et al. Outcomes of rigid night splinting and activity modification in the treatment of cubital tunnel syndrome. *J Hand Surg Am.* 2013;38(6).

28. Hershman EB. Brachial plexus injuries. *Clin Sports Med.* 1990;9(2):311-329.

29. Macnicol MF. The results of operation for ulnar neuritis. *J Bone Joint Surg Br.* 1979;61-B(2):159-164.

30. Conway JE, Jobe FW, Glousman RE, et al. Medial instability of the elbow in throwing athletes. Treatment by repair or reconstruction of the ulnar collateral ligament. *J Bone Joint Surg Am.* 1992;74(1):67-83.

31. Heithoff SJ. Cubital tunnel syndrome does not require transposition of the ulnar nerve. *J Hand Surg.* 1992;24:898-905.

32. Macadam SA, Gandhi R, Bezuhly M, et al. Simple decompression versus anterior subcutaneous and submuscular transposition of the ulnar nerve for cubital tunnel syndrome: a meta-analysis. *J Hand Surg Am.* 2008;33(8).

33. Danoff JR, Lombardi JM, Rosenwasser MP. Use of a pedicled adipose flap as a sling for anterior subcutaneous transposition of the ulnar nerve. *J Hand Surg Am.* 2014;39(3):552-555.

34. Thompson WH, Jobe FW, Yocum LA, et al. Ulnar collateral ligament reconstruction in athletes: muscle-splitting approach without transposition of the ulnar nerve. *J Shoulder Elbow Surg.* 2001;10(2):152-157.

35. Vitale MA, Ahmad CS. The outcome of elbow ulnar collateral ligament reconstruction in overhead athletes: a systematic review. *Am J Sports Med.* 2008;36(6):1193-1205.

36. Jobe F, Stark H, Lombardo S. Reconstruction of the ulnar collateral ligament in athletes. *J Bone Joint Surg Am.* 1986;68(8):1158-1163.

37. Vitale MA, Ahmad CS. Ulnar nerve complications following ulnar collateral ligament reconstruction of the elbow: a systematic review. *Am J Sports Med.* 2018:363546518765139.

38. Watson JN, McQueen P, Hutchinson MR. A systematic review of ulnar collateral ligament reconstruction techniques. *Am J Sports Med.* 2014;42(10):2510-2516.

39. Purcell DB, Matava MJ, Wright RW. Ulnar collateral ligament reconstruction: a systematic review. *Clin Orthop Relat Res.* 2007;455:72-77.

40. Maruyama M, Satake H, Takahara M, et al. Treatment for ulnar neuritis around the elbow in adolescent baseball players: factors associated with poor outcome. *Am J Sports Med.* 2017;45(4):803-809.

41. Boatright JR, D'Alessandro DF. Nerve entrapment syndromes at the elbow. In: Jobe FW, Pink MM, Glousman RE, Kvitne ZN, eds. *Operative Techniques in Upper Extremity Sports Injuries.* 1996:518-537.

42. Rokito AS, Iviciviahon PJ, Jobe FW. Cubital tunnel syndrome. *Oper Tech Sports Med.* 1996;4(1):15-20.

43. Del Pizzo W, Jobe FW, Norwood L. Ulnar nerve entrapment syndrome in baseball players. *Am J Sports Med.* 1977;5(5):182-185.

44. Rettig AC, Ebben JR. Anterior subcutaneous transfer of the ulnar nerve in the athlete. *Am J Sports Med.* 1992;21(6):836-839 [discussion 839-840].

45. Aoki M, Kanaya K, Aiki H, et al. Cubital tunnel syndrome in adolescent baseball players: a report of six cases with 3-to 5-year follow-up. *Arthroscopy.* 2005;21(6):758.

46. Verveld CJ, Danoff JR, Lombardi JM, et al. An original study adipose flap versus fascial sling for anterior subcutaneous transposition of the ulnar nerve. *Am J Orthop.* 2016;45(2):89-94.

47. Robb A, Sajko S. Conservative management of posterior interosseous neuropathy in an elite baseball pitcher's return to play: a case report and review of the literature. *J Can Chiropr Assoc.* 2009;53(4):300-310.

48. Rodner CM, Tinsley BA, O'Malley MP. Pronator syndrome and anterior interosseous nerve syndrome. *J Am Acad Orthop Surg.* 2013;21(5):268-275.

49. Strohl AB, Zelouf DS. Ulnar tunnel syndrome, radial tunnel syndrome, anterior interosseous nerve syndrome, and pronator syndrome. *J Am Acad Orthop Surg.* 2017;25(1):e1-e10.

50. Harris JD, Lintner DM. Nerve injuries about the elbow in the athlete. *Sports Med Arthrosc.* 2014;22(3):e7-e15.

51. Stanley J. Radial tunnel syndrome: a surgeon's perspective. *J Hand Ther.* 2006;19(2):180-184.

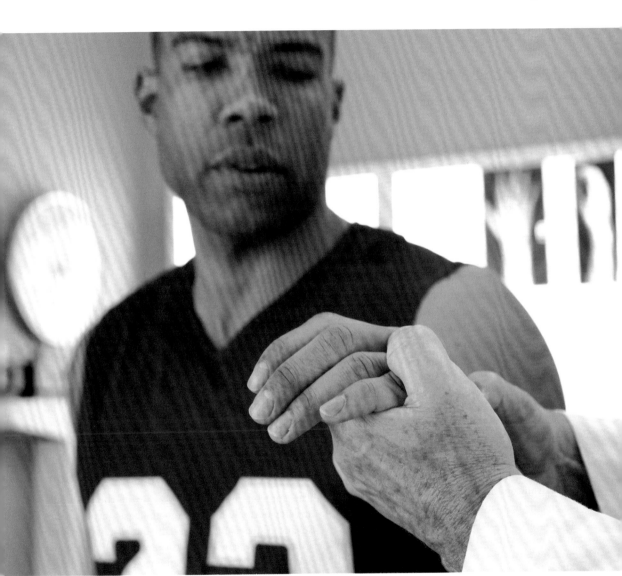

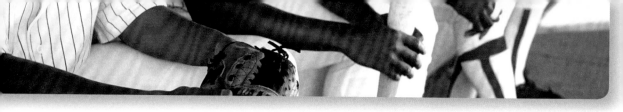

CHAPTER 13

Wrist Injuries and Baseball Players

Thomas J. Graham, MD

I believe anybody who is not afraid to fail is a winner.

—Joe Torre

INTRODUCTION

From the perspective of an upper extremity surgeon, few sports can rival baseball for presenting us with the volume and variety of clinical material. The unique demands of the throwing athlete have taught us all a great deal about how to diagnose and treat disorders if the shoulder and elbow, but the actions of fielding, hitting, and sliding, have provided an equivalent education regarding disorders of the wrist.

The full extent of multiplanar wrist motion is required for the tasks associated with most stick-and-ball sports, and baseball is no exception. Perhaps what compounds almost every challenge in the care of the baseball player is the length of the season; the 162-game schedule (not even taking into account spring training, playoffs, and off-season conditioning) is a marathon.

Over my quarter-century involved in the care of professional baseball players, I have seen a wide spectrum of acute and chronic injuries. Many of these considered uncommon in the general population are abundant in these athletes. For the purposes of this chapter, I have selected a representative sample of the common and complex that I believe comprise a portfolio with which those of you "in the game" should be familiar to affect return to the diamond.

The team doctor or hand surgery consultant will see practically everything if they remain around the game long enough.[1] Perhaps the sheer violence of football is not recapitulated in baseball, but complexity and competitive duration of this sport is practically unequaled; that is why it has been such a fascinating laboratory for many of us.

I hope to capture some of my personal enthusiasm for treating the baseball player and combine it with some of the lessons learned over the thousands of interactions I have had with these gifted athletes.

CLINICAL EVALUATION

Combining your wisdom derived from understanding the game of baseball with your skills as a physician will allow you to sort out almost any diagnostic dilemma. Judicious use of imaging and even differential injection (to be described) can corroborate your clinical suspicion.

For the hand surgeon, one of the advantages that baseball presents among the other North American team sports is time. The pace of the game and decision-making for its players are favorable. Understanding the rules surrounding the disabled lists makes you a more valuable asset to the player and the organization.

Salient History and Physical Examination

The surgeon involved in the care of these unique athletes not only has to know the basic (actually, the advanced) tenets of our specialty but also have to be a student of the game. Know the mechanics of the swing and the throwing motion—the violence of the head-first slide and collision—the vicissitudes introduced by thrown or batted projectiles moving at 100+ mph.

Common problems that affect fielding and throwing usually present through the normal course of following a team. Baseball is a contact sport, of course, with that contact between players or with a batted ball (or the wall) all contributing the normal bruises, sprains, and fractures. However, it is usually when the player is swinging the bat that the unique problems of the baseball athlete arise.

When gleaning the history, it happens "When I'm batting" is inadequate interrogatory; like the throwing motion, the hitting stroke has an almost infinite number of discreet positions of flexion, extension, radial- and ulnar-deviation, and pronosupination. Learning about the onset (and offset) of the symptom complex can lead one to even the most elusive diagnosis.

Ask (or better yet observe with a bat in your office or at the ballpark) whether a player follows-through 1- or 2-handed under normal circumstance.

Be knowledgeable enough to know the differences in top-hand and bottom-hand mechanics. Understand the forces generated in rapidly decelerating the immense angular velocity of the swing associated with "checking off" and their relationship to the player's complaints. Listen critically when a player tells you that he experiences discomfort on awkward or check swings but not when he "squares one up."

Learn how to listen (yes, listen) for the sound cutting of the bat through the air when your patient is finally rehabilitating to the point of regaining his stroke.

Regarding the examination outside of the usual thorough observation, palpation, and provocative maneuvers, I would emphasize the importance of developing a very meticulous ulnar-wrist examination and facility with the use of differential injection. Let us expound on that.

An inordinate number of the pathologies for which you will treat position players are ulnar-sided.[2] For this reason, a high level of concentration and a keen understanding of the regional pathologies are paramount.

Specifically, I would implore you to develop a comprehensive and reproducible mechanism to differentiate between the following pathologies. I have listed them along with the germinal examination maneuvers, which I have found to be most helpful to identify and segregate them from each other.

- Triquetral avulsion injury: You will see more than your share of vague dorsal wrist discomfort, especially on the ulnar side. Your anatomic knowledge, coupled with the assistance of fluoroscopy, can direct you to identify the point tenderness directly over the confluence of the dorsal radiocarpal and dorsal transverse intercarpal ligaments. Frankly, there is really almost nothing else that can reproduce the symptoms

- Lunatotriquetral (LT) sprain: It is admittedly rare, but sometimes a byproduct of head-first sliding, which loaded the pisotriquetral (PT) joint, transmitting forces across the LT interval. After ruling out pathologies of the PT joint and individual bones (such as body fractures) themselves, gaining a feel for the amount of dorsovolar translation by "shucking" or differentially loading the lunate and PT complex and ascertaining the level of discomfort—then comparing with the contralateral side—is effective. Although more difficult to detect than SL dissociation, looking for "uncoupled" or disconjugate motion of the lunate and triquetrum on live fluoroscopy on radial and ulnar deviation can assist in making the diagnosis

- Extensor carpi ulnaris (ECU) investment embarrassment: I have written extensively on almost all elements of ECU pathologies.[3,4] However, I can distill it here by directing the examiner to look for fusiform tumescence along the ECU indicating tendinitis, facile (and unequal) displacement of the ECU from the sulcus on direct manipulation, "snapping" indicating mechanical displacement on pronosupination, and "bowstringing" (again, unequal to the contralateral side) with resisted ulnar deviation

- Triangular fibrocartilage complex (TFCC) pathology: There are chapter and weekend conferences dedicated to the TFCC. There is little I shall elucidate here that the student of the ulnar wrist has not considered, but we shall describe its relevance to the baseball player. Many players will have either strains or sprains of the *limbi* (the dorsal and volar distal radioulnar joint [DRUJ] ligaments); **very** rarely will there be an attenuation of these structures that results in destabilization of the DRUJ relationship. More often, pathology about the TFCC will be related to a perforation of the articular disk that is identified by eliciting discomfort on direct palpation through the "volar portal"—the soft spot just ulnar to the FCU and just volar to the ulnar styloid

- Midcarpal impingement: This is the elusive one to which my colleagues and I have just started to call attention. It is a very real issue with athletes who generate huge angular velocities with a weighted bat and skillfully, but violently, transition from a radially deviated position ("open" ulnar midcarpal joint) to an ulnar-deviated position, closing the gap and impinging the hamate and triquetrum. The *sine quo non* is that the player experiences pain in the ulnar midcarpal "soft spot" just as they roll their hands through the hitting zone. As with a lot of pathologies related to batting, the discomfort is often greater when they swing and miss (or check or foul off) versus when they make solid contact

- Ulnocarpal abutment (UCA): Admittedly rare, this pathology can occur and is related to the interaction between the player's native anatomy and the demands of the sport. Judiciously combining physical examination with radiographs that almost always demonstrate a preternaturally long ulna will assist in the diagnosis. From a physical examination perspective, recognizing that the symptoms and findings of a TFCC tear may be an underlying component but when added to an often-vague central wrist "aching", they may point to abutment. This is 1 problem where an MRI (magnetic resonance imaging) is often the "tie breaker" that differentiates UCA from isolated components of its overall pathology
- Pisiform/pisotriquetral pathology: As rare as problems of the pisiform and PT joint are in the general population, they are a real concern in the stick-and-ball athlete, especially the aggressive defender and head-first slider. Determining subtle instability of the PT joint or the potential for cartilage shear injuries that may result in mechanical symptoms needs to be in the lexicon of the physician caring for baseball players. Pisiform subluxation, grinding or locking, and even the occasional pisiform or triquetral body fracture can be discovered through a dedicated examination
- Hamulus fracture: The modicum of embarrassment I feel by describing this to the advanced reader will pale in comparison with that one would feel if they missed a hook of the hamate fracture in the bottom hand of a baseball player—you simply cannot rest until you have ruled out this problem clinically and/or radiographically. Inquire about bat position on gripping and swinging and look for the batting callus that so many players develop. Aside from palpation, resisted flexion of the flexor digitorum profundus (FDP) to the small finger (and sometimes the ring finger) can help you avoid the cardinal sin of missing a hamate hook fracture when caring for the baseball athlete

We are all aware that pathologies are not isolated to the ulnar-sided structures, but the familiarity with examinations for scaphoid fracture (snuffbox tenderness), scapholunate ligament rupture (scaphoid shift test or "Watson maneuver"), and flexor carpi radialis (FCR) tendinitis (point tenderness at the scaphoid's distal pole and scaphotrapezial joint, exacerbated with resisted wrist flexion) are all well-known to our constituents.

Imaging

Plain Radiography and Arthrography

We are all familiar with the difficulty in diagnosing a fresh, nondisplaced scaphoid fracture, so let us just recognize that scenario and remember that repeated plain films or early use of cross-sectional imaging will usually address that challenge. When considering the more concerning "whiffs" I have seen with plain X-rays, I am really referring to the misdiagnosis of hamulus fractures on carpal tunnel views. Regardless of your experience, I challenge you to definitively diagnose a basilar hook of the hamate fracture reliably on this view.

First, there is probably no other view that is more variable in positioning and quality. The reasons range from the unusual subject positioning and vector of the beam to the fact that we are asking a patient/player with obvious wrist discomfort to adopt this contorted posture. Even when the quintessential carpal tunnel view is obtained, the midbody or basilar regions of the hamulus are obscured by osseous overlap or the angle of the fracture is not perfectly aligned with the beam to reveal its lucency.

Fortunately, the solution is exceedingly simple, especially if you adequately instruct your radiology technicians or have easy access to a fluoroscopy unit. Whether considered the "cup" or "butterfly" view, a lateral image taken through the first web space with the thumb widely abducted and the wrist in maximal radial deviation will allow amazing visualization of the hamulus and easy detection of a fracture of the tip, body, or base; it also gives an excellent opportunity to visualize the adequacy of the resected hamulus (Figure 13.1).

The last use of plain radiography I have chosen to highlight is for the purpose of determining the relative length of the radius and ulna. It usually distills down to a technical flaw, the most egregious stemming from an attempt to get both wrists imaged on the same plate.

I would simply advise the examiner to always get standard zero-rotation PA and lateral views every time any wrist problem is being evaluated. Then extend the basic series with images such as a pronated, grip, or ulnar deviation views. I have seen important data that may affect ultimate diagnoses related to relative radius and ulna length go undetected because of poor positioning.

As for arthrography, I will admit my bias against its use. I grew up in a time when it was the preferred, if not only, tool to determine certain internal derangements of the wrist, specifically those that could be characterized by the flow of contrast through the "path of least resistance."

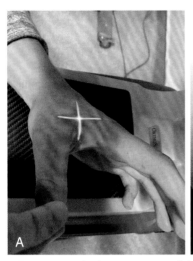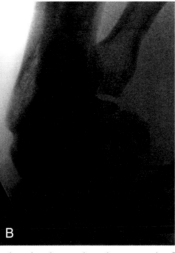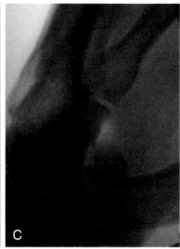

FIGURE 13.1 • A, The positioning of the hand radiographic plate or in the fluoroscopy beam to achieve visualization of the hamate hook is facile. Wide abduction of the thumb, radial deviation of the wrist, and slight pronation will bring the hamulus into view through the first web space. With the use of the butterfly, cup, or papillon view, fractures of the hamate hook are well visualized (B). The goal of the resection is to leave a smooth base that is approximately aligned with the base of the V metacarpal base (C).

With the ever-evolving sophistication of other cross-sectional imaging techniques, coupled with the discomfort and false-negative/-positive yields of dye studies, I have largely abandoned them. I simply learn more from a good physical examination and a corroboration with noncontrast studies.

Live Fluoroscopy

Whether it is simply the expedience, the magnification, the ability to see live motion, or anatomic localization, the use of low-dose fluoroscopy has afforded me a level of diagnostic capability that is decided advantageous.

Beside the extreme facility with characterizing fractures, especially those of the hamate, I believe the ability to watch for "conjugated" motion of the scaphoid and lunate (or lunate and triquetrum) is extremely valuable in determining the status of the respective intrinsic ligaments.

This may come down to expense over expedience in some organizations or clubhouses, but having access to live fluoroscopy to make "game time" decisions or even follow-up treatments or chronic issues is a luxury to which I have grown all too accustom.

Cross-sectional Imaging (Magnetic Resonance Imaging and Computed Tomography)

In a referral practice with a high concentration of focus on the care of professional athletes, it is almost rarer for a player to arrive without an MRI already having been performed. This is not a commentary about skill of prior examiners or some advocacy about fiscal responsibility in health care economics—it has just become commonplace to obtain this information.

I believe MRI has helped me most to (1) detect osseous edema (nondisplaced scaphoid fractures, hamate "stress fractures," and ulnocarpal abutment), (2) characterize the extent of TFC pathology, (3) grade tendinitis or extent of intrinsic tendon pathology in an unstable ECU situation, and (4) identify early lunatomalacia when vague wrist discomfort has been confounding. I have never hesitated to use it but again want to emphasize its corroborative role rather than that of a replacement for a thorough physical examination.

With the use of live fluoroscopy, and that of MRI to an extent, my reliance on computed tomography (CT) scanning has waned. It's role in following fracture healing or characterizing a complex distal radius fracture, for example, is valuable.

Miscellaneous (Bone Scan, Arteriography)

The use of "specialized studies" is somewhat rare in this age-group and activity cohort. Bone scans to detect subtle fracture of the scaphoid or hamate have been largely obviated.

There is a subset of players with vascular problems in whom contrast studies may be valuable. Catchers who are exposed to repetitive pounding or those players who exhibit vasospastic symptoms or splinter hemorrhages may be candidates for a workup of their vascular tree, especially the ulnar artery in Guyon canal.[5,6]

TREATMENT, REHABILITATION, AND RETURN TO PLAY

I selected an "all-star roster" about which I believe student of the game of baseball and the surgeon caring for these athletes should know. This portfolio is not exhaustive, as almost any wrist problem seen in the general population can also afflict the baseball player, but these are the ones that have either been most prevalent or problematic in my quarter-century of caring for this unique population.

- Hook of the hamate fractures
- Selected carpal fractures and intercarpal ligament injuries
- TFCC and DRUJ issues
- Midcarpal impingement
- Disorders of the ECU investments

I shall cover the therapeutic approach to these entities and expand the discussion to include the posttreatment rehabilitation and return to play projections.

Hook of the Hamate (Hamulus) Fractures

There is no real ambiguity around the treatment of the hook of the hamate fracture in the baseball player.[7] Except in the rare circumstances where a small tip fracture may present, the "standard" treatment is excision.

There is not a lot of education I can provide the experienced surgeon about approaching this region, but I have seen my share of problems encountered by those who may not find themselves as familiar with what some consider a "straightforward" operation.

Surgical Technique

Here are the basic tenets to which I abide when excising the fractured hamulus:

- One can localize the hamate utilizing any palpation, dermatoglyphics, or Kaplan cardinal line. I would encourage you to actually locate it with fluoroscopy, when available. Using a 25 gauge needle to exactly pinpoint the hook can be a worthwhile exercise and good teaching point if accompanied by residents or fellows

- Respect of the batting callus is a luxury, but one I try to accomplish. The skin of the palm is thick to begin with, and this coveted badge of honor is important to the athlete

- After I expose the ulnar neurovascular bundle, I characterize the anatomy and course of the motor branch of the ulnar nerve—it never ceases to amaze me how intimate this important branch is to the convex (ulnar) side of the hamulus

- I have always performed a complete release of the carpal tunnel; I want to make sure that there is no tendon attrition, fragment of the hamulus, or chance that a postoperative, acute carpal tunnel could evolve

- There are 2 absolutely critical technical aspect of this surgery: (1) intimate subperiosteal dissection of the pisohamate ligament and enveloping soft tissues from the convex side of the hook and (2) resecting (or smoothing) of the base of the hamate back to about the level of the volar face of the V metacarpal

I tell most players/trainers/teams that this is about a 6 to 8 week process before return to elite level play. About 25% of players will return before week 6, 50% between weeks 6 to 8, and the remaining players by weeks 10 to 12. Bat modification (knob structure) or glove padding can assist in return to play.

Results and Complications

Fortunately, with the frequency with which this injury occurs in this specialized population, the results are uniformly outstanding. If intraoperative nerve injury is avoided and no tendon attrition is discovered, there are really only 2 complications that I have seen with enough frequency that they deserve attention.

The more obscure of the two is a resulting hypermobility of the pisiform. In my experience, this is somewhat unpredictable, and a player's flexibility (hyperelastic diathesis) may be a contributor. I do believe that careful dissection of the ulnar aspect of the hamate hook fragment may help minimize the chance of problems, but it has no guarantee. I do not believe that full carpal tunnel release is the culprit, as I have never encountered this in my practice and I have always performed the full transverse carpal ligament release to excise the hook (150+ cases). This problem can usually be managed nonsurgically, but considerable instability may occasion pisiform excision in rare circumstances.

The more worrisome, yet ultimately avoidable complication is incomplete excision of the fractured hook. Anecdotally, I believe this occurs more frequently with oblique fractures that are more distant (volar) from the base. I have seen both partial excisions and inadequate resections cause later problems requiring reoperation.

Manager's Tips

- Always think hamulus fracture with even vague discomfort of the volar (or even dorsal) ulnar wrist in the batter
- Careful identification and protection of the motor branch of the ulnar nerve is of paramount importance and is accomplished by meticulous periosteal dissection of the fragment
- Tendon attrition is rare in the acute setting but possible in the chronic case; complete carpal tunnel release enhances visualization of the fracture and allows identification and immediate reconciliation

Selected Carpal Fractures and Intercarpal Ligament Injuries

Baseball athletes are certainly not immune to sustaining any carpal fracture or combination injury. Instead of enumerating the litany of common or even obscure carpal bone injuries, I will just make brief commentary on a couple of the injuries that may be encountered, which present diagnostic, therapeutic, or return to play challenges in the context of the germinal element confronting the treating and team physician.

For the purpose of this contracted section, I have elected to cover 4 pathologies: scaphoid fracture, pisotriquetral pathologies, SL injuries, and LT ligament injuries. Of course, this is inadequate in scope, but because of the volume of literature that exists on all of these and other topics in this realm, a condensed coverage seems appropriate.

Scaphoid fracture: There are really no changes in the workup, surgical indications, or technique regarding management of scaphoid fractures. The surgeon who is facile with percutaneous fixation may elect that approach while others (including myself) opt for a minimally open technique strongly favoring the dorsal approach when possible to avoid any manipulation of the FCR tendon. The issue of emphasis here is just the rehabilitation/return to play strategy. I would simply encourage the earliest possible motion.

Our experience indicate that for the "run of the mill" mid-waist scaphoid fracture in the elite baseball athlete, the return to play statistics are as follows: 25% of players return before postoperative week 10, 50% return between weeks 10 to 14, and 25% return after week 14.

- **SL and LT ligament injuries:** I am addressing these separately and not venturing into the combined perilunate instability patterns, which are more appropriately covered in a wrist trauma text, not necessarily a chapter about caring for baseball players. This is pertinent because the surgeon will be assured of seeing the common SL injury, but because of the unusual demands of the sport, it will not be implausible to see the rare isolated LT rupture [8]

The reason I will cover this injury at all is to highlight a technical approach that has significantly changed my outcomes regarding return to play interval. It is the use of a terminally threaded screw to associate the adjacent bones (vs simple smooth K-wire fixation), which I believe both coapts the bones better and permits far earlier free motion. I cannot determine whether there has been a material effect on long-term clinical or radiographic results, but the shorter-term (less than 1 year or season) influence has been advantageous (Figures 13.2 and 13.3).

The following is a standard rehabilitation/return to play plan:

- First 2 weeks
  - Remain in operative dressing
  - Cardio work permitted—keep dressing clean and dry
- Week 2 to 4
  - Transition either to cast or custom orthosis for full-time or "23-hours" wear
- Week 4
  - Structured motion recovery work (A/AAROM = active/active-assisted range of motion)
    - First 3 to 5 days. Out 2 to 3 X/day for A/AAROM
    - Next 3 to 5 days. Out 4 to 6 X/day for A/AAROM
    - Next 3 to 5 days. Out 6 to 8 X/day for A/AAROM
    - Next 3 to 5 days. Out 8 to 10 X/day for A/AAROM
    - Next 3 to 5 days. Out 10 to 12 X/day for A/AAROM
    - Next 3 to 5 days. Out 13 to 15 X/day for A/AAROM
- Week 8 to 12 (approx)
  - If radiographs and clinical examination permit, increase strengthening efforts
  - Typically, when 75% of strengthening achieved, start basketball-related activity
  - Graduate through: Passing/receiving, all forms of shooting, defense, and battling

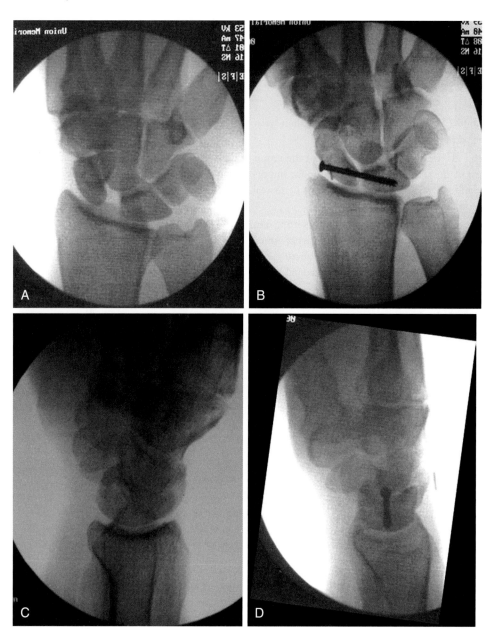

FIGURE 13.2 • In the preoperative (A) and postoperative (B) posteroanterior (PA) views, the coaptation of the scapholunate interval and securing it with a terminally threaded cancellous screw is demonstrated. The intercarpal and radiocarpal relationships in the preoperative (C) and postoperative (D) lateral views.

- Week 12 and beyond (approx)
  - SL screw removal followed by brief immobilization—target approximately 100 days
  - Resume baseball conditioning and drills
  - Usual outcomes: 25% before 16 W, 50% between 16 to 20 W, 25% after 20 W
- **PT Pathologies:** I have already mentioned the traumatic and iatrogenic PT instability, but there is another unusual pathology that I have seen almost exclusively in contact athletes—the loose-body-generating shear injury of the PT joint.

When a confounding diagnosis of mechanical symptoms of the wrist (including overt locking) is encountered, careful examination and imaging of the PT joint should be remembered. However, more troublesome is the fact that a cartilage fragment that may be blocking motion may remain radiographically undetectable

I have been faced with the unusual situation where I have seen a triquetral platform shear defect or an identifiable loose body in the PT joint (better yet when one can follow a mobile fragment on live fluoro) and

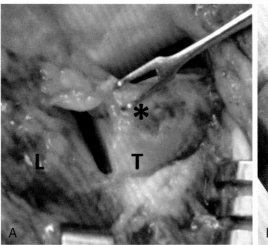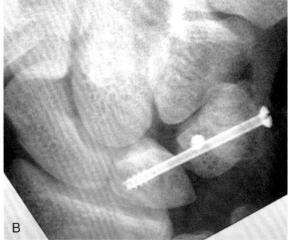

FIGURE 13.3 • The intraoperative photo (A) demonstrates both the lunatotriquetral (LT) ligament rupture (avulsed from the triquetrum) and an interesting finding of a triquetral avulsion fracture (*). In (B), the ligament is repaired with a suture anchor and the screw coapts the lunate and triquetrum.

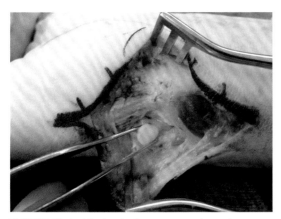

FIGURE 13.4 • Mechanical symptoms about the pisotriquetral (PT) joint can be caused by soft tissue laxity, by arthrosis, or rarely by a loose body. In this case, a small cartilaginous fragment is recovered after PT joint arthrotomy.

preoperatively prepared the patient either for loose body removal or even a pisiform excision, depending on the status of the articular cartilage. In the handful of these problems I have seen, I have only ever had to excise 3 pisiforms (2 baseball players and 1 hockey player) (Figure 13.4).

Manager's Tips

- As a parallel to the elbow (and maybe shoulder) in the thrower, the wrist is likely the most vulnerable anatomy in the batter
- Common and complex problems arise because of the multiple repetitions, the unpredictability of such a dynamic and violent process and the contact nature of the sport

- Regardless of the problem or its treatment, accelerating the motion-recovery phase is the difference-maker in the ultimate return to play journey, so therapeutic approach should consider this variable
- Rare problems can occur in this population, while some very common problems can affect the comfort and effectiveness in these elite athletes

Midcarpal Impingement

I have previously described that maintaining a very robust and sophisticated differential diagnosis list for ulnar-sided wrist problems in the baseball player is a necessity for those of us who are fortunate enough to take part in the care of these unique athletes.[9] Every once in a while even the most meticulous examiner becomes somewhat stumped by the presentation of a specific symptom complex until further focus, and even a bit of serendipity, begins to clarify a newly recognized problem that is inherent in a specific population.

Such was the case when my colleagues and I elucidated ulnar midcarpal impingement in the batter.[10] Admittedly, this may have been one of the pathologies that had "seen me, but I did not see it" in earlier stages of my career, but when I was repeatedly exposed to pinpoint midcarpal symptoms in the extreme of ulnar deviation with loading—essentially the hitting zone of the stroke—I started to dive more deeply and treat this as a "real" entity.

The true "eureka" moment happened when I had a well-known player manifest an impressive spurring from the hamate that actually excavated the corresponding aspect of the triquetrum (Figure 13.5). Characterizing this case fully was an exercise in

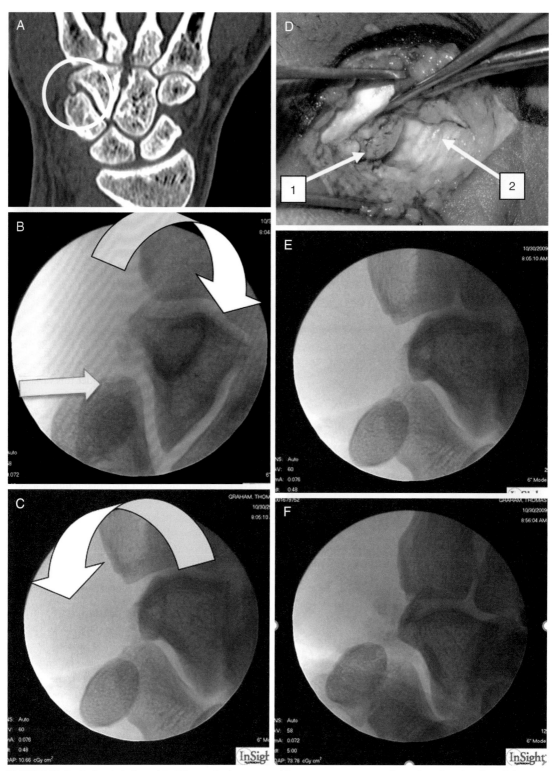

FIGURE 13.5 • A, Encircled on this CT scan is the unusual bone spur projecting from the ulnar border of the hamate at the midcarpal joint and the corresponding defect in the triquetrum. B and C, are the radial-deviation and ulnar-deviation views, respectively. The yellow arrow calls attention to the small triquetral defect, best revealed in radial-deviation but caused by impingement in ulnar-deviation. D, The osteophyte projection from the hamate (1) and the corresponding defect in the hamate (2) are highlighted. E and F, demonstrate ulnar-deviation images taken preoperatively (E) and postoperatively (F) highlighting the more generous space created after resection/ recontouring of the hamate's ulnar, midcarpal border.

defining the "screw home" mechanics of the triquetro-hamate joint, the intercarpal relationship through the batting stroke, and the spectrum of both the problem and treatments.[11-13]

Only the most extreme cases may manifest a "kissing" osteophytosis or even a noticeable "bone bruise" on MRI. The discomfort of midcarpal impingement is more likely to be related to capsular irritation/thickening and potentially some localized synovitis. In the majority of the cases, a "differential injection examination" (isolation of a specific anatomic structure or region thought to be the locus of discomfort with an anesthetic injection, followed by a cortisone injection, if the pain is ameliorated) is both diagnostic and therapeutic.

As demonstrated in the case featured in Figure 13.5, surgery may have role in selected circumstances. Often with the help of live fluoroscopy, the impingement can be appreciated, subtle bony changes identified, and the straightforward surgical decompression conducted.

Manager's Tips

- The triquetrum and hamate have a complex geometric relationship that may be prone to injury with violent closing of the midcarpal space as the wrists rotate through the hitting zone
- Whether solely a soft tissue problem or one with osseous manifestations, midcarpal impingement is a "real" pathology in this population
- Aside from meticulous physical examination, perhaps with the patient swinging a bat to further isolate the discomfort, the use of a differential injection examination is extremely helpful
- Surgical decompression will rarely be elected, but its requirement will present itself vividly, and its results are impressive

Pathologies of the Triangular Fibrocartilage Complex and Distal Radioulnar Joint

The shifting focus of specialties/subspecialties is interesting to monitor and largely tracks with the interests of the luminaries who are publishing in trusted journals and speaking at important meetings, perhaps multiplied by the emergence of new techniques and technologies. In hand surgery, there have been many of those waves that have seemingly reached a zenith of curiosity and contribution—tendon transfers, flexor tendon surgery, microsurgery, and wrist instability to name a few.

About 2 decades ago, one of the topics of preternatural interest was the TFCC and the DRUJ. I refer the reader to the voluminous information that has been contributed on these related topics that are subjects of books and courses themselves. In the interest of time and space, I shall simply try to provide a snapshot of what I think is relevant to the management of the baseball athlete by breaking the majority of the pathologies into 2 arbitrary but intersecting grouping set that I use: acute versus chronic and stable versus destabilizing. In descending order of frequency, here is how I see the problems and approaches present:

- **Chronic stable injuries: TFC perforation, ulno-carpal abutment, and DRUJ arthrosis**

    Baseball is a "war of attrition"; when you add spring training to the 162-game season to postseason (then off-season training, which has become a critical element of the player's regimen) it really is a marathon. That is why it is no surprise that so many players have resultant inflammation or central articular disk perforation of the TFC.

    It is exceedingly rare that I would end a player's season for TFCC irritation, instead managing it with oral anti-inflammatories or judicious use of injected cortisone after characterizing the extent of the tear on MRI (I prefer noncontrast examination to see the native anatomy clearly, but others may argue for a dye study). Seemingly, at the end of each season, we have a half-dozen players who present for an arthroscopic "cleanup"—not unlike those who come to my colleagues for elbow, knee, and shoulder procedures of similar types.

    Regarding the wrist, this means a thorough intra-articular inspection to rule out additional pathologies and a "radialization" of the central tear of the articular disk, so it does not propagate and potential encroach on the volar and dorsal radioulnar ligaments, or "limbi", the true DRUJ stabilizers. Uniformly, the arthroscopic debridements are successful and either do not require repeat treatment or only do so in a long enough interval that reinjury or extended interval degeneration is the culprit.

    However, there is a special subset of these players whose TFCC perforation is the result of ulnocarpal abutment. This adds an additional layer of more complex decision-making. The management of the positive ulna is itself a topic, and one would anticipate that continues attrition of the TFC and the bony manifestations of the lunate and ulna will persist if the abutment is not addressed.

    I shall give my unequivocal bias while respecting so many colleagues who hold a divergent view. I am not an advocate of ulnar shortening osteotomy in the professional athlete during their career. Whether it is the extended time to union or the potential for reinjury in this vulnerable region, I instead try simultaneous TFC debridement and recession of the ulnar pole through the TFC defect to relieve abutment—the so-called mini-open "Feldon wafer" procedure or its arthroscopic cousin[14] (Figure 13.6).

Moreover, falling primarily under the "stable" category, but with the potential to create malalignment or mechanical symptoms, is marginal osteophytosis of the DRUJ. I have seen an "apron" of spurring extend from the inferior articular margin of the ulnar seat. Rarely this will need debridement, but if it is elected, one must resect it in its full circumference, exposed through a dorsal incision by rotating the radius into a hyperpronated position to access the volar-most aspect of the ulna.

- **Acute stable injuries: acute TFC tears and DRUJ fractures**

The TFCC is equally as vulnerable to acute injuries as are the osseous structures about the DRUJ. Seldom do acute injuries result in unstable articulations, instead present as immediate points of discomfort that can linger longer than desired (often defined as the duration of the disabled list stay). The most common ones, beside the contusions from thrown and batter balls, are the acute TFC articular disk perforations and the subfailure DRUJ ligament attenuations. In both instances, I have had somewhat of a low threshold to inject these with cortisone if they are demonstrating that they do not represent a problem likely to progress to a more serious situation, yet ones in which they have shown the proclivity to linger for more than 3 or 4 weeks.

- **Acute and chronic destabilizing injuries: DRUJ ligament or TFC ruptures, destabilizing osseous injuries**

A collision/ballistic sport such as baseball will provide a sizable and varied litany of interesting acute injuries. Extremely few will lead to destabilizing injuries to the DRUJ, but it is possible. In my experience, these destabilizing injuries are not usually the isolated dorsal or volar DRUJ subluxations that may occur from an isolated limbus rupture but have been either a complete rupture of the TFCC from the radial aspect (an extremely rare circumstance I have seen twice, both resulting from collisions with the outfield wall [Figure 13.7]) or the more frequent basilar styloid fracture that untethers the foveal attachment of the TFCC, which can be isolated but usually accompanies a distal radius fracture.

There can also be the unusual injury where a player is hit by a pitch causing an ulnar styloid injury (or I have seen a line drive back to the pitcher cause an isolated ulnar styloid obliteration). That same mechanism can also cause a depressed fracture of the sigmoid fossa of the radius, which is an extremely rare and interesting occurrence that requires careful imaging and considerable decision-making. In one of my most memorable cases over the years, I elected not to operate on this injury and fortunately the player returned to finish a stellar career without sequelae (Figure 13.8).

Manager's Tips

- So much is written about the TFCC and DRUJ—almost all of it is pertinent to the care of the baseball athlete

- A large number of players will present at some time in their career with ulnar-sided wrist pain; TFCC-related pathology will be among one of the most frequent diagnoses, but few man-games will be lost if managed appropriately

- TFCC and DRUJ pathologies will range from the common to the complex, and an appreciation of that spectrum will benefit the consultant and the player

Pathologies of the Extensor Carpi Ulnaris and Its Investments

Admittedly, the other injuries and disorders that are covered in this chapter are well-known to most hand surgeons and sports medicine specialists. Nonetheless, I hope that I have elucidated some new perspectives and filled in some gaps.

However, the athletic wrist pathology that I have seen expand in its frequency of diagnosis and the fundamental understanding of anatomy/pathoanatomy are problems of the ECU tendon and its investments. I have tried to be a diligent student of this highly specialized and extremely relevant area because of my long history of caring for baseball athletes.

In this expanded section, I shall distill some of the many advancements we have made in understanding of this endemic problem to the baseball community.

Diagnostic Considerations and Classification

Pathologies of the ECU tendon and its investments can be broken down anatomically into 3 components, which sometimes conspire to create a multifactorial problem. The 3 culprits are

- Inflammatory: Tenosynovitis surrounding the ECU tendon

- Mechanical failure: Classic findings such as bowstringing and subluxation/dislocation of the ECU tendon

- Tendinopathy: Intrinsic damage or tendinosis of the ECU

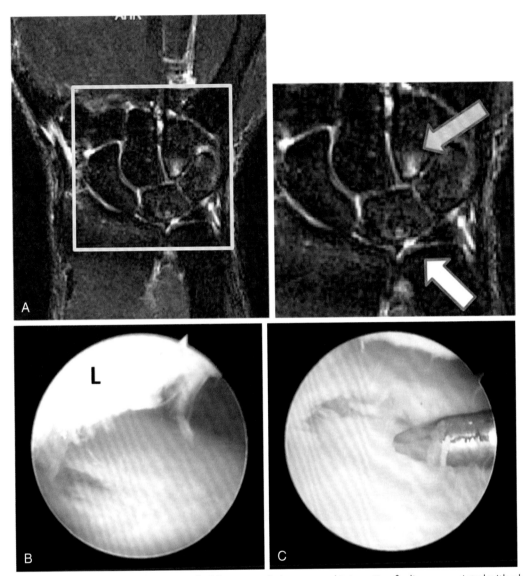

FIGURE 13.6 • A, This MRI and its magnified focus panel show several interesting findings associated with ulno-carpal abutment. The white arrow emphasizes the triangular fibrocartilage complex (TFCC) perforation and the edema in the lunate. The yellow arrow shows some edema in the hamate, presumably from the altered mechanics about the lunate and loading of the ulnar column, although the hamate facet of the lunate is not generous. In these arthroscopic images, the intra-articular derangement associated with ulnocarpal abutment is revealed. B, A complex tear of the TFCC and chondromalacia of the lunate (L) is seen. C, After "radialization" of the TFCC tear now exposes the distal end of the ulnar pole. D, There has already been eburnation of the lunate from chronic abutment. There are several mechanisms by which the ulnar pole can be decompressed. Beside formal ulnar shortening and mini-open "Feldon Wafer" resection of the distal ulna, arthroscopic decompression through the TFC defect is possible and beneficial. E, The full-radius burr is seen recessing the ulna through the TFC defect, and (F) an interesting view that shows the newly shortened ulna, the radialized TFC and the geographic lunate defect is also seen. G, These pre and postresection views demonstrate the recession of the ulnar pole that was achieved through the arthroscopic approach. Beside the key that the ulnar pole has been resected to alleviate the abutment, it is critical to maintain the DRUJ relationship by avoiding any encroachment on the ulnar seat and its relationship in the sigmoid fossa of the radius.

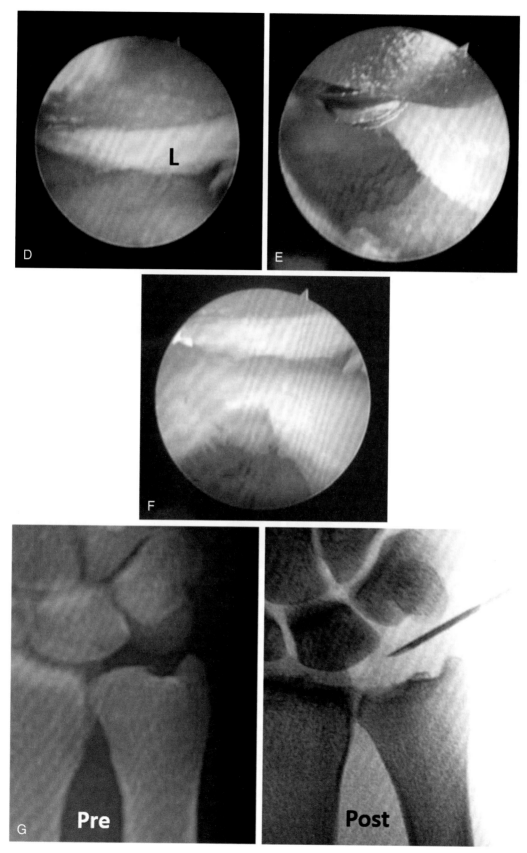

FIGURE 13.6—CONT'D

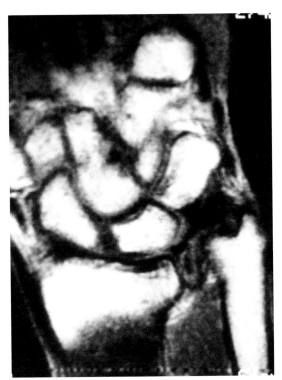

FIGURE 13.7 • This is a vivid example of the extremely rare radial-sided avulsion/rupture of the articular disc. In this example, the injury was sustained by an outfielder when he slammed against the wall attempting to make a catch and his forearm was forcibly compressed between his body and the wall. The articular disc was avulsed from its radial insertion and became intercalated between the radius and ulna, completely blocking forearm rotation before open reduction and reconstruction was performed.

The former 2 pathologies have overt physical examination findings that can be observed or elicited. Fullness about the length of the sheath, even including a stenosing tenosynovitis presentation with "squeaking," can occur.

Mechanical displacement on provocative testing has obvious implications related to failure of the anatomic constraints we have introduced above. Simply observing the prominence of the ECU while examining the patient's wrist in ulnar deviation while resisting a radial deviation force is valuable; this "bowstringing" can be subtle and should be compared with the contralateral side.

Patients with gross tendon instability can often demonstrate this in the office, even without a bat or club in their hand. By "rolling" their wrist, they can trap the tendon outside the sulcus, only to relocate it at the end of the maneuver with some modest radial deviation and flexion.

Intrinsic tendinopathy is inferred by a chronic pain, often described as "burning". This diagnosis can really only be made with cross-sectional imaging. An MRI, performed with or without any form of contrast, reveals valuable information of both the ECU tendon and its investments (Figure 13.9A). Perhaps one of the most comprehensive and contemporary treatments of the value of MRI in assessing ECU pathology was contributed in 2011 by Jeantroux and colleagues, who advocated for gadolinium contrast and dynamic pronation-supination sequences.[15]

Ultrasound may play an increasing role in the diagnosis of ECU pathology. Because it can be used in dynamic circumstances, I am encouraged about its future use as greater familiarity with the technology and techniques evolve.[16]

With the 3 hallmarks of ECU pathology firmly in mind, we can develop our admittedly arbitrary, but useful, classification system so that we can converse with patients, trainers and, fellow colleagues. I suggest this simple approach:

Mild: Swelling in sheath, no bowstringing, and no intrinsic abnormality (MRI).

Moderate: Bowstringing of ECU distal to ulnar styloid, possible intrinsic change (MRI), and no subluxation with pronosupination.

Severe: Bowstringing of ECU distal (and potentially proximal to) the ulna styloid, intrinsic (focal vs longitudinal) tendon embarrassment, and subluxation out of ulnar sulcus with pronosupination.

Strategies for Treating Pathologies of the Extensor Carpi Ulnaris and Investments

Nonoperative Treatment

I have already revealed my bias against deciding about surgical treatment of acute ECU problems. The reason behind this is simple and has been played out in my practice dozens of times over my 2-plus decades involved in the care of the elite athlete's wrist and hand. As my thesis has been one of initial nonoperative treatment, I have seen athletes trend toward 3 different outcomes.

- Complete or near-complete resolution of symptoms, with no lingering discomfort or mechanical manifestations
- Persistence of mechanical symptoms without significant discomfort or impairment of effective play at the elite level
- Continued discomfort and mechanical manifestations that prevent effective and safe play

Appertaining to the "conservative" philosophy and classification I have articulated, my protocol includes the following "phases".

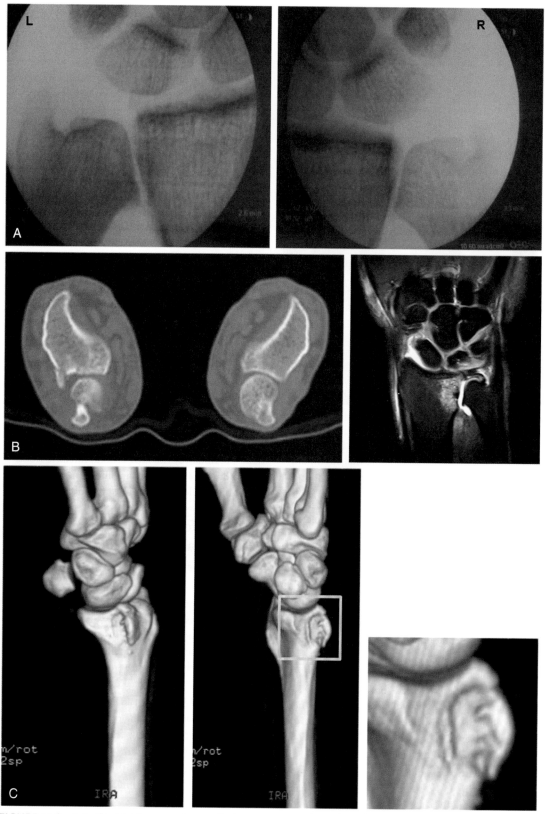

FIGURE 13.8 • A, In this highly unusual case, the batter was struck on the subcutaneous portion of the left distal ulna with a 100 mph fastball. Perhaps, slight irregularity about the inferior juxta-articular margin of the ulnar seat can appreciated on live fluoroscopy, but this finding is subtle. B, However, on further cross-sectional imaging, a depressed fracture of the sigmoid fossa is appreciated (left CT scan) and considerable intraosseous edema (right MRI) can be detected. C, Three-dimensional reconstructions begin to characterize the morphology of this unusual injury.

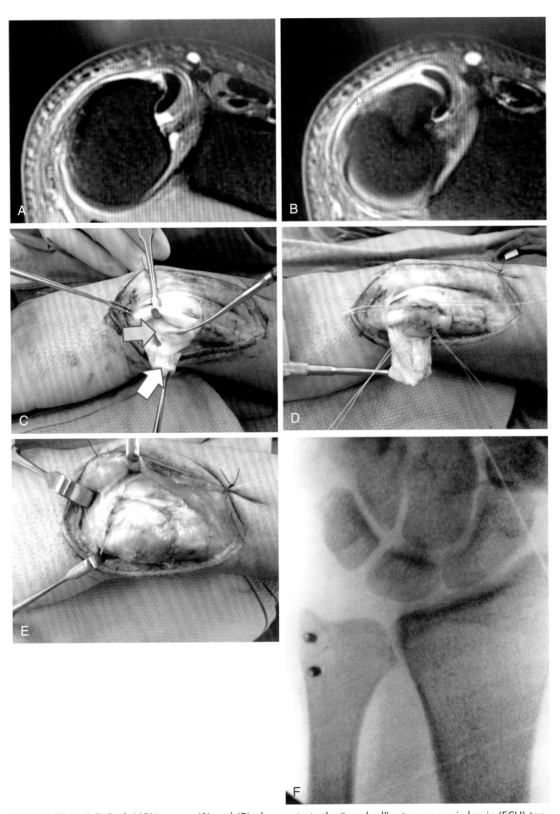

FIGURE 13.9 • A-E, Both MRI images, (A) and (B), demonstrate the "perched" extensor carpi ulnaris (ECU) tendon, which is demonstrating considerable mechanical instability and deformation. C, This intraoperative image shows the exposure achieved through an ulnar-based retinacular flap (white arrow) and the reflected subsheath (yellow arrow). Also interesting, the freer elevator shows a moderate "delamination" of the subsheath labrum from the ulnar pillar of the sulcus. These intraoperative images show the reconstructed subsheath and the reflected, ulnar-based retinacular flap (D) and the subsequent retinacular reinforcement (E). In (F), the intraoperative image is shown to emphasize the careful placement of the suture anchors. The key is to respect the basi-styloid region so that a stress riser is not created that may cause an ulnar styloid fracture.

Immobilization phase: Long-arm splint can be considered, but short-arm is usually effective. Wrist can be placed in neutral to slight flexion and radial deviation. Any cardio/leg work permitted per level of comfort.

- Mild: 5 to 7 days initial period of immobilization
- Moderate: 7 to 10 days initial period of immobilization
- Severe: 10 to 14 days initial period of immobilization

If in removable splint, may use ice or perform modalities such as iontophoresis. May be out for hygiene if taped around distal aspect of tendon. Consider dental bolster or elastomer mold longitudinal tendon support.

Motion recovery phase: After initial immobilization period, assess level of comfort. If pain and swelling persist with gentle motion, consider injection.

Start A/AAROM program to level of comfort along these guidelines:

- For 2 to 3 days, out 3 to 5 X/day for motion program (ECU taped)
- For next 2 to 3 days, out 6 to 8 X/day for motion program (ECU taped)
- For next 2 to 3 days, out 10 to 12 X/day for motion program (ECU taped)
- For next 2 to 3 days, out 13 to 15 X/day for motion program (ECU taped)

If motion exceeds 75%, may consider starting strengthening program. If at any time during motion recovery phase that symptoms dictate, injection could be considered; typically place in immobilization for 3 to 5 days postinjection, then resume motion recovery protocol.

Strength recovery phase: With ECU taped or splinted (Arnold Palmer–type splint), may commence strength recovery phase as directed by player experience and in collaboration with medical/training staff. When strength exceeds 75%, may start sports-specific preparation.

Sports-specific preparation phase (baseball): Obviously, this phase is largely conducted under the purview of the team's medical/training/coaching staff. In our experience, progression through the following stages has allowed appropriate monitoring and focus for this injury:

- Dry swinging with light or fungo bat
- Tee work
- Soft toss
- Cage BP @ 50% to 75% to 100%
- Field BP @ 50% to 75% to 100%
- Rehab assignment per individual team and player

RETURN TO PLAY

Individual decisions on return to play are the complete purview of the player's team. In our experience, the following guidelines can be useful in developing milestones and targets for resumption of elite level play at the Major League Baseball (MLB) level. Typically, even players in whom symptoms have not completely resolved can return in-season to safe and effective play—in that subset, end-of-season reconstruction (see subsequent sections) remains compatible with completion of the entire rehabilitation protocol so that participation in training camp can be accomplished.

- Mild: 25% of players typically return between 2 and 3 weeks, 50% between 3 and 4 weeks, and the remaining 25% after 4 weeks
- Moderate: 25% of players typically return between 3 and 4 weeks, 50% between 4 and 6 weeks, and the remaining 25% after 6 weeks
- Severe: 25% of players typically return between 4 and 6 weeks, 50% between 6 and 8 weeks, and the remaining 25% after 8 weeks

NB. There are a subset of players who have newly developed tendon subluxation after embarrassment of the ECU investments and remain relatively asymptomatic. These players can typically return to elite level play with taping safely and effectively, requiring symptom monitoring only.

Surgical Treatment of Extensor Carpi Ulnaris–Related Pathology: The "Modified Combined" Repair

The reasons we are comfortable recommending nonoperative treatment for problems of the ECU and its investments is that the same form of reconstructive surgery that we perform for acute cases is the same as we perform for remote cases. Stated alternatively, primary repair of the sheath, subsheath, or *linea jugata* is extremely unlikely, so some form of reconstruction and augmentation with a retinacular flap is usually likely for cases of ECU problems, especially tendon subluxation.

Almost every form of reconstruction described features a radially based retinacular flap that either is advanced over the ECU and secured on the ulnar aspect of the sulcus or creates a sling enveloping the tendon and also creating a barrier underneath the tendon, excluding it from the sulcus, which most authors advocate deepening to prevent subluxation.[17-21] There have even been authors who have advocated simple release and bone resection from the ulnar sulcus—I fear that this may not be applicable in a majority of elite athletes and would "burn a bridge" for later definitive reconstruction.[22]

I have several reasons why this was always somewhat illogical to me and why I have been performing a "modified combined" procedure for well over a dozen years now consisting of 3 basic components: (1) labral repair/reinforcement, (2) advancement of an ulnar-based flap of extensor retinaculum, and (3) "contouring" (not necessarily deepening) the ulnar sulcus.

First, I have already provided extreme focus on the unique architecture of the ulnar leaf of the subsheath. The stoutest portion, that which is longitudinally reinforced by the *linea jugata*, is almost always present and robust enough to accept sutures. I believe that this is the primary barrier to ulnarward subluxation of the ECU tendon under contractile force.

Second, I have described the anatomy and favorable mechanics of the extensor retinaculum, particularly, its resilience to mechanical failure. Personally, I have never seen a primary failure of this tissue (salvage after previous surgery will be discussed subsequently). This is completely compatible with the biomechanical studies quoted.[23] Therefore, I decidedly recommend against sectioning the lone tissue that is essentially intact. Furthermore, the strong septae, especially that between compartments 4 and 5, provides an excellent anchor when securing the radially advanced tissue.

Lastly, I certainly understand the intellectual appeal of simply deepening the ulnar sulcus to "capture" the ECU tendon and theoretically prevent recurrent subluxation after surgery. However, on too many occasions, I have seen 2 resulting problems: (1) if the ulnar buttress of the labrum and secure retinaculum is not reestablished in the presence of a deepened sulcus, the tendon actually has a greater proclivity to subluxate and "perch" on the ulnar lip of the deepened groove; this causes even more intrinsic tendon damage than originally was being experienced with the index pathology, and (2) weakening of the bone in the ulnar sulcus region where additional manipulation (such as placement of suture anchors) has been performed to advance a radially based flap—anything from soft tissue failure to rim fracture ensures and the entire reconstruction fails catastrophically.

Technique of the "Modified-Combined" Reconstruction

The accompanying figures (Figure 13.9B-D) tell a much more vivid story than I can project in words, but I shall summarize the key components in a checklist or "inventory" here:

- Carefully elevate an ulnar-based flap of retinaculum with its proximal extent where the transverse fibers can first be discerned and its distal
- Extent just at or slightly distal to the ulnar styloid. Importantly, I take the flap to include the healthy portion of the 4,5 septum (and of course, the 5,6 septum). This retinacular layer exposes the subsheath, which should not be disturbed at this time
- Inspect the subsheath to determine its status; typically, only the thicker region as it approaches the ulnar-sided labral attachment will be intact and useful for repair. Be sure to appreciate how the subsheath has been "delaminated" from the ulnar wall of the sulcus
- Appreciate the status of the ECU tendon itself, especially in comparison with the extensor digiti quinti proprius (EDQP) tendon that you have now exposed. Record photographically and/or in your operative note the intrinsic status of the tendon
- "Recontour" the ulnar wall of the sulcus. This is in contradistinction to deepening the concavity of the sulcus, which also creates a roughened surface against which the ECU would abrade. This creates a flatter, exposed region to which a combination of the labrum and the advanced retinaculum can be secured with a suture anchor
- Advance the ulnar-based retinacular flap radially. The amount of tensioning is dependent on individual anatomy, but the stout 4,5 septum allows flexibility to secure the flap to soft tissue or even to the radius through suture anchors. In a minority of cases, I have excluded the EDQP from its native location, electing instead to advance the flap underneath the tendon; I leave a generous amount of retinaculum distally, so this has never created a problem
- In cases where the EDQP has been relocated anatomically, I suture the proximal and distal edges of the advanced flap to local tissue

Typical Rehabilitation Plan After Modified-Combined Repair

- First 2 weeks: Maintain operative dressing (I use a "long" short-arm splint to about the maximum girth of the forearm)
  - Work on digital motion *ad lib*
  - Limited pronation/supination is permitted by splint to level of comfort

- At 2 weeks: Remove sutures, begin **motion recovery phase**
  - Fashion custom "long short-arm" splint
  - May begin A/AAROM program
  - For wrist flexion (F)/extension (E): Accelerate in this plane
    - Start with 20E/20F for 3 to 4 days
    - Then 30E-30F for 3 to 4 days
    - Then 40E-40F for 3 to 4 days
    - Then 50E-50F for 3 to 4 days
    - Then 60E-60F for 3 to 4 days
  - For pronation (P)/supination (S), follow similar plan
    - Start with 20P/20S for 3 to 4 days
    - Then 30P-30S for 3 to 4 days
    - Then 40P-40S for 3 to 4 days
    - Then 50P-50S for 3 to 4 days
    - Then 60P-60S for 3 to 4 days
- Next milestone is **strength recovery phase**, typically begun when motion exceeds 75% of normal/contralateral (collaboration with team)
- Next milestone is **sports-specific recovery phase**, typically begun when strength exceeds 75% of normal/contralateral (collaboration with team)
  - Wrist taping may be considered for comfort and support in practice and competition

Projected return to play is approximately 4 months, but if the reconstruction is performed at the end of the season, a slightly protracted rehabilitation can be favored before the start of spring training the following season. In our experience, 25% of athletes return between weeks 10 and 12, 50% return between weeks 12 and 16, and the remaining quarter resume play after week 16.

The catastrophic failure of the radially based flap approach lead me to develop a salvage procedure with which I have had success in returning players back to Major League competition. I have not elected to perform this reconstruction primarily, but having it in one's armamentarium if key tissues are found to be embarrassed prepares the surgeon for a variety of eventualities (Figure 13.10A and B).

In this salvage approach, a free tendon graft (*palmaris longus*, if available) is utilized to create both a buttress to ulnar subluxation of the tendon and also an investment of the tendon that provides volar and dorsal protection while allowing longitudinal excursion (Figure 13.10C and D). Slight variation of the technique can be elected intraoperatively depending on the surgeon's determination of the "environment in which he or she desires the tendon to reside"; protection from possible attrition on the osseous ulna can be affected by enveloping the ECU in tendon graft versus securing it in a more intimate position with the sulcus.

The rehabilitation times are usually lengthened by 10% to 25% in these salvage situations, but the repair is very sturdy and can be trusted through the rehabilitation phases once healed.

GENERAL COMPLICATIONS

Aside from the surgical complication profile we all accept, when performing open procedures, I should like to simply underscore 2 pertinent issues. First, the judicious initial surgical handling of the dorsal sensory branch of the ulnar nerve is important. The branch should cross the axial midline roughly at the midpoint between the ulnar styloid and the fifth metacarpal base, but this is variable. In almost all cases, I locate it and make sure it is both protected and in anatomic continuity at the terminus of the case.

The second complication is one I have seen about half a dozen times in over 2 decades of care of elite athletes—rupture of the ECU tendon. The etiology could have been attrition, weakening from chronic inflammation or the use of performance-enhancing substances or some iatrogenic manipulation (injection or surgical) (Figure 13.11). Regardless, I should close this chapter by relating that many of these turned to play at the highest levels. In most, not all, I have formally resected the tendon ends and "pseudotendon" that seems to bother players, who describe a "pulling" sensation.[24] The ability of these athletes to compensate is remarkable; although there must be weakness, by definition when you lose the influence of an important muscle, this is overcome by swing changes and other rehabilitation/strengthening techniques.[25]

Loss of the ECU does not necessarily translate into a career-ending event, but counseling and flexibility in approaching the craft of hitting will be required to regain playing status.

Manager's Tips

- Much has been learned about pathologies of the ECU and its investments in the last decade; it behooves the hand and wrist consultant to a baseball organization to have a refreshed understanding of this region with which many players will have problems
- Despite what appears to be significant initial injuries, a trial of nonoperative treatment is logical in many circumstances

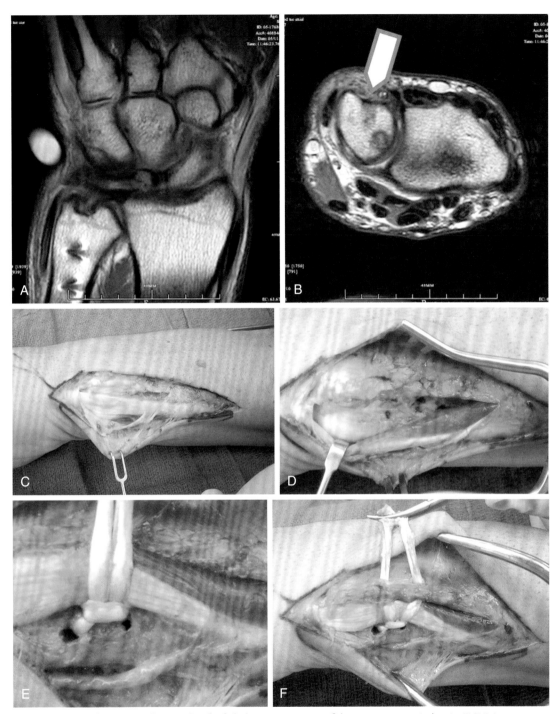

FIGURE 13.10 • This is a vivid example of a failed reconstruction of the extensor carpi ulnaris (ECU) investments (subsheath and retinaculum). In both (A) and (B), the ECU is clearly completely out of the ulnar sulcus. The arrow points to the "empty" sulcus. C, The intraoperative photo demonstrates the failure of the ECU stabilization procedure at approximately 8 weeks postoperative. The (green) sutures are easily seen. The reconstruction site is prepared by debriding the embarrassed tissues (D), then the ulna is drilled through and through, and then the tendon graft is looped to stabilize the ECU in the sulcus, which has been carefully recontoured (E). F, The tendon graft is secured by weaving it into the interseptal tissue or retinacular border. Careful tensioning allows sliding of the tendon while still securing it in the sulcus.

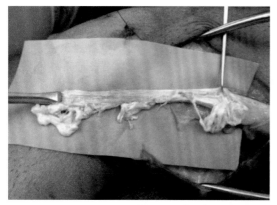

FIGURE 13.11 • A spectacular example of a rupture of the extensor carpi ulnaris (ECU) tendon. Potential contributors to this particular case included multiple steroid injections and even the potential use of performance-enhancing substances.

- The role of the ECU subsheath in native stability and reconstruction is critical, and it should be maintained or reconstructed
- Instability does not always result from a loss of anatomic continuity or rupture of the subsheath—instead, it is often "delaminated" or "peeled off" the ulnar wall of the ECU sulcus
- Understanding the anatomy and reconstructive utility of the ECU subsheath versus the extensor retinaculum is imperative

CONCLUSIONS

The number of potential pathologies of the wrist in the baseball player is abundant. I simply did not elect to cover vast topics such as distal radius fractures and Kienböck disease—both of which I have seen in MLB players. Instead, I tried to take the reader on a tour of my 2-plus decade career as a team physician and hand surgery consultant to MLB.

For many of us, baseball has been the ideal "laboratory" to learn and hone our craft. The volume and variety of pathology and the unique pace of the game have allowed us to learn so many things that we have now brought to the "everyday" practice of hand surgery. When you have highly motivated, extraordinary physical specimens backed by every possible resource, one can learn a great deal about the limits of our treatments to restore 100th percentile function to players and nonathletes alike.

Despite some progress in which we have participated, this is a dynamic field. We need to study more, exchange more, publish more, and learn more. I credit the editors and coauthors for stimulating that among this community of physicians who hold so much exceptional knowledge.

REFERENCES

1. Graham TJ, Mullen DJ. Athletic injuries of the adult hand. In: DeLee JC, Drez D Jr, Miller MD, eds. *DeLee and Drez's Orthopaedic Sports Medicine: Principles and Practice.* 2nd ed. Philadelphia, PA: Saunders; 2003:1381-1441.

2. Graham TJ. Problems about the distal end of the ulna. *Hand Clin.* 1998;14(2):155-330.

3. Graham TJ. Treatment of ECU injuries in professional baseball players. *Hand Clin.* 2012;28(3):357.

4. Graham TJ. Pathologies of the extensor carpi ulnaris (ECU) tendon and its investments in the athlete. *Hand Clin.* 2012;28:345-356.

5. Nuber GW, McCarthy WJ, Yau JS, Schafer MF, Suker JR. Arterial abnormalities of the athletes, *Am J Sports Med.* 1990;18(5):520-523.

6. Ginn TA, Smith AM, Snyder JR, Koman LA, Smith BP, Rishing J. Vascular changes of the hand in professional baseball players with an emphasis on digital ischemia in catchers. *J Bone Joint Surg Am.* 2005;87(7):1464-1469.

7. Parker RD, Berkowitz MS, Brahms MA, Bohl WR. Hook of the hamate fractures in athletes. *Am J Sports Med.* 1986;14(6):517-523.

8. Graham TJ. Perspective on scapholunate ligament injuries in baseball players. *Hand Clin.* 2012;28(3):261-264.

9. Grewal R, Faber KJ, Graham TJ, Rettig LA. Wrist and hand injuries: the diagnosis and management of ulnar wrist injuries in the athlete. In: Kibler WB, ed. *Orthopaedic Knowledge Update: Sports Medicine.* 4th ed. Rosemont, IL: American Academy of Orthopaedic Surgeons; 2009:69-80 [chapter 6].

10. Spangler JR, Bamberger HB, Graham TJ. Midcarpal impingement: a cause of ulnar-sided wrist pain in batters. *Abstract Amer Osteopath Acad Ortho.* 2013. Available at: http://meetings.aoao.org/meetings/annual/2013/posters/EPO11_Midcarpal_Impingement_A_Cause_of_Ulnar_sided_Wrist_Pain_in_Batters_Spangler-Jason.pdf

11. Kamal RN, Rainbow MJ, Akelman E, Crisco JJ. In vivo triquetrum-hamate kinematics through a simulated hammering task wrist motion. *J Bone Joint Surg.* 2012;94(385):1-7.

12. McLean J, Bain G, Eames M, Fogg Q, Pourgiezis N. An anatomic study of the triquetrum-hamate joint. *J Hand Surg.* 2006;31A:601-607.

13. Moritomo H, Goto A, Sato Y, Sugamoto K, Murase T, Yoshikawa H. The triquetrum-hamate joint: an anatomic and in vivo three-dimensional kinematic study. *J Hand Surg.* 2003;28A:797-805.

14. Feldon P, Terrono AL, Belsky MR. The "wafer" procedure: partial distal ulnar resection. *Clin Orthop Relat Res.* 1992(275):124-129.

15. Jeantroux J, Becce F, Guerini H, Montalvan B, Le Viet D, Drapé JL. Athletic injuries of the extensor carpi ulnaris subsheath: MRI findings and utility of gadolinium-enhanced fat-saturated T1-weighted sequences with wrist pronation and supination. *Eur Radiol.* 2011;21(1):160-166.

16. MacLennan AJ, Nemechek NM, Waitayawinyu T, et al. Diagnosis and anatomic reconstruction of extensor carpi ulnaris subluxation. *J Hand Surg.* 2008;33A:59-64.

17. Vulpius J. Habitual dislocation of the extensor carpi unlnaris tendon. *Acta Orthop Scand.* 1964;34:105-108.

18. Eckhardt WA, Palmer AK. Recurrent dislocation of extensor carpi ulnaris tendon. *J Hand Surg Am.* 1981;6(6):629-631.

19. Burkhart SS, Wood MB, Linscheid RL. Posttraumatic recurrent subluxation of the extensor carpi ulnaris tendon. *J Hand Surg Am.* 1982;7(1):1-3.

20. Rayan GM. Recurrent dislocation of the extensor carpi ulnaris in athletes. *Am J Sports Med.* 1983;11(3):183-184.

21. Rowland SA. Acute traumatic subluxation of the extensor carpi ulnaris tendon at the wrist. *J Hand Surg Am.* 1986;11(6):809-811.

22. Oka Y, Handa A. Recurrent dislocation of the ECU tendon in a golf player: release of the extensor retinaculum and partial resection of the ulno-dorsal ridge of the ulnar head. *Hand Surg.* 2001;6(2):227-230.

23. Iwamoto A, Morris RP, Andersen C, et al. An anatomic and biomechanical study of wrist extensor retinaculum septa and tendon compartments. *J Hand Surg.* 2006;31A:896-903.

24. Kiyono Y, Nakatsuchi Y, Saitoh S. Ulnar-styloid nonunion and partial rupture of extensor carpi ulnaris tendon: two case reports and review of the literature. *J Orthop Trauma.* 2002;16(9):674-677.

25. Wang C, Gill TJ, Zarins B, Herndon JH. Extensor carpi ulnaris Tendon Rupture in an ice hockey player: a case report. *Am J Sports Med.* 2003;31(3):459-461.

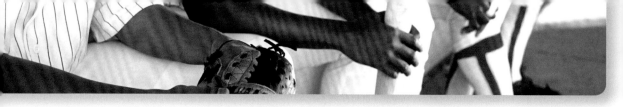

CHAPTER 14

Hand Injuries in Baseball

Joe Metz, MS, ATC, CSCS | Gary M. Lourie, MD

After I hit a home run I had a habit of running the bases with my head down. I figured the pitcher already felt bad enough without me showing him up rounding the bases.

—*Mickey Mantle*

INTRODUCTION

Injuries of the hand in baseball are common, complex, and unique to the game. If missed, they may result in significant morbidity to the player-athlete. Every facet of the game can place the hand at risk. The head first slide into second base, the violent swing of the bat, the foul tip striking the catcher's hand, and even the pitcher with an insignificant blister—all of these actions can result in morbidity. A recent MLB review of orthopedic injuries between 2010 and 2016 revealed the hand and wrist ranked third in frequency with only the shoulder and elbow listed higher (D'Angelo J. Unpublished MLB Data). Further analysis showed injury to the hand represented almost 10% of total days on the disabled list (DL), again ranking third to the shoulder and elbow (D'Angelo J. Unpublished MLB Data). Delay in diagnosis and treatment can have dramatic consequence not only in return to play but also in long-term morbidity. In 2016 the Atlanta Braves under the direction of Joe Metz, our Minor League coordinator, instituted a new protocol regarding early treatment of hamate hook fractures. These data were compared with the senior author's referred cohort of athletes with this injury. With heightened awareness, the Atlanta Braves hamate injury averaged only a 1- to 2-day delay in diagnosis, and with expedient surgery, return to play averaged 7.2 weeks. This compares favorably when matched with the outside cohort in which delay in diagnosis averaged 6.2 weeks, while return to play averaged up to 18 weeks owing to failure to institute treatment in a timely basis. Clearly accurate diagnosis with expedient treatment provides the best optimal chance for early return to play with minimal risk. The goal of this chapter is to provide a discussion of hand injuries in baseball, emphasizing, documenting, and describing the injuries particular to this game. Pertinent anatomy, mechanism of injury, clinical diagnosis, and radiographic imaging, along with treatment to allow early return to play with minimal risk, will be highlighted. The continued importance of a team approach including the athletic trainer, the physical therapist, and other health care personnel will be emphasized. Ligament, tendon, bone, nerve, vascular, and soft tissue will be covered. Injuries located from the tip of the finger to the base of the metacarpal will be covered with the wrist discussed in chapter 13 (Table 14.1).

DISTAL TIP INJURIES (NAIL BED, SOFT TISSUE, DISTAL PHALANX FRACTURES)

A well-padded, sensate, and mobile distal tip of the finger is vital in the baseball player. Injury can result from the digit being struck by a line drive, a head first slide into the base, or even seemingly innocuous friction from the pitcher's necessary grip on the baseball. The clinical anatomy of this small, ostensibly insignificant organ is vital to the baseball.[1-4] The tip compromises the region distal to the distal interphalangeal joint (Figure 14.1). The flexor digitorum attaches to the base of the volar aspect of the distal phalanx, while the terminal tendon attaches to the dorsal aspect, with the former flexing and the latter extending the tip. The skin of the volar tip is richly innervated and anchored to the bone through multiple septae that allow for efficient pinch, vital to the pitcher. Equally important is the stability

TABLE 14.1 Hand Injuries Particular to Baseball

Distal Tip Injuries (Nail Bed, Fractures)

Soft tissue injuries
  Blisters
Bony injuries
  Bony mallet
Tendon injuries
  Jersey finger FDP avulsion (with and without fracture)
  Annular pulley (A4 rupture)
Ligament/joint injuries/soft tissue
  Thumb metacarpophalangeal ligament injuries
  Radial collateral ligament injuries index finger metacarpophalangeal (MP) joint
  Adductor jamming web space injury

Vascular Injuries in the Hand

Nerve injuries
  Injury posterior branch medial antebrachial cutaneous nerve UCL reconstruction
  Dynamic nerve compression in the elbow of the pitcher
  Ulnar nerve dysfunction in excision of the hook of the hamate
  Superficial radial nerve injury in thumb RCL MP injuries
  Perineural fibrosis (Bowler's Thumb)

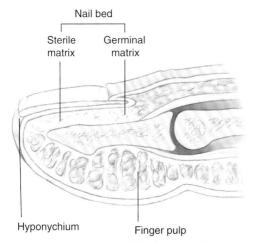

FIGURE 14.1 ⚬ Anatomy of the distal tip of the digit.

provided by the dorsum of the tip, housed by the nail bed, secured by the nail plate comprising the germinal and sterile matrix, and anchored by the nail folds at each periphery.[2] Injury to this essential structure can be the result of blunt axial force seen with a head first slide or being struck by a pitch or hard hit ground ball. Hyperflexion of the digit can result in extensor tendon rupture (mallet injury); however, an extensor force subjected to the flexed digit, as seen when caught in a jersey, can result in rupture of the flexor digitorum profundus (FDP) (jersey finger). The injury can be complex and involve some or all parts of this specialized structure. Failure to assess and treat all components may produce a dystrophic stiff painful digit.

FLEXOR DIGITORUM PROFUNDUS AVULSION (JERSEY FINGER)

The FDP is the deeper of the 2 flexors in the digit, attaching to the distal phalanx and producing flexion, vital to grasp. For the pitcher, as well as the batter, its intact function is crucial. The mechanism of injury and hence its name "jersey finger" occurs commonly when the flexed finger is caught in a jersey and the extension force ruptures the tendon. Grabbing the base in a steal attempt or being caught in a chain link fence or a catcher's mask will affect the same result. The ring finger is the most common digit involved. The player will be unable to flex the distal interphalangeal joint. Often ecchymosis will be present on the volar tip and digit. It is important not only to obtain an accurate history but also to assess for flexion at the distal joint. Failure will result in delay of treatment and adversely affect outcome. The classification by Leddy demonstrates the need for expedient diagnosis.[5,6] The injury can be designated into 4 types. In the type I presentation, the flexor is torn and retracts into the palm and, without vascular and synovial nutrition, must be repaired within 7 to 10 days. In the type II injury, the flexor retracts to the proximal interphalangeal joint and, with retained synovial nutrition present, can be repaired in up to 6 to 8 weeks. In the type III injury, the flexor remains at the distal interphalangeal attached to a piece of bone and can be repaired up to 8 weeks. Type IV can be complex, as there is a piece of bone similar to

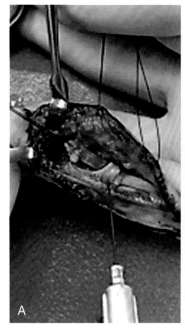
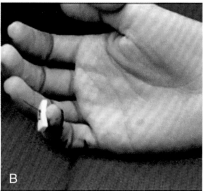

FIGURE 14.2 • A, Rupture of the flexor digitorum profindus, the placed suture in the tendon. B, Repair of the flexor digitorum profundus, the tendon secured by a button.

type III, but on exploration the tendon has torn from the bone and retracted to the palm, signifying the need for early repair. Expedient assessment and referral by the trainer allows for proper treatment and successful return to baseball. Successful repair with a supervised rehabilitation program allows full return at 4 to 6 months. The retention of independent flexion at this joint is imperative for the baseball player, and although there are reconstructive procedures for missed injury, prompt diagnosis with heightened awareness of the morbidity of the missed injury provides the best outcome (Figure 14.2).

ANNULAR PULLEY INJURIES

The annular pulleys serve an important role in tendon function, and injury can result loss of motion, dexterity, and power. Found on the volar surface of the finger, the pulleys are fibrous bands that overlay the synovial flexor tendon sheath and function to keep the tendons close to the bone and help in the transfer of linear force of muscle contraction into an efficient flexion moment at the joints.[7] There are 5 annular pulleys, 3 cruciate pulleys, and the palmar aponeurotic pulley. The odd-numbered pulleys (A1, A3, A5) are found at the metacarpophalangeal (MP) joint, the proximal interphalangeal (PIP) joint, and the distal interphalangeal (DIP) joint, respectively.[7] The A2 and A4 pulleys are located over the proximal

and middle phalanges; their prime role is preventing bowstringing and optimizing flexion force. Their injury can have pronounced morbidity if not treated in an expedient manner.

Closed traumatic rupture of the annular pulley has been reported in the rock climber where recommended grips place the digits in adverse positions of eccentric force predisposing to injury. Typically, the injury in the climber occurs during a difficult passage and a sudden force is directed to the digit exceeding physiologic limits. The diagnosis of rupture can be made clinically if bowstringing is present, which usually signifies multiple pulley rupture. In more subtle cases (ie, single pulley), localized palmar tenderness, swelling, and pain against flexion resistance confirm injury. The ring finger is the most common digit affected, while A2 is the most frequently injured pulley followed by the combined A2 and A4 presentation. Treatment is dependent on the extent of involvement, and a useful classification to dictate therapeutic guidelines is based on the number of pulleys injured. A single pulley injury can be treated conservatively, whereas multiple pulley disruption requires open reconstruction with a variety of techniques described, most using a tendon graft (Figure 14.3).

The senior author has described a unique presentation of pulley injury in the pitcher.[8] Our report described the presentation and treatment of 4 professional baseball pitchers with ruptures of the A4 pulley.

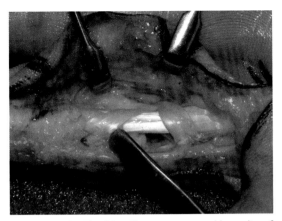

FIGURE 14.3 • The A2 pulley reconstructed by a slip of the superficialis tendon.

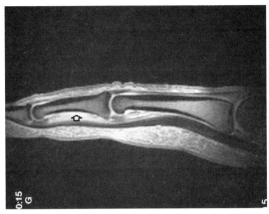

FIGURE 14.4 • MRI sagittal image showing tendon bone interval (TBI) >1 mm suggesting tear of pulley. The arrow represents the tendon displacement.

The history is prodromal soreness localized to the middle phalanx of the middle finger, usually seen with the fastball and experienced at release of the ball as the tip of the finger leaves the seams. Other pitches such as the curve do not aggravate the middle finger and are less prone to cause the injury, likely due to decreased stress placed on the tip of the middle finger with gripping the ball. The soreness culminates with a "pop," which signifies the rupture of the A4 pulley.

The pitcher will present with swelling, ecchymosis, and tenderness over the middle phalanx, often more over the lateral margins of the bone at the origin of the pulley. Weakness and pain with resisted flexion is present, but bowstringing is rarely present owing to the presence of 1 pulley injured. Radiographs are recommended to rule out fracture. Although computed tomography (CT) and ultrasound have been advocated to confirm diagnosis, magnetic resonance imaging (MRI) remains the gold standard. A tendon bone interval (TBI) > 1 mm of anterior displacement of the tendon from the volar surface of the bone on sagittal views is confirmatory of pulley rupture (Figure 14.4).

Once the diagnosis of pulley rupture is made, successful conservative treatment has been effective in returning the player to preinjury status. Initial management includes placement of an orthoplast pulley protector or taping full time for 2 weeks to achieve motion. Next long toss with the thumb and index finger gripping the ball is started. At 1 month, an interval throwing program is initiated with full return usually at 3 months, even though abbreviated protocols have seen earlier return since publication. The A4 isolated injury is unique to the baseball pitcher, and its awareness can avoid prolonged recovery.[8] Other pulleys, however, can be involved. Figure 14.5 shows an MLB player who sustained a combined A2 pulley and MP collateral ligament injury due to slippage of the bat requiring operative repair.

MALLET INJURY (DISTAL EXTENSOR TENDON WITH OR WITHOUT BONY DISRUPTION)

The injury in which the extensor tendon is disrupted from its attachment is termed the "mallet" injury. The extensor tendon that attaches to the dorsal aspect of the distal phalanx is responsible for its extension (Figure 14.1). Anatomic studies have shown that the distance between the insertion of the tendon and the origin of the nail bed is less than 2 mm.[9] This precarious location with minimal skin coverage explains the potential combined injury of these structures often seen. These accompanying injuries will be discussed subsequently.

The mechanism of injury in the mallet injury is forced flexion to the extended digit. In baseball this can occur with a head-first slide, an errant pitch striking the digit in the batter, or a mishandled hit by the nongloved hand seen on a bad hop. Often, this injury can occur with minimal trauma with the patient only later noticing a flexed position of the distal tip.[10,11] The examination reveals inability to extend the distal joint. The injury can be closed or open with skin disruption. It can involve the tendon or a bony fragment, which can dictate treatment. The initial evaluation should confirm the flexed position of the digit with inability to extend the distal joint. The clinician should also inspect the distal tip for laceration and/or involvement of the nail bed, as these injuries frequently involve soft tissue. Radiographs should be obtained to rule out fracture. If not present, the injury is termed a "tendinous mallet," and full-time splinting of the distal joint in extension

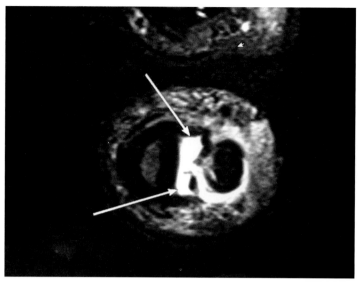

FIGURE 14.5 • MRI showing combined tear A2 pulley and collateral ligament. Both arrows represent rupture and interposition of the torn ends of the pulley.

for 6 weeks followed by nighttime splinting for 6 weeks will produce a satisfactory outcome.[12] The splint can be aluminum, commercial, or fabricated orthoplast, but it is important to educate the player on compliance. In cases in which the patient cannot tolerate a splint, placing an internal pin across the joint is a viable option, but this treatment would not be advocated in the baseball player owing to high risk of pin breakage.

If the radiographs reveal a fracture of the distal phalanx, the injury is termed a "bony mallet." Treatment is dependent on the percentage of bone involved. Historically, when the fragment involved more than 40% of the joint surface and/or subluxation is present, open operative stabilization was advocated. Many long-term studies have proven this treatment not only unnecessary but fraught with complications such as infection and stiffness.[11] Still in certain cases such as a large fragment untreated with late presentation, operative intervention with less invasive means may yield an excellent result.[13] The distal joint is splinted in extension for 4 to 6 weeks and the pin is removed when radiographs confirm bony healing (Figure 14.6A and B).

Early return to play with the mallet injury is dependent on the digit involved; the type of mallet, ie, tendinous versus bony; the position played; and the treatment that was instituted. These considerations must be weighed against future morbidity, ie, long-term stiffness, pain, or even posttraumatic arthritis. Playing with a mallet injury treated with pins can be fraught with complications and should be avoided. If pins were used, placement on the DL should be recommended. Playing with a splint, however, may be allowed, but the splint must be full

time and requires vigilance to ensure player compliance. Obviously, the digit involved and the position played dictate early return to play. In the dominant hand, especially the index or middle finger of a pitcher, it is not realistic to expect early return. However, a position player or designated hitter may be able to play in low-profile splint, but each case should be evaluated by the athletic trainer.

NAIL BED INJURIES/TIP TRAUMA

As stated, many injuries in baseball result from blunt trauma to the tip of the digit. The distal tip is the first portion of the upper extremity to engage in many aspects of baseball, making it prone to injury. An intact distal tip and nail plays a vital role by protecting the dorsal surface of the distal phalanx, maximizing pinch, and improving sensory perception and further has a cosmetic role. These characteristics are important in the pitcher, which relies on grip and sensory feedback, but can be just as important in fielding the ball and holding the bat. These injuries, therefore, often involve disruption, tip amputation, and laceration of the nail bed and plate, necessitating early recognition, treatment, and referral by the athletic trainer. Failure to recognize the coexistence of these injuries can result in significant morbidity and decreased athletic performance. The anatomy of this structure begins at the insertion of the FDP and the extensor tendon.[2] The nail complex can be separated into specific regions: the nail plate, nail bed, and the surrounding skin attachments including the eponychium (cuticle),

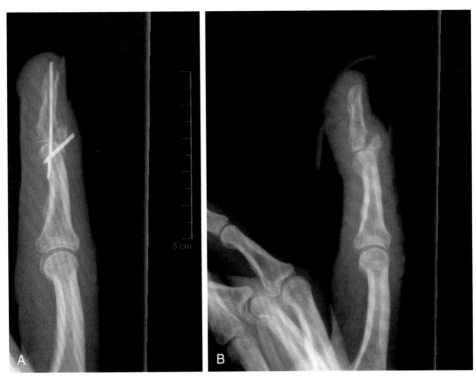

FIGURE 14.6 • A, Bony mallet secondary to extensor tendon disruption. B, Fixation achieved with K-wire fixation.

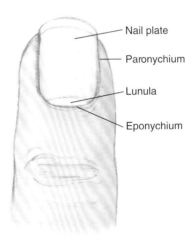

Nail plate

Paronychium

Lunula

Eponychium

FIGURE 14.7 • Anatomy of the nail, nail plate, and surrounding structures.

perionychium, and the hyponychium (Figure 14.7). The nail bed is divided into the germinal and sterile matrix; the germinal provides the cells to make the nail plate, while the sterile matrix adds thickness to the nail and allows for its adherence to the bed.[1] The lunula, which is present at the base of the bed and is "moon shaped," is the boundary between the germinal and sterile sites. The nail plate is composed of a hardened keratin substance that serves as a barrier to the bed and an efficient pivot point for pinch. The eponychium and the paronychium make up the proximal and lateral specialized areas of the skin that attach to the nail, while the hyponychium is located distally and with its thickened keratin helps secure the nail attachment. All these structures make up the dorsal aspect of the tip, while the volar pulp is composed of a richly innervated, firmly secured area of skin that with an intact dorsal nail complex provides stable pinch.

The mechanism of injury to this structure in baseball is multifactorial with crush, laceration, and avulsion all possible. Specific treatment protocols are outside the scope of this chapter, but general guidelines along with desired goals will be discussed. The goal of treatment in distal tip injury in the ballplayer is to maximize length while providing for a mobile, well-padded, and sensate tip.[14] It is our opinion that this goal should be achieved in the most expedient, well-planned manner that avoids prolonged time out of competition. Evaluation of an open injury requires knowledge of its mechanism followed by a thorough examination supplemented with radiograph. Initial bacterial cultures should be obtained of the open area, along with antibiotics including MRSA (methicillin-resistant *Staphylococcus aureus*) coverage if suspected. Thorough cleansing of the wound along with a sterile dressing should be done before referral.

Upon referral, the clinician should assess the structures injured, ie, the nail, the nail bed, the volar skin pulp and its loss, the surrounding skin, the bone involved and whether it is exposed, along with function of the tendons, and the neurovascular status. Each injured structure must be treated. After adequate anesthesia is obtained, usually through a digital block utilizing a local anesthetic, simple skin lacerations should be closed with fine suture. The nail bed should be addressed next. Debate exists over removal of the nail and repair of the nail bed laceration versus simple trephination, and the reader is advised to study the references included. If the decision is made to repair the nail bed laceration, fine absorbable suture should be used, and recent studies have advocated the use of skin adhesives to supplement the repair. Replacement of the nail or a commercial silastic strut has been advocated to protect the repair through the use of permeable soft gauze or nothing at all has yielded satisfactory results.[14] A recent study by the senior author has shown good results using type II bovine collagen to resurface loss of sterile matrix in complex injuries.[15] Fractures of the distal phalanx can be addressed in several ways. Simple comminuted but nondisplaced fragments often heal well with soft tissue treatment alone. Displaced fractures especially in the proximal to middle aspect of the bone may require pin fixation. Finally, when skin loss occurs either from crush or amputation, repair and reconstruction is often necessary to achieve the stated goals. The use of a classification for distal tip injuries can be useful and help in guiding treatment. We have found the Allen classification useful[16] (Figure 14.8). Type 1 involves loss of skin and soft tissue, usually volar, with no exposed bone and heals well with wound care. Full healing, depending on the size of the defect, occurs within 7 to 10 days, and early return to play depending on the digit involved and the position played can be considered during the healing phase. If the size of the defect is considerable (>50% of the pulp), a full-thickness skin graft, usually from the hypothenar eminence, provides a durable graft. Type 2 is designated by loss of skin including part of the nail bed but importantly no exposed bone. Treatment is similar to type 1 injuries including wound debridement, closure of lacerations, followed by healing by secondary intention versus skin grafting if the defect is large. The time to heal is 10 to 14 days, slightly longer than in type 1. The minimal loss of nail bed is usually inconsequential, but 2 situations deserve discussion. With nail bed loss, the added maceration may precipitate the formation of "proud flesh," more accurately called a pyogenic granuloma (Figure 14.9). This friable proliferative hemorrhagic mass is benign but should be recognized and responds well to silver nitrate topical treatment. In addition, nail bed loss is usually minor, but in certain cases where the defect may impair pinch

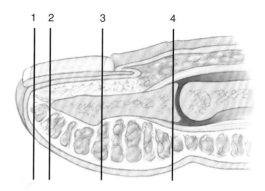

FIGURE 14.8 ● Allen classification distal tip/nail bed injury. 1, Injury involves skin and subcutaneous tissue only. 2, Injury involves skin, subcutaneous tissue and nailbed. 3, Injury involves skin, subcutaneous tissue, nailbed and bone but distal to the lunula. 4, Injury similar to #3 but proximal to the lunula.

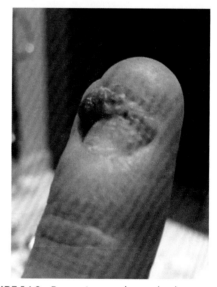

FIGURE 14.9 ● Pyogenic granuloma also known as "proud flesh."

such as in a pitcher, then reconstruction may be indicated. Split-thickness grafting for nail bed loss has been advocated; however, the senior author advocates the use of dermal allograft collagen in these instances[15] (Figure 14.10). In type 3 injuries, there is skin loss, exposed bone, and nail bed with the level of loss distal to the lunula, an important factor. Usually this level demands treatment, as coverage with supple skin can maintain useful motion and strength. It is beyond the scope of this chapter to recommend the specific flap or technique used, but the level and obliquity of the tissue loss helps to determine the choices. Included references serve as an excellent review.[2] More recent specialized flaps that rely on a specific blood vessel

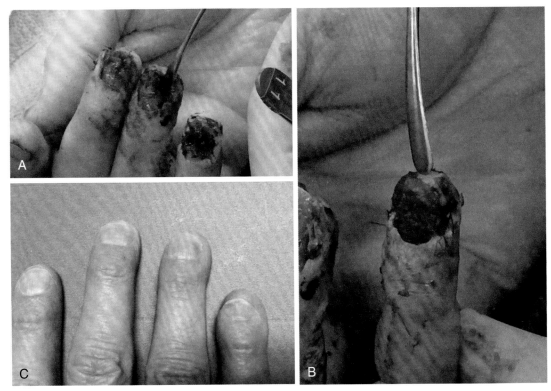

FIGURE 14.10 • A-C, Reconstruction of nail bed loss with dermal regenerate.

(homodigital) are available, but our treatment scheme is to learn these techniques and to strive to keep it simple and understand the player's innate ability to heal. An age-old principle is thorough debridement, and when needed, skin grafts and local flaps have worked well. A recent example is shown (Figure 14.11). In the type 4 injury, the level of loss includes skin loss, exposed bone, and nail bed with the tissue loss level proximal to the lunula, an injury that if repaired or reconstructed may yield a very short residual distal tip and phalanx. Many would advocate revision amputation; however, in the baseball player that relies on this joint, this may be disadvantageous; therefore, attempted replantation with or without vessel repair could be recommended. The specialized training in hand and microvascular surgery should be available to the medical staff. Again, the goals in all these distal tip injuries remain steadfast; thorough debridement of devitalized tissue along with coverage using healthy sensate skin by established means available is important.

One further injury pattern deserves recognition. In the pediatric skeletally immature population, the injury to the distal tip can often involve the fracture or trauma to the distal phalanx growth plate. Termed the "Seymour fracture," this injury can involve entrapment of the torn nail bed into the fracture defect and if unrecognized lead to impaired nail bed and plate growth and even worse osteomyelitis. Awareness and prompt recognition and treatment avoid these complications[17,18] (Figure 14.12).

FRICTION BLISTERS

In the normal population, a friction blister may be harmless with minimal aggravation. In the baseball pitcher, this can result in significant pain, prolonged healing, time on the DL, and even infection. In compiled MLB data reaching back to 2010, 6 players made up 7 stints on the DL adding up to 151 days out of baseball (D'Angelo J. Unpublished MLB data). This innocuous injury can be catastrophic in the professional pitcher. Much of the knowledge on the pertinent anatomy of the blister, the mechanism of injury, evaluation, and treatment come from the military literature.[19] Application of this knowledge in the pitcher is important to avoid mistreatment and prolonged recovery.

The anatomy of the friction blister involves the thickened epidermis found in the soles of the feet and volar tips of the digits. The epidermis in this area is more specialized being composed of the stratum corneum, the stratum lucidum, the stratum granulosum, and the deepest layer the stratum spinosum[20,21] (Figure 14.13). Rubbing models to simulate blister formation reveal a predictable series of events.[19] As the friction force (Ff) increases in cycles, the first manifestation

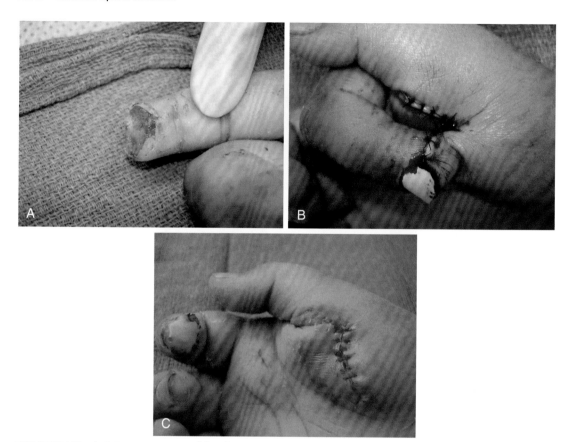

FIGURE 14.11 • A-C, Reconstruction of distal tip partial amputation with local flap and healing by secondary intention.

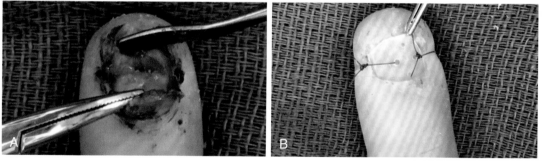

FIGURE 14.12 • A, Seymour fracture in which nail bed becomes entrapped in fracture. B, After extraction and repair.

is erythema at the point of rubbing. This is located at the stratum corneum and is referred to as a "hot spot" owing to the localized pain experienced by the player. With continued rubbing, the localized area becomes pale and elevated as the fluid blister develops. Studies performed on the blister show that the fluid pocket forms deeper, specifically the stratum spinosum with the roof of the blister composed of the intact stratum corneum and the stratum granulosum[19] (Figure 14.14). Contributing factors such as

the magnitude of forces and number of rubbing cycles applied have been studied to show that the higher the Ff, the less the cycles necessary to produce the blister. Moist skin increases the Ff, whereas dry or very wet skin decreases the Ff and lowers the chance of blister formation.[20,21]

This pathologic sequence of blister formation can be applied to the baseball pitcher.[20] Similar changes found in military recruits have been described in the pitcher where the digit meets the seams of the baseball. The transmitted forces disrupt the stratum spinosum where the fluid accumulates with the roof of the blister initially undisrupted.[20] Contributing factors such as moist skin rather than dry or wet along with higher ambient temperatures predispose to formation of the blister. In the pitcher the heightened Ffs seen where primarily the index and finger meet the seams of the baseball explain the incidence of these digits involved. The thumb is rarely involved owing to its function as a post unlike the index and middle, which transmit force to the ball to give it its "action."

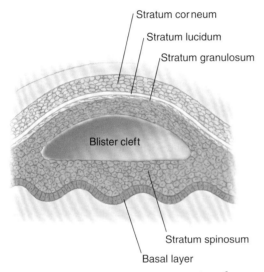

FIGURE 14.13 • Diagrammatic representation of blister formation.

Blister prevention in the high-level pitcher is of importance to avoid impaired performance. Data are scant, and many therapeutic methods are anecdotal and based on little scientific support, as evidenced by reports of pickle juice, superglue, and miscellaneous topicals, even urine to "toughen" the blister skin and prevent its development. The control of precipitating factors is important. Minimizing moisture and sweat with towels, rosin bags, and use of a rice bucket can help. Maintaining nail length and contouring are essential, as the nail protects the digital skin by "elevating" the ball from the skin and protecting it.[20] Proper contour with use of nail clippers and an emery board to avoid sharp edges prevents trauma. Similarly, proper maintenance of callus formation is imperative, as an enlarged callus will increase the Ff contacting the baseball seam.

Once the blister forms, expedient treatment can prevent prolonged morbidity. In a study by Cortese et al,[22] a model of blister formation was used to study the natural history of healing compared with treatment with and without blister debridement. Results showed that early preservation of the blister roof with careful drainage with a needle or surgical blade within the first 24 hours allowed for adherence of the top skin, resulting in the least discomfort as well as protection from secondary infection. Early removal of the roof, however, yielded the greatest discomfort, higher chance of infection, and prolonged morbidity. The Atlanta Braves treatment regimen follows the recommendations of McNamara et al[20] In contained blisters, early aspiration with a fine-tipped needle with retention of the blister roof is performed. The free-edge entrance

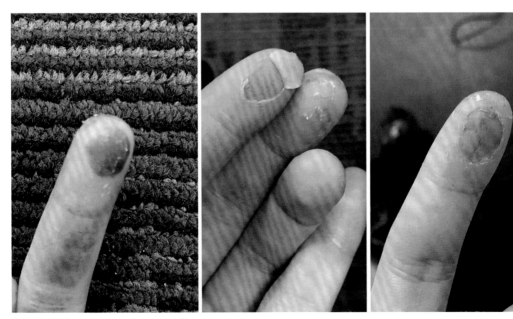

FIGURE 14.14 • Pitcher with early blister formation.

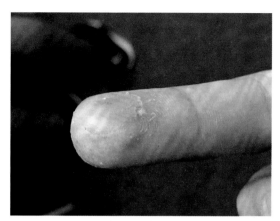

FIGURE 14.15 • Final stage of blister healing.

site can be secured with surgical glue adhesive, and the author often will add a small amount of zinc oxide as a skin barrier. In the small contained blister, this plan, in a starting pitcher, may prevent more than only 1 missed start. In the larger blister or one that has already separated, more treatment may be required. Loose devitalized tissue must be debrided with the raw bed treated with topical antibiotic for the first 5 days. Once early reepithelization forms, application of surgical adhesive or other agents such as benzoin tincture will help augment skin healing. Oral antibiotics are recommended only if secondary infection has developed. This more involved presentation leads to prolonged recovery and lost performance time often with placement of the pitcher on the DL (Figure 14.15).

THUMB METACARPOPHALANGEAL COLLATERAL LIGAMENT INJURY

The thumb MP joint is susceptible to injury in the baseball player. Any radial- or ulnar-directed stress can injure these ligaments and if not treated appropriately result in long-term instability, pain, arthritis, and impaired athletic performance. The head-first slide that traps the thumb on the base, the aggressive swing in which the bat slips into the thumb web space, the gloved thumb that is struck by a line drive or a fall to the ground, and the outfielder who falls into the wall with direct trauma to the thumb are only a few of the mechanisms that the ballplayer is subjected to in the game.

Understanding the anatomy of the thumb MP joint and distinct differences between the radial collateral ligament (RCL) and ulnar collateral ligament (UCL) is important in initiation of proper care in this injury.[22] The MP joint of the thumb shares anatomical

properties of both a condyloid and a ginglymus articulation, an advantage that allows for motion not only in flexion-extension but also in abduction-adduction and pronation-supination. Our data have confirmed variability of motion at the MP joint with these differences due to the sphericity of the metacarpal head, which predisposes to higher risk of injury.[22] Clearly this increased motion allows for better prehension, pinch, and overall function but does place the thumb, particularly this joint at risk for more injury.

The stability of the MP joint is based on bony support, ligaments, and intrinsic muscles, along with the capsule. The prime stabilizers, however, are the RCL and UCL. The proper portion, which is tight in maximal flexion, originates from the dorsal aspect of the metacarpal condyle and courses in an oblique volar direction to insert on the volar third of the proximal phalanx through a bony insertion. The accessory portion, tight in extension, arises more volarly on the metacarpal head and inserts into the volar plate and both the radial and ulnar sesamoid.[22] The volar plate, a fibrocartilaginous structure, forms the floor of the joint with further dynamic stability contributed by the intrinsic musculature. The adductor pollicis and the deep head of the flexor pollicis brevis (FPB) insert into the ulnar sesamoid, the adductor extensor aponeurosis, and the base of the proximal phalanx. The abductor pollicis brevis (APB) and the superficial head of the FPB insert into the radial sesamoid, the abductor extensor aponeurosis, and the base of the proximal phalanx.[22] There are important anatomical differences between the RCL and UCL that affect clinical presentation and treatment. The APB on the radial side is dorsal to the axis of the joint, completely covers the RCL, and courses parallel to the ligament. On the ulnar side, the adductor is more volar in its course, does not cover the UCL, and approaches the joint in a direction perpendicular to the joint. This is important clinically because when the UCL is torn off its distal insertion (most common), it can become displaced and entrapped outside the adductor aponeurosis (Stener lesion).[22] On the radial side, this finding is exceedingly rare, as the aponeurosis runs parallel, the ligament tears proximally, and in its midsubstance more commonly than distally, both factors that make a radial "Stener lesion" improbable.

ULNAR COLLATERAL LIGAMENT INJURIES THUMB MP JOINT

The incidence of UCL versus RCL injury favors the ulnar injury in a 2/3 to 1/3 ratio. The mechanism of injury in the thumb UCL injury involves a radial

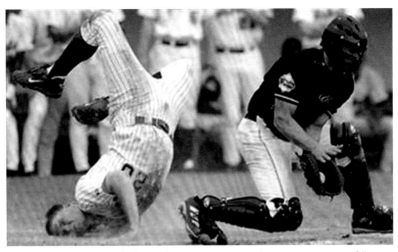

FIGURE 14.16 • The thumb metacarpophalangeal (MP) joint is at risk in many aspects of the game.

stress to the ulnar side of the joint, usually seen in an acute manner. In our experience, the head-first slide in which the thumb gets trapped by the leading edge of the base and a fall lunging for a line drive in which the thumb is driven into the ground (both gloved and nongloved hand) represent the 2 most common mechanisms (Figure 14.16).

The evaluation should include a history followed by examination assessing for tenderness and stability. Radiographs, if possible, should be taken before stability testing to determine if a fracture is present and avoid its iatrogenic displacement. If a player is seen in the first 24 hours after injury, it may be possible to palpate a Stener lesion, manifested as a distinct swelling proximal and superficial to the adductor aponeurosis and confirms a complete tear. Often the radiograph will show a small fragment of bone in the ulnar soft tissue signifying a Stener lesion (Figure 14.17). Without a fracture present, usual stability testing should be performed in maximal flexion and extension. Flexion testing assesses the proper portion of the UCL, whereas testing in extension, the accessory portion. It is important for the examiner to grasp the metacarpal head at the metaphyseal flare with the nondominant hand while placing a radial stress to the joint to avoid excess motion and inaccurate results. If the player is splinting from pain, injecting the joint with a local anesthetic from the radial side of the joint can allow for better stability testing. Further, extravasation felt on the ulnar subcutaneous region may confirm a complete tear. The author feels that greater than 35° of laxity in maximal flexion or greater than 15° compared with the uninjured side is indicative of a complete tear. The absence of an endpoint on testing further confirms a complete tear.

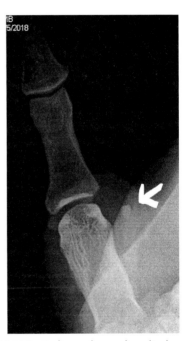

FIGURE 14.17 • Radiograph revealing displaced fleck of bone indicative of a Stener lesion. Arrow represents avulsed ligament with fleck of bone.

Diagnostic imaging should be performed; plain radiographs will rule out a fracture and allow for stress testing. We have recently observed that the morphology of the metacarpal head can dictate injury pattern and may have therapeutic advantages.[23] In comparing the sphericity of the metacarpal head, it is apparent that the square head has less motion and a higher incidence of a complete tear. The round head in our study was found to have less incidence of a complete tear; our hypothesis is that the increased motion "protects" the ligament with injury (Figure 14.18). Biomechanical

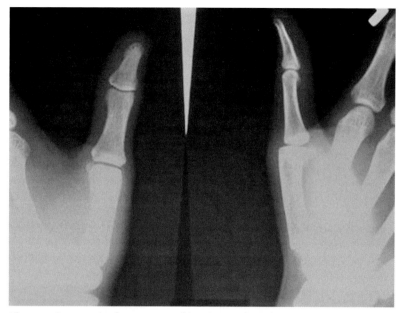

FIGURE 14.18 ◦ The round versus the flat metacarpal head may play role in injury.

testing in a load-to-failure model supported this observation, showing that the round head UCL elongated 3 times the distance before rupture when compared with the flat head.[23] Thenar strengthening with possible taping or prophylactic bracing may help protect the ballplayer with the at-risk square metacarpal head, especially when he reaches base and is attempting to steal. Advanced imaging such as MRI has been advocated routinely in the high-level ballplayer, although the author believes that a thorough examination can diagnose a complete tear. There are 2 instances where an MRI may help in dictating treatment. The scan may confirm a complete tear but not the presence of a Stener lesion and allow for conservative treatment. The second follows a recent publication that proposes an algorithm based on displacement of the ligament.[24] In their analysis, a complete tear less than 3 mm displaced from its insertion healed well with casting; however, displacement greater than 3 mm resulted in a poorer outcome with surgical repair recommended.[24] Once the ligament becomes interposed by the adductor, primary healing will not occur without extraction and operative repair. The incidence of the Stener lesion in a complete tear of the UCL is high, so the usefulness of this protocol may be limited.

The classification of these ligament injuries is that used in other joint afflictions. Grade I represents a stretch injury with conservative treatment successful, with full return at 2 to 3 weeks. Protective taping or bracing may be necessary up to 8 to 12 weeks. Grade II represents a partial tear with a firm endpoint. Treatment is similar to grade I, although prolonged

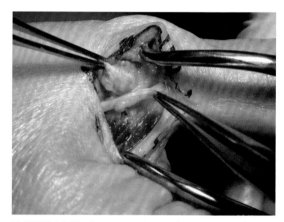

FIGURE 14.19 ◦ Intraoperative exploration revealing torn ulnar collateral ligament (UCL) and important anatomy.

return to play may be seen. Grade III represents a complete tear. As the incidence of an accompanying Stener lesion is high, our recommended treatment is almost universally operative repair.[22] Technical detail to extract the ruptured UCL from the interposed adductor aponeurosis, along with avoiding inadvertent damage to the distal medial branch of the superficial radial nerve (SRN), is important (Figure 14.19). We have instituted an accelerated postoperative protocol with initial immobilization for 3 to 4 weeks followed by protective splinting. Range of motion is begun at 4 weeks with the thumb placed in the palm to avoid stress to the repaired ligament. At 6 weeks, the thumb is brought out of the palm with passive motion and gentle strengthening initiated. Full return with

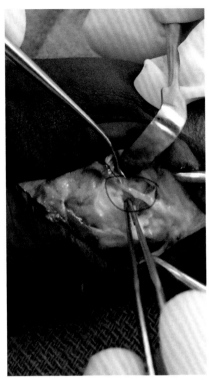

FIGURE 14.20 · Chronic thumb radial collateral ligament (RCL) metacarpophalangeal (MP) joint with osteophyte compressing superficial nerve.

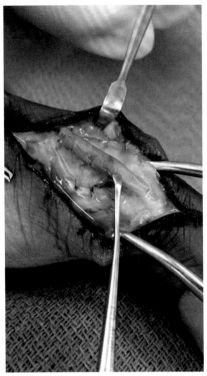

FIGURE 14.21 · Repaired thumb radial collateral ligament (RCL) metacarpophalangeal (MP) joint with excision of osteophyte and wrapping of nerve.

protective taping and low-profile bracing is allowed at approximately 8 weeks. In treatment of the grade III injury, it is advocated to perform early repair, as the UCL associated with a Stener component will often shorten and fibrose at this point making primary repair difficult.

Treatment of the thumb RCL injury is based on a similar grading system as its UCL counterpart with important differences. Grade I and grade II are the same. The grade III complete ligament tear is not associated with a Stener component owing to anatomical differences previously discussed. A case could be made, therefore, that a complete tear could be handled conservatively. We do advocate, however, that in the high-level baseball player this injury should be repaired. A recent report from our institution did describe a triad of clinical findings with partial RCL injury associated with osteophyte formation and entrapment of the distal lateral branch of the SRN (Dhulipala S. Lourie, GM. Submitted Publication) (Figure 14.20). In this series of baseball players, a chronic injury to the RCL healed with minimal instability associated with an osteophyte located at the distal dorsal radial aspect of the MC head. This spur was found to compress the distal lateral branch of the SRN, resulting in chronic pain and dysfunction. Recognition of the

neural entrapment in this scenario allows for better treatment. Preoperative anesthetic block of the nerve helps confirm the diagnosis. Successful return to play was achieved with addressing all 3 components: (1) treatment of RCL, usually "tightening" or plication is all necessary; (2) neurolysis of the lateral branch of the SRN in the area compressed by osteophytes with an extracellular matrix wrap to prevent rescarring; and (3) removal of the osteophyte (Figure 14.21). Recognition of these potential sequelae seen in this injury may prevent morbidity in the high-level baseball player.

RADIAL COLLATERAL LIGAMENT INJURY INDEX FINGER MP JOINT

An injury to the RCL of the index finger MP joint can often be missed and, like the neglected complete tear of the UCL of the thumb, result in pain, instability, and weakness. In the baseball player, this can have adverse consequences.[25] The anatomy of the RCL of the index finger MP joint is similar to that of the UCL of the thumb with both a proper and accessory component. An acute ulnar stress to the radial side of the index MP joint in the baseball player often seen in the errant slide or collision with the wall can impart

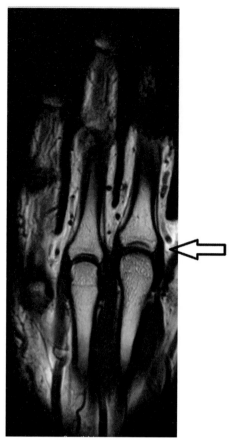

FIGURE 14.22 • Grade III index finger radial collateral ligament (RCL) metacarpophalangeal (MP) joint injury, similar consequences ulnar collateral ligament (UCL) thumb MP. Arrow represents partially torn ligament.

injury. The player will present with pain, tenderness, and ecchymosis over the radial aspect of the joint. In a publication from our institution, we reported on the significance of this injury if missed or undertreated.[25] Grade I to grade II injuries fared better in follow-up with initial splinting, even casting for 4 to 6 weeks to allow for optimal ligament healing and retention of important pinch and strength. It is imperative to assess for stability as a complete grade III tear, in the author's opinion, should be treated in the athlete with surgical repair much like the complete UCL injury in the thumb (Figure 14.22). Immobilization for 3 to 4 weeks followed by range of motion and strengthening allows for protected return at 6 to 8 weeks.[25] Chronic missed cases will lead to reduced motion of the index finger, pain, deformity, and weakness and may require reconstruction with tendon autograft to allow for return to play in the baseball player. As in most ligament injuries, early recognition of the injury in the acute state with prompt treatment minimizes morbidity.

ADDUCTOR POLLICIS JAMMING INJURY

A rare but potentially disabling injury that can be confused with the more common thumb MP ligament injury is the adductor pollicis jamming injury. This injury is unique to the baseball player and is imperative for the clinician to be aware of its existence. Altobelli et al published a case series that introduces and reviews this injury.[26] The adductor pollicis is a powerful muscle found in the thumb web space that arises off the metacarpals and attaches to the base of the proximal phalanx, the adductor aponeurosis, and the ulnar sesamoid. Its function is to produce strong adduction of the thumb, important in grip and pinch. The authors described the injury in which the butt of the bat was impacted into the web space during an eccentric contraction of the muscle. The top hand is usually involved. The injury pattern ranged from intramuscular strain to frank rupture at the tendinous insertion. The players presented with swelling and ecchymosis in the thumb web space along with weak adduction and pain with passive abduction. Collateral ligament testing was stable. Radiographs were negative and MRI scanning documented the type and severity of injury (Figure 14.23). Conservative treatment with rest, ice, compression, and edema control followed by custom splinting will be successful in the partial injury. In complete disruption, operative repair may allow better return to preinjury status. This injury may be underdiagnosed, and it is prudent for the athletic trainer and hand surgeon to be aware of its occurrence to prevent potential prolonged morbidity.

VASCULAR INJURY IN THE HAND

There are few sports other than baseball that place such a repetitive impact to the hand that blood vessel injury can occur. Publications report on this trauma and have been described in the gloved hand of the catcher, the hypothenar eminence of the hitter, and the tip of the finger in the pitcher.[27] The continued prevalence of tobacco use with its nicotinic vasospastic effects can further aggravate not only large (axillary) vessels but also small (ulnar artery) vessels and digital (microvascular) vessels too. This cumulative effect can result in significant morbidity; hence, it is important for the trainer to have a high index of suspicion for vascular injury when the player presents with symptoms as innocuous as an ulcer on the tip of the finger. Other manifestations such as cold intolerance, Raynaud's phenomenon, digital hypersensitivity, index finger

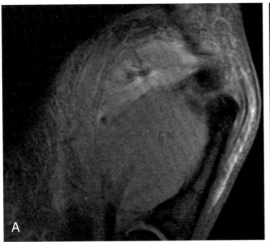
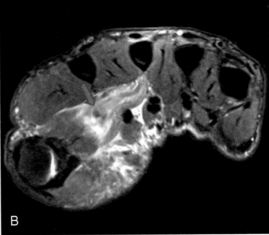

FIGURE 14.23 • Adductor jamming injury thumb web space MRI revealing extent of injury. All arrows represent the different presentations of adductor pollicis injury.

hypertrophy, fatigue, and heaviness of the arm deserve attention. Their recognition is crucial, as they may be harbingers of ensuing catastrophic trauma as seen, for example, in the pitcher presenting with acute thrombosis of the axillary artery, often a surgical emergency. Just as important is the knowledge that vessel trauma can exist at every level from the upper arm involving the axillary vessels to the fingertip involving the digital vessels. As commonly the existence of trauma at any level will result in clinical findings at the hand, this chapter will cover multilevel presentation.

In the pitcher the arm may be subjected to continued trauma by the position of abduction, external rotation, and extension. This repetition with time can compress the axillary artery and vein by the pectoralis muscles and the humeral head, which can produce thrombosis, embolism distal, or even aneurysm.[27,28] The pitcher will present with a spectrum of symptoms ranging from early fatigue, a sense of heaviness, cold intolerance, paresthesia, numbness, color changes ranging from cyanosis to ischemia, and often embolic phenomenon. On presentation, a detailed history is mandatory, including the temporal sequence of complaints along with the use of tobacco products, caffeine-related products, and sports drinks. These products can contribute to a vasospastic state and aggravate symptoms. Also, playing early in the season or in colder climates, especially at night, will often exacerbate the symptoms. The examination should include inspection of the upper extremity noting vascular findings such as ischemia, cyanosis, or presence of petechiae (Figure 14.24). Pulses should be assessed and compared with the asymptomatic contralateral side. Palpation for thrills in the axilla along with auscultation for bruits may indicate vascular intimal damage.

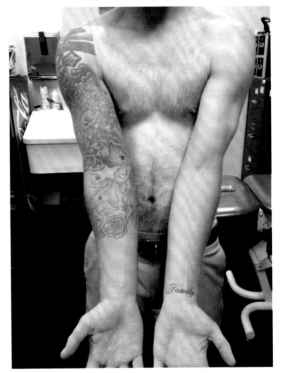

FIGURE 14.24 • Photograph swollen right upper extremity pitcher with axillary artery thrombosis.

Provocative testing such as the Adson test and the EAST (extension, abduction stress test) can help clarify the vascular insult and have been described, along with the shortcomings of these maneuvers.[27,28]

Standard radiographs should be obtained directly not only at the upper extremity but also at the cervical spine looking for a cervical rib and the chest if indicated. Advanced imaging may be necessary to document the extent and level of vessel injury. Noninvasive vascular studies measuring pressure can be carried out at standard levels in the upper extremity and used to compare with that of the uninjured. Computed ratios that can detect a possible structural problem are helpful. The gold standard, however, remains angiography, but less invasive methods such as MRI, which can include angiography and/or CT, can be used with adequate sensitivity and specificity.[27,28] Once the diagnosis of upper arm axillary vessel injury is made, a vascular consultation is recommended. Treatment protocols are beyond the scope of this chapter; however, anticoagulation by oral route, use of injected thrombolytic agents, angioplasty with or without stenting, and surgical resection with interposition grafting have all been advocated.[27] A recent protocol published by DiFelice et al advocates successful treatment in effort-related thrombosis of the axillary artery with initial transluminal catheter-directed thrombolysis, followed by first rib resection, and systemic anticoagulation for 3 months.[29] Our organization has adopted this protocol with similar success.

Hypothenar hammer syndrome in which repetitive trauma imparted by the butt of the bat to the bottom hand resulting in ulnar artery thrombosis has been described elsewhere in this textbook, specifically the hook of the hamate sequelae, and the reader is directed to that chapter. The clinician, however, must be vigilant; as in the axillary vessel injury, the ulnar artery injury too may manifest itself in the digits and thus be knowledgeable in the differential of digital vascular ischemic symptoms.

Repetitive trauma subjected to the hand, most commonly in the index finger of the gloved hand in the catcher and the pitching hand in the pitcher, is not uncommon. It is significant to note that structural changes in the small and microvessels of the hand have been documented even in asymptomatic players, highlighting the importance of the clinician to understand the significance of this repetitive trauma. Ginn et al, in investigating these deleterious effects on the microvascular level, evaluated 36 asymptomatic baseball players at the minor league level comparing catchers with outfielders, infielders, and pitchers.[30] Each player underwent history, examination, along with Doppler ultrasound, times Allen test, digital brachial indices, and ring sizing of the fingers. Although this was a small sample size, catchers compared with the other positions showed important findings. These findings are significant, especially when noted that no subjects reported significant pretesting complaints of ischemia, ie, cold intolerance, cyanosis, or ulcers. All advanced testing in the catcher showed decreased vascular supply to the ring finger in both the gloved and throwing hand. Furthermore, 7 of 9 catchers also showed hypertrophy of the index finger thought to be soft tissue overgrowth due to trauma.[30] The authors felt that better protective padding of the glove may help alter these changes. It is our experience with the Atlanta Braves that limiting nicotine and caffeine products can help alleviate the magnitudes of these symptoms. Clearly the fact that this study documented vascular changes in the asymptomatic player dictates increased vigilance necessary in all players, especially the catcher.

The pitcher is also at risk for vascular trauma at the small and microvascular level. More proximal causes such as axillary vessel trauma must be assessed; however, causes have been described at the digital level. Itoh et al reported a case series in which compression of digital vessels by thickened normal cutaneous ligaments (Cleland ligaments) in the finger and compression of palmar vessels by thickened palmar fascia in the palm resulted in ischemia, cold intolerance, and ulcer formation.[31] Each of the pitchers returned to preinjury play status with surgical release of the offending anatomical structures. In our pitchers with vasospastic symptoms involving the index or middle finger, once a true anatomic compressive structure is ruled out, successful alleviation of ischemic symptoms can be treated successfully with avoidance of nicotine and excessive caffeine products along with minimizing exposure to cold temperatures often seen early season. If this fails, empirical treatment with aspirin and vasodilators (if needed) can be used. In a limited number of our catchers seen with recalcitrant symptoms and failure to improve with conservative treatment, digital sympathectomy in which surgical stripping of the adventitia of the artery results in a permanent vasodilatory effect has been successful in curing ischemic symptoms.

In summary, the ballplayer seen with upper extremity ischemic symptoms should undergo a thorough history including exposure to nicotine and caffeine products. Recent use of energy booster drinks should be questioned owing to their high-caffeine content. A thorough examination of the upper extremity and cardiovascular assessment should be performed with specific attention to the axillary vessel in the pitcher. Similarly, the examination should target the hypothenar region and digits, especially the catcher who is at risk for more symptoms. Specific maneuvers on the examination including the Adson and Allen test are useful in locating the possible anatomic source of vascular compromise. Ancillary testing and vascular consultation may be necessary along with advanced imaging such as angiography. This coordinated approach along with rehabilitation and preventive support (protective padding, etc) offered by the athletic trainer is vital to returning the player to preinjury status and avoidance of prolonged morbidity.

NERVE INJURIES IN THE HAND

Symptoms of nerve compression and injury are not uncommon in the baseball player. More proximal etiology of these conditions can include the cervical spine, thoracic outlet region, axilla, elbow, forearm, and wrist and are discussed elsewhere in this text. There are, however, sequelae of soft tissue injury in the arm that may manifest themselves in the hand of the baseball player and require discussion. In addition, there are specific nerve conditions intrinsic to the hand in the ballplayer that the clinician and trainer should be aware of to allow for successful treatment.

Injury to the Posterior Branch Medial Antebrachial Cutaneous Nerve

Reconstruction of the UCL of the elbow in the high-level pitcher yields up to a greater than 90% success in return to play. There are adverse occurrences; injury to the posterior branch of the medial antebrachial cutaneous nerve can occur during operative exposure. Knowledge of its anatomy is imperative to avoid iatrogenic damage. Most commonly this nerve arises from the medial cord of the brachial plexus and in the distal arm divides into an anterior and posterior branch. An anatomic study performed at our institution revealed that the medial antebrachial cutaneous nerve becomes superficial to the fascia an average of 9 cm proximal to the medial epicondyle.[32] At approximately 6 cm proximal to the medial epicondyle, it splits into its anterior and posterior branch. From this point, the posterior branch runs most commonly posterior to the basilica vein and anterior to the medial intermuscular septum (Figure 14.25). It usually split into 1 to 4 branches at the level of the medial epicondyle providing cutaneous sensation to the posterior olecranon region. Iatrogenic damage to this nerve can result in a symptomatic neuroma, in some causing persistent dysesthesias and avoidance of placing the posterior elbow on any hard surface. In the pitcher recovering from UCL reconstruction, this can delay rehabilitation and impair recovery. With our study's findings in a pitcher seen with this neuroma, a subcutaneous block using a local anesthetic and corticosteroid approximately 6 cm proximal to the medial epicondyle, anterior to the medial intermuscular septum, and posterior to the basilica vein may be not only diagnostic in confirming injury but also therapeutic in alleviating symptoms.[32]

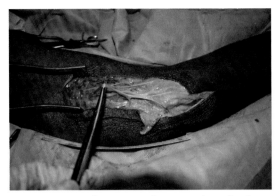

FIGURE 14.25 • Illustration of posterior branch of medial antebrachial cutaneous nerve.

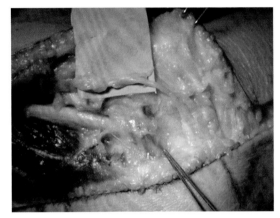

FIGURE 14.26 • Reconstruction neuroma posterior branch medial antebrachial cutaneous nerve.

Nerve desensitization techniques performed by the trainer may help in addition. If conservative treatment fails to lessen the neuroma symptoms, surgical exploration and transposition of the neuroma using the anatomic guidelines described by Tanaka and Lourie can help diminish the neuritic pain[32] (Figure 14.26).

Dynamic Nerve Compression Syndrome

Compressive peripheral neuropathies such as cubital and carpal syndrome have been well described. In the high-level athlete, especially the pitcher, awareness of a dynamic presentation due to anomalous or hypertrophied musculature is important. In these players, symptoms are rarely present at rest but with exertion may become present even disabling. In a preliminary study by the senior author, a case series of professional pitchers were treated with classic cubital symptoms, ie, numbness in the ring and small finger along with intrinsic weakness, not at rest but after 2 to 3 innings of pitching.[33] Drop in velocity and control was present. Pre- and postpitching intrinsic muscle testing of ulnar-innervated musculature showed profound

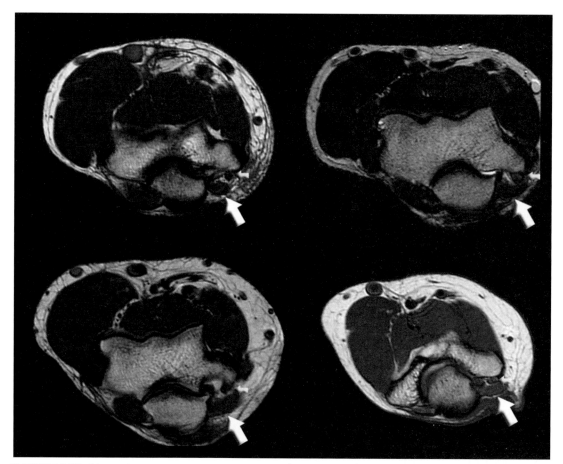

FIGURE 14.27 • Magnetic resonance imaging (MRI) revealing anconeus epitrochlearis muscle. All arrows represent different variations of anconeus epitrochlearis.

dynamic weakness. In addition, pre- and postexercise nerve conduction studies revealed consistent decrease in velocity and prolonged latency across the elbow after exercise. MRI revealed presence of an enlarged anconeus epitrochlearis, a rare accessory muscle found on the medial side of the elbow[33] (Figure 14.27). Excision of this muscle and decompression of the ulnar nerve resulted in return of velocity and control and restitution of preinjury status (Figure 14.28). In a larger series (7 cases), we have described this dynamic presentation in the high-level pitcher due to different muscles (VonBergen T. Lourie, GM. Submitted Publication). In addition to an anconeus epitrochlearis, in this series compression of the musculocutaneous nerve between the biceps and brachialis at the level of the elbow required, surgical decompression and 3 cases of dynamic compression of the posterior interosseous nerve (PIN) were described (Figure 14.29). The authors emphasize the importance of an accurate history confirming the dynamic presentation with examination to identify the nerve involved. Pre- and postexercise nerve studies will document the decreased

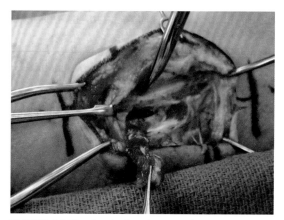

FIGURE 14.28 • Surgical exploration decompression ulnar nerve with planed excision anconeus.

nerve conduction velocity and prolonged latency and confirm the diagnosis. These syndromes are rarer than the established compressive neuropathies, but because of their potential morbidity in the pitcher, a heightened awareness of their presence by the trainer and clinician is important.

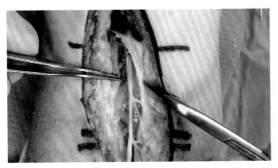

FIGURE 14.29 • Dynamic compression musculocutaneous nerve between 2 muscle arms.

Ulnar Nerve Dysfunction With Hook of Hamate Excision

Fractures of the hamate, specifically the hook, are rare in frequency in the general population seen in less than 1% with the scaphoid, triquetrum, and the trapezium more common. The baseball player, however, is more at risk for this fracture; usually the bottom hand where the butt of the bat impacts trauma to the hypothenar eminence resulting in its injury. The recommended treatment is excision with usual reported return to play at approximately 6 weeks. It is, however, our experience and that of others, specifically Bansal et al, that complications of this procedure do exist and not only may return take up to 8 to 10 weeks but also other adverse occurrences exist.[34] In a published cohort of 81 patients, there was a 25% incidence of complications with the majority being transient ulnar nerve dysfunction. The deep branch of the ulnar nerve courses perilously close to the hook, and it is imperative for the surgeon to identify and protect it to prevent its damage[34] (Figure 14.30). Even with attention to its presence transient, ulnar nerve dysfunction can still exist, and this should be discussed with the player.

Superficial Radial Nerve Dysfunction With Thumb MP Joint Injury

Injury to the thumb MP joint along with its diagnosis and treatment in the baseball player has been previously discussed with mention of the RCL and nerve association. We have recently described a series of ballplayers seen with injury to RCL associated with compression of the lateral branch of the SRN by a posttraumatic osteophyte at the metacarpal head. Anatomic cadaver studies confirmed its course, its closeness to the joint, and its innervation of the joint (Dhulipala S. Lourie, GM. Submitted Publication). It was postulated that the RCL may heal with overall stability, but microlaxity, with formation of a posttraumatic osteophyte, may compress the lateral branch of

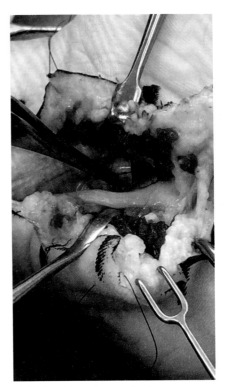

FIGURE 14.30 • Motor branch in close proximity to hook of hamate.

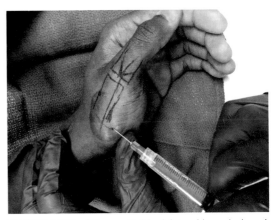

FIGURE 14.31 • Diagnostic block lateral branch dorsal radial sensory nerve.

the SRN causing persistent deep aching and weakness in pinch and prehension.[26] Diagnostic block proximal to the joint along the course of the lateral branch of the nerve confirms the nerve dysfunction syndrome (Figure 14.31). Often corticosteroid injection will "free" up the nerve and lessen the neuritic pain. If this is unsuccessful, operative intervention with plication of the RCL, neurolysis of the lateral branch of the SRN, and debridement of the osteophyte will allow return to preinjury play status[26] (Figure 14.32).

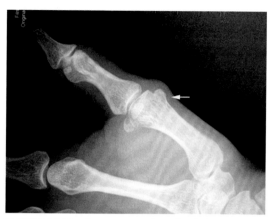

FIGURE 14.32 • Compression dorsal radial sensory nerve due to osteophyte (arrow) and ligament metacarpophalangeal (MP) injury.

Perineural Fibrosis (Bowler's Thumb)

In 1970 and 1972 Howell and Dobyns et al in 2 publications described the development of perineural fibrosis of the ulnar digital nerve in bowlers.[35,36] It was postulated that repetitive impact of the border of the hole of the ball on the ulnar aspect of the thumb causes fibrosis within and surrounding the nerve. This is manifested clinically by pain, sensitivity, and often dysesthesias within the distribution of the nerve. We have seen and treated hitters with this syndrome in which perineural fibrosis can also affect the ulnar digital nerve. The top hand is most commonly involved, and the mechanism is similar to the adductor jamming injury already described. Repetitive at bats, often aggravated by a check swing, result in impact trauma to the ulnar digital nerve. As seen in the bowler, perineural fibrosis can result. In our experience, a conservative approach including edema control, desensitization, and protective padding usually will be successful. Recurrent symptoms may occur, and judicious use of a corticosteroid injection can be used to decrease scarring, but care must be taken to avoid subcutaneous atrophy, a potential side effect of steroid injection. This could further aggravate the underlying condition. Rarely is surgery necessary; however, the senior author has, in limited cases, achieved resolution of neuritic pain with neurolysis and wrapping with an extracellular matrix tube.

MANAGER'S TIPS

- Hand injuries in the baseball players are specific and particular to the sport
- The hand is subjected to not only significant acute injury but also repetitive impact trauma

- The position played, the specific hand involved, and levels of play are just some of the many factors that can influence early return to play without undue risk
- It is imperative for the clinician to work closely with the training staff to best treat baseball players

REFERENCES

1. Peterson SL, Peterson EL, Wheatley MJ. Management of fingertip amputations. *J Hand Surg Am.* 2014;39:2093-2101.
2. Bickel KD, Dosanjh A. Fingertip reconstruction. *J Hand Surg.* 2008;33A:1417-1419.
3. Fehrenbacher V, Blackburn E. Nail bed injury. *J Hand Surg Am.* 2015;40:581-582.
4. Mignemi ME, Unruh KP, Lee DH. Controversies in the treatment of nail bed injuries. *J Hand Surg.* 2013;38A:1427-1430.
5. Leddy JP, Packer JW. Avulsion of the profundus tendon insertion in athletes. *J Hand Surg.* 1977;2(1):66-69.
6. Netscher DT, Badal JJ. Closed flexor tendon ruptures. *J Hand Surg Am.* 2014;39:2315-2323.
7. Marino JT, Lourie GM. Boutonniere and pulley rupture in elite athletes. *Hand Clin.* 2012;28:437-445.
8. Lourie GM, Hamby Z, Raasch WG, et al. Annular flexor pulley injuries in professional baseball pitchers. *Am J Sports Med.* 2011;39(2):421-424.
9. Cheah AE, Yao J. Hand fractures: indications, the tried and true and new innovations. *J Hand Surg Am.* 2016;41:712-722.
10. Lin JD, Strauch RJ. Closed soft tissue extensor mechanism injuries (mallet, boutonniere, and sagittal band). *J Hand Surg Am.* 2014;39:1005-1011.
11. Leinberry C. Mallet finger injuries. *J Hand Surg.* 2009;34A:1715-1717.
12. Altan E, Alp NB, Baser R, et al. Soft-tissue mallet injuries: a comparison of early and delayed treatment. *J Hand Surg Am.* 2014;39:1982-1985.
13. Hofmeister EP, Mazurek MT, Shin AY, et al. Extension block pinning for large mallet fractures. *J Hand Surg.* 2003;28A(3):453-459.
14. Mignemi ME, Unruh KP, Lee DH. Controversies in the treatment of nail bed injuries. *J Hand Surg.* 2013;38A:1427-1430.
15. Fiedler DK, Barrett JE, Lourie GM. Nail bed reconstruction using single-layer bovine acellular dermal matrix. *J Hand Surg Am.* 2017;42:e67-e74.
16. Yeo CJ, Sebastin SJ, Chong AKS. Fingertip injuries. *Singapore Med J.* 2010;51(1):78-86.
17. Krusche-Mandl I, Kottstorfer J, Thalhammer G, et al. Seymour fractures: retrospective analysis and therapeutic considerations. *J Hand Surg.* 2013;38A:258-264.
18. Abzug JM, Kozin SH. Seymour fractures. *J Hand Surg.* 2013;38A:2267-2270.

19. Knapik JJ, Reynolds KL, Duplantis KL, et al. Friction blisters. Pathophysiology, prevention and treatment. *Sports Med.* 1995;20(3):136-145.

20. McNamara AR, Ensell S, Farley TD. Hand blisters in major league baseball pitchers: current concepts and management. *Am J Orthop.* 2016;45(3):134-136.

21. Cortese TA, Fukuyama K, Epstein W, et al. Treatment of friction blisters. An experimental study. *Arch Derm.* 1968;97:717-721.

22. Gaston RG, Lourie GM. Thumb metacarpophalangeal joint collateral ligament injuries. In: Seitz EW, ed. *Fractures and Dislocations of the Hand.* ASSH: E-Publishing; 2013 [Chapter 10].

23. Le M, Lourie GM, Gaston G. Relationship of surgically repaired ulnar collateral ligament injury of the thumb to the morphology of the metacarpophalangeal joint of the thumb. *J Hand Surg Eur.* 2017;1(1):1-2.

24. Milner CS, Manon-Matos Y, Thirkannad SM. Gamekeeper's thumb - a treatment-oriented magnetic resonance imaging classification. *J Hand Surg Am.* 2015;40:90-95.

25. Gaston RG, Lourie GM, Peljovich AE. Radial collateral ligament injury of the index metacarpophalangeal joint: an underreported but important injury. *J Hand Surg.* 2006;31A(8): 1355-1361.

26. Altobelli GG, Ruchelsman DE, Belsky MR, et al. Adductor pollicis jamming injuries in the professional baseball player: 2 case reports. *J Hand Surg.* 2013;38A:1181-1184.

27. Trehan SK, Weiland AJ. Baseball and softball injuries: elbow, wrist, and hand. *J Hand Surg Am.* 2015;40:826-830.

28. Schneider K, Kasparyan NG, Altchek DW, et al. An aneurysm involving the axillary artery and its branch vessels in a major league baseball pitcher. *Am J Sports Med.* 1999;27(3):370-375.

29. DiFelice GS, Paletta GA, Phillips BB, et al. Effort thrombosis in the elite throwing athlete. *Am J Sports Med.* 2002;30(5):708-712.

30. Ginn TA, Smith AM, Snyder JR, et al. Vascular changes of the hand in professional baseball players with emphasis on digital ischemia in catchers. *J Bone Joint Surg.* 2005;87-A(7):1464-1469.

31. Itoh Y, Wakano K, Takeda T, et al. Circulatory disturbances in the throwing hand of baseball pitchers. *Am J Sports Med.* 1987;15(3):264-269.

32. Tanaka SK, Lourie GM. Anatomic course of the medial antebrachial cutaneous nerve: a cadaveric study with proposed clinical application in failed cubital tunnel release. *J Hand Surg Eur.* 2013;XXE(X):1-2.

33. Morgenstein A, Lourie G, Miller B. Anconeus epitrochlearis muscle causing dynamic cubital tunnel syndrome: a case series. *J Hand Surg Eur.* 2014;XXE(X):1-2.

34. Bansal A, Carlan D, Moley J, et al. Return to play and complications after hook of the hamate fracture surgery. *J Hand Surg Am.* 2017;42:803-809.

35. Howell AE, Leach RE. Bowler's thumb. Perineural fibrosis of the digital nerve. *J Bone Joint Surg.* 1970;52-A(2): 379-381.

36. Dobyns JH, O'Brien ET, Linscheid RL, Farrow GM. Bowler's thumb: diagnosis and treatment. *J Bone Joint Surg.* 1972;54-A(4):751-755.

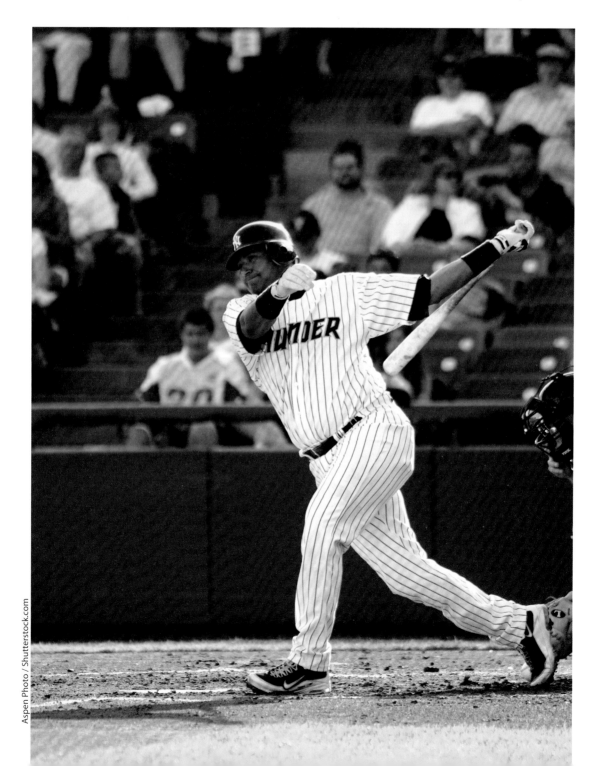

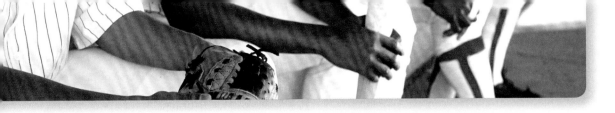

CHAPTER 15

Rotator Cuff Tears in Baseball Players

Eric C. Makhni, MD, MBA | Neal S. ElAttrache, MD | Christopher S. Ahmad, MD

Today, I consider myself the luckiest man on the face of the earth.

—Lou Gehrig

INTRODUCTION

Owing to the highly dynamic and stressful nature of the throwing motion, the shoulder[1] and its soft tissue structures experience enormous repetitive force and stress that predispose it to injury. One common cause of pain and disability in baseball players is injury to the rotator cuff. Interestingly, rotator cuff tears may also be found in players with no pain or symptoms whatsoever.[2] Therefore, successful management of these injuries requires a comprehensive understanding of the underlying anatomy, pathology, symptoms, and treatment options available.

In the overhead athlete, the shoulder may be vulnerable to injury either owing to intrinsic deficiencies of the shoulder girdle or owing to imbalanced mechanics elsewhere in the kinetic chain[3,4] (eg, core musculature, spin, and lower extremity). Therefore, shoulder injury in the overhead athlete must be evaluated not only in context of the shoulder girdle and scapula but also with respect to the entire kinetic chain and throwing motion. Special emphasis must also be placed on ensuring that the pitcher has appropriate throwing mechanics to avoid such injury.

PATHOANATOMY

The rotator cuff consists of 4 distinct muscles about the shoulder girdle: the subscapularis, supraspinatus, infraspinatus, and teres minor. Together, these muscles form a collective unit that provides stability and strength to the shoulder girdle.

During the throwing motion, the rotator cuff has been found to both concentrically and eccentrically contract.[5] In the beginning of the throwing motion, during windup, the activation is largely silent. As the

pitcher goes from early cocking to late cocking, the posterosuperior rotator cuff (consisting of the supraspinatus, infraspinatus, and teres minor) concentrically contracts, bringing the shoulder into external rotation. As the acceleration phase begins, the subscapularis, along with other shoulder internal rotators, contracts. During follow-through, the posterosuperior cuff again activates. However, at this time the shoulder is an internally rotated position; therefore, the posterosuperior cuff works to aid in deceleration in an eccentric manner.

There are numerous causes for rotator cuff failure that have been identified.

One cause may be due to the excessive tensile forces on the posterosuperior cuff, as it helps the shoulder decelerate during the follow-through motion.[5] Over time, the rotator cuff may fail owing to the excessive stresses experienced during this eccentric contraction in the throwing motion. The rotator cuff may also be vulnerable owing to posterior capsule contracture leading to GIRD (glenohumeral internal rotation deficit). This is commonly seen in overhead athletes and results in relative anterior translation of the humeral head and stretching of the inferior glenohumeral ligaments, as the shoulder moves into the abducted and externally rotated position as seen in the throwing motion. As a result, the undersurface (articular aspect) of the posterior supraspinatus and anterior infraspinatus comes into contact with the posterior superior glenoid, resulting in articular-sided posterior supraspinatus and anterior infraspinatus tears. This is referred to as internal impingement (Figure 15.1).[3,6] These are commonly referred to as PASTA (partial articular-sided tendon avulsion) lesions. Recent biomechanical studies have additionally indicated that this posterior contraction

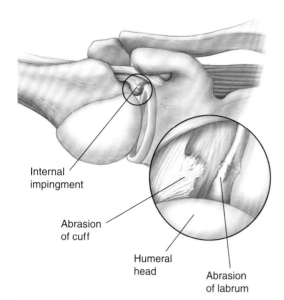

Internal
impingment

Abrasion
of cuff

Humeral
head

Abrasion
of labrum

FIGURE 15.1 • Internal impingement: In the throwing motion, as the shoulder goes into external rotation and abduction, the posterior supraspinatus and anterior infraspinatus may experience impingement with the posterosuperior glenoid and labrum, leading to articular-sided tear.

can lead to increased forces between the rotator cuff and the coracoacromial ligament superior, further leading to rotator cuff pathology.[7]

As our understanding of rotator cuff pathology in the throwing athlete expands, so does our recognition that many of these "injuries" may actually represent normal, adaptive changes in the overhead athlete. In a recent study by Lesniak and colleagues, the study team found that rotator cuff tears were found in pitchers who had absolutely no symptoms whatsoever of shoulder pain or weakness. Moreover, the authors reported that pitchers with higher cumulative innings pitched appeared to have higher likelihood of demonstrating rotator cuff tears on magnetic resonance imaging (MRI) findings.[2] This lends credence to the notion that rotator cuff tears, particularly articular-sided, may represent an adaptive change with time that allows the athlete's shoulder to accommodate the extremes of motion required for a successful throwing motion. Therefore, the presence of imaging findings of rotator cuff pathology in the asymptomatic athlete warrants no treatment or intervention.

CLINICAL EVALUATION

With throwing athletes, the chief complaint may not necessarily only be pain and/or weakness. With regard to the throwing shoulder, athletes may additionally complain of early fatigue in the course of practice or game or even a loss of accuracy. The symptoms may be corroborated or clarified by the player's coaches or family members.

The provider must ask additional questions related to the thrower's training regiment and risk for overuse injury to the shoulder. These include recent changes in throwing mechanics or schedules, adherence to pitch/inning counts, and compliance with taking rest days in-between games or practice sessions. Overuse of the pitcher may place additional risk to the athlete for injury, especially to the throwing shoulder and elbow. Finally, the provider must ask about additional symptoms not related to the shoulder, such as hip pain, back pain, or injury to the core musculature. Either of these (along with other areas of pain/injury) may lead to compromise in the throwing motion kinetic chain, further predisposing the thrower to shoulder injury. Moreover, failure to address these areas of deficiency will likely result in continued injury or lack of treatment success.

Following the detailed history, the provider must then perform a thorough physical examination. For any suspected shoulder injury in a throwing athlete, the provider must perform an assessment of the spine, beginning with the cervical spine and extending through the lumbar spine, assessing for range of motion deficits, asymmetric pain, or neurologic deficits. Any complaints of core, hip, or other lower extremity pain should also be examined.

Focused examination of the shoulder consists of assessment of appearance, palpation, range of motion, strength, and provocative maneuvers. First, the provider must assess the patient from anterior and posterior with the entire shoulder girdle exposed and the shirt off. Visual inspection should assess for side-to-side differences in the appearance of the shoulder, thoracic spine, scapula, and other bony landmarks, with special emphasis placed on any areas of atrophy that may be noted. Selective atrophy of the supraspinatus and/or infraspinatus fossa may represent suprascapular nerve compression, which may be due to a spinoglenoid or suprascapular notch cyst. This may manifest with symptoms similar to rotator cuff tear, thus underlying the importance of the visual examination. Scapula dyskinesis should also be assessed for all throwing athletes with shoulder pain and is evident by asymmetric position or protraction of the scapula with range of motion. The provider should then palpate relevant surface landmarks to assess for points of tenderness. These include the acromioclavicular joint, the sternoclavicular joint, and the biceps tendon.

Following visual inspection and palpation, range of motion should then be assessed, ideally in the supine position. The provider should note any side-to-side differences in range of motion in forward elevation (in the scapular plane), external and internal rotation at the side, abduction, and external and internal rotation in the abducted position. GIRD will be evident in the setting of increased external rotation in abduction, typically in the throwing shoulder, compared with the contralateral shoulder, along with a corresponding decrease in internal rotation in abduction. The total arc of rotation in abduction will be symmetric for both sides. The provider may also simultaneously assess strength in these planes of motion as well, taking note to compare asymmetry with the contralateral side.

The physical examination concludes with a variety of provocative maneuvers focused on various structures of the shoulder. Traditional impingement (abutment of the bursal aspect of the rotator cuff with the undersurface of the acromion or coracoacromial [CA] ligament) is performed with the Neer and Hawkins maneuvers. Lag signs indicating massive rotator cuff tears are typically absent in these athletes. Next, labral pathology is assessed through a variety of maneuvers. Anteroinferior labral tears or instability is accompanied by positive findings of anterior apprehension. Superior labral pathology is suspected with deep pain on O'Brien active compression testing. Speed and Yergason testing—aimed at eliciting biceps pathology—should also be tested, as these findings can be present with superior labral tears (type II SLAP). Posterior labral examinations, such as Kim and Jerk testing, are also routinely conducted. While rotator cuff tears may result in significant objective weakness on manual muscle testing or even lag signs, these findings are typically only seen in large tears. In overhead athletes, the rotator cuff tear is generally not large enough to cause significant weakness on examination. Instead, findings of impingement may be noted if there is outlet narrowing of the supraspinatus (eg, due to impingement with a subacromial spur or CA arch), and this would manifest as positive findings on Neer and Hawkins impingement testing. Patients with articular, undersurface tears due to internal impingement demonstrate range of motion findings consistent with GIRD as hallmark by decrease of internal rotation in the abducted position. There may be some mild weakness to resisted strength testing with the supraspinatus as well.

Finally, imaging may be used to confirm the diagnosis. Plain films are routinely taken, consisting of standard Grashey, axillary, and scapular Y views to rule out any obvious bony abnormalities. If rotator cuff pathology is suspected, ultrasound may be used and

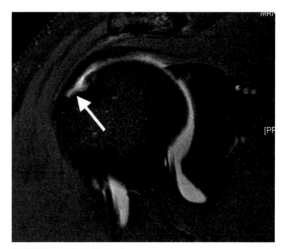

FIGURE 15.2 • MRI arthrogram demonstrating partial articular rotator cuff tear (arrow).

is an excellent screening tool (provided technician and radiologist are skilled in musculoskeletal ultrasound). The mainstay imaging modality, however, remains the MRI scan. Noncontrast imaging is sufficient to detect rotator cuff pathology, while arthrograms are typically used to detect labral pathology. Figure 15.2 is a coronal MRI arthrogram of the shoulder that demonstrates articular-sided partial tear of the rotator cuff at the posterior supraspinatus.

Management

Initial management of overhead athletes with rotator cuff tear follows principles of other treatment protocols for upper extremity injury in these patients. This consists of initial attempt at nonoperative treatment. While details of rehabilitation will be discussed elsewhere in this text, nonoperative treatment follows a multimodal, multidisciplinary approach. This consists of pain control through modalities such as ice, rest, and anti-inflammatory treatment, as well as a structured return-to-throwing program. Such a program permits advancement through the stages of rehabilitation only when the player can exhibit pain-free completion of each preceding stage. Moreover, the entire kinetic chain must be addressed, as opposed to solely focusing on the shoulder, and requires strength training of the lower extremities, core, and upper extremities as well. Additionally, proper throwing mechanics must be emphasized throughout the rehabilitation process.

Selective injections may be useful for overhead athletes, with rotator cuff tear attempting nonoperative treatment. The type and location of injection depends on the underlying pathology. In athletes who have evidence of external impingement, with bursal-sided pathology of the rotator cuff, a subacromial cortisone

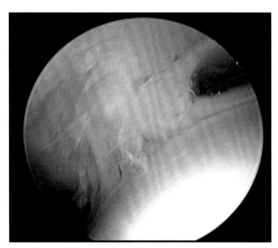

FIGURE 15.3 • Arthroscopic view of articular partial rotator cuff tear.

injection may provide a strong anti-inflammatory benefit that aids in pain control. It is the authors' opinion that many baseball players with shoulder pain from subacromial bursitis may develop dysfunction of the rotator cuff, further predisposing the athlete to injury through altered (and improper) imbalance of kinematics during the throwing motion. Therefore, subacromial injection may help relieve symptoms due to bursitis and thus restore proper throwing mechanics, minimizing progression to rotator cuff tear. For athletes with intra-articular pathology, such as PASTA lesions, an intra-articular injection may alternatively be useful. Biologic injections, such as platelet-rich plasma, may also be a useful option for intra-articular pathology; unfortunately, there is a lack of high-quality research regarding efficacy of these injection types.

Surgical treatment is reserved for patients who cannot adequately return to throwing following a comprehensive nonoperative treatment program. The type of surgical treatment depends on the underlying injury severity. In general, for patients with partial articular tears that comprise less than 50% of the tendon thickness, treatment is directed toward debridement of the tear down to stable margins, along with debridement of inflamed synovial tissue and subacromial bursitis. Figure 15.3 demonstrates an intraoperative picture of an articular-sided partial rotator cuff tear.

Specific to overhead athletes, the rotator cuff may exhibit an intralaminar tear, usually at the posterior aspect of the supraspinatus tendon. These are commonly referred to as "PAINT" lesions (partial-thickness articular surface intratendinous tears). This is compared with traditional rotator cuff tears, in which the tendon avulses from the bony footprint. The surgeon must be careful to repair these tears in a manner as

to avoid overtensioning the rotator cuff, which can lead to tightness in abduction and external rotation. Such a limitation is especially debilitating for the overhead athlete, resulting in pain and/or stiffness. The authors' preferred technique for managing these injuries can be seen in Figure 15.4. The underlying treatment strategy is to perform a side-to-side repair of the delaminated portion of the rotator cuff without anchoring the repair down to the bone. In this fashion, the tear may be treated without risk of overtensioning or tightening. When the rotator cuff exhibits a higher-grade injury, such as a tear of the anterior cable of the rotator cuff or a partial-thickness tear of greater than 50% of the footprint width,[8] a formal repair down to the bony footprint may be necessary. In fact, recent biomechanical evidence suggests that a partial-thickness articular-sided tear comprising >50% of the rotator cable can adversely alter glenohumeral kinematics.[9] In these instances, care must be taken to anatomically repair the rotator cuff to avoid overtightening of the shoulder.

TRIP TO THE MOUND

The goal of surgery for treatment of rotator cuff pathology in the overhead athlete is to adequately treat the underlying pathology while respecting the anatomical functional adaptations related to pitching. Knowledge of the location of the rotator cuff attachment on the greater tuberosity is needed to restore the proper anatomy during the repair. For tears that comprise less than 50% tendon width, successful treatment may include debridement of the tear without a formal repair. When encountering PAINT lesions, the surgeon must repair the delamination in a side-to-side manner without overtensioning the rotator cuff. Repair to the bone with traditional suture anchor repair is not necessary and may in fact cause overtensioning and loss of necessary adaptive footprint changes. Care must also be taken to investigate the anterior attachment (rotator cable) of the supraspinatus. If this is torn, an anatomic repair is necessary to preserve shoulder function postoperatively.

Following treatment, regardless of technique, guided rehabilitation is necessary to ensure optimal outcomes. Regardless of the level of competition—from Little League through Major League—rehabilitation must be guided by professionals knowledgeable with caring for

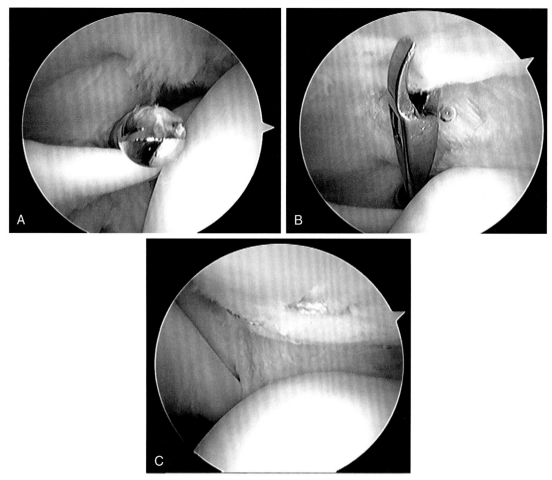

FIGURE 15.4 • Debridement and repair of partial rotator cuff tear (PAINT) lesion. A, Debridement of partial tear using an arthroscopic shaver. B, Following debridement, a delaminated tear is evident. C, Repair of delaminated tear with nonabsorbable sutures.

overhead athletes. Typically, return-to-throwing protocols follow structured guidelines with regard to progression of throwing. These protocols will accommodate for different surgical treatments (namely a debridement vs formal repair or reconstruction)[10] and precautions.

Outcomes in baseball players with rotator cuff tears vary according to the underlying pathology. Historically, those with full-thickness tears have had low rates of return to preinjury levels of competition, especially if treated with an open approach.[11] Those treated with arthroscopic repair may experience higher rates of return to sport, which was reported as >80% return to competition but unfortunately with decreased performance.[12] However, in patients with concomitant superior labral tears, presence of partial-thickness rotator cuff tear was associated with decreased return to competition despite good outcomes on patient-reported outcome scores.[13] Continued research is needed to better understand

factors promoting successful return after treatment of rotator cuff injury in this high-demand patient population.

SCOUTING REPORT

- Owing to the highly stressful and dynamic overhead throwing motion, the rotator cuff in baseball players may experience significant stress and strain
- This strain may cause internal impingement, resulting in undersurface (articular) rotator cuff tears
- Pitchers commonly have asymptomatic partial-thickness rotator cuff tears, and these tears may be adaptive to high-level throwing
- Injury to the rotator cuff in baseball players can be partial thickness or full thickness
- Nonoperative treatment is still the preferred initial management option

- Surgery is indicated if nonoperative treatment fails
- When requiring repair, care must be taken to anatomically restore the rotator cuff while respecting the anatomic adaptive changes relative to pitching
- Excessive tension or tightening of the rotator cuff during repair may cause stiffness and pain in the postoperative period, potentially impairing ability to return to sport
- Postoperative rehabilitation is necessary and is tailored to the treatment performed

REFERENCES

1. Sabick MB, Torry MR, Kim YK, Hawkins RJ. Humeral torque in professional baseball pitchers. *Am J Sports Med.* 2004;32:892-898.

2. Lesniak BP, Baraga MG, Jose J, Smith MK, Cunningham S, Kaplan LD. Glenohumeral findings on magnetic resonance imaging correlate with innings pitched in asymptomatic pitchers. *Am J Sports Med.* 2013;41:2022-2027.

3. Burkhart SS, Morgan CD, Kibler WB. The disabled throwing shoulder: spectrum of pathology Part I: Pathoanatomy and biomechanics. *Arthroscopy.* 2003;19:404-420.

4. Burkhart SS, Morgan CD, Kibler WB. The disabled throwing shoulder: spectrum of pathology Part III: The SICK scapula, scapular dyskinesis, the kinetic chain, and rehabilitation. *Arthroscopy.* 2003;19:641-661.

5. Williams GR, Kelley M. Management of rotator cuff and impingement injuries in the athlete. *J Athl Train.* 2000;35:300-315.

6. Greiwe RM, Ahmad CS. Management of the throwing shoulder: cuff, labrum and internal impingement. *Orthop Clin North Am.* 2010;41:309-323.

7. Shiota Y, Yamamoto N, Kawakami J, et al. Contact pressure of the coracoacromial arch in shoulders with joint contracture: a cadaveric study. *J Orthop Sci.* 2017;22(6):1031-1041.

8. Mazzocca AD, Rincon LM, O'Connor RW, et al. Intra-articular partial-thickness rotator cuff tears: analysis of injured and repaired strain behavior. *Am J Sports Med.* 2008;36:110-116.

9. Pinkowsky GJ, ElAttrache NS, Peterson AB, Akeda M, McGarry MH, Lee TQ. Partial-thickness tears involving the rotator cable lead to abnormal glenohumeral kinematics. *J Shoulder Elbow Surg.* 2017;26(7):1152-1158.

10. Makhni EC, Webwe AE, Ball B. Thomas A. Principles of postoperative shoulder rehabilitation in throwing athletes. *Oper Tech Sports Med.* 2016;24:223-225.

11. Mazoue CG, Andrews JR. Repair of full-thickness rotator cuff tears in professional baseball players. *Am J Sports Med.* 2006;34:182-189.

12. Dines JS, Jones K, Maher P, Altchek D. Arthroscopic management of full-thickness rotator cuff tears in major league baseball pitchers: the lateralized footprint repair technique. *Am J Orthop (Belle Mead NJ).* 2016;45:128-133.

13. Neri BR, ElAttrache NS, Owsley KC, Mohr K, Yocum LA. Outcome of type II superior labral anterior posterior repairs in elite overhead athletes: effect of concomitant partial-thickness rotator cuff tears. *Am J Sports Med.* 2011;39:114-120.

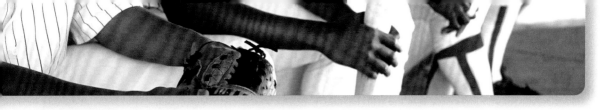

CHAPTER 16

SLAP Lesions and the Biceps in Baseball Players

Justin W. Griffin, MD | Anthony A. Romeo, MD

INTRODUCTION

The physical demands of repetitive overhead throwing can contribute to significant shoulder pain in baseball players. In high-level pitchers, the throwing speed and torque generated leads to forces regularly in excess of 1000 N with a maximum internal rotation velocity up to 7700°/s.[1] In response to these forces, internal compensatory changes gradually occur as well as potential internal derangement of the biceps-labrum complex.[2] Superior labral anterior posterior (SLAP) tears, first described by Andrews et al in 1985 and further classified by Snyder et al and later others, have become an increasingly common diagnosis and cause for shoulder arthroscopy among baseball players in the United States.[3-6] Despite well-defined classification system, a better understanding of pathologic versus adaptive changes, and an improved understanding of the role of the superior labrum, management of SLAP lesions remains controversial.

Repetitive overhead throwing is largely regarded as the reason for injury, although multiple specific mechanisms have been suggested.[5,7-9] The end result is detachment of the superior glenoid labrum with potential involvement of the biceps tendon along its course. Associated shoulder instability and significant glenohumeral dysfunction is not uncommon in athletes with lesions of the biceps-labral complex.[2] Currently there is little evidence that preventative programs have any effect on decreasing the incidence of SLAP tears in baseball players. Among baseball players, superior labral changes may often represent nonpathologic, adaptive findings advantageous to throwing.[4]

CLINICAL EVALUATION

History

Repetitive overhead throwing is the most common cause of a superior labral tear or biceps tendinopathy in baseball players.[8] Players often present with diminished athletic performance and vague deep-seated shoulder pain with provocative overhead activity. It is not uncommon for pitchers to experience a decrease in velocity, strength, and location. Players with pathologic SLAP lesions often complain of superior pain that radiates posteriorly.[10] One aspect of the history that can be particularly helpful to identify a traumatic or pathologic tear, as compared with more adaptive changes, is the recall of a specific event preceding their pain. Anterior shoulder pain around the biceps groove with mechanical symptoms can represent a biceps tendon lesion. However, overlap in symptoms with concomitant shoulder pathology may limit diagnostic accuracy and obscure clinical decision-making.[11]

Physical Examination

A thorough physical examination is paramount to establishing the diagnosis of a problematic SLAP lesion. Range of motion should be carefully assessed taking into account decreased internal rotation, which in many baseball players is adaptive. Changes in arc of rotational motion even as little as 5° may contribute to heightened risk of SLAP lesion and internal impingement.[12] In addition to range of motion, strength, and neurovascular testing, several examination maneuvers may be utilized to confirm SLAP tears in combination, as one single test has not proven to be definitive. Five clinical tests are widely used in the diagnosis of SLAP tears. These include the active compression or O'Brien test, the biceps load II, the dynamic labral shear or O'Driscoll test, the Speed test, and the labral tension test.[13] Cook et al evaluated the accuracy of these 5 clinical tests in diagnosis of SLAP tears recently.[13] They reported that SLAP tear could not be independently ruled in or out with the use of a single test. In a meta-analysis of selected tests, Meserve et al demonstrated that Crank test, O'Brien test, and Speed test were the best tests for identifying a SLAP tear.[14]

Long head of the biceps tendon pathology can be identified by several clinical tests as well. Pain may be elicited by the Speed or Yergason test, but still the most utilized test is simply tenderness to palpation over the proximal biceps groove. Tenderness in the biceps groove should be distinguished by pressing on both sides simultaneously, as this can be a painful spot for many patients. To perform Speed test, the examiner positions the patient's arm with the elbow extended and forearm supinated having the patient forward elevate the shoulder against resistance.[10,14-16] A positive test is when the patient has pain localized in the bicipital groove. In addition, one needs to closely scrutinize scapulothoracic and glenohumeral range of motion, which should be done in the supine position to stabilize the scapula.[10]

Recently, the "3-pack" examination as initially defined by O'Brien has demonstrated value in the clinical assessment of the biceps-labrum complex.[17] The 3-pack test includes examination maneuvers performed in sequence: the active compression test, throwing test, and bicipital tunnel palpation (need to describe positive and negative tests). Taylor et al demonstrated that the 3-pack had high interrater reliability, sensitivity and negative prognostic value—if the test were negative, there was not lesion of the biceps-labral complex.[17] Importantly, arthroscopically hidden and often poorly visualized on magnetic resonance imaging (MRI), extra-articular bicipital tunnel disease can be excluded based on a lack of tenderness to palpation and a negative O'Brien sign.

Imaging

Standard radiographic evaluation begins with Grashey, outlet, and axillary views of the shoulder. This allows for evaluation of early degenerative changes, loose bodies, bone reaction such as osteopenia of the posterior greater tuberosity, or other pathology such as a Bennett lesion. In most cases, advanced imaging is necessary to clearly define the the site of pathology when the player is unable to throw or is unable to return to prior performance. Noncontrast MRI is most commonly performed, despite the fact that this test may have variable sensitivity depending on the technique and quality of the study, owing to high specificity for identifying SLAP tears (Figure 16.1).[18,19] MR arthrogram (MRA) can also be used for diagnosis of SLAP tears, with several studies showing comparably higher sensitivity and specificity than other imaging modalities. In an evaluation of 40 patients with recurrent symptoms after prior labral repair, Probyn et al found that MRA results directly correlated with results of second-look surgical evaluation with specificity of MRA 85.7%.[20] Baseball players have a high false-positive rate for pathologic SLAP tears, as abnormal MRI signals have been noted in up to half of all MRIs of asymptomatic pitchers or throwers, reminding the treating physician

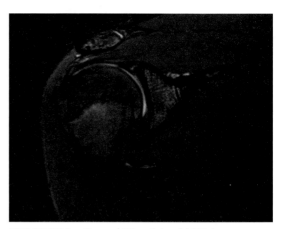

FIGURE 16.1 • Coronal T2-weighted MRI demonstrating a SLAP (superior labral anterior posterior) tear.

that MRI must be interpreted carefully and synchronized with the history and clinical examination findings.[18,21] MRI can also help to identify other injuries, including rotator cuff tears, capsular tears, articular cartilage abnormalities, and reactive bone changes. Correlation with clinical examination and patient history is essential to develop the correct treatment plan.

TREATMENT

Nonoperative

The initial treatment of most athletes with injuries to the biceps-labrum complex consists of nonoperative care, especially for in-season players. Athletes will often respond to a period of therapeutic rest and activity modification, especially after a period of increasing throwing activity. Nonsteroidal anti-inflammatory medication, ice, and stretching can be helpful to manage in-season players. When pain is significant and may interfere with physiotherapy, a localized corticosteroid injection may help the athlete comply with the exercise program. Physical therapy and strengthening programs can be initiated to work on scapular mechanics, motion deficits, and disruption of the broader kinetic chain of throwing, once the initial pain has subsided. The "sleeper stretch" works on passive internal rotation performed when lying on the affected side and is commonly utilized to diminish GIRD (glenohumeral internal rotation deficit) to within 20° of the contralateral shoulder.[7] Cross-body adduction can also be valuable to stretch the posterior capsule. Pectoralis minor tightness, when recognized, can be managed through passive stretching and progressive strengthening from closed to open chain.[7] As the symptoms at rest and with exercise subside, the more advance rehabilitation and return to sport activities focus on a return throwing program and endurance. Several studies have demonstrated some success with nonsurgical rehabilitation of symptomatic SLAP lesions with players able to return to play (RTP) in up to 40% to 66%,[12,22] and therefore nonoperative management remains the first effort in most baseball players. Return to prior performance, however, is far less promising, at 22%, so the response of the athletes to rehabilitation and their sports-related goals including full return to sport will play a role in the decision for operative management.

Operative

Surgical fixation of SLAP tears is indicated for athletes with persistent symptoms unable to RTP or unable to return to their same level of performance despite an appropriate rehabilitation program. This is entirely different than recommendations for nonoverhead athletes with more degenerative SLAP lesions.[23] Simple debridement is usually all that is needed in certain tears that are not unstable such as in type I lesions. Type II lesions are the most commonly surgically treated tears where there is separation of the labrum from the superior glenoid with at least 5 mm of excursion.[24] Evaluation by the surgeon intraoperatively for a peel-back lesion by placing the arm in abduction, external rotation, as opposed to a sulcus of 1 to 2 mm, may confirm the presence of a true pathologic type II SLAP tear.[5,25] Instability and direction of tear propagation is important to consider as well. Type III lesions can present a decision-making challenge. This is where there is an intact biceps-labral complex but a bucket-handle tear of the superior labral complex. A type IV tear includes additional extension of the tear into the biceps tendon, which may be more reliably treated with tenodesis in our experience.[23,25,26] Despite well-defined classification systems, management of SLAP lesions remains controversial. Biceps tenodesis until recently was not in the surgical algorithm for overhead athletes but has been more recently demonstrated a consideration in athletes owing to the fact that one of the most common symptoms that occur after SLAP repairs that fail to achieve the expected result of the athlete and surgeon is persistent anterior shoulder pain often attributed to the biceps tendon.

Surgical Options

Arthroscopic limited debridement can be considered for certain lesions that fail nonsurgical care. When indicated, fixation of SLAP tears can be safely and effectively achieved through modern arthroscopic techniques. This allows for complete assessment of any concomitant pathology, especially to the remaining labrum, the biceps tendon, and the rotator cuff. Knotless or knotted fixation can achieve stable fixation of the superior labrum and associated labral pathology. Biceps tenodesis can be considered in select patients when clinically indicated. In baseball players with no bicipital groove pain, or signs of severe tendinopathy or biceps tendon tearing, we favor an arthroscopic SLAP repair. If symptomatic biceps pathology exists, we prefer a subpectoral biceps tenodesis for optimal maintenance of the length tension relationship and mitigation of groove pathology, although increasingly all-arthroscopic techniques have been used by surgeons treating this condition.

AUTHORS' PREFERRED SURGICAL TECHNIQUE

Preoperative Planning

For isolated SLAP repair or biceps tenodesis, MRI is reviewed for planned fixation and any concomitant lesions. Anesthesia and patient positioning are carried out according to surgeon preference. The patient may be positioned beach chair or lateral decubitus. If concomitant labral repair anterior or posterior is planned, lateral decubitus positioning may be advantageous based on recent literature.[27] We prefer lateral decubitus positioning in all cases to allow for addressing all labral pathology with appropriate tensioning with well-placed portals (Figure 16.2). The lateral position, as well as the beach position, allows full assessment and treatment of pathology of the rotator cuff and biceps tendon. In all cases, a preoperative interscalene nerve block is performed under ultrasound guidance by an experienced anesthesia team.

Equipment Needed

- 4.0-mm 30° arthroscope, 3.5- and 4-mm mechanical shavers
- Covered burr or bone-cutting shaver for labral rim preparation and grasping instruments
- 8.25-mm cannula, as well as percutaneous metal or clear cannula (4.5-5.0 mm) for transrotator cuff portal
- Switching sticks
- Labral elevators (15° and 30°)
- Power drill
- Left and right suture shuttling device depending on the side, as well as a crescent-shaped suture shuttling device
- Knotless anchors with associated high-strength suture and suture tape
- Arthroscopic suture cutter
- If biceps tenodesis is being performed, open instruments are needed along with appropriate sized drills and either a tenodesis screw or other method of secure fixation such as a metal button

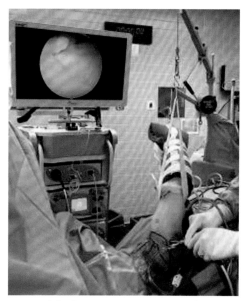

FIGURE 16.2 • Viewing a SLAP (superior labral anterior posterior) tear from a high-posterior portal.

Technique, Step by Step

- The authors' preferred method is the lateral decubitus position with the arm held in a 2-point suspension system

- Anatomic landmarks are carefully marked and planned portals are marked out

- The shoulder is initially accessed for diagnostic arthroscopy through a high posterior-superior border just off the posterolateral edge of the acromion. This portal placement allows for full inspection of the shoulder joint and can be converted to a working portal for fixation of the posterior-superior labrum when indicated

- The joint is systematically evaluated with regard to the rotator cuff and biceps as well as comprehensive labral evaluation

- An anterior portal is made in an outside-in technique and an 8.25-mm cannula is inserted. If posterior or anterior labral work is needed, a 7-o'clock portal is also established and cannulated

- Dynamic evaluation intraoperatively for a peel-back lesion by placing the arm in abduction, external rotation, as opposed to a sulcus, may confirm the presence of a type II SLAP tear. This can be critical for decision-making

- Next the SLAP tear is evaluated, and decisions are made regarding ideal anchor placement if a repair is indicated. With type I tears or a tear that does not require fixation, debridement is carried out

- If repair is indicated, a labral elevator is used to mobilize the tear for repair

- Next, a covered burr or bone-cutting shaver is used to prepare the repair site down to bone to encourage a better biologic healing environment

- In many cases, a Wilmington portal is created utilizing a smaller 4.5- or 5.0-mm percutaneous cannula

- Next, using a more traditional approach, a suture shuttling device is brought in from the anterior portal, and horizontal mattress suture is created with high-strength suture with tails facing the articular surface (Figure 16.3). Careful attention is paid to avoid incorporation of superior capsule tissue. A Neviaser portal may be utilized with a spinal needle for suture shuttling with a PDS suture

- An appropriate location is chosen for drilling through the Wilmington portal

- Increasingly, knotless fixation is utilized to repair the SLAP tear with appropriate tensioning techniques to avoid overtensioning the labrum. Low-profile knotless fixation is achieved, and sutures cut flush with the articular surface. An inverted mattress technique to avoid any prominence of synthetic material on the periphery of the labrum may avoid future abrasion on the humeral articular cartilage

- If posterior extension is present. Anterior viewing with posterior instrumentation through the previously made high posterior-superior portal can be utilized for anchor insertion with passage utilizing a crescent or angled passer

- Upon completion of the arthroscopic surgery, the fluid is evacuated from the cannula and the portals

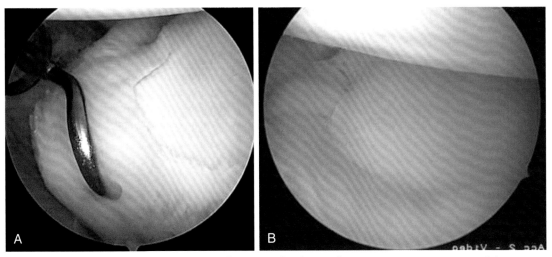

FIGURE 16.3 • A 45° crescent suture passing device is utilized to perform a mattress suture repair of the superior labrum from the anterior portal (A). Finished knotless repair of a SLAP (superior labral anterior posterior) repair (B).

are closed with 3-0 Prolene suture. Sterile dressings are applied, and the patient is then placed into a shoulder abduction sling

- In baseball players with no bicipital groove pain, or signs of gross tendinopathy, we favor an arthroscopic SLAP repair. If biceps pathology exists, we have preferred a subpectoral biceps tenodesis for optimal maintenance of the length tension relationship and mitigation of groove pathology

- Fixation of the tendon can be accomplished in multiple ways, including soft tissue tenodesis, interference screw fixation, and surface anchors. We prefer to utilize a tenodesis screw in the subpectoral location as outlined by Mazzocca et al.[28] This includes a 2-cm incision in Langer lines once identifying the inferior border of the pectoralis major tendon. Following, the biceps is retrieved and a whipstitch is placed to include the musculotendinous junction and a small segment of the tendon. The remaining proximal tendon is excised. Next, the groove is exposed and an 8.0-mm tunnel is drilled unicortically. One limb of the whipstitch is placed through the screw. The tendon is inserted into the cortical hole and then securely fixed in this location with the interference screw followed by tying the 2 limbs of the suture. This incision is closed with monocryl 2-0, running 3-0, and then dermabond is used to seal the skin

POSTSURGICAL REHABILITATION

Patients are maintained in a sling for 4 weeks. Internal rotation is avoided initially with forward elevation allowed up to 90° and external rotation at the side to 40°. Resisted forward flexion or biceps flexion is avoided for 6 weeks postoperatively to avoid stressing the biceps origin. After 6 weeks, range of motion is increased, and strengthening is initiated within the range of motion guidelines. At 3 months after surgery, eccentric strengthening is added to the program and may include an ergometer. Advanced conditioning and sport-specific training is initiated at this point with return to throwing typically at 4.5 months if the shoulder is now pain free at rest and during range of motion activities. Throwing from a pitcher's mound begins at 6 months if the throwing progression over the previous 6 weeks has been uneventful.

RESULTS

Although various methods exist, SLAP repair most commonly consists of repairing the superior labrum, which often includes part of biceps anchor. Management of type II SLAP lesions remains controversial owing to the fact that numerous studies have demonstrated challenges with returning overhead athletes to their same level of performance after SLAP repair, and more recent studies have suggested that biceps tenodesis is an effective alternative in older recreational athletes. Several prospective studies have demonstrated improved overall outcomes after SLAP repair.[29-31] Other series have demonstrated less promising outcomes including dissatisfaction with persistent pain and inability to return to throwing.[32-35] A recent systematic review reported that the percentage of patients who return to reinjury level of play was only 64%.[34] Overhead throwing athletes' results were even worse with only 22% to 60% able to return to their previous level of play. Challenging the concept of SLAP repair alone, more recently satisfactory outcomes have been reported with combined SLAP repair and biceps tenodesis.[36]

Not surprisingly, position players have a higher RTP than pitchers treated for SLAP tear.[12] In a recent study of Major League Baseball (MLB) pitchers, 62.5% were able to RTP at the MLB level after SLAP repair surgery; however, there was a noted statistically significant decrease in innings pitched.[35] While SLAP repair has historically been the standard, biceps tenodesis presents a surgical option with low complication rates, consistent method of secure fixation, and low revision rates, although results have varied.[37] As additional data regarding glenohumeral kinematics and outcomes in young athletes are revealed, improved decision-making algorithms will likely follow. It is likely that true pathologic SLAP lesions in baseball players that are fixed securely and without overtensioning the shoulder will remain the key to returning to prior levels of performance owing to the critical role that a 360° intact labrum has with glenohumeral stability; however, some of these cases may have improved outcomes if the biceps tendon is also treated at the same procedure.

A recent study by Chalmers et al evaluated pitchers utilizing surface EMG and motion analysis in 6 players after SLAP repair, 5 after biceps tenodesis, and 7 uninjured controls. The analysis revealed that the biceps tenodesis group appeared to more closely restore the normal pattern of muscular activation than the SLAP repair group.[38] More recent evidence suggests professional pitchers may have a lower rate of RTP than position players after biceps tenodesis; however, the majority of these athletes were treated with a biceps tenodesis after failing previous surgery.[39,40] For failed SLAP repair in baseball players, debridement of the labrum and any loose or prominent fixation material combined with biceps tenodesis is the preferred treatment of choice, as it reliably alleviates preoperative pain, although return to sport at the same level of performance remains challenging.[9,41,42]

COMPLICATIONS

Perhaps the most obvious complication is failure to RTP or failure to achieve the preinjury level of performance. Reasons for failure of SLAP repair remain unclear.[33] Labral repair may result in permanent alterations in pitching biomechanics, leading to inability to regain velocity and command after SLAP repair or biceps tenodesis.[26,36,43] While loss of external rotation is a concern with SLAP fixation, studies have also suggested the athlete's shoulder may remain unstable even after repair.[2] Hardware complications are a grave concern in baseball players. Suture anchor pullout, iatrogenic cartilage damage, or reactive changes from suture anchors can occur and may lead to irreversible changes that affect the athlete beyond the playing field.[44-49] Prominent knots can lead to devastating cartilage damage or rotator cuff impingement (Figure 16.4). For this reason, knotless fixation has been increasingly used for SLAP and other labral repairs, showing comparable strength and fixation with traditional suture anchor fixation.[49-51] Lack of healing is another reason for SLAP failure owing to poor vascular supply to the superior labrum. Persistent

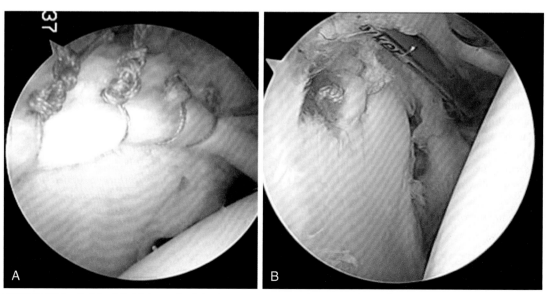

FIGURE 16.4 • Finished SLAP (superior labral anterior posterior) repair utilizing knots (A) can overconstrain the biceps and lead to cartilage damage (B).

biceps tendinopathy is an increasingly recognized cause of persistent pain after SLAP repair.[9,23,52]

Postoperative stiffness remains a significant problem after SLAP repair, which may occur owing to over tensioning and poor anchor placement; this is particularly concerning for pitchers as loss of 5° to 10° of external rotation may lead to an inability to achieve preinjury velocity and result in the conclusion of their career. Reduction in overhead motion noted in other sports and recreational activities can be tolerated but is far less acceptable in overhead throwing athletes.[33,53] As for biceps tenodesis, neurovascular injury, loss of fixation, and humerus fracture are among the most feared complications, have been reported, and fortunately are rare.[54-57]

MANAGER'S TIPS

- Careful patient selection is required to surgically treat only those athletes with persistent symptomatic SLAP tears despite a carefully developed rehabilitation program, with clinical findings corresponding to MRI findings

- A thorough history, physical examination, and advanced imaging are required to avoid fixing changes in the superior labrum that are interpreted as SLAP tears but in fact represent the natural adaptation to repetitive throwing activities

- The articular cartilage must be protected both by careful cannula insertion and preferably the utilization of knotless fixation (Figure 16.5)

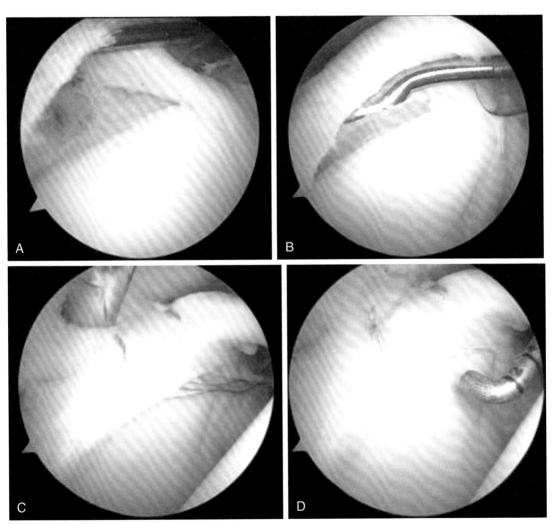

FIGURE 16.5 • Type II SLAP (superior labral anterior posterior) tear with posterior extension in a pitcher (A). The glenoid is prepared to maximize biologic healing (B). High-strength suture is passed in a mattress configuration. The Wilmington portal is demonstrated in this figure as well (C). Finished knotless vertical mattress SLAP repair (D).

- Attention must be paid to avoid overtensioning of the biceps-labral anchor and the anterior-superior labrum, which will result in restricted external rotation

- When clinically indicated, biceps tenodesis has been shown to be a safe and effective option without deleterious effects, resolving anterior shoulder pain and providing an acceptable RTP[40]

REFERENCES

1. Fleisig GS, Andrews JR, Dillman CJ, Escamilla RF. Kinetics of baseball pitching with implications about injury mechanisms. *Am J Sports Med.* 1995;23(2):233-239. doi:10.1177/036354659502300218.

2. Mihata T, McGarry MH, Tibone JE, Fitzpatrick MJ, Kinoshita M, Lee TQ. Biomechanical assessment of type II superior labral anterior-posterior (SLAP) lesions associated with anterior shoulder capsular laxity as seen in throwers: a cadaveric study. *Am J Sports Med.* 2008;36(8):1604-1610. doi:10.1177/0363546508315198.

3. Snyder SJ, Banas MP, Karzel RP. An analysis of 140 injuries to the superior glenoid labrum. *J Shoulder Elbow Surg.* 1995;4(4):243-248. doi:10.1016/S1058-2746(05)80015-1.

4. Snyder SJ, Karzel RP, Pizzo Del W, Ferkel RD, Friedman MJ. SLAP lesions of the shoulder. *Arthroscopy.* 2010;26(8):1117. doi:10.1016/j.arthro.2010.06.004.

5. Morgan CD, Burkhart SS, Palmeri M, Gillespie M. Type II slap lesions: three subtypes and their relationships to superior instability and rotator cuff tears. *Arthroscopy.* 1998;14(6):553-565. doi:10.1016/S0749-8063(98)70049-0.

6. Andrews JR, Carson WG, Mcleod WD. Glenoid labrum tears related to the long head of the biceps. *Am J Sports Med.* 1985;13(5):337-341. doi:10.1177/036354658501300508.

7. Burkhart SS, Morgan CD, Kibler WB. The disabled throwing shoulder: spectrum of pathology part III: the SICK scapula, scapular dyskinesis, the kinetic chain, and rehabilitation. *Arthroscopy.* 2003;19(6):641-661. doi:10.1016/S0749-8063(03)00389-X.

8. Burkhart SS, Morgan CD, Ben Kibler W. The disabled throwing shoulder: spectrum of pathology Part I: pathoanatomy and biomechanics. *Arthroscopy.* 2003;19(4):404-420. doi:10.1053/jars.2003.50128.

9. Gupta AK, Bruce B, Klosterman E, McCormick F, Harris JD, Romeo AA. Subpectoral biceps tenodesis for failed type II SLAP repair. *Orthop J Sport Med.* 2013;1(4). doi:10.1177/2325967113S00088.

10. Ben Kibler W, Sciascia AD, Hester P, Dome D, Jacobs C. Clinical utility of traditional and new tests in the diagnosis of biceps tendon injuries and superior labrum anterior and posterior lesions in the shoulder. *Am J Sports Med.* 2009;37(9):1840-1847. doi:10.1177/0363546509332505.

11. Thorsness RJ, Romeo AA. Diagnosis and management of the biceps-labral complex. *Instr Course Lect.* 2017;66:65-77.

12. Fedoriw WW, Ramkumar P, McCulloch PC, Lintner DM. Return to play after treatment of superior labral tears in professional baseball players. *Am J Sports Med.* 2014;42(5):1155-1160. doi:10.1177/0363546514528096.

13. Cook C, Beaty S, Kissenberth MJ, Siffri P, Pill SG, Hawkins RJ. Diagnostic accuracy of five orthopedic clinical tests for diagnosis of superior labrum anterior posterior (SLAP) lesions. *J Shoulder Elbow Surg.* 2012;21(1):13-22. doi:10.1016/j.jse.2011.07.012.

14. Meserve BB, Cleland JA, Boucher TR. A meta-analysis examining clinical test utility for assessing superior labral anterior posterior lesions. *Am J Sports Med.* 2009;37(11):2252-2258. doi:10.1177/0363546508325153.

15. Bennett WF. Specificity of the Speed's test: arthroscopic technique for evaluating the biceps tendon at the level of the bicipital groove. *Arthroscopy.* 1998;14(8):789-796. doi:10.1016/S0749-8063(98)70012-X.

16. Holtby R, Razmjou H. Accuracy of the Speed's and Yergason's tests in detecting biceps pathology and SLAP lesions: comparison with arthroscopic findings. *Arthroscopy.* 2004;20(3):231-236. doi:10.1016/j.arthro.2004.01.008.

17. Taylor SA, Newman AM, Dawson C, et al. The "3-Pack" examination is critical for comprehensive evaluation of the biceps-labrum complex and the bicipital tunnel: a prospective study. *Arthroscopy.* 2017;33(1):28-38. doi:10.1016/j.arthro.2016.05.015.

18. Connor PM, Banks DM, Tyson AB, Coumas JS, D'Alessandro DF. Magnetic resonance imaging of the asymptomatic shoulder of overhead athletes: a 5-year follow-up study. *Am J Sports Med.* 2003;31(5):724-727. doi:10.1177/03635465030310051501.

19. Davidson PA, Rivenburgh DW. Mobile superior glenoid labrum: a normal variant of pathologic condition? *Am J Sports Med.* 2004;32(4):962-966. doi:10.1177/0363546503259348.

20. Probyn LJ, White LM, Salonen DC, Tomlinson G, Boynton EL. Recurrent symptoms after shoulder instability repair: direct MR arthrographic assessment—correlation with second-look surgical evaluation. *Radiology.* 2007;245(3):814-823. doi:10.1148/radiol.2453061329.

21. Lesniak BP, Baraga MG, Jose J, Smith MK, Cunningham S, Kaplan LD. Glenohumeral findings on magnetic resonance imaging correlate with innings pitched in asymptomatic pitchers. *Am J Sports Med.* 2013;41(9):2022-2027. doi:10.1177/0363546513491093.

22. Edwards SL, Lee JA, Bell J-E, et al. Nonoperative treatment of superior labrum anterior posterior tears: improvements in pain, function, and quality of life. *Am J Sports Med.* 2010;38:1456-1461. doi:10.1177/0363546510370937.

23. Griffin JW, Leroux TS, Romeo AA, et al. Management of proximal biceps pathology in overhead athletes management of proximal biceps pathology in overhead athletes. 2016:1-4.

24. Keener JD, Brophy RH. Superior labral tears of the shoulder: pathogenesis, evaluation, and treatment. *J Am Acad Orthop Surg.* 2009;17(10):627-637. doi:10.5435/00124635-200910000-00005.

25. Nho SJ, Strauss EJ, Lenart BA, et al. Long head of the biceps tendinopathy: diagnosis and management. *J Am Acad Orthop Surg.* 2010;18(11):645-656.

26. Mccormick F, Bhatia S, Chalmers P, Gupta A, Verma N, Romeo AA. The management of type II superior labral anterior to posterior injuries. *Orthop Clin North Am.* 2014;45(1):121-128. doi:10.1016/j.ocl.2013.08.008.

27. Frank RM, Saccomanno MF, McDonald LS, Moric M, Romeo AA, Provencher MT. Outcomes of arthroscopic anterior shoulder instability in the beach chair versus lateral decubitus position: a systematic review and meta-regression analysis. *Arthroscopy.* 2014;30(10):1349-1365. doi:10.1016/j.arthro.2014.05.008.

28. Mazzocca AD, Rios CG, Romeo AA, Arciero RA. Subpectoral biceps tenodesis with interference screw fixation. *Arthroscopy.* 2005;21(7):896. doi:10.1016/j.arthro.2005.04.002.

29. Brockmeier SF, Voos JE, Williams RJ, et al. Outcomes after arthroscopic repair of type-II SLAP lesions. *J Bone Joint Surg Am.* 2009;91(7):1595-1603. doi:10.2106/JBJS.H.00205.

30. Boileau P, Parratte S, Chuinard C, Roussanne Y, Shia D, Bicknell R. Arthroscopic treatment of isolated type II slap lesions: biceps tenodesis as an alternative to reinsertion. *Am J Sports Med.* 2009;37(5):929-936. doi:10.1177/0363546508330127.

31. Denard PJ, Ldermann A, Burkhart SS. Long-term outcome after arthroscopic repair of type II slap lesions: results according to age and workers' compensation status. *Arthroscopy.* 2012;28(4):451-457. doi:10.1016/j.arthro.2011.09.005.

32. Provencher MT, McCormick F, Dewing C, McIntire S, Solomon D. A prospective analysis of 179 type 2 superior labrum anterior and posterior repairs: outcomes and factors associated with success and failure. *Am J Sports Med.* 2013;41(4):880-886. doi:10.1177/0363546513477363.

33. Katz LM, Hsu S, Miller SL, et al. Poor outcomes after SLAP repair: descriptive analysis and prognosis. *Arthroscopy.* 2009;25(8):849-855. doi:10.1016/j.arthro.2009.02.022.

34. Gorantla K, Gill C, Wright RW. The outcome of type II SLAP repair: a systematic review. *Arthroscopy.* 2010;26(4):537-545. doi:10.1016/j.arthro.2009.08.017.

35. Smith R, Lombardo DJ, Petersen-Fitts GR, et al. Return to play and prior performance in major league baseball pitchers after repair of superior labral anterior-posterior tears. *Orthop J Sport Med.* 2016;4(12). doi:10.1177/2325967116675822.

36. Chalmers PN, Monson B, Frank RM, et al. Combined SLAP repair and biceps tenodesis for superior labral anterior–posterior tears. *Knee Surg Sports Traumatol Arthrosc.* 2016;24(12):3870-3876. doi:10.1007/s00167-015-3774-6.

37. Griffin JW, Cvetanovich G, Kim J, et al. Biceps tenodesis is a viable option for management of proximal biceps injuries in patients less than 25 years of age. *Arthroscopy.* 2018;5(3 suppl3).

38. Chalmers PN, Trombley R, Cip J, et al. Postoperative restoration of upper extremity motion and neuromuscular control during the overhand pitch: evaluation of tenodesis and repair for superior labral anterior-posterior tears. *Am J Sports Med.* 2014;42(12):2825-2836. doi:10.1177/0363546514551924.

39. Chalmers PN, Erickson BJ, Verma NN, D'Angelo J, Romeo AA. Incidence and return to play after biceps tenodesis in professional baseball players. *Arthroscopy.* 2017. doi:10.1016/j.arthro.2017.08.251.

40. Waterman B, Newgren J, Richardson C, Romeo AA. Return to sporting activity among overhead athletes with subpectoral biceps tenodesis for type II SLAP tear manuscript _cat's edits (1). *Arthroscopy.* 2018.

41. Werner BC, Brockmeier SF, Miller MD. Etiology, diagnosis, and management of failed SLAP repair. *J Am Acad Orthop Surg.* 2014;22(9):554-565. doi:10.5435/JAAOS-22-09-554.

42. McCormick F, Nwachukwu BU, Solomon D, et al. The efficacy of biceps tenodesis in the treatment of failed superior labral anterior posterior repairs. *Am J Sports Med.* 2014;42(4):820-825. doi:10.1177/0363546513520122.

43. Erickson BJ, Chalmers PN, Waterman BR, Griffin JW, Romeo AA. Performance and return to sport in elite baseball players and recreational athletes following repair of the latissimus dorsi and teres major. *J Shoulder Elbow Surg.* 2017;26(11):1948-1954. doi:10.1016/j.jse.2017.05.015.

44. Park MJ, Hsu JE, Harper C, Sennett BJ, Huffman GR. Poly-L/D-lactic acid anchors are associated with reoperation and failure of SLAP repairs. *Arthroscopy.* 2011;27(10):1335-1340. doi:10.1016/j.arthro.2011.06.021.

45. Lembeck B, Wülker N. Severe cartilage damage by broken poly-L-lactic acid (PLLA) interference screw after ACL reconstruction. *Knee Surg Sports Traumatol Arthrosc.* 2005;13(4):283-286. doi:10.1007/s00167-004-0545-1.

46. Wilkerson JP, Zvijac JE, Uribe JW, Schürhoff MR, Green JB. Failure of polymerized lactic acid tacks in shoulder surgery. *J Shoulder Elbow Surg.* 2003;12(2):117-121. doi:10.1067/mse.2003.16.

47. Sassmannshausen G, Sukay M, Mair SD. Broken or dislodged poly-L-lactic acid bioabsorbable tacks in patients after SLAP lesion surgery. *Arthroscopy.* 2006;22(6):615-619. doi:10.1016/j.arthro.2006.03.009.

48. Freehill MQ, Harms DJ, Huber SM, Atlihan D, Buss DD. Poly-L-lactic acid tack synovitis after arthroscopic stabilization of the shoulder. *Am J Sports Med.* 2003;31(5):643-647. doi:10.1177/03635465030310050201.

49. Yang HJ, Yoon K, Jin H, Song HS. Clinical outcome of arthroscopic SLAP repair: conventional vertical knot versus knotless horizontal mattress sutures. *Knee Surg Sports Traumatol Arthrosc.* 2016;24(2):464-469. doi:10.1007/s00167-014-3449-8.

50. Uggen C, Wei A, Glousman RE, et al. Biomechanical comparison of knotless anchor repair versus simple suture repair for type II SLAP lesions. *Arthroscopy.* 2009;25(10):1085-1092. doi:10.1016/j.arthro.2009.03.022.

51. Yian E, Wang C, Millett PJ, Warner JJP. Arthroscopic repair of SLAP lesions with a bioknotless suture anchor. *Arthroscopy.* 2004;20(5):547-551. doi:10.1016/j.arthro.2004.01.036.

52. Nho SJ, Reiff SN, Verma NN, Slabaugh MA, Mazzocca AD, Romeo AA. Complications associated with subpectoral biceps tenodesis: low rates of incidence following surgery. *J Shoulder Elbow Surg.* 2010;19(5):764-768. doi:10.1016/j.jse.2010.01.024.

53. Werner BC, Pehlivan HC, Hart JM, et al. Increased incidence of postoperative stiffness after arthroscopic compared with open biceps tenodesis. *Arthroscopy.* 2014;30(9):1075-1084. doi:10.1016/j.arthro.2014.03.024.

54. Ma H, Van Heest A, Glisson C, Patel S. Musculocutaneous nerve entrapment: an unusual complication after biceps tenodesis. *Am J Sports Med.* 2009;37(12):2467-2469. doi:10.1177/0363546509337406.

55. Beason DP, Shah JP, Duckett JW, Jost PW, Fleisig GS, Cain EL. Torsional fracture of the humerus after subpectoral biceps tenodesis with an interference screw: a biomechanical cadaveric study. *Clin Biomech.* 2015;30(9):915-920. doi:10.1016/j.clinbiomech.2015.07.009.

56. Dein EJ, Huri G, Gordon JC, Mcfarland EG. A humerus fracture in a baseball pitcher after biceps tenodesis. *Am J Sports Med.* 2014;42(4):877-879. doi:10.1177/0363546513519218.

57. Reiff SN, Nho SJ, Romeo AA. Proximal humerus fracture after keyhole biceps tenodesis. *Am J Orthop (Belle Mead NJ).* 2010;39(7):E61-E63. http://www.ncbi.nlm.nih.gov/pubmed/20844775.

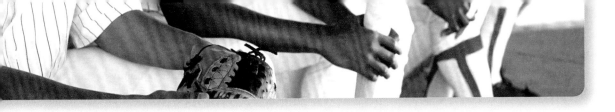

CHAPTER 17

Traumatic Shoulder Instability and Baseball Players

Jeffrey R. Dugas, MD | Michael K. Ryan, MD

INTRODUCTION

The glenohumeral joint exhibits the greatest range of motion (ROM) for any joint in the body, allowing for near-circumferential placement of the upper extremity in space. This vast motion is a result of minimally restrictive bony architecture with static and dynamic restraints, which provide checkreins at the extremes of the arc of motion.[1] Baseball players benefit significantly from the shoulder's mobility, which allows for extreme external rotation up to 175° without loss of joint contact, which maximizes torque, upward of 52 N/m and rotational velocity, up to 7000°/s, imparted during the throwing motion.[2] However, the trade-off to this great freedom of motion is the susceptibility of the joint to pathologic instability, and any failure of the static or dynamic checkreins frequently results in symptomatic glenohumeral instability. Glenohumeral instability has been described in various forms, including directional (anterior, posterior, or multidirectional), etiology (traumatic or atraumatic), and frequency (primary or recurrent). This chapter will discuss the incidence, assessment, treatment, and outcomes of traumatic glenohumeral instability in baseball players.

Traumatic glenohumeral instability is one of the more common shoulder injuries affecting young athletes.[3,4] The majority of traumatic glenohumeral instability is anterior, affecting the anterior capsulolabral complex, causing a Bankart lesion in 86% to 100% of athletes after an anterior subluxation or dislocation.[5-11] Bony injuries of the humeral head (Hill-Sachs lesion) and glenoid frequently occur with traumatic anterior dislocations and increase in frequency and size with recurrent instability.[9,12] Hill-Sachs lesions have been described in 48% to 100% of anterior glenohumeral dislocations, and glenoid deficiency is seen in 20% to 41% of primary and 66% to 87% of recurrent instability.[9,12-19]

Although relatively rare in the urban population at an incidence of 1.7% or 0.082 to 0.24 per 1000 person-years, traumatic glenohumeral instability is seen at a much higher rate 0.12 to 0.21 per 1000 athlete exposures (AE) among the athletic population and is significantly higher in contact or collision athletes.[3,4,20-22] Although the shoulder is the most frequently injured joint in baseball players at all levels accounting for an injury rate of 1.39 per 10,000 AEs, the incidence of traumatic glenohumeral instability is significantly lower, as capsulolabral injury is more frequently microtraumatic in nature.[3,23-29] When traumatic glenohumeral instability does occur in baseball players, it generally only represents 1.9% to 16% of all shoulder injuries in baseball players and is typically a result of a collision with another object or player or sustained after sliding into a base.[3,12,20,28-31] Sliding alone accounts for an injury incidence of 4.87 injuries per 1000 game exposures (or 6.0-9.5/1000 slides), and of those, shoulder and clavicle injuries account for 12% to 20% of all sliding injuries, 23% of which result from head-first slides.[27,30,31] Shoulder injuries alone account for 21% of missed time in Major League Baseball players and 26% of total disabled list days.[25] One report demonstrated that shoulder subluxations and dislocations sustained after a sliding injury account for the overwhelming majority (92%) of time lost.[31]

In addition to being less common, glenohumeral instability in baseball players typically demonstrates less severe bony defects (70% demonstrating no glenoid defect) and smaller average glenoid defects compared with other sports, including rugby and football (4.5% vs 12% and 8.9%, respectively) and has fewer large glenoid defects (>20%) as well (7% vs 22% and 16%, respectively).[12] More rarely, a humeral avulsion of the glenohumeral ligament involving the axillary pouch (APHAGL) was reported in 4 pitchers who developed pain after "hard throwing" emphasizes the infrequency of traumatic anterior instability.[32]

Despite the infrequency of traumatic glenohumeral instability in baseball players, this injury can be severely functionally limiting, frequently fails nonoperative treatment, regularly requires surgical intervention, and requires significantly longer return to sport when compared with other athletes and sports.[33] Although baseball is a noncontact or noncollision sport, the throwing motion positions the upper extremity in abduction and maximal external rotation, the position most susceptible to anterior dislocation. Throwing athletes therefore require proper treatment to return to play at preinjury levels without recurrence. Nonoperative treatment of traumatic anterior glenohumeral instability in young athletes has demonstrated very high recurrence rates, ranging from 41% to 73%.[34-36] Surgical management of traumatic glenohumeral instability tightens the ligamentous checkreins of the shoulder, specifically the anterior band of the inferior glenohumeral ligament, and restores normal anterior labral contour, restoring depth and anterior stability. Unfortunately, surgical stabilization of the anterior capsulolabral complex frequently causes decreased external rotation postoperatively.[34,37] For a throwing athlete depending on maximal, stable, external rotation of the shoulder to achieve optimal velocity and accuracy, traumatic glenohumeral instability and the necessary surgical treatment may cause significant delay in return to play or may severely limit throwing function in the long-term.[38]

CLINICAL EVALUATION

Traumatic shoulder instability is typically caused by an acute injury resulting in a subluxation or frank dislocation event. In baseball players, this most frequently occurs during a collision (with another player or stationary object or wall), while diving to catch a ball (with the upper extremity in maximal forward flexion), or while sliding into a base head first (with the arms stretched out in front of the player).[26,30,31] The player will report acute, severe pain deep within the shoulder and will have pain with active motion of the shoulder immediately after the injury. During a subluxation event, the player frequently reports the shoulder "came out" or "popped out" and "went back in", while a frank dislocation requires manual traction, by either the player or medical staff, to reduce the shoulder. Pain typically persists until after initial phase of recovery, when active ROM and full strength have returned. Although pain frequently abates, many players continue to have symptoms of apprehension.

As throwing places the upper extremity in abduction, extension, and maximal external rotation, this motion places the glenohumeral joint in an at-risk position with the potential for recurrent subluxation or dislocation. Players who experience this may have apprehension or pain while throwing and may lose velocity or distance to altered mechanics and loss of external rotation.

Physical Examination

In the acute setting, patients with a subluxation will have a normal-appearing shoulder girdle, with no obvious deformity or signs of trauma, but will typically hold the arm against the chest wall, often supporting it with the contralateral arm, to limit motion. Alternatively, players with an acute dislocation demonstrate loss of the normal contour of the shoulder with squaring and prominence of the acromion, flattening of the deltoid, and possible prominence of the anterior aspect of the shoulder, representing the dislocated humeral head. Tenderness along the anterior aspect of the shoulder joint is common, but this is a vague finding. Active and passive ROM are typically guarded and limited by pain. When placed in abduction and external rotation, patients frequently experience apprehension with the sensation of instability and fear of possible subluxation or dislocation. In the acute setting, the apprehension test is frequently too painful and usually not possible. A thorough neurovascular examination is necessary after a traumatic instability event because neurovascular injuries can occur with primary glenohumeral dislocations.[20,39] Nerve injury has been reported in (5%-48%) of primary shoulder dislocations, with the axillary nerve most commonly affected 42% of the time, although other brachial plexus injuries, including radial nerve palsies have been reported.[20,40] Additionally, vascular injuries have also been reported after primary glenohumeral dislocations, emphasizing the need for a thorough neurovascular examination.[39]

In the chronic setting, patients have typically regained normal motion and strength, and any capsulolabral injury has had time to scar, reducing guarding and pain typically seen in the acute setting. This allows for a much more focused and thorough examination. The majority of patients with traumatic instability demonstrate normal shoulder anatomy, but any signs of atrophy in the deltoid or rotator cuff should be concerning for a peripheral nerve injury and should be thoroughly investigated. Tenderness is typically not present in the chronic setting. Active ROM is expected to be normal for forward elevation, abduction, extension, and internal and external rotation, although

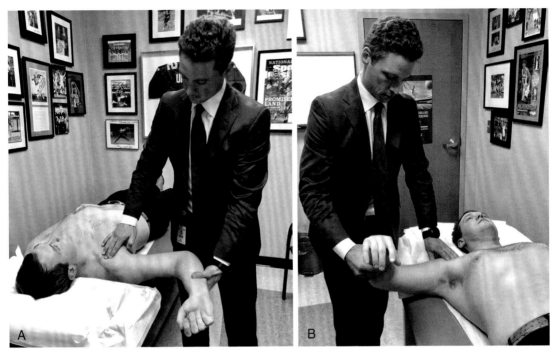

FIGURE 17.1 • Supine passive range of motion assessment. With stabilization of the scapula and palpation of the coracoid process, true passive range of motion can be accurately assessed. As the glenohumeral joint reaches extremes of internal and external rotation in the plane of the scapula, the scapula will begin to rotate, which can be palpated when the coracoid process begins to move. Glenohumeral external rotation in baseball players is usually greater on the dominant side (A). Internal rotation is often decreased compared with the contralateral side, but the overall arc of rotation is equal in healthy shoulders (B).

slight differences in external rotation with the arm in abduction may be noted. Passive ROM should be normal (Figure 17.1). Motor strength testing of the rotator cuff and deltoid should also be normal. A variety of examination maneuvers have been developed to assess instability and provoke symptoms based on the location of the injury. Anterior instability can be assessed with the patient seated upright or laying supine. With the patient seated, the load and shift test can be performed by stabilizing the scapula with 1 hand, centering the humeral head by placing an axial load, and translating the humeral head anteriorly to assess the degree of translation and laxity (Figure 17.2).[41,42] With the patient supine at the edge of a table, the apprehension test can be performed by placing the upper extremity in 90° of abduction and 90° of external rotation, supporting the shoulder blade (Figure 17.3A). If the patient experiences apprehension or pain, the test is considered positive, although the sensation of apprehension has demonstrated better specificity compared with pain.[43-46] The Jobe relocation test is an addition to the apprehension test and performed by placing a posterior-directed force on the proximal humerus with the arm in the position described in the apprehension

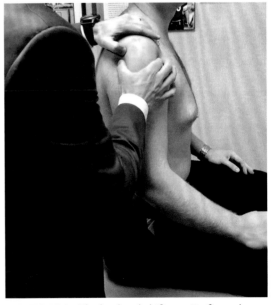

FIGURE 17.2 • The load and shift test. Performed with the patient sitting upright; the patient's right scapula is stabilized with the examiner's left hand, and the right hand is used to place an axial load on the humeral head, which is then translated anterior to assess the degree of instability.

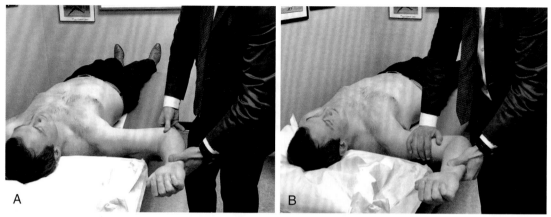

FIGURE 17.3 • The apprehension (A) and Jobe relocation (B) tests. With the patient supine, the examiner abducts the arm to 90°, and then gradually externally rotates the arm to 90°. The test is considered positive if the patient experiences apprehension with the sensation that the shoulder will subluxate or dislocate. Pain may also be present in this position but is not as sensitive an indicator of instability. If apprehension and/or pain is relieved after application of a posterior force on the shoulder, the Jobe relocation test is considered positive.

test, translating the humeral head posterior (Figure 17.3B). If the patient experiences decreased apprehension or pain during this maneuver, it is considered positive, and similarly, improvement of apprehension has demonstrated better specificity compared with improvement in pain.[43-46] Glenohumeral translation can also be assessed with the patient supine, by holding the arm in 90° of external rotation, 70° of abduction, and 20° of forward flexion (in plane with the glenoid) with 1 hand and manually translating the humeral head anteriorly toward the glenoid rim with the other hand (Figure 17.4). This modified anterior drawer test as described by Gerber and Ganz describes the degree of anterior translation by anatomic location and is classified as follows: grade 1—to the anterior glenoid rim; grade 2—over the rim, but humeral head spontaneously reduces; and grade 3—over the rim, does not spontaneously reduce.[47] Using this test, 30% of baseball players have demonstrated slightly increased anterior translation, 83% of which were in the dominant arm, although translation was neither pathologic nor significant.[48] A sulcus test can also be performed with the patient seated, by pulling axial traction on the humerus toward the floor, noting the distance of separation between the lateral acromion and humeral head. The sulcus test is an assessment of inferior instability and the integrity of the superior glenohumeral ligament and is frequently positive, and bilateral, in baseball pitchers (61%) and position players (47%).[49] In conjunction with a thorough patient

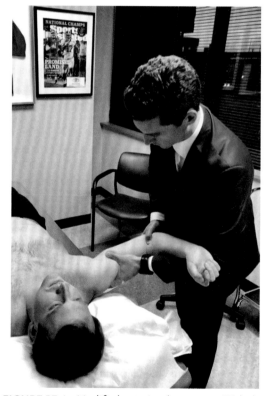

FIGURE 17.4 • Modified anterior drawer test. With the patient supine and the scapula stabilized, the arm is placed in 90° of abduction, 90° of external rotation, and 20° of forward flexion (in the plane of the glenoid), and then an anterior force is placed on the humeral head, translating it forward.

history, a detailed examination including active and passive ROM, strength, and provocative instability testing will properly diagnose anterior glenohumeral instability.

Imaging

Imaging after a traumatic glenohumeral event begins with standard radiographs. A standard anteroposterior (AP) of the glenohumeral joint and an axillary view are essential to assess joint congruency, joint space, and the presence of any fractures (Figure 17.5). Additional AP internal and external humeral rotation and scapular-Y views are useful to assess the greater and lesser tuberosities, the coracoid, and acromion and help rule out any associated fractures. With a standard subluxation or dislocation event, most of the above radiographs will appear normal, with a reduced, well-maintained glenohumeral joint space, without any associated fractures. However, as indicated, Hill-Sachs lesions and anterior glenoid rim fractures, "bony Bankart," and chronic glenoid bone loss frequently occur with traumatic instability events and should be assessed on standard radiographs. Additional, specialized radiographic views should also be obtained for athletic patient with traumatic instability, which improve the assessment of the bony architecture of the proximal humerus and glenoid. The Stryker notch view is used to assess the posterior-superior aspect of the humeral head, specifically Hill-Sachs impaction lesions acquired at the time

of injury (Figure 17.6). This view is obtained by lying the patient supine with the cassette behind the affected shoulder, and then having the patient place his hand behind his head (arm flexed to approximately 135°), and the beam is centered over the coracoid process angled 10° cephalad.[50,51] The AP view with 45° internal rotation combined with the Stryker notch view can identify 92% to 100% of Hill-Sachs lesions reliably.[52] For assessment of acute bony Bankart lesions and chronic, attritional glenoid bone loss in patients, the West Point view provides a dedicated view of the anteroinferior glenoid. This view is obtained by placing the patient prone on the X-ray table with the affected arm resting flat, abducted to 90° with the elbow flexed, allowing the forearm and hand to hang off of the table. The patient's head is turned and tilted away from the arm, and the X-ray cassette is placed perpendicular to the table and superior and parallel to the shoulder, and then the beam is centered on the axilla, angled 25° downward from the horizontal plane and 25° lateral from the midline.[53] The West Point view has been shown to have a diagnostic accuracy of 70%, when assessing the anteroinferior glenoid.[19] Standard and supplemental radiographic views of the shoulder are essential diagnostic tools, which provide a comprehensive picture of the osseous pathology in patients with anterior glenohumeral instability. Magnetic resonance imaging (MRI) can significantly augment standard radiographs by providing multiplanar imaging of

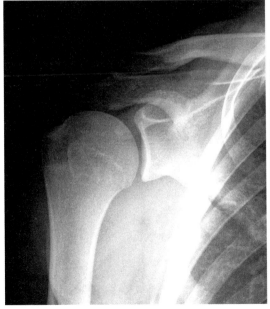
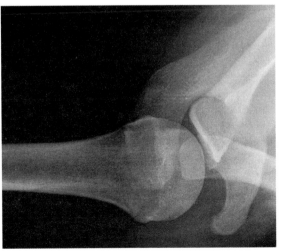

FIGURE 17.5 • Standard radiographs used to assess bony architecture after a traumatic shoulder subluxation or dislocation. Included here are an anteroposterior (AP) and axillary of a baseball player who sustained a traumatic dislocation. No significant bony defects are seen on either view.

osseous structures but more importantly demonstrate labral, capsular, ligamentous, articular, and musculotendinous pathology in much greater detail.

Advanced imaging is recommended after traumatic glenohumeral instability to more thoroughly assess the location and degree of soft tissue and capsulolabral injury, specifically labral tears and Bankart lesions (Figure 17.7). Both standard MRI and MRA, performed by injecting intra-articular gadolinium, provide superior assessment of labral tears when compared with computed tomography (CT) arthrography, detecting 93% and 96% of labral tears, respectively.[54] However, MRA demonstrates superior ability to detect detached labral tears compared with MRI and CT arthrography (96% vs 46% and 52%, respectively) and exhibits the highest sensitivity of all 3 modalities

for detection of labral tears, detached labral fragments, and labral degeneration.[54] Compared with noncontrast studies, MRA demonstrates superior sensitivity and specificity for diagnosing glenoid labral lesions (76% and 87% vs 88% and 93%, respectively).[55] With the addition of the abduction-external rotation (ABER) sequence to MRA, whereby the patient is positioned with the upper extremity in an abducted and externally rotated position during the scan; the sensitivity for detecting anteroinferior labral lesions has been shown to be higher when compared with MRA in the neutral position (92% to 96% vs 48% to 83%).[56,57] When used simultaneously, neutral MRA and ABER MRA demonstrate sensitivity and specificity for anteroinferior labral tears of 96% and 97%, respectively.[56] The combination of standard and specialized radiographs and neutral and ABER MRA provide abundant information concerning the osseous and soft tissue structures about the shoulder. If no significant osseous deficiency (Hill-Sachs or glenoid deficiency) is noted on these images, no additional imaging is needed, but if acute or attritional bone loss of the humeral head or glenoid is of concern, a CT scan is recommended to obtain a more comprehensive assessment of the osseous architecture.

CT scans of the shoulder provide excellent assessment of the bony architecture, facilitating identification and quantification of Hill-Sachs lesions and measurement of anterior glenoid bone loss and assessing any possible small or comminuted fractures. This is an important component to glenohumeral instability imaging, as shoulders with glenohumeral bone loss have significantly higher failure rates after arthroscopic Bankart repair.[58] Three dimensional (3D) reconstructions are also very helpful for assessing overall bony deficiency in the setting of glenohumeral instability. The degree of "critical" bone loss is currently evolving,

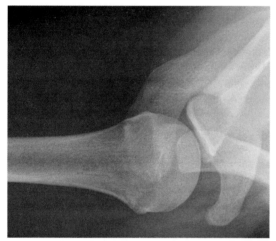

FIGURE 17.6 • Additional radiographs include the Stryker view to assess bony impaction injury of the posterior humeral head (Hill-Sachs lesion). No significant Hill-Sachs lesion is noted in this baseball player who sustained a traumatic dislocation.

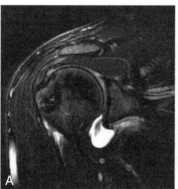
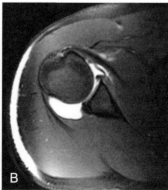
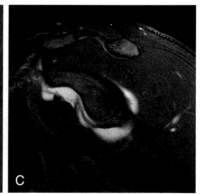

FIGURE 17.7 • Magnetic resonance arthrogram of a right shoulder demonstrating coronal (A), axial (B), and sagittal (C) images of a Bankart lesion with fraying of the anteroinferior labrum and separation of the chondrolabral junction.

but it is clear that anterior glenoid bone loss is a risk factor for failure of surgical stabilization in high-risk athletes, and bipolar lesions are also a risk factor for failure of surgical stabilization.[58,59] The presence and extent of glenoid bone loss can alter the surgical procedure, so a valid assessment of bone stock is essential in the acute setting where a fracture or large Hill-Sachs is noted or in the chronic, recurrent instability setting.

TREATMENT

Nonoperative

Nonoperative treatment of fist time traumatic shoulder instability is typically best reserved for in-season athletes participating in contact or overhead sports. Treatment typically involves pain control, edema reduction, focus on return of painless full ROM, and regaining full strength. In NCAA division I athletes, this has proven successful in 73% of players, allowing them to return to season (including 2 baseball players in the study), despite a high rate of recurrent instability events seen in 64% of players who return.[35] Other reports have demonstrated recurrence rates with nonoperative treatment ranging from 25% to 92%.[34,60-62] Unfortunately, this approach may not prove as successful in baseball players given the abduction, extension, and extreme external rotation required during the throwing motion, a position that can be avoided or limited in contact athletes by bracing. Bracing effectively limits abduction and external rotation, preventing the glenohumeral joint from entering a position of potential subluxation or dislocation, but bracing is not practical for baseball athletes. In the setting of traumatic glenohumeral instability in the baseball player, nonoperative treatment has a relatively limited role, as most of these athletes are unable to function effectively as an overhead throwing athlete with symptomatic instability.

Operative

The main indication for operative treatment of traumatic instability for baseball players is reserved for those who fail nonoperative management after a primary, traumatic subluxation or dislocation or those who experience symptomatic recurrent instability. Relative indications include participation in overhead or contact sports, injury at the end of the season without sufficient rehabilitation time, greater than 13.5% glenoid bone loss, and age less than 20 years.[37] Our preferred technique in baseball players is an arthroscopic Bankart repair, which is also the primary technique performed in the United States for those undergoing initial surgical treatment, but other options involving bone block techniques should be considered if significant bone loss is present.

Surgical Options

A variety of surgical options exist for management of traumatic instability. These include the historic gold standard, open Bankart repair, the arthroscopic Bankart repair, the open Latarjet, the arthroscopic Latarjet, open bone block procedures (distal tibial allograft or iliac crest), and other auxiliary procedures including the inferior capsular shift and thermal capsulorrhaphy. Each of these procedures has its proper indications based on the patient, pathoanatomy, chronicity, bone stock, and surgeon preference, but in the baseball player, this decision must take into the account the demand required during the throwing motion. The most commonly performed surgery for overhead and contact athletes in the United States is the arthroscopic Bankart repair.[63] This is likely multifactorial owing to concern the for decreased postoperative ROM noted with open procedures, which require at least partial release or splitting of the subscapularis, prolonged rehabilitation time with open procedures compared with arthroscopic procedures, and surgeon preference. There is currently ongoing debate concerning the young, high-risk athlete, as many in Europe espouse the success of the Latarjet procedure (either open or arthroscopic), as some studies have shown decreased dislocation rates in this population of athletes.[64] However, few (number) of the athletes in this cohort were baseball players; therefore the difference in recurrence and return to same level of play may not apply to the throwing athlete.

Authors' Preferred Surgical Technique

In the setting of traumatic glenohumeral instability without significant bony defects, our preferred surgical technique is the arthroscopic Bankart with suture anchor repair. Additionally, we prefer to perform all shoulder arthroscopy, especially glenohumeral instability surgery, in the lateral decubitus position. This allows for optimal visualization of and access to the anteroinferior aspect of the glenoid using gentle axial traction. Additionally, a recent meta-analysis has demonstrated significantly better results after arthroscopic stabilization of anterior instability when performed in the lateral position.[65]

We use a standard operating table with a bean bag positioner, axillary roll, arm board for the contralateral arm, safety strap, and several pillows to pad the patient's legs. The operative arm is protected with a well-padded sleeve, which is then suspended from a standard traction boom with 10 to 15 pounds of weight (10 for females, 15 for males). A shoulder drape with suction pockets is helpful to prevent pooling of water and distraction of the drapes. A standard arthroscopic setup, including a 4 mm, 30° arthroscope with shoulder-length metal cannulas and light, suction, inflow, and outflow tubing are used in all shoulder arthroscopies and instability cases. Blade-down and blade-up soft tissue liberators are used to elevate the capsulolabral tissue, and a 4.5 mm full-radius shaver on foot control is used for glenoid preparation. A variety of suture anchors may be used to treat glenohumeral instability, but we prefer to use 1.5 mm all-suture suture anchors, which generate only a small pilot hole, allow for use of a curved drill guide, are inert and will not cause cystic resorption, and demonstrate excellent pull-out strength. Sutures are passed using a 45° or 70° suture passer with a deployable lasso, typically through an 8.5 mm cannula. Occasionally, a bird beak (straight, 15°, 22° and 45° curved) will be used to pass sutures, so having these instruments available is helpful. The anchors are then tied and cut using a standard knot pusher and an open, end-cutting suture cutter. After draping, have a second Mayo stand positioned from opposite side of the patient, over patient's hip, to allow all cords to run off of the feet.

Technique, Step by Step

After standard sterile skin prepping and draping, mark out the scapular spine, acromion, acromioclavicular (AC) joint, coracoid, clavicle, and coracoacromial (CA) ligament. Position a standard posterior portal is about 2 to 3 cm inferior and a 1 to 2 cm medial to posterolateral corner of acromion, palpating for the soft spot between the humeral head and glenoid. Insert an 18 g spinal needle into the glenohumeral joint, and inject 30 to 60 cc of sterile saline. The arm will internally rotate as capsule distends, indicating proper positioning of the needle. Incise skin with a #11 blade, and insert the arthroscope trocar and sheath and then insert the camera. Create an anterior portal under direct visualization and use an 18 g spinal needle to localize. Our starting point for the anterior portal is located just lateral to the coracoid and just lateral to a line representing the CA ligament, drawn from the tip of the coracoid to the anterolateral corner of the acromion—staying lateral to this line avoids injuring the acromial branch of the coracoacromial artery, reduces bleeding, and optimizes visualization. We then perform a diagnostic arthroscopy to assess intra-articular pathology. Create a systematic, reproducible way

to assess the glenohumeral joint so that all structures are seen every time the joint is assessed. We use this order: anterior labrum, subscapularis, subscapularis recess and middle glenohumeral ligament (MGHL), glenohumeral articular surfaces, anteroinferior labrum, inferior labrum, axillary pouch, posterior labrum, posterior-superior labrum, long head of the biceps, rotator cuff, and posterior-superior humeral head (assess for Hill-Sachs). If needed, the camera should be switched to the anterior portal to obtain a better view of the posterior labrum and capsule, as well as a better view of the subscapularis recess.

After a labral tear or Bankart lesion has been identified and repair indicated, the labrum is mobilized and the glenoid rim is prepared (Figure 17.8). Debride all loose labral tissue initially with a 4.5 mm shaver. Then use the elevators to separate residual labrum and capsule from glenoid. This is a key step—if tissue is not properly mobilized, it cannot be properly positioned back up to the rim and the fixation will likely fail owing to improper tensioning of the glenohumeral ligaments and improper restoration of the labral depth and contour. Proper mobilization of the capsulolabral tissue is achieved when the muscle belly of the subscapularis can be seen between the capsule and the glenoid neck. To achieve this, a plane is developed between the capsulolabral tissue and glenoid neck using an elevator and then the tissue is peeled off by levering against the elevator shaft against the glenoid neck. Perform this in a controlled fashion, not aggressively, as the elevator can break. Once

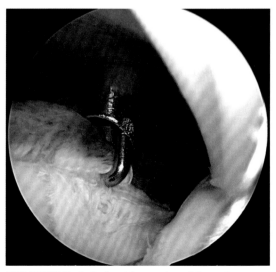

FIGURE 17.8 • Left shoulder as viewed from the posterior portal via the axillary recess (inferior) demonstrating a Bankart lesion of the anteroinferior labrum with a bucket-handle component.

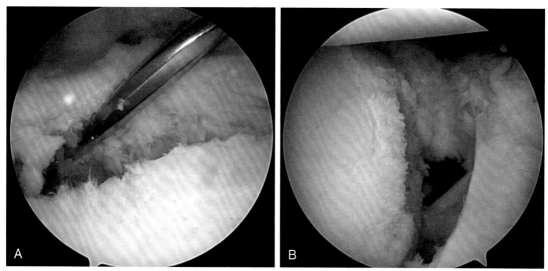

FIGURE 17.9 • Posterior view of a left shoulder after adequate mobilization of the capsulolabral complex with an elevator (A) and bony preparation of the anterior glenoid with a shaver (B). Note the deep border of the subscapularis can be seen deep to the capsule (dark triangle).

the capsulolabral tissue is mobilized adequately, use a 4.5 mm shaver to remove residual tissue from the anterior glenoid neck, and then gently decorticate the rim and anterior neck until bone is seen along the entire repair site (Figure 17.9).

After proper glenoid and labral prep, anchors can then be placed. To assist in suture passing and knot tying, an 8.5 mm cannula is inserted through the anterior portal. An accessory anterior portal is created to provide a better angle for anchor insertion at the 6 o'clock position. We prefer to use a transsubscapularis portal, positioned 4 to 5 cm inferomedial to the standard anterior portal. Use an 18 g needle for localization, aiming to enter the joint just above or through the subscapularis, ensuring that the trajectory easily accesses the inferior-most aspect of the glenoid. We typically modify this portal by inserting the drill guide and passer through the subscapularis tendon but place a second 8.5 mm cannula just above the superior border of the subscapularis to avoid placing a larger bore cannula through the tendon.

The first anchor to be placed is the 6:00 anchor (the most inferior), which is key, as this sets the tension of the anterior band of the inferior glenohumeral ligament (IGHL) and the remaining sutures as the repair proceeds proximally on the glenoid face (Figure 17.10). Ensure that placement of this anchor is optimal. Use the accessory anterior portal as described above and place the drill guide at the 6:00 position at the chondral margin. Placing the anchor too far off the chondral margin will secure the labrum down off of the glenoid rim, potentially decreasing the tension

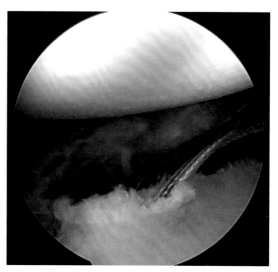

FIGURE 17.10 • Left shoulder viewed through the posterior portal showing an anchor placed at the 6:00 position at the articular margin.

needed for a good repair. Have an assistant to lift up and back on the arm, translating the humeral head laterally and posteriorly to more easily access the 6:00 position. Place the tip of the guide on the articular margin and then lever your hand up (laterally) and distal (inferiorly) to make sure the angle is correct, so as not to drill too posterior or too shallow. Err toward putting the anchor slightly more on the glenoid face (articular surface) than down the rim. Drill and then insert the anchor, testing it by pulling on it to ensure it does not pull out. Insert the 70° suture passer through the accessory portal, through the subscapularis and grab a good bite of the capsulolabral tissue, making sure not to grab more than 1 cm of tissue off the rim at this site, as the axillary nerve runs deep to the capsule in this location. Push the tip of the passer through the capsule first before rotating the passer and then drop hand distally (toward foot) to prevent the passer from existing too posterior. Walk the tip of the passer up the glenoid neck and exit at the chondrolabral junction. In some cases, this first pass may be easier if passed from the posterior portal (viewing from the anterior portal). Once the tip of the passer is in the correct position, deploy the loop and shuttle 1 suture through the loop and the pull the passer out of the joint, shuttling the suture through the capsule and labrum. This step is repeated to create a mattress stitch at the 6:00 position. Adjust the location of the next pass to optimize the fixation and position of the tissue repair at

this position. Retrieve both sutures out of the passing cannula, and tie using a sliding knot. We prefer to use alternating half hitches. Cut the sutures, leaving a small tail. Repeat these steps, moving up the clockface, placing 1 anchor per hour on the clockface. We prefer to alternate between mattress and simple sutures for the first 4 anchors and then use simple sutures after. Starting at the 3 o'clock position, most of the remaining anchors can be placed, passed, and tied via the anterior portal. When tying, make sure knots are off edge of the rim and push up a good labral bumper each time (Figure 17.11). After all anchors have been placed, passed, and tied, obtain final images and then remove the arthroscope. We close all portals with 3-0 nonabsorbable monofilament, place dry dressings, and position the operative extremity in a sling with a side pillow.

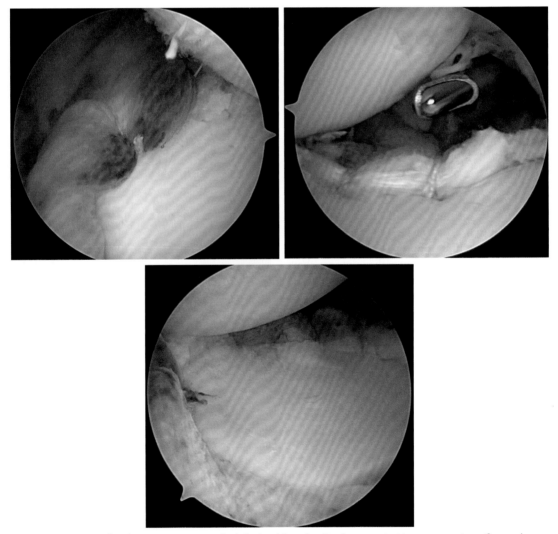

FIGURE 17.11 ▪ Final arthroscopic images of a left shoulder after Bankart repair. Note restoration of capsular tension at the anteroinferior aspect of the shoulder and restoration of the labral bumper.

POSTSURGICAL REHAB

Our typical postsurgical rehabilitation protocol for throwing athletes begins on postoperative day 1 and progresses in 5 phases with gradually increasing focus on motion, neuromuscular control, balance, strength, functional motion and strength, and finally sport-specific activity. Phase 1 is the immediate postoperative phase, focusing on "restrictive motion" taking place from weeks 0 to 6. The goal of this phase is to protect the surgical repair, reduce pain and inflammation, limit detrimental effects of immobilization, and promote dynamic stability and proprioception. During this phase, a sling and shoulder immobilizer are worn during all daily activities and during sleep for the first 4 weeks (longer if indicated by the physician based on the pathology seen during surgery). Therapy focuses on regaining motion with gentle passive and active ROM exercises, with the goal to reach 160° of forward flexion, and progressive internal and external rotation with increasing abduction, up to 90° by the end of the sixth week. Hand, wrist, and elbow motion, along with gripping exercises and submaximal shoulder isometrics are also added. A Thrower's Ten strengthening program is started at the conclusion of week 6. Phase 2 (weeks 7-14) is a moderate protection phase with the goals of preserving the integrity of the surgical repair, regaining full ROM, enhancing neuromuscular control, and restoring muscular strength and balance. ROM is progressed to 180 of flexion and 115° of external rotation with the arm in 90° of abduction. Thrower's Ten exercises are continued, and isotonic strengthening and progressive plyometrics are added near the end of this phase. Provided full, painless ROM and progressing strength and neuromuscular control, a hitting program can begin near the end of this phase. The third phase (weeks 15-20) is the minimal protection phase, which focuses on maintaining full ROM, improving muscular strength, power, and endurance, gradually initiating functional activities, and initiating an interval throwing program. The Thrower's Ten exercises are continued, and manual resistance, endurance training, and restricted sport activities are started during this phase. For baseball players and other overhead athletes, an interval throwing program typically begins at week 16. Phase 4 (weeks 21-24) is the advanced strengthening phase, which focuses on maintaining shoulder mobility, enhancing muscular strength, power, and endurance, and progressing functional activities. Flexibility exercises, isotonic strengthening, plyometrics for neuromuscular control, and interval sport programs are all continued and progressed. Pitchers may begin throwing off of a mound beginning at weeks 22-24. Phase 5 is the return to activity phase (months 7-9) and includes continued focus on strength, mobility and stability, and gradual return to unrestricted sporting activities.

RESULTS

When assessing the results of a surgical procedure in high-level athletes, several measures must be taken into account. The first is recurrence of instability. Recurrent instability after surgical stabilization is the primary indicator of failure of the procedure and frequently indicates a poor indication, a missed diagnosis, an inadequate surgical stabilization, or recurrent trauma. Overall, surgical treatment of traumatic glenohumeral instability demonstrates good clinical results with relatively low recurrence rates, good outcomes scores, and good return to play rates. In general, recurrence rates for arthroscopic Bankart repairs range from 2.4% to 21%, outcome scores range from 85 to 92.3 for Rowe scores and 84.1 to 91.2 for ASES scores, and return to same level of play rates range from 71% to 90% at an average of 5.3 to 9.8 months[13,60,66-72] Outcomes after open Bankart repairs, the historical gold standard, demonstrate similar return to play at same level rates, ranging from 53% to 82%, at an average of 6 months after surgery, with recurrence rates ranging from 6.7% to 12%.[67,73] The Latarjet procedure demonstrated similar return to play at same level rates (73%) 6 months after surgery but demonstrated a lower recurrence rate (0%-10%).[64,67,74] Return to play timing has been shown to be similar for both arthroscopic Bankart and Latarjet procedures (5-6 months) but is typically longer for open Bankart repair.[33,73,75] Thus, surgical stabilization for anterior glenohumeral instability for all athletes demonstrates acceptable clinical outcomes, with high return to play rates, moderate return to same level rates, and recurrence rates that have decreased over the years, but with variations based on sport and activity type. However, the demand placed on the glenohumeral joint by a baseball player requires a different level of scrutiny.

Specifically focusing on baseball and overhead throwing athletes, results of surgical management of anterior glenohumeral instability demonstrates significantly inferior results concerning return to play and return to play at same level. This has been a long-understood sequelae of anterior shoulder instability in the throwing athlete. Bergfeld noted, in 1983, the ability of surgical correction to properly treat glenohumeral instability, but regaining full throwing function after surgery was rare.[38] Part of this limitation is likely related to a loss of external rotation noted in many studies. Average external rotation deficits after surgical treatment of anterior instability range from 2° to 15° (range 0°-30°) with only 48% to 69% regaining full external rotation, but this external rotation deficit severely limits a thrower's ability to maximize torque during the throwing motion, which can have significant effects on velocity and distance.[34,37,60,66,68-70,75-78] Loss of external rotation has proven the main cause of failure to return to play in throwing athletes, compared with recurrent instability, which causes failure to return to play in contact athletes.

Several studies assessing open and arthroscopic techniques have demonstrated lower return to play rates and lower return to same level rates in throwing and baseball athletes when compared with all athletes undergoing surgical stabilization. Clinical outcomes typically demonstrate significant improvements in noncollision, overhead, and throwing athletes with Constant scores up to 91.2% and Rowe scores ranging from 62% to 93.2%[66] Additionally, dislocation rates are similar for noncollision, overhead, and throwing athletes when compared with contact athletes, ranging from 5.9% to 6.7%.[66,68] While clinical outcomes and recurrence rates are similar to most other groups, throwing athletes demonstrate return to play rates ranging from 64% to 100%, with return to same level dropping precipitously to 50% to 68% in all throwers and as low as 33% to 69% in high-level (varsity and professional) baseball players.[33,68,78-80] Throwing athletes typically experience prolonged return to play as well, ranging from 8.1 to 24 months, which is significantly longer compared with nonthrowing athletes.[33,68]

In the late 1970s, before the open Bankart becoming the standard, throwing athletes undergoing a Magnuson-Stack or Bristow procedure were found to be incapable of returning to high-level performance.[81] Shortly thereafter, Rowe published one of the first studies to describe outcomes in throwing athletes after an open Bankart repair, reporting only 33% (10/30) were able to throw at the same level.[16] As a follow-up to that initial study, Rowe and Zarins reported that only 64% of those undergoing open Bankart on the dominant arm were able to return to forceful throwing.[82] One of the first assessments specifically focusing on overhead athletes, performed by Frank Jobe, included 20 baseball players, 11 of whom were professional and 8 of whom were pitchers, who underwent open anterior capsulolabral reconstruction, a modification of the Bankart procedure with an inferior capsular shift.[33] His report found an overall return to same level of 72% (18/25) in all overhead athletes. All 7 players who did not return to sport were baseball players, who retired owing to loss of ROM, velocity, noncompliance, or personal reasons. Of the 12 pitchers in the study, only 50% returned to their former competitive level, including 38% (3/8) of professional pitchers returned to their preoperative level of play. Of these 3 professional pitchers, only 1 was still competing after 2 years of play. The average return to play for all overhead athletes was 14 months (15 months for pitchers, 14 for nonpitchers). Despite the low return to play rates found in this analysis, all were satisfied with the procedure, which successfully alleviated their pain, stabilized their shoulder, and achieved near full ROM.

A few years later, Jobe subsequently published a larger cohort of baseball players undergoing the anterior capsulolabral reconstruction, which demonstrated slightly better results, but these were still inferior to those seen in nonthrowing athletes.[80] Fifty-two baseball players, 35 pitchers, were evaluated an average of 33 months after surgery, and 64% of all players, 69% of all pitchers, and 60% of professional pitchers were able to return to same level of competition. In 2004, Ide et al evaluated 55 patients undergoing arthroscopic Bankart repair with suture anchors, reporting good overall results with a mean Rowe score of 92.3, a 7.7% recurrence rate, and an 80% return to sport with no limitations.[68] Importantly, overhead throwing athletes in this group demonstrated a 68% return to same level of play rate at a mean time of 8.1 months, both of which were significantly lower and longer, respectively, than nonoverhead athletes. Similarly, Ozturk et al demonstrated an overall return to play rate of 87% after arthroscopic anterior stabilization in patients under 25 years of age, with 75% returning to same level. Of those, only 66% of the noncontact athletes (of which 7 were baseball players) were able to return to same level of play.[72]

Additionally, in athletes with a large, engaging Hill-Sachs lesions and a glenoid deficiency less that 20%, the addition of an arthroscopic remplissage is frequently added to reduce recurrent instability. Unfortunately, this can lead to a loss of external rotation postoperatively and can limit throwers from achieving a normal, full throwing motion. In their study, Garcia et al reported that 65.5% of all throwers (softball, baseball, football) had issues with throwing due to surgery and 58.6% could not normally windup.[83] Additionally, 34.5% of throwers reported decreased velocity, 17.2% reported pain with throwing, and 58.6% reported stiffness, with an overall return to sport rate of 51.7%, demonstrating a significant difference and severe limitation in throwing athletes undergoing arthroscopic Bankart repair and remplissage.

Although surgical fixation of traumatic glenohumeral instability in the general and contact athletic population demonstrates good clinical outcomes and return to play rates in the 80% to 90% range, overhead athletes and baseball players, in particular, experience inferior return to same level of play rates. The supraphysiologic glenohumeral external rotation required for optimal velocity in elite baseball players is frequently compromised, even if only be a few degrees. Any loss of external rotation can cause significant difficulty, pain, loss of velocity, or stiffness that can prevent baseball players from returning to their prior level of play. Should nonoperative modalities fail to alleviate instability and the symptoms associated with it, instability surgery for baseball players should be approached cautiously and with full disclosure of the potential risks for loss of motion and subsequent difficulty regaining full throwing motion and velocity.

COMPLICATIONS

The rate of complications after traumatic glenohumeral instability and subsequent surgical repair are relatively low. While axillary neuropraxia can be seen in 5% to 35% of patients sustaining a shoulder dislocation, 87% will resolve spontaneously within 12 months, despite up to 51% experiencing residual decreased deltoid function.[20,41,84] Neurovascular injury has also been reported as a surgical complication but more frequently occurs with open Bankart repairs, capsular shifts, and Latarjet procedures.[84,85] The Latarjet procedure has been shown to have a higher overall complication (up to 30%) and revision surgery rate (up to 7%) when compared with open and arthroscopic Bankart repairs, although more recent reports indicate that this is likely not significantly higher.[85-87]

Recurrent instability is a well-known complication after surgery for glenohumeral instability. Overall, recurrence rates have been shown to be lower with Latarjet when compared with arthroscopic fixation, with up to 21% and 12% experiencing recurrent instability with arthroscopic Bankart and Latarjet, respectively.[86]

Additionally, loss of ROM has been consistently reported in many outcomes studies, which significantly affects baseball players. As mentioned above, average external rotation deficits can range from 2° to 15° after arthroscopic Bankart repairs, which is enough to cause limitations in throwing.[65,83]

After arthroscopic Bankart, other complications including infection, nerve palsy, and stiffness have been reported at less than 1% for each.[65]

CONCLUSION

Traumatic glenohumeral instability in baseball players is relatively rare when compared with other overhead and contact athletes. Unfortunately, as with other athletes sustaining a traumatic subluxation or dislocation, nonsurgical treatment demonstrates relatively low success rate in young, athletic populations. Surgical management of glenohumeral instability has demonstrated good results for contact athletes and some overhead athletes, but baseball players and pitchers, in particular, experience inferior results and significantly lower return to same level rates. These results are correlated to a lack of external rotation that is frequently associated with arthroscopic and open Bankart repair and Latarjet procedures. Although the arthroscopic Bankart repair is the treatment of choice for those baseball players with good glenoid and humeral head bone stock, return to same level rates are still lower than other sports. Focus on external rotation during postoperative rehab is important, but despite this, full return to play may be difficult to achieve. This potential and expectation must be discussed with the player before surgery, as this can significantly affect their ability to return to the same level of play.

MANAGER'S TIPS

- Traumatic glenohumeral instability in baseball players is relatively rare, but it most commonly occurs after contact with another object or person or with sliding into a base or diving for a ball
- While nonoperative treatment of traumatic glenohumeral instability has high recurrence rates, this should be emphasized early and initially after a shoulder subluxation or dislocation with the goal of returning to sport after full ROM and strength are achieved
- If nonoperative therapy fails, surgical treatment should be considered. The authors' recommended surgical treatment is arthroscopic Bankart repair, provided glenoid bone loss is subcritical and there is no large or engaging Hill-Sachs lesion
- With surgical treatment, athletes must be informed of the potential for loss of external rotation and subsequent loss of velocity, which may prevent them from returning to their prior level of play
- After the initial healing phase, physical therapy should focus on regaining full external rotation to maximize the rotation arc and provide the best chance of return to play at the same level

REFERENCES

1. Halder AM, Itoi E, An KN. Anatomy and biomechanics of the shoulder. *Orthop Clin North Am.* 2000;31(2):159-176.

2. Pappas AM, Zawacki RM, Sullivan TJ. Biomechanics of baseball pitching. A preliminary report. *Am J Sports Med.* 1985;13(4):216-222.

3. Kerr ZY, Collins CL, Pommering TL, Fields SK, Comstock RD. Dislocation/separation injuries among US high school athletes in 9 selected sports: 2005-2009. *Clin J Sport Med.* 2011;21(2):101-108.

4. Owens BD, Agel J, Mountcastle SB, Cameron KL, Nelson BJ. Incidence of glenohumeral instability in collegiate athletics. *Am J Sports Med.* 2009;37(9):1750-1754.

5. Bankart ASB. Recurrent or habitual dislocation of the shoulder-joint. *Br Med J.* 1923;2(3285):1132-1133.

6. Coughlin L, Rubinovich M, Johansson J, White B, Greenspoon J. Arthroscopic staple capsulorrhaphy for anterior shoulder instability. *Am J Sports Med.* 1992;20(3):253-256.

7. Goss TP. Anterior glenohumeral instability. *Orthopedics.* 1988;11(1):87-95.

8. Norlin R. Intraarticular pathology in acute, first-time anterior shoulder dislocation: an arthroscopic study. *Arthroscopy.* 1993;9(5):546-549.

9. Taylor DC, Arciero RA. Pathologic changes associated with shoulder dislocations. Arthroscopic and physical examination findings in first-time, traumatic anterior dislocations. *Am J Sports Med.* 1997;25(3):306-311.

10. Thomas SC, Matsen FA. An approach to the repair of avulsion of the glenohumeral ligaments in the management of traumatic anterior glenohumeral instability. *J Bone Joint Surg Am.* 1989;71(4):506-513.

11. Knapik DM, Voos JE. Magnetic resonance imaging and arthroscopic correlation in shoulder instability. *Sports Med Arthrosc Rev.* 2017;25(4):172-178.

12. Nakagawa S, Ozaki R, Take Y, Mizuno N, Mae T. Enlargement of glenoid defects in traumatic anterior shoulder instability: influence of the number of recurrences and type of sport. *Orthop J Sports Med.* 2014;2(4):2325967114529920.

13. Nakagawa S, Mae T, Sato S, Okimura S, Kuroda M. Risk factors for the postoperative recurrence of instability after arthroscopic bankart repair in athletes. *Orthop J Sports Med.* 2017;5(9):2325967117726494.

14. Calandra JJ, Baker CL, Uribe J. The incidence of Hill-Sachs lesions in initial anterior shoulder dislocations. *Arthroscopy.* 1989;5(4):254-257.

15. Fox JA, Sanchez A, Zajac TJ, Provencher MT. Understanding the Hill-Sachs lesion in its role in patients with recurrent anterior shoulder instability. *Curr Rev Musculoskelet Med.* 2017;10(4):469-479.

16. Rowe CR, Patel D, Southmayd WW. The Bankart procedure: a long-term end-result study. *J Bone Joint Surg Am.* 1978;60(1):1-16.

17. Griffith JF, Antonio GE, Yung PSH, et al. Prevalence, pattern, and spectrum of glenoid bone loss in anterior shoulder dislocation: CT analysis of 218 patients. *AJR Am J Roentgenol.* 2008;190(5):1247-1254.

18. Edwards TB, Boulahia A, Walch G. Radiographic analysis of bone defects in chronic anterior shoulder instability. *Arthroscopy.* 2003;19(7):732-739.

19. Pavlov H, Warren RF, Weiss CB, Dines DM. The roentgenographic evaluation of anterior shoulder instability. *Clin Orthop Relat Res.* 1985(194):153-158.

20. Burra G, Andrews JR. Acute shoulder and elbow dislocations in the athlete. *Orthop Clin North Am.* 2002;33(3):479-495.

21. Zacchilli MA, Owens BD. Epidemiology of shoulder dislocations presenting to emergency departments in the United States. *J Bone Joint Surg Am.* 2010;92(3):542-549.

22. Simonet WT, Melton LJ, Cofield RH, Ilstrup DM. Incidence of anterior shoulder dislocation in Olmsted County, Minnesota. *Clin Orthop Relat Res.* 1984(186):186-191.

23. Altchek DW, Dines DM. Shoulder injuries in the throwing athlete. *J Am Acad Orthop Surg.* 1995;3(3):159-165.

24. Collins CL, Comstock RD. Epidemiological features of high school baseball injuries in the United States, 2005-2007. *Pediatrics.* 2008;121(6):1181-1187.

25. Conte S, Camp CL, Dines JS. Injury trends in major league baseball over 18 seasons: 1998-2015. *Am J Orthop.* 2016;45(3):116-123.

26. Darrow CJ, Collins CL, Yard EE, Comstock RD. Epidemiology of severe injuries among United States high school athletes: 2005-2007. *Am J Sports Med.* 2009;37(9):1798-1805.

27. Dick R, Sauers EL, Agel J, et al. Descriptive epidemiology of collegiate men's baseball injuries: National Collegiate Athletic Association Injury Surveillance System, 1988-1989 through 2003-2004. *J Athl Train.* 2007;42(2):183-193.

28. McFarland EG, Wasik M. Epidemiology of collegiate baseball injuries. *Clin J Sport Med.* 1998;8(1):10-13.

29. Saper MG, Pierpoint LA, Liu W, Comstock RD, Polousky JD, Andrews JR. Epidemiology of shoulder and elbow injuries among United States high school baseball players: school years 2005-2006 through 2014-2015. *Am J Sports Med.* 2018;46(1):37-43.

30. Camp CL, Curriero FC, Pollack KM, et al. The epidemiology and effect of sliding injuries in major and minor league baseball players. *Am J Sports Med.* 2017;45(10):2372-2378.

31. Hosey RG, Puffer JC. Baseball and softball sliding injuries. Incidence, and the effect of technique in collegiate baseball and softball players. *Am J Sports Med.* 2000;28(3):360-363.

32. Chang EY, Hoenecke HR, Fronek J, Huang BK, Chung CB. Humeral avulsions of the inferior glenohumeral ligament complex involving the axillary pouch in professional baseball players. *Skeletal Radiol.* 2014;43(1):35-41.

33. Jobe FW, Giangarra CE, Kvitne RS, Glousman RE. Anterior capsulolabral reconstruction of the shoulder in athletes in overhand sports. *Am J Sports Med.* 1991;19(5):428-434.

34. Dickens JF, Rue JP, Cameron KL, et al. Successful return to sport after arthroscopic shoulder stabilization versus nonoperative management in contact athletes with anterior shoulder instability: a prospective multicenter study. *Am J Sports Med.* 2017;45(11):2540-2546.

35. Dickens JF, Owens BD, Cameron KL, et al. Return to play and recurrent instability after in-season anterior shoulder instability: a prospective multicenter study. *Am J Sports Med.* 2014;42(12):2842-2850.

36. Buss DD, Lynch GP, Meyer CP, Huber SM, Freehill MQ. Nonoperative management for in-season athletes with anterior shoulder instability. *Am J Sports Med.* 2004;32(6):1430-1433.

37. Elsenbeck MJ, Dickens JF. Return to sports after shoulder stabilization surgery for anterior shoulder instability. *Curr Rev Musculoskelet Med.* 2017;10(4):491-498.

38. Anderson T, Bergfeld J. Common throwing injuries of the shoulder. *Mediguide Orthop.* 1983;4:1-5.

39. Shah R, Koris J, Wazir A, Srinivasan SS. Anterior humeral circumflex artery avulsion with brachial plexus injury following an isolated traumatic anterior shoulder dislocation. *BMJ Case Rep.* 2016;2016:bcr2015213497.

40. Visser CPJ, Coene LN, Brand R, Tavy DLJ. The incidence of nerve injury in anterior dislocation of the shoulder and its influence on functional recovery: a prospective clinical and EMG study. *J Bone Joint Surg Br.* 1999;81-B(4):679-685.

41. Silliman JF, Hawkins RJ. Classification and physical diagnosis of instability of the shoulder. *Clin Orthop Relat Res.* 1993;291:7-19.

42. Bahk M, Keyurapan E, Tasaki A, Sauers EL, McFarland EG. Laxity testing of the shoulder: a review. *Am J Sports Med.* 2007;35(1):131-144.

43. Owens BD, Duffey ML, Nelson BJ, DeBerardino TM, Taylor DC, Mountcastle SB. The incidence and characteristics of shoulder instability at the United States Military Academy. *Am J Sports Med.* 2007;35(7):1168-1173.

44. Safran O, Milgrom C, Radeva-Petrova DR, Jaber S, Finestone A. Accuracy of the anterior apprehension test as a predictor of risk for redislocation after a first traumatic shoulder dislocation. *Am J Sports Med.* 2010;38(5):972-975.

45. Lo IK, Nonweiler B, Woolfrey M, Litchfield R, Kirkley A. An evaluation of the apprehension, relocation, and surprise tests for anterior shoulder instability. *Am J Sports Med.* 2004;32(2):301-307.

46. Farber AJ, Castillo RM, Clough M, Bahk M, McFarland EG. Clinical assessment of three common tests for traumatic anterior shoulder instability. *J Bone Joint Surg Am.* 2006;88(7):1467-1474.

47. Gerber C, Ganz R. Clinical assessment of instability of the shoulder. With special reference to anterior and posterior drawer tests. *J Bone Joint Surg.* 1984;66-B(4):551-556.

48. Ellenbecker TS, Bailie DS, Mattalino AJ, et al. Intrarater and interrater reliability of a manual technique to assess anterior humeral head translation of the glenohumeral joint. *J Shoulder Elbow Surg.* 2002;11(5):470-475.

49. Bigliani LU, Codd TP, Connor PM, Levine WN, Littlefield MA, Hershon SJ. Shoulder motion and laxity in the professional baseball player. *Am J Sports Med.* 1997;25(5):609-613.

50. Hall RH, Isaac F, Booth CR. Dislocations of the shoulder with special reference to accompanying small fractures. *J Bone Joint Surg Am.* 1959;41-A(3):489-494.

51. Garth WP, Slappey CE, Ochs CW. Roentgenographic demonstration of instability of the shoulder: the apical oblique projection. A technical note. *J Bone Joint Surg Am.* 1984;66(9):1450-1453.

52. Danzig LA, Greenway G, Resnick D. The Hill-Sachs lesion. An experimental study. *Am J Sports Med.* 1980;8(5):328-332.

53. Engebretsen L, Craig EV. Radiologic features of shoulder instability. *Clin Orthop Relat Res.* 1993(291):29-44.

54. Chandnani VP, Yeager TD, DeBerardino T, et al. Glenoid labral tears: prospective evaluation with MRI imaging, MR arthrography, and CT arthrography. *Am J Roentgenol.* 1993;161(6):1229-1235.

55. Smith TO, Drew BT, Toms AP. A meta-analysis of the diagnostic test accuracy of MRA and MRI for the detection of glenoid labral injury. *Arch Orthop Trauma Surg.* 2012;132(7):905-919.

56. Cvitanic O, Tirman PF, Feller JF, Bost FW, Minter J, Carroll KW. Using abduction and external rotation of the shoulder to increase the sensitivity of MR arthrography in revealing tears of the anterior glenoid labrum. *AJR Am J Roentgenol.* 1997;169(3):837-844.

57. Tian C-Y, Cui G-Q, Zheng Z-Z, Ren A-H. The added value of ABER position for the detection and classification of anteroinferior labroligamentous lesions in MR arthrography of the shoulder. *Eur J Radiol.* 2013;82(4):651-657.

58. Burkhart SS, Beer JFD. Traumatic glenohumeral bone defects and their relationship to failure of arthroscopic Bankart repairs: significance of the inverted-pear glenoid and the humeral engaging Hill-Sachs lesion. *Arthroscopy.* 2000;16(7):677-694.

59. Shin S-J, Kim RG, Jeon YS, Kwon TH. Critical value of anterior glenoid bone loss that leads to recurrent glenohumeral instability after arthroscopic bankart repair. *Am J Sports Med.* 2017;45(9):1975-1981.

60. Arciero RA, Wheeler JH, Ryan JB, McBride JT. Arthroscopic Bankart repair versus nonoperative treatment for acute, initial anterior shoulder dislocations. *Am J Sports Med.* 1994;22(5):589-594.

61. Jakobsen BW, Johannsen HV, Suder P, Søjbjerg JO. Primary repair versus conservative treatment of first-time traumatic anterior dislocation of the shoulder: a randomized study with 10-year follow-up. *Arthroscopy*. 2007;23(2):118-123.

62. Kirkley A, Werstine R, Ratjek A, Griffin S. Prospective randomized clinical trial comparing the effectiveness of immediate arthroscopic stabilization versus immobilization and rehabilitation in first traumatic anterior dislocations of the shoulder: long-term evaluation. *Arthroscopy*. 2005;21(1):55-63.

63. Zhang AL, Montgomery SR, Ngo SS, Hame SL, Wang JC, Gamradt SC. Arthroscopic versus open shoulder stabilization: current practice patterns in the United States. *Arthroscopy*. 2014;30(4):436-443.

64. Bessière C, Trojani C, Carles M, Mehta SS, Boileau P. The open latarjet procedure is more reliable in terms of shoulder stability than arthroscopic bankart repair. *Clin Orthop Relat Res*. 2014;472(8):2345-2351.

65. Frank RM, Saccomanno MF, McDonald LS, Moric M, Romeo AA, Provencher MT. Outcomes of arthroscopic anterior shoulder instability in the beach chair versus lateral decubitus position: a systematic review and meta-regression analysis. *Arthroscopy*. 2014;30(10):1349-1365.

66. Cho NS, Hwang JC, Rhee YG. Arthroscopic stabilization in anterior shoulder instability: collision athletes versus noncollision athletes. *Arthroscopy*. 2006;22(9):947-953.

67. Ialenti MN, Mulvihill JD, Feinstein M, Zhang AL, Feeley BT. Return to play following shoulder stabilization: a systematic review and meta-analysis. *Orthop J Sports Med*. 2017;5(9):2325967117726055.

68. Ide J, Maeda S, Takagi K. Arthroscopic Bankart repair using suture anchors in athletes: patient selection and postoperative sports activity. *Am J Sports Med*. 2004;32(8):1899-1905.

69. Wheeler JH, Ryan JB, Arciero RA, Molinari RN. Arthroscopic versus nonoperative treatment of acute shoulder dislocations in young athletes. *Arthroscopy*. 1989;5(3):213-217.

70. Petrera M, Dwyer T, Tsuji MRS, Theodoropoulos JS. Outcomes of arthroscopic Bankart repair in collision versus noncollision athletes. *Orthopedics*. 2013; 36(5):e621-e626.

71. Gerometta A, Rosso C, Klouche S, Hardy P. Arthroscopic Bankart shoulder stabilization in athletes: return to sports and functional outcomes. *Knee Surg Sports Traumatol Arthrosc*. 2016;24(6):1877-1883.

72. Ozturk BY, Maak TG, Fabricant P, et al. Return to sports after arthroscopic anterior stabilization in patients aged younger than 25 years. *Arthrosc J Arthrosc Relat Surg*. 2013;29(12):1922-1931.

73. Kjeldsen SR, Tordrup PJ, Hvidt EP. Return to sport after a Bankart operation of the shoulder using the Mitek anchor system. *Scand J Med Sci Sports*. 1996;6(6):346-351.

74. Blonna D, Bellato E, Caranzano F, Assom M, Rossi R, Castoldi F. Arthroscopic bankart repair versus open Bristow-latarjet for shoulder instability: a matched-pair multicenter study focused on return to sport. *Am J Sports Med*. 2016;44(12):3198-3205.

75. Pavlik A, Csépai D, Hidas P, Bánóczy A. Sports ability after Bankart procedure in professional athletes. *Knee Surg Sports Traumatol Arthrosc*. 1996;4(2):116-120.

76. Levine WN, Richmond JC, Donaldson WR. Use of the suture anchor in open bankart reconstruction: a follow-up report. *Am J Sports Med*. 1994;22(5):723-726.

77. Rosenberg BN, Richmond JC, Levine WN. Long-term followup of bankart reconstruction: incidence of late degenerative glenohumeral arthrosis. *Am J Sports Med*. 1995;23(5):538-544.

78. Rubenstein DL, Jobe FW, Glousman RE, Kvitne RS, Pink M, Giangarra CE. Anterior capsulolabral reconstruction of the shoulder in athletes. *J Shoulder Elbow Surg*. 1992;1(5):229-237.

79. Bigliani LU, Kurzweil PR, Schwartzbach CC, Wolfe IN, Flatow EL. Inferior capsular shift procedure for anterior-inferior shoulder instability in athletes. *Am J Sports Med*. 1994;22(5):578-584.

80. Kvitne RS, Jobe FW, Jobe CM. Shoulder instability in the overhand or throwing athlete. *Clin Sports Med*. 1995;14(4):917-935.

81. Aamoth GM, O'Phelan EH. Recurrent anterior dislocation of the shoulder: a review of 40 athletes treated by subscapularis transfer (modified Magnuson-Stack procedure). *Am J Sports Med*. 1977;5(5):188-190.

82. Rowe CR, Zarins B. Recurrent transient subluxation of the shoulder. *J Bone Joint Surg Am*. 1981;63(6):863-872.

83. Garcia GH, Wu H-H, Liu JN, Huffman GR, Kelly JD. Outcomes of the remplissage procedure and its effects on return to sports: average 5-year follow-up. *Am J Sports Med*. 2016;44(5):1124-1130.

84. Perlmutter GS, Apruzzese W. Axillary nerve injuries in contact sports: recommendations for treatment and rehabilitation. *Sports Med*. 1998;26(5):351-361.

85. Bokshan SL, DeFroda SF, Owens BD. Comparison of 30-day morbidity and mortality after arthroscopic bankart, open bankart, and latarjet-Bristow procedures: a review of 2864 cases. *Orthop J Sports Med*. 2017;5(7). Available at https://www.ncbi.nlm.nih.gov/pmc/articles/PMC5518960/. Cited January 22, 2018.

86. An VVG, Sivakumar BS, Phan K, Trantalis J. A systematic review and meta-analysis of clinical and patient-reported outcomes following two procedures for recurrent traumatic anterior instability of the shoulder: latarjet procedure vs. Bankart repair. *J Shoulder Elbow Surg*. 2016;25(5):853-863.

87. Griesser MJ, Harris JD, McCoy BW, et al. Complications and re-operations after Bristow-Latarjet shoulder stabilization: a systematic review. *J Shoulder Elbow Surg*. 2013;22(2):286-292.

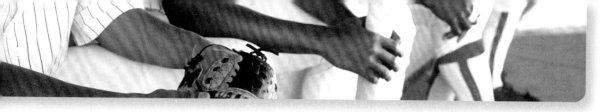

CHAPTER 18

The Batter's Shoulder

Frank J. Alexander, MS, ATC | Christopher S. Ahmad, MD

You hit home runs not by chance, but by preparation.

—*Roger Maris*

INTRODUCTION

The baseball pitcher receives more clinical attention and research compared with position players because of the enormous frequency of injuries to his throwing shoulder and elbow. Hitting a baseball, however, is considered one of the most challenging tasks in sport and has unique injury patterns.[1] Recently, greater attention has been directed to batters and their specific injury pathology. An increasingly recognized injury hitters suffer is posterior glenohumeral instability in the lead (front) shoulder due to the forceful repetitive microtrauma associated with hitting. This posterior instability with labral tearing has come to be known as batter's shoulder.

Similar to throwing, hitting uses a kinetic chain sequence that is initiated in the legs.[1,2] Tremendous force is generated in the larger lower half of the body that moves up through the core to the smaller shoulders, upper extremities, and the bat itself. Therefore, hitting places great demands on the shoulder. Although these demands are less than that of throwing, the frequency of swings taken by a hitter can be high.[2]

When considering instability in the general athletic population, posterior instability accounts for 2% to 12% of all shoulder instability cases.[3,4] The batter's lead shoulder specifically experiences a posterior humeral head force with the arm positioned in relative adduction (Figure 18.1). Shoulder adduction is increased when a player swings at pitch that is on the outside portion of home plate, which increases the posterior force. The symptoms of instability may present insidiously or with acute pain with a single swing.

> **TRIP TO THE MOUND**
>
> Although the majority of position players throw right handed, switch hitters and left-handed batters are of special interest because their lead hitting shoulder experiences the additional stress of throwing. Hitting-related shoulder injuries can therefore create throwing-related symptoms, and corrective posterior instability surgery needs to avoid overtightening the posterior capsule. Posterior capsular contracture is a recognized problem for pitchers.

The hitting motion can be broken into 5 different phases (Figure 18.2). The process of hitting is initiated when there is front foot elevation. During this phase, weight is transferred to the back leg. Moreover, the hips, trunk, and upper body begin coiling. The coiling phase is where the body rotates away from the approaching baseball. The lead shoulder is in maximum internal rotation and adduction during the coiling phase. As the front leg approaches contact, the hips begin their uncoiling rotation while the shoulders continue their coiling rotation.[6] This allows for the maximum force generation through an uncoiling process to transfer energy through the kinetic chain.[2]

At foot contact, upper body uncoiling begins. It is believed that the bodyweight transfer from the back foot to front foot is necessary to successfully hit the ball by promoting proper timing and dynamic balance.[1] At this point, hitting becomes a closed chain energy transfer.[6] As the hips rotate toward the ball, the trunk remains relatively neutral and the shoulders continue toward maximum rotation. The upper extremities begin their rotation forward as the trunk rotates toward the ball in an attempt to maximize the angular velocity of the bat as it approaches ball contact. This process of the hitter initiating his swing to the point where his bat crosses the plate is about 0.2 seconds.[7] Once contact is made with the ball, the batter must decelerate the bat's velocity during the follow-through.

Throughout the hitting motion, much of the force generated in the batter's shoulder is over the posterior portion of the lead shoulder. Just before ball contact, there is over 500 pounds of force directed posteriorly on the shoulder.[2] As the activity of the posterior deltoid increases during acceleration of the swing, large forces are directed on the humeral head. The humeral head is already in a posteriorly directed position, as it is adducted and internally rotated. Forces may change depending on pitch location. The front shoulder is more adducted and flexed during a swing on an outside pitch. Players swinging at and missing an outside pitch (Figure 18.3) are also in a position where their lead shoulder is more adducted and flexed. This position puts players at higher risk for posterior labrum injury when compared with swings taken on pitches elsewhere in the strike zone (Figure 18.4).

If the player makes contact, kinetic energy from the bat is transferred into the ball and additional stabilizing muscles are recruited, dissipating the total amount of energy the body must stop during the follow-through. If the player swings and misses, they must stop the energy of the bat during the follow-through. The lead shoulder does most of the work in slowing the bat down during a follow-through on a missed pitch, and the stresses placed on the posterior shoulder may be increased owing to the lack of recruited stabilizing muscles.[8]

As the bat moves toward the front of the batter, there is an increased posteriorly directed force that can exceed the ability of the soft tissue restraints containing the humeral head. This can lead to posterior subluxations of the humeral head, damaging the posterior labrum and other tissues.

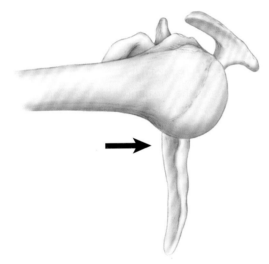

FIGURE 18.1 • The shoulder in relative adduction demonstrating the posterior forces occurring during the phases of hitting (arrow).

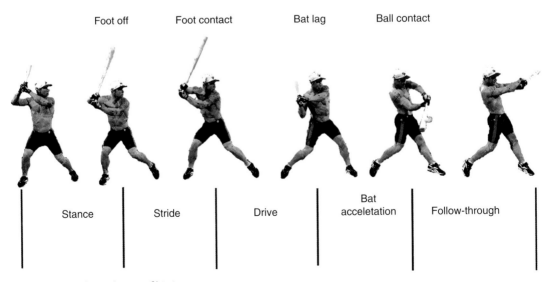

FIGURE 18.2 • The 5 phases of hitting.

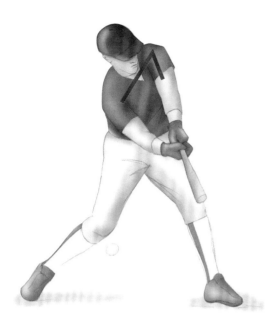

FIGURE 18.3 • The lead shoulder in a more adducted position, demonstrated by the red lines, when swinging and missing a pitch low and away.

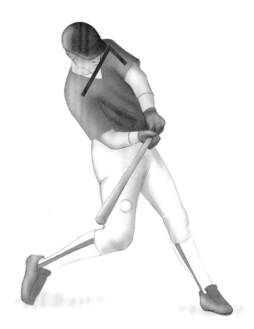

FIGURE 18.4 • When swinging at pitches at other locations in the strike zone, the shoulder still experiences posterior forces, but adduction is not as great when compared with pitches low and away. Note the adduction angle demonstrated by the red lines.

The follow-through also stresses the anterior capsule and labrum, especially when the player finishes his swing one-handed.

CLINICAL EXAMINATION

History

Players often report a sensation of glenohumeral instability during a swing-and-miss or reaching for an outside pitch.[8] Hitters may describe continued difficulty, pain, and apprehension with swinging at pitches that are outside, typically low-and-away or up-and-in. Symptoms are exacerbated by swinging and missing because no energy is dissipated to the ball. Players may have sensations of subluxation when swinging.

Physical Examination

Physical examination demonstrates pain with strength testing of the posterior cuff. Specific tests of the posterior labrum include the load and shift, Jerk (Figure 18.5), Kim (Figure 18.6), and active compression testing. One or all of these special tests may be considered positive when pain is elicited or a clunk or click is felt or heard. Provocative positions including forward flexion, adduction, and internal rotation may also increase pain and discomfort.[8] When the Kim and Jerk tests are performed in conjunction with each other, there is 97% sensitivity in detecting a posteroinferior labral lesion.[9,10]

Imaging

X-rays obtained include glenohumeral anteroposterior views with the arm in internal and external rotation, scapular Y views, and axillary views. These radiographs are typically normal but should be performed to rule out any intra-articular loose bodies and bone pathology, such as a reverse Hill-Sachs lesion, and determine glenohumeral version. Magnetic resonance imaging (MRI) generally demonstrates a posterior labral tear (Figure 18.7). MRI may also help depict any additional pathology such as a chondral lesions or rotator cuff tears. Players' throwing and lead shoulder may have increased glenoid retroversion leading to greater risk for posterior instability.

TREATMENT

Nonoperative Treatment

Treatment of the batter's shoulder should initially be nonoperative. Players undergo a period of complete rest from swinging. Rehabilitation should be direct at reducing symptoms through optimization of shoulder range of motion, improving rotator cuff and periscapular strength. A course of nonsteroidal anti-inflammatory drugs may be prescribed in addition to physical therapy. Once symptoms are alleviated, a swing progression is initiated with an emphasis on proper

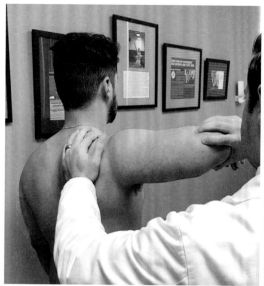
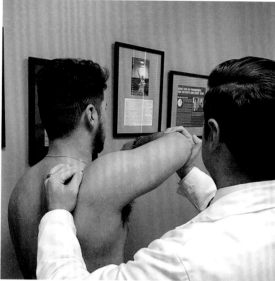

FIGURE 18.5 • Jerk test: The examiner holds the elbow and stabilized the scapula. An axial force is applied to the arm in 90° of abduction and internal rotation, and the patient's arm is there horizontally adducted while the axial load is maintained. (Courtesy of Christopher Ahmad.)

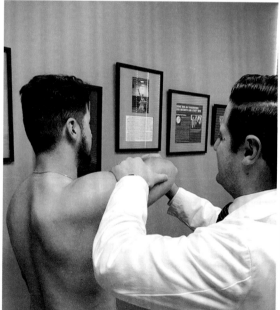
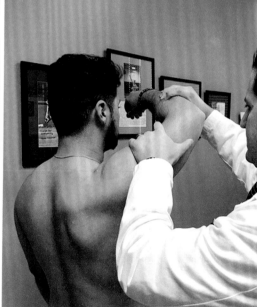

FIGURE 18.6 • The Kim test: The examiner holds the elbow and lateral aspect of the proximal arm. An axial loading force is applied. The arm is then elevated upward on a 45° angle and a downward and proximal force is applied. (Courtesy of Christopher Ahmad.)

mechanics. Should the lead shoulder and throwing shoulder be the same, return to throwing and hitting should be staggered. This will help alleviate the amount of stress put on the shoulder simultaneously and prevent a setback. A nonoperative approach may take as long as 12 weeks to determine failure.

Operative Treatment

Surgical intervention is indicated with failure of nonoperative treatment. However, some athletes may wish to avoid failure of nonoperative treatment and elect for earlier surgical intervention based on seasonal and career timing.

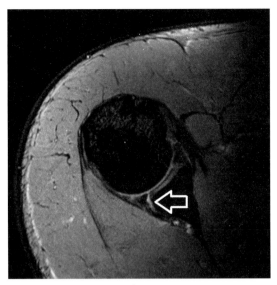

FIGURE 18.7 • MRI scan demonstrating posterior labrum tear (arrow). (Courtesy of Christopher Ahmad.)

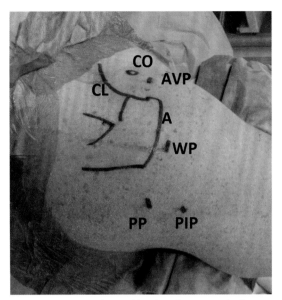

FIGURE 18.8 • Traditional landmarks are marked out. CL, clavicle; CO, coracoid; AVP, anterior viewing portal; A, acromion; WP, Wilmington portal; PP, posterior portal; PIP, posteroinferior portal. (Courtesy of Christopher Ahmad.)

TABLE 18.1 Surgical Equipment

• Lateral arm positioner	• Bean bag
• 4.0-mm mechanical shaver	• Electrocautery device
• Switching stick(s)	• Standard 4-mm arthroscope
• Probe	• 7 mm clear cannula
• Suture anchors	• Nonserrated loop grasper
• Labral tape (polyethylene tape)	• 10cc syringe with lidocaine
• 2.9-mm knotless suture anchor	• Elevator

AUTHOR'S PREFERRED SURGICAL TECHNIQUE

Preoperative Planning

Preoperative planning should include a review of MRI and any other imaging obtained. Size and location of the tear should be identified on imaging, although diagnostic arthroscopy is the gold standard. Surgical instruments are listed in Table 18.1.

Surgical Technique, Step by Step

Surgical repair of posterior labrum tears is performed arthroscopically with the patient positioned lateral decubitus. Examination under anesthesia is performed, and posterior instability magnitude is determined. Traction is then pulled on the arm and a bump is placed in the axilla. The arm is placed in 40° to 45° of abduction and 10° to 20° of forward elevation for improved global visualization and access to the labrum and capsule.[11]

Traditional landmarks, including the acromion, clavicle, coracoid, and portals, are marked out (Figure 18.8). The posterior viewing portal is established just lateral to the lateral edge of the acromion. A more lateral position facilitates improved instrumentation and access to the posterior labrum. Diagnostic arthroscopy evaluates the entire labrum as well as the articular-sided rotator cuff.[11] An anterior portal is created lateral to the coracoid with a spinal needle introduced through the rotator interval, and a cannula is placed. A probe is introduced and used to assess the integrity of the labral attachment to the glenoid (Figure 18.9). Any undersurface rotator cuff partial tearing is debrided. The scope is placed into the anterior cannula, and the posterior capsulolabral complex is better visualized.

All labral tissues requiring repair are mobilized and adjacent glenoid surfaces are abraded with a shaver or rasp to enhance healing (Figure 18.10). We prefer a knotless repair technique. A percutaneous approach allows placement of suture passing devices (Figure 18.11) to shuttle suture tape around the capsulolabral complex (Figure 18.12). The extent of capsule incorporated in the repair depends on the degree of instability. If the lead shoulder is also the throwing shoulder, then overtightening the capsule

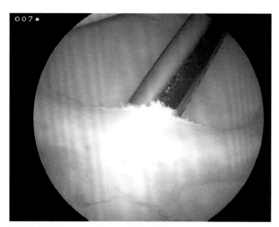

FIGURE 18.9 • Probing of the labrum to assess integrity. (Courtesy of Christopher Ahmad.)

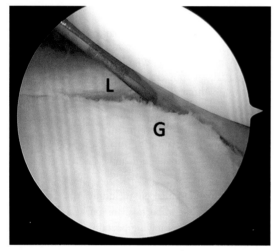

FIGURE 18.10 • The labrum (L) and adjacent glenoid (G) are abraded and ready for repair. (Courtesy of Christopher Ahmad.)

is avoided. A drill guide and drill are used to create a hole at the articular margin of the glenoid (Figure 18.13). The suture tape is placed through the eyelet of the anchor. The anchor is then placed in the pre-drilled glenoid hole, and tension is applied to the tape (Figure 18.14). The anchor is then advanced securing the tape, and excess tape is cut. The suture passing and fixation process is repeated as needed to complete the repair (Figure 18.15).

POSTSURGICAL REHABILITATION

The player is immobilized in a sling with slight external rotation, which will be used for 6 weeks. The sling may be removed throughout the day only for light daily activities. Physical therapy is initially aimed at restoring range of motion while avoiding posterior stress. Once range of motion is restored, resistance training and plyometric exercises are initiated.

A return to hitting program is initiated 4 months postoperatively. Should the lead shoulder and throwing shoulder be the same, a throwing program is initiated at 4 months and a hitting program is delayed. This delay is built-in to the player's rehabilitation program as to not overstress the repaired labrum. Once a return to play is initiated, it is suggested that players continue to maintain the strength of the rotator cuff.

Return to hitting begins on a tee. Once the player successfully completes a phase of hitting off a tee, he may progress to soft toss and live batting practice. Should a throwing program be necessary, it should be initiated 6 weeks after the hitting progression begins. Players may return to competition at 5 to 6 months

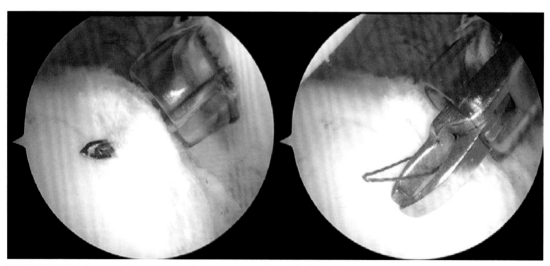

FIGURE 18.11 • A suture lasso passes the suture tape through the labrum. (Courtesy of Christopher Ahmad.)

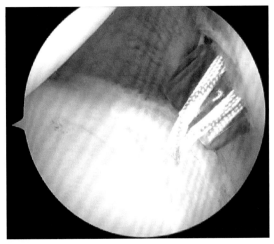

FIGURE 18.12 • The sutures are passed through the labrum and are readied for anchoring. (Courtesy of Christopher Ahmad.)

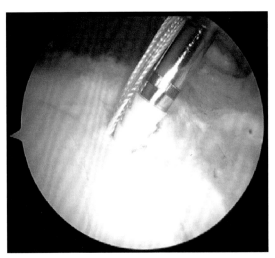

FIGURE 18.14 • The pushlock placed in the pre-drilled glenoid hole with tension applied to the tape. (Courtesy of Christopher Ahmad.)

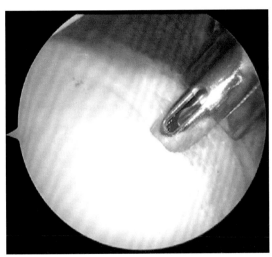

FIGURE 18.13 • A drill and drill guide are used to create a hole in the glenoid for the pushlock to be placed. (Courtesy of Christopher Ahmad.)

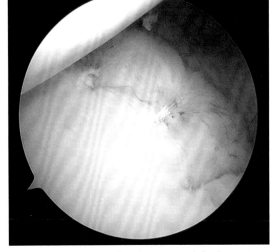

FIGURE 18.15 • Completed posterior labral repair utilizing knotless sutures for batter's shoulder as viewed from the anterior portal. (Courtesy of Christopher Ahmad.)

postoperatively, although timelines vary for each patient. For specific protocol strategies, please refer to chapter 36.

RESULTS

Players who undergo posterior labrum repairs are able to return to play. Research in this area indicates that arthroscopic treatment of posterior instability is an effective and reliable means to help elite athletes back to unrestricted activity. Nevertheless, surgical intervention for posterior instability has been inconsistent and resulted in unreliable functional outcomes.

Studies show that 84% of the overhead throwing athletic population is able to return to play after an arthroscopic stabilization procedure. It has been reported that overhead throwing athletes were able to return to their preoperative playing level 58% of the time after an arthroscopic stabilization[3,5]; however, these results may have utilized older surgical techniques. Newer surgical techniques may increase an athlete's ability to return to preoperative playing levels. Overall, greater than 90% of patients with posterior labral repairs were satisfied with their outcomes postoperatively.[3,5]

Although there is a fair amount of literature focused on posterior labral repairs, there is only 1 study that specifically identified surgical treatment of batter's shoulder.[4] Wanich et al[4] retrospectively reviewed the cases of 14 players: 4 professional players, 6 collegiate players, and 4 players at the varsity level in high school. All players underwent initial trial of nonoperative treatment, and 2 of the 14 players succeeded without needing further treatment.[4] Of the remaining 12 players, 11 (92%) returned to play at the same level of play.[4] The players who underwent surgery returned to batting at an average of 5.9 months and returned to play at an average of 6.5 months.[4] The lone surgical patient who did not return to play had additional pathology at the time of surgery. Wanich et al[4] noted their limitations including small sample size of patients and potential for selection bias. Further research of the batter's shoulder is recommended.

COMPLICATIONS

Surgical complications may include infection, stiffness, anesthesia-related complications, and injury to surrounding nerves, vessels, and/or soft tissue. Moreover, complications of posterior labral repairs may not result in issues that arise from the surgical procedure itself. Complications may include players not returning to their desired level of competition and failure of the repair if the player returns to play prematurely.

MANAGER'S TIPS

- Batter's shoulder affects the lead shoulder of the batter and results in symptomatic labral tearing
- Greater consideration for avoidance of overtightening the posterior shoulder is required for players whose lead hitting shoulder and throwing shoulder are the same, so throwing-related symptoms are avoided
- Initial treatment should be nonoperative, but surgical treatment may be elected earlier owing to seasonal and career timing
- Operative treatment is indicated after failure of nonoperative treatment

- A knotless technique is preferred
- Players return to live hitting around 5 to 6 months postoperatively

REFERENCES

1. Fortenbaugh D, Fleisig G, Onar-Thomas A, et al. The effect of pitch type on ground reaction forces in the baseball swing. *Sports BioMech*. 2011;10(4):270-279.
2. Dugas JR. The batter's shoulder. In: Dines JM, Altchek DW, Andrews J, et al, eds. *Sports Medicine of Baseball*. Philadelphia, PA: Lippincott Williams & Wilkins; 2012:15-19.
3. Bradley JP, McClincy MP, Arner JW, et al. Arthroscopic capsulolabral reconstruction for posterior instability of the shoulder: a prospective study of 200 shoulders. *Am J Sports Med*. 2013;41(9):2005-2014.
4. Wanich T, Dines J, Dines D, et al. 'Batter's Shoulder': can athletes return to play at the same level after operative treatment? *Clin Orthop Relat Res*. 2012;470:1565-1570.
5. DeLong JM, Jiang K, Bradley JP. Posterior Instability of the Shoulder: a systematic review and meta-analysis of clinical outcomes. *Am J Sports Med*. 2015;43(7):1805-1817.
6. Welch CM, Banks SA, Cook FF, et al. Hitting a Baseball: a biomechanics description. *J Orthop Sports Phys Ther*. 1995;22(5):193-201.
7. Adair RK. The physics of baseball. *Phys Today*. 1995;48(5):26-31.
8. Kang RW, Mahony GT, Harris TC, et al. Posterior instability caused by batter's shoulder. *Clin Sports Med*. 2013;32(4):797-802.
9. Kim SH, Park JS, Jeong WK, et al. The Kim test: a novel test for posteroinferior labral lesion of the shoulder – a comparison to the jerk test. *Am J Sports Med*. 2005;33(8):1188-1192.
10. Provencher MT, LeClere LE, King S, et al. Posterior instability of the shoulder: diagnosis and management. *Am J Sports Med*. 2011;39(4):874-886.
11. Vance DD, Ahmad CS. Arthroscopic treatment of posterior-inferior multidirectional instability of the shoulder. In: Lee D, Neviaser R, eds. *Operative Techniques: Shoulder and Elbow Surgery*. Philadelphia, PA: Elsevier; 2019:179-190.

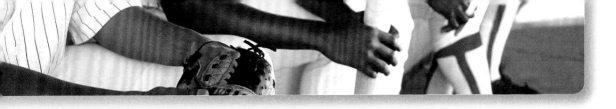

CHAPTER 19

Posterior Capsular Contracture and Bennett Lesion Treatment

Gregory L. Cvetanovich, MD | Eamon D. Bernardoni, MS | Nikhil N. Verma, MD

Pitching is the art of instilling fear.

—*Sandy Koufax*

INTRODUCTION

Evaluation and management of the painful throwing shoulder presents a unique challenge for the sports medicine physician. The overhead athlete's shoulder experiences substantial forces as a result of transfer of energy through the kinetic chain to the upper extremity,[1-3] which can lead to a variety of acute and chronic overuse injuries of the thrower's shoulder and elbow.[4] In response to the repetitive stresses, the thrower's shoulder undergoes osseous and soft tissue adaptations during physical maturation resulting in increased external rotation and decreased internal rotation. The adaptive external rotation increase and internal rotation decrease are usually both approximately equal and on the order of 15°, such that the total arc of shoulder rotation is unchanged in the well-functioning throwing shoulder.[5,6] Osseous adaptation has been implicated in the shift of rotation arc in throwers, and humeral retroversion in the professional pitcher has been reported to be 17° compared with the nonthrowing arm, with glenoid retroversion correlating in approximately a 2:1 ratio.[7,8] There are mixed reports implicating adaptive capsular laxity in throwing shoulders, with some reports suggesting greater anteroposterior translation and other studies finding no difference in translation.[9,10]

Posterior capsular contracture and Bennett lesion are 2 common findings in evaluation of the throwing athlete, and both are potential causes of shoulder pain in this population. In throwers, the posterior band of the inferior glenohumeral ligament (PIGHL) commonly undergoes hypertrophic changes in response to repeated loads.[11] Several aspects of throwing mechanics have been proposed to be key factors causing microtrauma and, subsequently, the development of the contracture of the posteroinferior capsule. During the late cocking phase, the humeral head translates posteriorly with the arm in abduction and external rotation, causing increased stress on the posterior capsule. With hypertrophy and contraction of the posterior capsule, there is loss of internal rotation. This is important in the follow-through phase of the pitch as the humerus internally rotates and tensions the PIGHL during deceleration, compounding the microtrauma of the PIGHL.[11,12] The Bennett lesion is an exostosis of the posteroinferior glenoid rim. Although this lesion's etiology is not clearly defined in the literature, it is thought to result from traction of the PIGHL, generally in the setting of a PIGHL contracture. The Bennett lesion has been shown to be radiographically present in 22% to 32% of baseball players regardless of symptoms.[13,14]

To develop the forces needed to throw a pitch, the shoulder requires major contributions from the entire body. This is referred to as the kinetic chain. The ground, legs, and trunk help generate the energy that is delivered to the shoulder and arm for the pitch. Well-balanced coordination and synchronization of the kinetic chain is necessary to deliver and dissipate the energy of the pitch without placing excessive force on the shoulder components.[15] Alterations in any segment of the kinetic chain such as muscle imbalance or flexibility can force the pitcher to use suboptimal pitching mechanics to compensate, which ultimately may lead to pathology of the shoulder including the posterior capsule.

SICK scapula syndrome (scapular malposition, inferior medial border prominence, coracoid pain and malposition, and dyskinesis of scapular movement) is another common condition found in symptomatic shoulders. This is thought to be an overuse muscular fatigue syndrome that produces altered kinematics of the scapula during throwing.[15] Posteroinferior capsular tightness has been shown to accompany the SICK scapula, and stretching of the posterior capsule is one of the main aspects of rehabilitation of a SICK scapula.

Treatment of patients with posterior capsular contracture and Bennett lesion requires comprehensive clinical and radiographic evaluation to determine the contributing factors to the athlete's shoulder pain and disability as opposed to findings representing asymptomatic pathology and adaptive changes. Treatment is nonoperative in the majority of cases, and steps toward injury prevention are critical. In patients who have failed extensive nonsurgical management, arthroscopic posterior capsular release and excision of the Bennett lesion can successfully restore overhead athletes to competition.

CLINICAL EVALUATION

History

The history is critical to the evaluation of the overhead athlete with shoulder complaints. Patients may present with loss of control or velocity, a "dead arm," posterior shoulder pain with throwing, and fatigue. History should assess whether there was an acute event or whether symptoms are gradual in onset and suggestive of chronic overuse. Discussion with the patient as well as trainers and coaches may help to determine if there have been changes in pitch count, pitching mechanics, or development of a new pitch. Neurologic and mechanical symptoms should be elicited. Timing of pain during delivery should be elicited and is most commonly worst during late cocking. The patient should be asked about prior treatment modalities, history of injury to the shoulder or elbow, and injuries elsewhere in the kinetic chain including the hip, trunk, and lumbar spine.

Physical Examination

Examination should be comprehensive given the complex interplay of shoulder mechanics with the remainder of the kinetic chain including lower extremities and trunk. Any muscle tightness, weakness, or imbalance in the lower extremities and trunks is critical to identify and address early because these issues can lead to alterations of throwing mechanics, placing greater stress on the shoulder and predisposing to injury.

Next, a comprehensive shoulder examination is performed. The scapula is evaluated for evidence of scapular dyskinesis or SICK scapula syndrome. Visual inspection for muscular atrophy or asymmetry is performed. Palpation of the shoulder is performed to assess for any focal areas of pain. Neurovascular function of the upper extremity is assessed. Rotator cuff strength, as well as tests of shoulder laxity and provocative tests for other associated shoulder pathology to the biceps, superior labrum, and acromioclavicular joint, are determined.

Shoulder range of motion is assessed actively and passively with the arm at the side as well as abducted 90°. The normal adaptive increased external rotation and decreased internal rotation for the throwing shoulder is generally on the order of 15° with preserved total arc of rotation.[5,6] Loss of internal rotation of the shoulder greater than 20° compared with the nonthrowing shoulder is defined as glenohumeral internal rotation deficit (GIRD), which has been associated with shoulder injury in pitchers.[16] Furthermore, the total rotational motion (TRM) arc of the shoulder is generally within 5° of the nonthrowing shoulder, with loss of TRM of over 5° associated with shoulder injuries.[16] Identification of GIRD and loss of TRM on examination are suggestive of posterior capsular contracture, particularly of the posteroinferior capsule and posterior band of the inferior glenohumeral ligament. To measure internal and external rotation, the patient is placed supine on the examination table to ensure scapular stabilization with the arm abducted to 90° off the edge of the table. The patient is moved through passive internal rotation until motion in the scapula is detected. Maximum external range of motion was measured at end range, as the table appropriately blocks the scapula with the patient in supine (Figure 19.1).

Imaging

Initial workup of the symptomatic thrower's shoulder involves radiographs, anteroposterior, axillary, Stryker notch, and scapular Y views, to evaluate for bony pathology (Figure 19.2). Stryker notch and West Point views can be added and may provide further useful information. In particular, the Stryker notch view (Figure 19.2D) allows for improved identification of a Bennett lesion or posteroinferior glenoid rim exostosis,[12] but it may also be seen in an axillary view (Figure 19.2C).

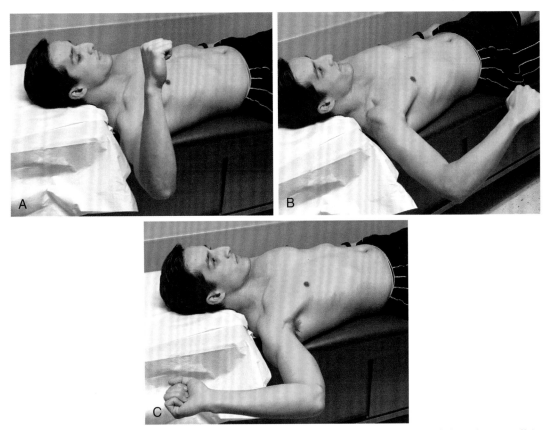

FIGURE 19.1 • The patient is placed supine to ensure scapular stabilization with the arm abducted to 90° off the edge of the table (A), and then, the arm is moved through passive internal rotation (B) and external rotation (C).

Radiographs are frequently normal for the symptomatic overhead athlete's shoulder, and MRI (magnetic resonance imaging) or MR arthrography is the study of choice for more detailed investigation of soft tissues including the rotator cuff and labrum (Figure 19.3). MR arthrography offers improved sensitivity and specificity in identifying superior labral tears from anterior to posterior (SLAP) lesions compared with standard MRI.[17] Furthermore, MR arthrography with the abduction external rotation view (ABER) allows superior ability to identify subtle partial rotator cuff tears of the articular surface and delaminated tears.[18] MRI may reveal the size of the Bennett lesion, although capsular contracture is difficult to assess on advanced imaging. Computed tomography (CT) scan is not routinely used in evaluation of throwing shoulder but could be used if additional delineation of Bennett lesion 3-dimensional shape and size was needed for preoperative planning (Figure 19.4A and B). CT would also be the gold standard for glenoid and humeral version, although increased retroversion is generally considered to be adaptive and not addressed surgically.

Complicating image interpretation, there is a high rate of asymptomatic pathology in the thrower's shoulder that must be considered when evaluating and treating these patients, with MRI of asymptomatic pitchers revealing evidence of labral abnormality in 79% and partial- or full-thickness rotator cuff tears in 52%.[19,20] Correlation of imaging findings with clinical examination is critical in developing a treatment plan, as addressing adaptive changes or asymptomatic pathology in the thrower's shoulder may lead to inability to return to the same level of competition.

TREATMENT

Nonoperative

Nonoperative treatment is the first-line treatment for posterior capsular contracture and Bennett lesion in the throwing shoulder, including rest, activity modification, and rehabilitation. Rest from throwing is used while rehabilitation is initiated to allow the shoulder to rest while initial rehabilitation occurs. Rehabilitation addresses the entire kinetic chain including lower extremities and trunk, with

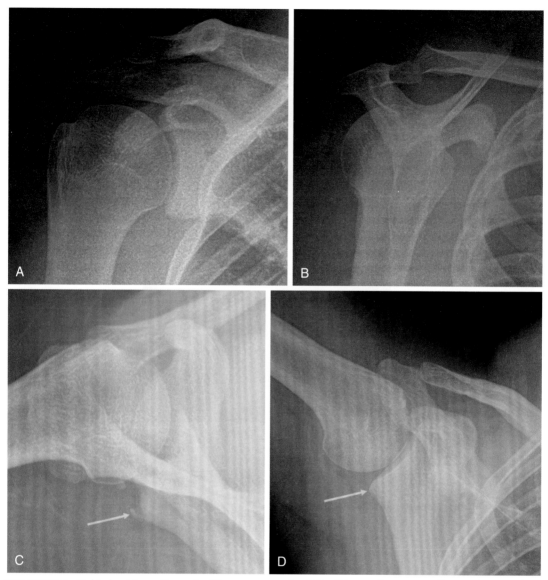

FIGURE 19.2 • Right shoulder radiographs (A) anteroposterior (AP), (B) scapular Y, (C) axillary, and (D) Stryker views. Axillary and Stryker views demonstrate Bennett lesion from posterior inferior glenoid rim (arrow).

special focus on any abnormalities identified on comprehensive examination as well as assessment by physical therapists and trainers. Scapular and dynamic stabilizers of the shoulder are addressed including rotator cuff strengthening, strengthening of scapular musculature, and addressing scapular dyskinesis or SICK scapula syndrome. In addition, modalities to decrease pain and inflammation are often used including nonsteroidal anti-inflammatory drugs (NSAIDs), injection, ice, iontophoresis, and heat.

Critical to addressing posterior capsular contracture and Bennett lesion is stretching of the postero-inferior capsule. The sleeper stretch is performed with

the patient lying on the ipsilateral side with the shoulder flexed and elbow 90°, and the shoulder is passively internally rotated by the contralateral arm toward the table (Figure 19.5). The crossed body adduction stretch is also used.

Using these concepts, Wilk et al described a 4-phase rehabilitation plan for overhead athletes including acute phase, intermediate phase, strengthening phase, and return to throwing phase.[21] The return to throwing process begins in the strengthening phase with an interval throwing program once patient has exhibited return to normal TRM arc, relief of pain, and improved strength and neuromuscular control throughout the kinetic chain. The interval throwing program progresses slowly over 6 to 12 weeks, with any recurrent symptoms treated by rest and return to the prior phase. Any flaws in throwing mechanics are identified and corrected by trainers and coaches. Once the athlete returns to competition, pitch counts should be carefully monitored and rest periods should be enforced combined with ongoing preventative stretches and strengthening exercises to prevent recurrent symptoms.

Operative

Indications (Include Contraindications)

Nonoperative treatment is successful in the majority of throwing athletes in returning them to

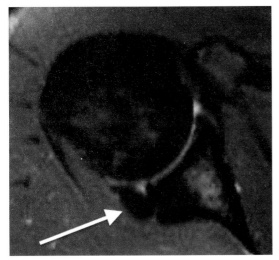

FIGURE 19.3 • Axial MRI showing Bennett lesion (arrow) of the posterior inferior glenoid.

competition.[15,22,23] Surgical treatment is reserved for athletes who are unable to return to play despite extensive nonoperative management. Patients should be counseled that there is no guarantee they will be able to return to pitching after surgery. Harris et al conducted a systematic review finding 68% rate of return to sport at 12 months following throwing shoulder surgery for pitchers and 22% of Major League Baseball (MLB) pitchers failing to return to play in MLB.[24]

Surgical Options

Arthroscopic posteroinferior capsular release is the treatment of choice for the rare patient with posterior capsular contracture who fails to respond to extensive conservative treatment. Bennett lesion is similarly treated arthroscopically with posteroinferior capsular release and removal of the exostosis with a burr. The goal in both cases is to release the contracted posterior band of the IGHL.

Authors' Preferred Surgical Technique

Preoperative Planning

History, examination findings, and imaging studies are reviewed to establish a surgical plan. The size and shape of the Bennett lesion is assessed with radiographs and advanced imaging, with location on the glenoid corresponding to the posterior band of the IGHL. The contributions of other pathology to the patient's shoulder dysfunction should be considered including internal impingement, partial- and full-thickness rotator cuff tears, SLAP tears, and instability.

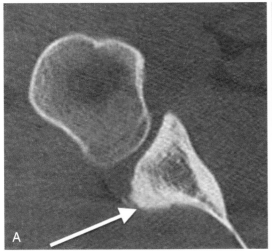
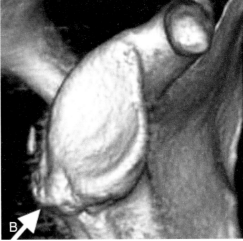

FIGURE 19.4 • A, Axial CT showing Bennett lesion (arrow) of the posterior inferior glenoid. B, Three-dimensional CT reconstruction showing the Bennett lesion (arrow) of the same patient.

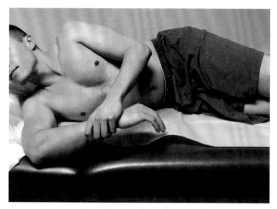

FIGURE 19.5 • The sleeper stretch is performed with the patient lying on the ipsilateral side with 90° of elbow and glenohumeral flexion and the shoulder passively internally rotated by the contralateral arm toward the table.

Equipment Needed

Arthroscopic instrumentation is needed including 30° arthroscope. The patient is positioned in the lateral decubitus position, which requires the use of lateral positioning devices. We prefer the Spider Limb Positioner and lateral distraction device (Smith and Nephew). At times a 70° arthroscope can be used to allow improved visualization of the Bennett lesion around the posterior glenoid. An arthroscopic shaver (Dyonics 4.5 mm Incisor Plus Platinum Blade, Smith and Nephew), radiofrequency device (Super Turbovac 90, Smith and Nephew), and arthroscopic burr (5.5 mm Bonecutter Platinum Blade, Smith and Nephew) are used.

Technique, Step by Step

The patient is anesthetized via an interscalene block and placed in the lateral decubitus position with intravenous sedation. Examination under anesthesia is performed including range of motion and stability examination compared with the contralateral shoulder. The Spider Limb Positioner is used (Smith and Nephew). We feel that lateral position provides improved joint distraction and visualization of the posteroinferior glenoid, labrum, and capsule (Figure 19.6A and B).

Next, diagnostic arthroscopy is performed beginning with a posterior viewing portal off the posterolateral corner of the acromion followed by an anterior rotator interval portal established via spinal needle. Any additional pathology is diagnosed and addressed as indicated.

After diagnostic arthroscopy, the arthroscope is moved to view from the anterior portal and the posterior portal is used as a working portal. The posteroinferior capsule is generally contracted and thickened. An arthroscopic shaver is placed through the posterior portal to open the posteroinferior capsule just lateral to the glenoid labrum. Care is taken not to violate the posterior labrum or underlying posterior rotator cuff. The release should be carried out just lateral to the glenoid rim and not be performed any farther laterally owing to concerns of proximity of the axillary nerve. The capsular release is carried using electrocautery and arthroscopic shaver from the posterior 9-o'clock position to inferior 6-o'clock position to release the contracted capsule and posterior band of the IGHL (Figure 19.7). At the inferior extent of the release, we prefer to use an arthroscopic basket owing to the proximity of the axillary nerve. Complete capsular release is confirmed by visualization of rotator cuff muscle fibers.

If a Bennett lesion is present, the camera remains in the anterior portal and instruments, in the posterior portal. In some cases, changing to a 70° arthroscope improves visualization of the exostosis around the posteroinferior glenoid rim. The exostosis is palpated using the arthroscopic shaver or a probe and is located on the posteroinferior glenoid rim. Exposure can be carried out using a radiofrequency device. A burr is used to remove the Bennett lesion without damaging the normal glenoid (Figure 19.8). The capsule and labrum are generally not repaired in this location because the exostosis is felt to be the result of traction from tight posterior band of the IGHL and posteroinferior capsular contracture. Final images are captured (Figure 19.9).

After completion of the release, the arm is released from traction and gentle manipulation is performed to confirm that internal rotation has been restored in comparison with the preoperative examination under anesthesia.

Postsurgical Rehabilitation

Rehabilitation depends on the exact procedures performed. Concomitant procedures such as SLAP repair or rotator cuff repair would often necessitate a delayed rehabilitation protocol for 4 to 6 weeks to protect the soft tissue repair during early healing. For isolated posterior capsular release or excision of Bennett lesion, postoperative rehabilitation can be aggressive with initial sling for comfort and early range of motion exercises with physical therapy and home exercises starting in the first day after surgery. Active assisted and passive range of motion can be initiated in the first few postoperative days along with isometric strengthening exercises. Sleeper stretch and similar stretches can be utilized postoperatively starting on postoperative day

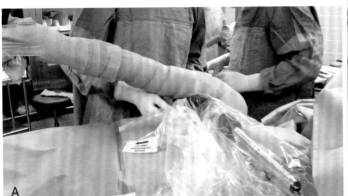
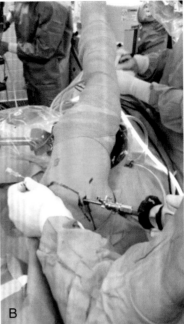

FIGURE 19.6 • The Spider Limb Positioner (Smith and Nephew) is used to hold the arm while the patient is in the lateral decubitus position. This position provides improved joint distraction and visualization of the postero-inferior glenoid, labrum, and capsule. (A) Shows an anterior view of lateral positioning. (B) Shows a superior view of the shoulder in lateral positioning, along with initial posterior viewing portal placement and spinal needle localization of an anterior rotator interval portal.

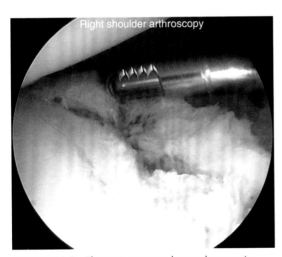

FIGURE 19.7 • Electrocautery and an arthroscopic shaver are used to release the contracted capsule and posterior band of the inferior glenohumeral ligament (IGHL) from the posterior 9-o'clock position to inferior 6-o'clock position.

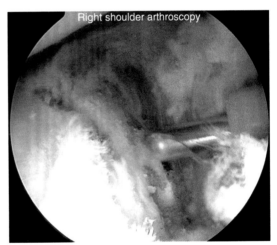

FIGURE 19.8 • After identifying the exostosis on the posteroinferior glenoid rim by palpating it with an arthroscopic shaver or a probe, a burr is used to remove the Bennett lesion without damaging the normal glenoid.

1 to maintain internal rotation. The goal is full passive range of motion by postoperative week 4.

Rotator cuff and scapular strengthening is performed with isotonic exercises and active range of motion, beginning in week 4. Strengthening and range of motion is performed as tolerated. Once full motion and strength have returned without pain, the patient can begin an interval throwing program around postoperative week 12. Progression of return to throwing occurs around 5 to 6 months from surgery for isolated capsular release and excision of Bennett lesion. Longer rehabilitations are common if other pathology is concomitantly addressed such as SLAP repair or rotator cuff repair.

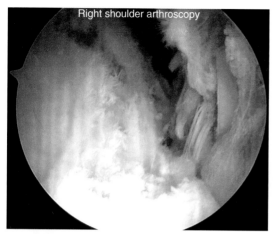
Right shoulder arthroscopy

FIGURE 19.9 • Final appearance following capsular release and removal of the Bennett lesion.

RESULTS

Andrews et al reported 22 throwing athletes with Bennett lesion; average length of symptoms before surgery was 2.3 years. Patients underwent debridement of the Bennett lesion in 50% of cases, no debridement of the Bennett lesion in 50% of cases. Associated procedures included debridement of a rotator cuff partial-thickness tear in 21 patients (95%) and debridement of labral tears in 19 patients (86%). Of those available for follow-up, 10/18 patients (55%) were able to return to their preoperative level of competition for at least 1 year after surgery. Average time to return to sport was 5 months after surgery.[25] Increased morbidity and failure to return to sport was found with exostosis greater than 100 mm.[2]

Park et al assessed player characteristics and the association of Bennett lesion found on MRI by retrospectively analyzing 388 male baseball players.[14] They found that players with MRI evidence of a Bennett lesion had played baseball an average of 10.6 years compared with those without a lesion playing 8.8 years, $P < .001$. No difference in Bennett lesion incidence was found between pitcher and nonpitcher groups. There was no difference in pain visual analog scale, American Shoulder and Elbow Surgeons (ASES) score, and posterior joint line tenderness between those players with Bennett lesion on MRI and those without. Owing to the Bennett lesion often being present without symptoms, it is difficult to determine if it is the cause of pain in patients with symptoms and a Bennett lesion.

The surgical indications for treatment of a symptomatic Bennett lesion are not thoroughly established. In a study carried out by Yoneda et al, 16 baseball players with symptomatic Bennett lesions were treated

TABLE 19.1 Characteristics of a Symptomatic Bennett Lesion Defined by Yoneda et al[26]

Detection of a bony spur at the posterior glenoid rim on plain radiographs
Posterior shoulder pain during throwing, especially in the follow-through phase
Tenderness at the posteroinferior aspect of the glenohumeral joint
Reduction of throwing pain by an injection of lidocaine into the Bennett lesion

with arthroscopic Bennett-plasty.[26] To determine who qualified for surgical intervention, they developed a set of criteria to determine what constitutes a symptomatic Bennett lesion as shown in Table 19.1. At a minimum of 1 year follow-up, they reported 11 of the 16 players (69%) were able to return to sport at their pre-injury level and 14 of the 16 (88%) were satisfied with their outcome. Of the players, 10 had no throwing pain after the surgery while the other 6 had less pain postoperation. When patients for surgery are appropriately selected, good outcomes can be achieved.

COMPLICATIONS

Complications of the procedure are uncommon and similar to arthroscopic shoulder surgery more generally, including infection, risks of anesthesia, and damage to neurovascular structures. Neuropraxia can occur from prolonged traction or traction in excess of 10 to 15 lbs. In addition, the axillary nerve is in close proximity to the inferior glenoid and inferior capsule and can be damaged during capsular release without careful technique. Postoperative stiffness could occur without appropriate postoperative physical therapy and home exercise program. Although not a complication per se, patients must understand that return to high-level throwing after shoulder surgery is not guaranteed, so patient expectations are critical.

MANAGER'S TIPS

- Posterior capsular contracture and Bennett lesion are common findings in throwing athletes
- Detailed history and evaluation of the entire kinetic chain and scapula are critical for diagnosis and treatment planning
- Stryker notch view can be used to improve diagnosis of Bennett lesion radiographically
- MRI, particularly MR arthrogram in ABER, can allow identification of associated labral and rotator cuff pathology

- Nonoperative treatment is the first-line treatment for posterior capsular contracture and Bennett lesion, with surgery as a last resort, given the high success rates in nonoperative treatment and variable return to prior level of pitching after shoulder surgery
- Sleeper stretch of the posteroinferior capsule and posterior band of the IGHL is a mainstay of nonoperative treatment, preventing recurrent symptoms
- Arthroscopic treatment with posteroinferior capsular release from 9-o'clock to 6-o'clock position is the treatment of choice. Bennett lesions are addressed with a burr when present
- An arthroscopic basket is used to perform the most inferior component of the release owing to the proximity of the axillary nerve
- A 70° arthroscope may improve visualization of bony pathology in Bennett lesions
- Postoperative rehabilitation includes early range of motion and sleeper stretches, with progression to strengthening, an interval throwing program, and return to competition around 5 to 6 months postoperatively. Recovery is adjusted and may take longer for cases with SLAP or rotator cuff repair

REFERENCES

1. Fleisig GS, Andrews JR, Dillman CJ, Escamilla RF. Kinetics of baseball pitching with implications about injury mechanisms. *Am J Sports Med.* 1995;23(2):233-239. doi:10.1177/036354659502300218.

2. Fleisig GS, Barrentine SW, Zheng N, Escamilla RF, Andrews JR. Kinematic and kinetic comparison of baseball pitching among various levels of development. *J Biomech.* 1999;32(12):1371-1375.

3. Sabick MB, Torry MR, Kim Y-K, Hawkins RJ. Humeral torque in professional baseball pitchers. *Am J Sports Med.* 2004;32(4):892-898. doi:10.1177/0363546503259354.

4. Limpisvasti O, ElAttrache NS, Jobe FW. Understanding shoulder and elbow injuries in baseball. *J Am Acad Orthop Surg.* 2007;15(3):139-147.

5. Bigliani LU, Codd TP, Connor PM, Levine WN, Littlefield MA, Hershon SJ. Shoulder motion and laxity in the professional baseball player. *Am J Sports Med.* 1997;25(5):609-613. doi:10.1177/036354659702500504.

6. Meister K, Day T, Horodyski M, Kaminski TW, Wasik MP, Tillman S. Rotational motion changes in the glenohumeral joint of the adolescent/Little League baseball player. *Am J Sports Med.* 2005;33(5):693-698. doi:10.1177/0363546504269936.

7. Wyland DJ, Pill SG, Shanley E, et al. Bony adaptation of the proximal humerus and glenoid correlate within the throwing shoulder of professional baseball

pitchers. *Am J Sports Med.* 2012;40(8):1858-1862. doi:10.1177/0363546512452720.

8. Crockett HC, Gross LB, Wilk KE, et al. Osseous adaptation and range of motion at the glenohumeral joint in professional baseball pitchers. *Am J Sports Med.* 2002;30(1):20-26. doi:10.1177/03635465020 300011701.

9. Sethi PM, Tibone JE, Lee TQ. Quantitative assessment of glenohumeral translation in baseball players: a comparison of pitchers versus nonpitching athletes. *Am J Sports Med.* 2004;32(7):1711-1715. doi:10.1177/0363546504263701.

10. Borsa PA, Wilk KE, Jacobson JA, et al. Correlation of range of motion and glenohumeral translation in professional baseball pitchers. *Am J Sports Med.* 2005;33(9):1392-1399. doi:10.1177/0363546504273490.

11. Bach HG, Goldberg BA. Posterior capsular contracture of the shoulder. *J Am Acad Orthop Surg.* 2006;14(5):265-277.

12. Andrews JR, Dugas JR, Hackel JG, Reinold MM, Wilk KE. The Thrower's exostosis pathophysiology and management. *Tech Shoulder Elbow Surg.* 2004;5(1):44.

13. Wright RW, Paletta GA. Prevalence of the Bennett lesion of the shoulder in major league pitchers. *Am J Sports Med.* 2004;32(1):121-124. doi:10.1177/0363546503260712.

14. Park J-Y, Noh Y-M, Chung S-W, Moon S-G, Ha D-H, Lee K-S. Bennett lesions in baseball players detected by magnetic resonance imaging: assessment of association factors. *J Shoulder Elbow Surg.* 2016;25(5):730-738. doi:10.1016/j.jse.2015.11.062.

15. Burkhart SS, Morgan CD, Kibler WB. The disabled throwing shoulder: spectrum of pathology Part III: the SICK scapula, scapular dyskinesis, the kinetic chain, and rehabilitation. *Arthroscopy.* 2003;19(6):641-661.

16. Wilk KE, Macrina LC, Fleisig GS, et al. Correlation of glenohumeral internal rotation deficit and total rotational motion to shoulder injuries in professional baseball pitchers. *Am J Sports Med.* 2011;39(2):329-335. doi:10.1177/0363546510384223.

17. Arirachakaran A, Boonard M, Chaijenkij K, Pituckanotai K, Prommahachai A, Kongtharvonskul J. A systematic review and meta-analysis of diagnostic test of MRA versus MRI for detection superior labrum anterior to posterior lesions type II-VII. *Skeletal Radiol.* 2017;46(2):149-160. doi:10.1007/s00256-016-2525-1.

18. Qiu W, Tang X, Li Y, Ji Y, Xu W. Abduction external rotation position in magnetic resonance arthrography for the diagnosis of rotator cuff tears. *J Orthop Sci.* 2016;21(4):446-451. doi:10.1016/j.jos.2015.12.019.

19. Miniaci A, Mascia AT, Salonen DC, Becker EJ. Magnetic resonance imaging of the shoulder in asymptomatic professional baseball pitchers. *Am J Sports Med.* 2002;30(1):66-73. doi:10.1177/036354 65020300012501.

20. Lesniak BP, Baraga MG, Jose J, Smith MK, Cunningham S, Kaplan LD. Glenohumeral findings on magnetic resonance imaging correlate with innings pitched in asymptomatic pitchers. *Am J Sports Med.* 2013;41(9):2022-2027. doi:10.1177/0363546513491093.

21. Wilk KE, Obma P, Simpson CD, Cain EL, Dugas JR, Andrews JR. Shoulder injuries in the overhead athlete. *J Orthop Sports Phys Ther.* 2009;39(2):38-54. doi:10.2519/jospt.2009.2929.

22. Burkhart SS, Morgan CD, Kibler WB. The disabled throwing shoulder: spectrum of pathology Part I: pathoanatomy and biomechanics. *Arthroscopy.* 2003;19(4):404-420. doi:10.1053/jars.2003.50128.

23. Burkhart SS, Morgan CD, Kibler WB. The disabled throwing shoulder: spectrum of pathology. Part II: evaluation and treatment of SLAP lesions in throwers. *Arthroscopy.* 2003;19(5):531-539. doi:10.1053/jars.2003.50139.

24. Harris JD, Frank JM, Jordan MA, et al. Return to sport following shoulder surgery in the elite pitcher: a systematic review. *Sports Health.* 2013;5(4):367-376. doi:10.1177/1941738113482673.

25. Meister K, Andrews JR, Batts J, Wilk K, Baumgarten T, Baumgartner T. Symptomatic thrower's exostosis. Arthroscopic evaluation and treatment. *Am J Sports Med.* 1999;27(2):133-136. doi:10.1177/03635465990 270020301.

26. Yoneda M, Nakagawa S, Hayashida K, Fukushima S, Wakitani S. Arthroscopic removal of symptomatic Bennett lesions in the shoulders of baseball players: arthroscopic Bennett-plasty. *Am J Sports Med.* 2002;30(5):728-736. doi:10.1177/036354650203000 51701.

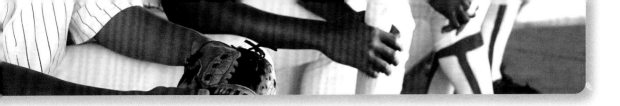

CHAPTER 20

Latissimus Dorsi and Teres Major Muscle Injuries in Pitchers

Brandon J. Erickson, MD | Christopher S. Ahmad, MD | Anthony A. Romeo, MD

Tomorrow's another day.

—*David Wright*

INTRODUCTION

While much attention is paid to the shoulder girdle and the elbow in the throwing athlete, there are less common injuries that can often be overlooked and amount to significant disability for an overhead athlete. Tears of the latissimus dorsi (LD) and teres major (TM) muscles are one such injury that can be seen in high-level athletes and, when missed, can prevent these athletes from successfully returning to sport.[1,2] The LD originates from the spinous processes of the lower 6 thoracic vertebrae, lower ribs, and iliac crest and, after externally rotating 90°, inserts on the floor of the intertubercular groove of the humerus (Figure 20.1).[3,4] The TM originates on the dorsal surface of the inferior angle of the scapula and inserts on the medial lip of the intertubercular of the humerus. The TM runs deep and superior to the LD, and several cadaveric studies have shown that LD/TM tendons are often adherent to one another, and, on occasion, the TM tendon can actually insert into the LD tendon.[3,5-7] Both these muscles are strong internal rotators of the humerus and are most active during the late cocking and acceleration phases of the pitching cycle, with slightly less activation seen in the deceleration phase of the pitching cycle.[8,9]

TRIP TO THE MOUND
One Strike or Two?
In evaluating pitchers with suspected LD/TM tendon injuries, it can be difficult to differentiate between single tendon and dual tendon tears. The anatomy of these muscles is such that they can be confluent before their insertion on the humerus, and because they are so intimately related, oftentimes if one of these tendons is injured, the other is injured as well. At this time, the treatment of these injuries does not vary based on whether the injury involves one or both muscles.

The LD/TM are important structures in translating the force generated from the lower extremity and trunk to the humerus and upper extremity during the overhead pitch and play a role in both protecting the shoulder from excess shear and in creation of pitch speed. The primary function of the LD/TM is humeral extension, adduction, and internal rotation, which correlates to several important functions of the LD/TM during the overhead pitch. First, the LD/TM eccentrically contract at the end

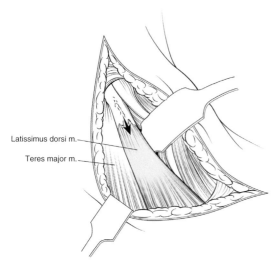

Latissimus dorsi m.

Teres major m.

FIGURE 20.1 • Anatomy of the latissimus dorsi and teres major. Note the close proximity of the axillary nerve to these muscles.

of the late cocking phase to decelerate the arm and halt shoulder eternal rotation. This prevents hyper-rotation that can lead to stretching and tearing of the anterior capsule. The LD/TM concentrically contract during acceleration phase to produce humeral internal rotation. The LD/TM also play a role in decelerating the arm in the deceleration/follow-through phase. Therefore, when a baseball pitcher sustains a complete tear involving the LD/TM, he often cannot continue to compete at a high level without some kind of intervention. Although injuries to the LD and TM are most commonly seen in overhead athletes (specifically baseball pitchers), they can also be seen in other sporting activities including water skiing, wakeboarding, tennis, and rock climbing.[10-12]

CLINICAL EVALUATION

History

Unlike problems with the rotator cuff, ulnar collateral ligament (UCL), and shoulder labrum, the presenting symptoms of baseball players with an LD/TM tear are oftentimes nonspecific. The athlete may remember a discrete throw where they felt a pop or the acute onset of pain in their shoulder. Sometimes, the athlete may also complain of early fatigue in the shoulder/back region with loss of velocity and control seen in pitchers. Unlike UCL tears, it is more common for pitchers who sustain

a tear of the LD/TM to remember a specific pitch where they developed pain in the upper arm and posterior axillary region during the late acceleration/deceleration phase.[9] Pitchers will often complain of pain beginning in the late cocking/early acceleration phases of the pitching cycle that continues throughout the rest of the pitch. Finally, it is important to obtain a complete history from athletes including prior injuries, prior surgeries, and whether or not they have been shut down for a period before their office visit. This will give clinicians an idea of where they are in their treatment, and whether this injury has been going on for some time or was it a recent, acute occurrence.

Physical Examination

Physical examination of the shoulder should begin by adequately exposing the shoulder, maintaining modesty in females. Any areas of bruising, swelling, or atrophy should be noted. Asymmetry of the posterior axillary fold can be seen when there is a humeral avulsion of the LD/TM with some retraction. Occasionally, the TM will demonstrate medial retraction. In an athlete with a suspected LD/TM tear, bruising can sometimes be seen in the postero-medial arm, axilla, or back at the level of the inferior angle of the scapula. The shoulder girdle should be palpated for any areas of tenderness. The entire course of the LD and TM, especially the insertion onto the humerus, should then be palpated, as patients with injuries of these structures will often be tender in the posterior axillary fold or at the humeral insertion of the LD/TM.

The shoulder is then taken through active and passive range of motion (ROM) and compared with the noninjured side. LD/TM tears do not typically cause abnormalities in ROM, unless the ROM is limited secondary to pain. The strength of the athlete's shoulder is then tested. Players with tears of the LD/TM should have normal muscle strength of the rotator cuff muscles but may be weak in shoulder adduction and extension and, to a lesser degree, in internal rotation. Pain is often reproduced with resisted shoulder extension and adduction. This examination can be performed in the prone position, which can allow more control, especially in tall athletes. Other sources of pathology in the thrower's shoulder should be tested for as well. The function of the radial nerve should be tested, as this lies in close proximity to the LD/TM and may be injured in traumatic injuries.

Imaging

All players who present to the office with complaints of shoulder pain should obtain a complete 4-view shoulder radiographic series (anteroposterior [AP], scapular Y, axillary, and Grashey). These radiographs are typically normal but occasionally will show concomitant pathology. Advanced imaging is critical to accurately diagnose and define the extent of an LD/TM tear. Magnetic resonance imaging (MRI) or magnetic resonance arthrogram (MRA) studies can evaluate the LD/TM over the entire course of the muscle-tendon unit. The MRI/MRA of a player with an LD/TM tear can demonstrate a discontinuous tendon or muscle and can quantify the amount of retraction that is present (if any). Increased fluid on T2-weighted images often surrounds the area of the injury and can often track down the muscle (Figure 20.2).

When ordering an MRI or MRA to evaluate for an LD/TM tear, it is crucial to communicate a desire to visualize the entire LD/TM, so the MRI technician expands the field of view to go more inferior than a standard shoulder MRI. If a standard shoulder MRI is ordered, the entire course of the LD/TM is unlikely to be well visualized and the diagnosis can be missed.[9] To help ensure images that are orthogonal to the entire length of the LD and TM, one method of acquiring images that are more recognizable to orthopedic surgeons who do not evaluate this area commonly is to ask the radiology technician for a standard MRI of the shoulder with an MRI of the lateral chest wall. Rarely, if very subtle injuries are important to diagnose, which is rare, then it may be beneficial to obtain a MRI of the bilateral shoulder girdles to evaluate for any subtle differences between the affected and unaffected sides.[13] An ultrasound may also be used to evaluate the LD/TM; although this imaging modality is operator dependent, it may not be routinely available, and the algorithm for ultrasound imaging of an LD/TM injury has not been established.[14]

TREATMENT

Nonoperative

An initial trial of nonoperative treatment is recommended for most athletes who present with injury of the LD/TM. The early phase involves rest, control of symptoms using cryotherapy, anti-inflammatory medications, other palliative modalities, and a complete shutdown from throwing. Once the player's pain is controlled, they begin to work on regaining ROM as well as core muscle and lower body strengthening, as weakness of the core muscles can contribute to altered throwing mechanics and shoulder injuries in pitchers.[15] Shoulder ROM should be restored to preinjury levels before progressing to the strengthening stage. Generally, once the pain is controlled, the ROM that returns at this condition does not directly affect the capsule of the glenohumeral joint. The program initially focuses on isometric strengthening of the LD/TM and progresses to resistance exercises as the athlete regains his strength.

Once the pitcher has regained his normal full arc of motion and strength, he is progressed through a throwing program. The throwing program begins with lofted long toss, followed by long toss on a line, and finally flat ground throwing. Once this progression of throwing is completed, the pitcher is allowed to throw from the mound first in practice and then in competition. The length of time for each phase varies by player, but the overall time frame for return to competition after the successful nonoperative treatment of an LD/TM injury is around 3 months but can be longer.[9] There are currently no reports in the literature of using platelet-rich plasma (PRP) or other biologics (bone marrow aspirate concentrate, etc) to augment the healing of LD/TM tears in players treated nonoperatively. However, the authors have used PRP in this setting without complications with the hope of relieving pain from inflammation and providing a stimulus to a better healing environment.

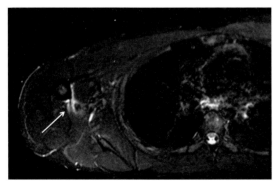

FIGURE 20.2 • Axial MRI (taken from an MRI of the chest) demonstrating a tear of the latissimus dorsi (white arrow) without significant retraction.

> **TRIP TO THE MOUND**
> **Fastball or Changeup?**
> Many athletes who sustain a tear of the LD and/or TM can be successfully treated nonoperatively. However, there are some patients who require surgical intervention. Studies have shown no significant difference in clinical outcomes for pitchers and other athletes who underwent surgery acutely versus those who had surgery in a delayed fashion. The surgical procedure is technically more challenging and demanding in the chronic setting; however, the results after surgery are still expected to be excellent in both the acute and chronic setting. If the outcome clearly favors surgical management, such as a complete avulsion with retraction, earlier intervention is better for both the surgeon and the patient.

Operative Indications

The current literature suggests that a 3- to 6-month trial of nonoperative treatment is warranted in athletes who present with tears of the LD/TM.[2,9] These recommendations have been based on a high incidence of return to throwing after this injury. However, thorough analysis of the level of return to play, effectiveness, and longevity have not factored into the decision. Furthermore, there have been some anecdotal discussions that surgical repair of any tendon around the shoulder of a throwing athlete has a great risk of not accomplishing the ability to return to sport (RTS) at the same level as before injury. Currently, based on experience, if these athletes are unable to RTS at their preinjury level and desire a chance to continue to compete at a high level, surgical repair of the LD/TM should be offered. Other surgical indications include significant tendon retraction that should be treated acutely, persistent pain despite comprehensive nonoperative treatment, and significant soft tissue fullness of the posterior shoulder. If the athlete has decided to end his career or is able to RTS (often through compensation of shoulder extension, adduction, and internal rotation by other muscles), without significant pain, soreness, or cramping, then surgical repair is not indicated.

Surgical Options

There are 2 surgical approaches when performing a repair of the LD/TM. These options include the 2-incision repair performed in the supine or beach chair position and the 1-incision repair performed in the lateral decubitus position. The 2-incision technique utilizes a standard deltopectoral approach to expose the footprint of the LD/TM on the humerus and a second posterior axillary incision to expose and liberate the retracted tendon stump. The single-incision technique is performed in the lateral decubitus position using a posterior axillary incision approach. The surrounding neurovascular structures are relatively close to the surgical site and footprint of the LD/TM, including the radial nerve, axillary nerve, and posterior brachial cutaneous nerve. A complete understanding of their position based on the selected approach is critical to avoid neurovascular complications. Once the tendon is retrieved in either technique, it should be anatomically restored to the humeral footprint with proven methods of fixation, preferably cortical buttons loaded with high-strength suture or suture tape.

Authors' Preferred Surgical Technique

The authors' preferred surgical technique when performing a repair of the LD/TM is via the posterior 1-incision technique using cortical buttons with single-cortex fixation loaded with high-strength suture and suture tape.

Preoperative Planning

- Equipment needed:
  - Shoulder positioner (Trimano, Arthrex, Naples, FL)—positioned on the opposite side of the surgical site, with the forearm brace placed upside down on the forearm; this allows for the positioner to statically hold the arm abducted, forward flexed, and internal rotated
  - Beanbag and lateral post for secure positioning and protection of any potential pressure points
  - Axillary roll to take pressure off and protect the opposite extremity brachial plexus
  - Large chandler (smooth) bone retractor
  - Pointed Hohmann (medium and large)
  - Variety of right-angled retractors
  - 3.2-mm diamond-tipped drill bit
  - Free Mayo needles, medium
  - Pec Button Kit (Arthrex, Naples, FL)
  - High-tensile suture/tape (FiberWire/FiberTape—Arthrex, Naples, FL)

Patient Setup

- Patient positioning is important, and great attention to detail is required to ensure adequate exposure during the case

- The patient is given combined regional and general anesthesia and then placed in the lateral decubitus position with use of a beanbag, axillary roll, and adjustable shoulder positioner (Trimano, Arthrex, Naples FL)
  - The Trimano is placed on the opposite end of the bed, proximal to where the arm board for the down arm is placed
  - This will allow >90° of abduction, forward flexion, and maximal internal rotation without damaging the down arm (Figure 20.3)
- A lateral post is placed posteriorly at the level of the scapula to prevent the patient from leaning backward during the case
- Preoperative examination under anesthesia (EUA) is performed before prepping and draping to confirm a palpable deformity and/or loss of contour of the posterior axillary fold, as well as confirming unrestricted shoulder motion
- A wide area is prepped and draped, and the arm is placed in the positioner such that the radial border of the forearm is directed toward the floor
- The shoulder is placed in 90° of abduction and maximum internal rotation while the elbow is placed in 90° of flexion; abduction is increased during exposure of the humeral footprint but reduced when securing the tendon to the bone
- The forearm is maximally pronated and the arm is placed in the arm positioner, 180° opposite of its typical orientation used when a patient is in the beach chair position (Figure 20.4)

Step-by-Step Procedure

- The posterior aspect of the axillary fold overlying the palpable defect and retracted muscle belly is identified
- A curvilinear, hockey stick incision 6 to 8 cm in length is marked out along the palpable defect (Figure 20.5A and B); the length of the incision for the humeral exposure remains relatively constant; however, the length of the incision on the flank side can be shortened when there is minimal retraction of the tendon or lengthened as needed for severe retraction of the tendon distally
- Local injection with 1% lidocaine with epinephrine is used before incision to aid in dissection and hemostasis
- The incision is taken sharply down to fascia, taking care to avoid the posterior brachial cutaneous nerve
  - The incision is often somewhat posterior, so flaps are raised anteriorly and posteriorly to facilitate exposure and adequate visualization; ideally, both the exposure should allow the surgeon to visualize the full extent of the LD/TM muscle group, with the LD tendon clearly visualized at the anterior extent of the exposure and the muscular appearance of the TM seen at the posterior extent of the exposure
- There is a variable appearance to the LD/TM
  - Sometimes the tendon is retracted and is readily visible
  - Sometimes the tendon is torn but has attempted to heal itself back to the insertion or at least

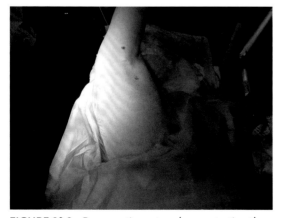

FIGURE 20.3 • Preoperative setup demonstrating the proper position for the patient and the arm positioner. A wide area is prepped and the patient is held in the lateral decubitus position such that he is not leaning forward or backward.

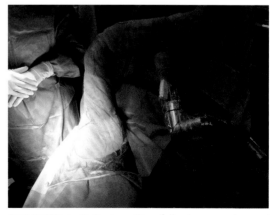

FIGURE 20.4 • Patient position following prepping and draping, and connection of the arm to the Trimano arm holder. This allows abduction and internal rotation of the arm to facilitate exposure of the latissimus and teres tendons.

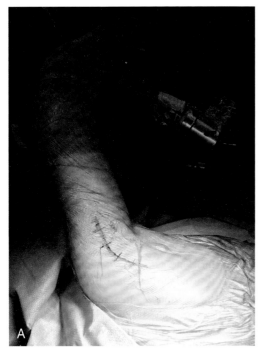

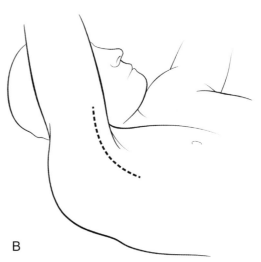

FIGURE 20.5 • Intraoperative image (A) and drawing (B) demonstrating the proposed incision that is along the latissimus tendon in the posterior axillary fold.

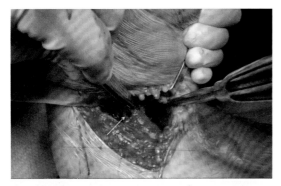

FIGURE 20.6 • Intraoperative image demonstrating the latissimus dorsi (LD) tendon (held in the forceps) and teres major (TM) tendon (white arrow) that have been torn off their insertion.

bridge the gap such that fibrous tissue (and occasionally calcified scar tissue) is holding the LD/TM tendons from more extensive retraction
- The LD/TM tendon stump is then identified and separated from the neotendon, scar tissue, and seroma cavity (Figure 20.6A and B). In many cases, this requires the LD tendon to be separated from the TM muscle; in other injuries, both insertions are involved to various degrees, and this can only be identified and separated out when the exposure is completed from the insertion point of the LD and TM tendons (where

some of the tendon may remain intact in partial injuries) to the level of actual retracted part of the tear
- Care is taken to preserve the epimysium of the LD/TM muscle belly
- The LD/TM tendon stump is mobilized using blunt dissection until it can readily be approximated to the insertion footprint
  - Alice clamps or holding sutures are placed on the torn edge of the tendon to allow tension on the muscle-tendon unit during dissection (Figure 20.7)
- The medial ridge or lip of the intertubercular groove (humeral insertion) of the LD/TM is then exposed by placing the humerus in maximal internal rotation with the shoulder in approximately 90° of abduction
- A Hohmann is placed anteriorly between the pectoralis major and the biceps to retract these tissues away from the exposure
  - This retractor is used to protect the biceps tendon as well as expose the insertion site of the LD/TM tendons
  - This retractor also protects against injury to the radial nerve
- A large chandler is placed on the lateral side of the humerus to retract the triceps

- A right-angled retractor (eg, Richardson) is placed distally at the apex of the incision to facilitate exposure

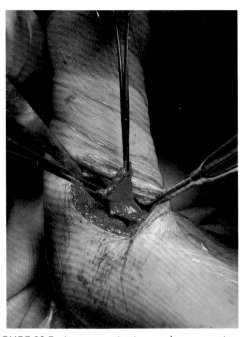

FIGURE 20.7 • Intraoperative image demonstrating the isolated latissimus dorsi (LD) tendon held by 2 Alice clamps. Adequate mobilization of the LD tendon has been achieved as evidenced by the excursion seen in this image.

- The LD/TM footprint is gently prepared using a high-speed burr, elevator, and/or rasp to obtain a bleeding surface (Figure 20.8A and B)
- The insertion is then evaluated to determine the number of cortical buttons (Pec Button, Arthrex, Naples, FL) that will be used to repair the tendon; for a complete tear, typically 3 buttons are used: 1 proximal, 1 distal, and 1 in-between
  - These buttons should be approximately 8 to 10 mm apart to achieve secure fixation along the entire footprint
  - The locations for the Pec Button insertion are then marked with an electrocautery or marking pen
- A 3.2-mm diamond-tipped guide pin is then drilled unicortically on the prepared footprint (Figure 20.9A), preferably with a slight angle to the flat surface of the cortex
- Ideally, there should be room for 2 to 3 cortical buttons (Pec Button, Arthrex, Naples, FL)
- These buttons are preloaded with both high-tensile, #2 or #5 nonabsorbable suture (FiberWire, Arthrex, Naples, FL) and 2-mm tape (FiberTape, Arthrex, Naples, FL)
- Each button is then pushed into the prepared pilot hole until it makes contact with the opposite cortex. The chamfer of the button should be oriented so that additional advancement will deflect the

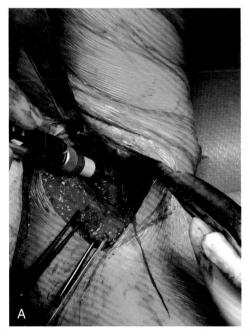

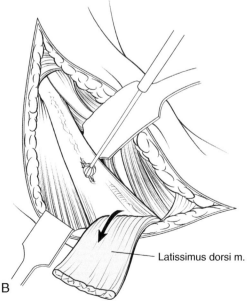

Latissimus dorsi m.

FIGURE 20.8 • Intraoperative image (A) and drawing (B) demonstrating the use of a burr to decorticate the insertion site of the latissimus dorsi (LD)/teres major (TM) to create a favorable repair bed.

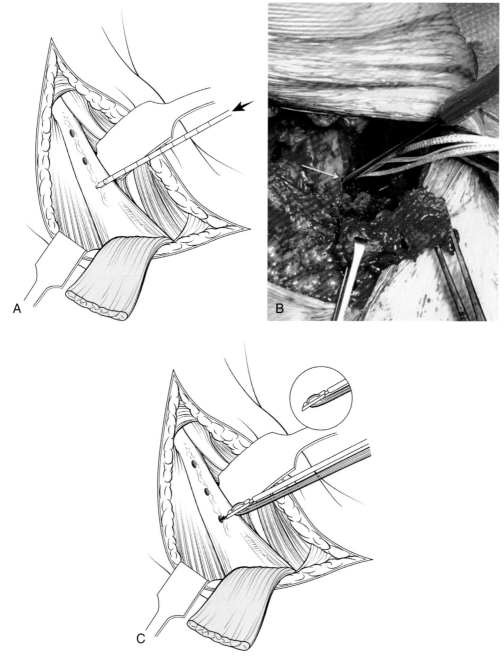

FIGURE 20.9 ▪ A, Drawing representing the 3 drill holes placed in the humerus for the unicortical buttons that will be used to reattach the latissimus dorsi (LD)/teres major (TM). Intraoperative image (B) and drawing (C) demonstrating the insertion of the first endosteal button (white arrow) into the LD/TM insertion site. The LD tendon is held in the 2 Alice clamps. D, Drawing representing the technique to properly deploy and flip the unicortical button within the intramedullary canal.

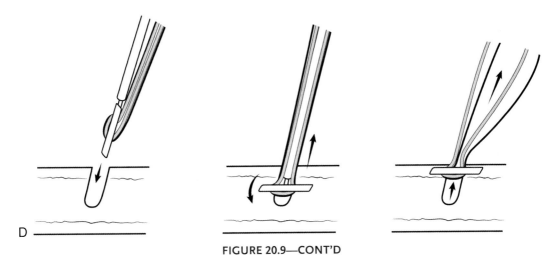

FIGURE 20.9—CONT'D

button off the opposite cortex. Once the button makes contact with the opposite cortex, the surgeon backs the button up 1 to 2 mm, disengages the button from the central inserter, then pushes the inserter forward while applying toggling traction on the attached sutures to spin the button, and lock it under the dense cortical bone (Figure 20.9B and C)

- Once the button makes gentle contact with the second cortex, back up the button 1 to 2 mm, then unscrew/disengage the inserter
- Maintain constant pressure on the inserter, and gently advance forward while pulling up on the sutures to flip the button; often, a palpable shift in the inserter is felt as the button goes from parallel to perpendicular to the inserter
- Once the button is flipped, keep tension on the sutures while slowly removing the inserter; once the button engages the endosteal surface of the first cortex, pull hard on the sutures to ensure the button is flipped and stable (Figure 20.9D)
- All buttons are be placed unicortically (Figure 20.10A and B)
  - Stable fixation of the buttons should be confirmed by a forceful pull on the sutures after the inserter has been removed
- One limb of the high-tensile suture is used to prepare the tendon in a locking Krackow configuration (Figure 20.11A-E)
  - This will be the nonpost limb for tying the suture
- The opposite limb of the high-tensile suture is then passed from the deep to superficial aspect of

the tendon; this allows the knot to be tied on the superficial surface of the tendon

- This limb of the suture serves as the post, delivering the tendon to its attachment by pulling only this limb of the suture, using the tension-slide technique
- The post limb is marked with a scribe for identification
- For reinforcement, the same steps are repeated using high-tensile tape
- The other buttons are prepared in the same manner
- After all sutures are passed, the arm is positioned with less abduction to improve the ease of reducing the tendon to the repair site and then marked post limbs are sequentially tensioned, thereby bringing the entire tendon into place
- The sutures are sequentially tied using standard knot tying technique; for some cases, an arthroscopic knot tying instrument can facilitate knot tension deep in the wound
- The suture should be cut short to prevent irritation (Figure 20.12A and B)
- When there is a combined injury of the LD and TM, the surgical repair can be performed in a way that allows both tendons to be fixed together on the medial slope of the medial intertubercular ridge. When there is a differential disruption with a complete tear of the LD, and a partial tear of the TM, the TM can be repaired back to the LD using heavy suture after the LD is fixed (Figure 20.13)
- The normal contour of the posterior axillary fold is restored with anatomic fixation of the LD/TM injury

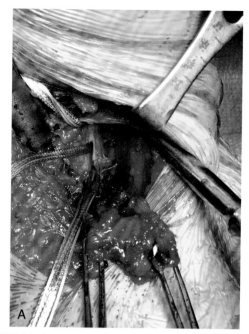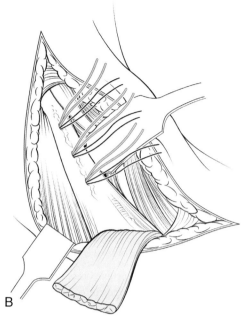

FIGURE 20.10 ● Intraoperative image (A) and drawing (B) showing placement of all 3 endosteal buttons at the insertion site of the latissimus dorsi (LD)/teres major (TM), with sutures coming out of each hole.

- The fascial layer is closed with 2-0 monofilament suture
  - Care should be taken to avoid excessive suturing of this layer with a resultant irregular contour of the axillary soft tissues
- Dermal and subcuticular layers are closed using monofilament suture, and topical skin adhesive is applied to create an impervious, watertight closure and avoid the superficial irritation and potential blistering that can occur with Steri-Strips

POSTSURGICAL REHABILITATION

The postoperative rehabilitation course begins with immobilization in a sling with a 4-inch abduction pillow (used to place the shoulder in internal rotation and slight abduction) for 6 weeks. The primary purpose of the sling is to protect the athlete from a sudden movement of his arm, especially resisted adduction or excessive abduction. During this time, the patient is permitted to perform gentle shoulder pendulum exercises and elbow/hand/wrist ROM once or twice per day. Passive ROM exercises begin at 2 weeks with discontinuation of the sling at 6 weeks. Passive and active ROM exercises are continued until full ROM of the shoulder is achieved, which usually occurs by 8 to 12 weeks after surgery. During this time, light isometric and stretching

exercises can also be performed. A throwing program is initiated between 12 and 16 weeks depending on the resolution of postoperative pain and response to the ROM and strengthening program, with progression through each phase dictated by the individual athlete's response to activity. RTS is delayed until at least 6 months (and possibly longer depending on tissue integrity, repair quality, and anticipated at-risk physical demands).[16]

TRIP TO THE MOUND

Going Back on Short Rest

There are limited data regarding timing of RTS after operative and nonoperative treatment of LD/TM injuries. If pitchers are successful in RTS after nonoperative management, they can often pitch competitively by 3 to 5 months. In pitchers who undergo surgical repair of the LD/TM, the timing of RTS is longer, with pitchers able to compete around 6 months after surgery but likely to sense full recovery around 9 to 12 months. Each player will progress through his or her rehabilitation program at a different pace. The information provided should act as a guide, with every player treated on an individual basis.

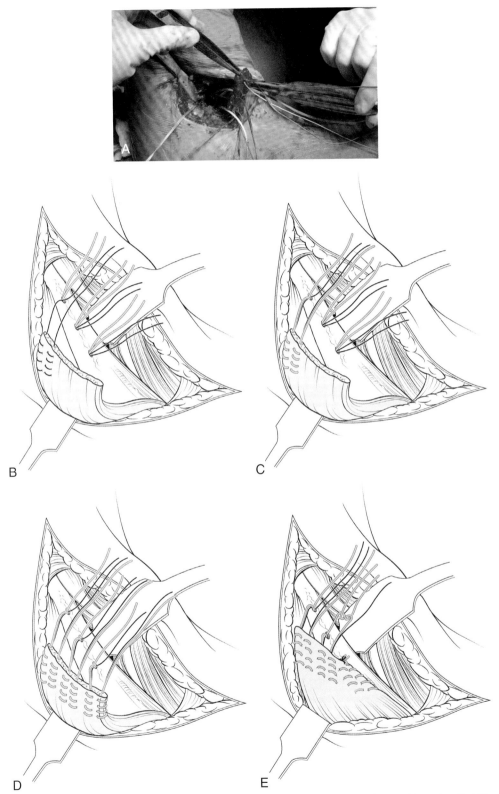

FIGURE 20.11 • A, Intraoperative image demonstrating the prepared latissimus dorsi (LD) tendon (held by the Alice clamp). All sutures from all buttons have been passed. The post limb of all sutures will be pulled up on sequentially to bring the tendon down to bone using a tension-slide technique. B-E, Drawing representations of how the LD/teres major (TM) tendons are prepped using running, locking sutures with the sutures from the previously placed unicortical buttons. The tendons are prepped from proximal to distal end.

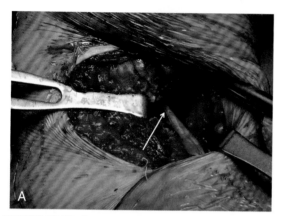
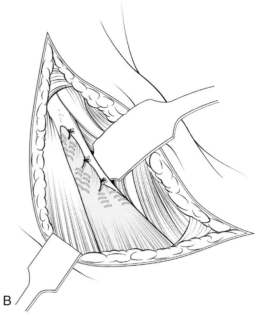

FIGURE 20.12 • Intraoperative image (A) and drawing (B) of the repaired latissimus dorsi (LD) tendon (white arrow).

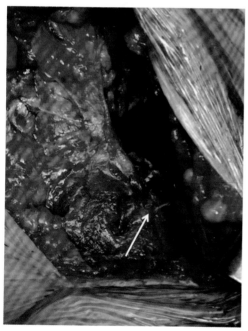

FIGURE 20.13 • Intraoperative image following closure of the latissimus dorsi (LD)/teres major (TM) interval heavy suture (white arrow).

RESULTS

Tears of the LD/TM are uncommon, and therefore the literature surrounding the results of operative and nonoperative treatment of these injuries is limited to small case series and case reports. Schickendantz et al

reported on the nonoperative management of 10 Major League Baseball (MLB) players who sustained an injury to their LD/TM.[9] All but 1 player were able to RTS at the same level as before injury in the same season the injury occurred (9 of the 10 players RTS at 3 months). One player suffered a recurrence at 6 months after he had RTS and was successfully treated nonoperatively the second time. Nagda et al performed a similar study where 16 professional baseball pitchers with LD/TM tears were managed nonoperatively and found 94% were able to RTS at the same or higher level.[2] These authors found a similar time to RTS as the average time to throwing was 35.6 days, average time to pitching was 61.9 days, and average time lost for athletes who were able to RTS the same season was 82.4 days. In this series, 56% of the injuries were season ending. Similar to the prior study, 2 players sustained a recurrent injury. Also of note, complete disruptions of the LD were associated with poorer results in terms of RTS.

The largest operative series to date reported on 11 athletes (8 of whom were baseball pitchers, 1 weight lifter, 1 kite surfer, and 1 wakeboarder) who underwent surgical repair of the LD/TM tendons at an average of 389 ± 789 days (range, 8-2555 days) from the date of injury.[17] Outcomes after surgery were excellent with 100% of athletes able to RTS at the same level. All patients had good to excellent clinical outcome scores and shoulder ROM with no evidence of residual shoulder weakness. Furthermore, when the authors isolated the performance of the baseball pitchers using modern detailed metrics, no significant differences were seen between any of the preoperative and postoperative performance metrics. No complications were reported. This study is consistent with earlier, smaller cases series and reports of surgically treated patients.[6,16,18,19]

COMPLICATIONS

Complications after nonoperative and operative treatment of LD/TM injuries are uncommon. One complication that can occur after nonoperative treatment of LD/TM injuries is a re-tear or re-strain of these muscles.[2,9] This often required another trial of nonoperative treatment, with surgical repair offered for players who are unable to RTS. While a theoretical risk to the radial nerve and axillary nerve exists during surgical repair of LD/TM injuries, no reports of permanent injuries to these nerves exist in the literature.

MANAGER'S TIPS

- Injuries to the LD and TM are underrecognized causes of disability in high-level athletes, specifically baseball pitchers
- A high level of suspicion for a tear of the LD/TM should be maintained in pitchers who present with pain in the axilla or posterior aspect of their arm and flank during the acceleration, deceleration, and follow-through phases of the pitching cycle
- MRI and MRA are the imaging studies of choice to diagnose an LD/TM tear (remember to communicate to the imaging department the clinical suspicion of an LD/TM tear so the MRI extends inferiorly to adequately image both muscles, or specifically request an addition of an MRI of the lateral chest wall to supplement the standard shoulder MRI)
- Nonoperative management should be attempted in most athletes for a period of 3 to 6 months, especially for strains, partial tears, or complete tears with minimal retraction
- Athletes who fail to RTS after a period of nonoperative management and who wish to RTS at a high level should be offered surgical repair of the LD/TM, with an understanding that full recovery after surgical repair and appropriate rehabilitation is likely to take 9 to 12 months

REFERENCES

1. Mehdi SK, Frangiamore SJ, Schickendantz MS. Latissimus dorsi and teres major injuries in major league baseball pitchers: a systematic review. *Am J Orthoped.* 2016;45(3):163-167.

2. Nagda SH, Cohen SB, Noonan TJ, Raasch WG, Ciccotti MG, Yocum LA. Management and outcomes of latissimus dorsi and teres major injuries in professional baseball pitchers. *Am J Sports Med.* 2011;39(10):2181-2186.

3. Pearle AD, Kelly BT, Voos JE, Chehab EL, Warren RF. Surgical technique and anatomic study of latissimus dorsi and teres major transfers. *J Bone Jt Surg Am.* 2006;88(7):1524-1531.

4. Pouliart N, Gagey O. Significance of the latissimus dorsi for shoulder instability. I. Variations in its anatomy around the humerus and scapula. *Clin Anat.* 2005;18(7):493-499.

5. Beck PA, Hoffer MM. Latissimus dorsi and teres major tendons: separate or conjoint tendons? *J Pediatr Orthop.* 1989;9(3):308-309.

6. Lim JK, Tilford ME, Hamersly SF, Sallay PI. Surgical repair of an acute latissimus dorsi tendon avulsion using suture anchors through a single incision. *Am J Sports Med.* 2006;34(8):1351-1355.

7. Pearle AD, Voos JE, Kelly BT, Chehab EL, Warren RF. Surgical technique and anatomic study of latissimus dorsi and teres major transfers. Surgical technique. *J Bone Jt Surg Am.* 2007;89(suppl 2 Pt 2):284-296.

8. Jobe FW, Tibone JE, Perry J, Moynes D. An EMG analysis of the shoulder in throwing and pitching. A preliminary report. *Am J Sports Med.* 1983;11(1):3-5.

9. Schickendantz MS, Kaar SG, Meister K, Lund P, Beverley L. Latissimus dorsi and teres major tears in professional baseball pitchers: a case series. *Am J Sports Med.* 2009;37(10):2016-2020.

10. Hapa O, Wijdicks CA, LaPrade RF, Braman JP. Out of the ring and into a sling: acute latissimus dorsi avulsion in a professional wrestler: a case report and review of the literature. *Knee Surg Sports Traumatol Arthrosc.* 2008;16(12):1146-1150.

11. Hiemstra LA, Butterwick D, Cooke M, Walker RE. Surgical management of latissimus dorsi rupture in a steer wrestler. *Clin J Sport Med.* 2007;17(4):316-318.

12. Park JY, Lhee SH, Keum JS. Rupture of latissimus dorsi muscle in a tennis player. *Orthopedics.* 2008;31(10).

13. Leland JM, Ciccotti MG, Cohen SB, Zoga AC, Frederick RJ. Teres major injuries in two professional baseball pitchers. *J Shoulder Elbow Surg/American Shoulder and Elbow Surgeons [et al].* 2009;18(6):e1-e5.

14. Grosclaude M, Najihi N, Ladermann A, Menetrey J, Ziltener JL. Teres major muscle tear in two professional ice hockey players: cases study and literature review. *Orthop Traumatol Surg Res.* 2012;98(1):122-125.

15. Erickson BJ, Sgori T, Chalmers PN, et al. The impact of fatigue on baseball pitching mechanics in adolescent male pitchers. *Arthroscopy.* 2016;32(5):762-771.

16. Ellman MB, Yanke A, Juhan T, et al. Open repair of an acute latissimus tendon avulsion in a major league baseball pitcher. *J Shoulder Elbow Surg/American Shoulder and Elbow Surgeons [et al].* 2013;22(7):e19-e23.

17. Erickson BJ, Chalmers PN, Waterman BR, Griffin JW, Romeo AA. Performance and return to sport in elite baseball players and recreational athletes following repair of the latissimus dorsi and teres major. *J Shoulder Elbow Surg/American Shoulder and Elbow Surgeons [et al]*. 2017;26(11):1948-1954.

18. Gregory JM, Harwood D, Sherman SL, Romeo AA. Surgical repair of a subacute latissimus dorsi tendon rupture. *Tech Shoulder Elbow Surg*. 2011;12(4):77-79.

19. Cox EM, McKay SD, Wolf BR. Subacute repair of latissimus dorsi tendon avulsion in the recreational athlete: two-year outcomes of 2 cases. *J Shoulder Elbow Surg/American Shoulder and Elbow Surgeons [et al]*. 2010;19(6):e16-e19.

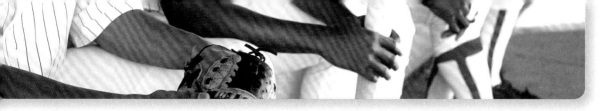

CHAPTER 21

Acromioclavicular Injuries in Overhead Athletes

Mark Schickendantz, MD | Megan Flynn, MD

Love is the most important thing in the world, but baseball is pretty good, too.

—*Yogi Berra*

INTRODUCTION

The incidence of acromioclavicular (AC) joint injuries and disorders in throwing athletes is not known but anecdotally represents a relatively small percentage of the total number of injuries seen in this population. Although some athletes will experience a single traumatic injury, more commonly the onset of AC joint pain is insidious. Accurate diagnosis and appropriate treatment depend on a thorough history, detailed physical examination, and high-quality imaging. An understanding of the complex anatomy and biomechanics of the AC joint is critically important when evaluating these athletes.

ANATOMY AND BIOMECHANICS

The AC joint is a diarthrodial joint with an articular surface made of hyaline cartilage and surrounded by a joint capsule located between the medial facet of the acromion and lateral aspect of the clavicle.[1] Motion is limited in the AC joint, and the majority of motion comes from the associated osseous anatomy. The clavicle rotates 40° to 50° posteriorly with shoulder elevation resulting in 8° of rotation through the AC joint.[2] Stability of the AC joint is provided by both static and dynamic structures. Three static stabilizers exist and provide stability in different planes.

The AC ligament primarily provides anterior-posterior stability to the AC joint. It is comprised of superior, inferior, anterior, and posterior components, the strongest of which is the superior component.

The trapezoid and conoid ligaments, also referred to as the coracoclavicular (CC) ligaments, provide superior–inferior stability.[2] The CC ligaments span from the inferior clavicle to the base of the coracoid process and are the strongest static stabilizers of the AC joint. The trapezoid ligament inserts 3 cm from the distal end of the clavicle and provides resistance to AC joint compression. It is 0.8 to 2.5 cm in length and 0.8 to 2.5 cm in width and attaches anterolaterally to the conoid ligament on the coracoid process, extending superiorly to the undersurface of the clavicle.[3] The conoid ligament is 0.7 to 2.5 cm in length and 0.4 to 0.95 cm in width and cone shaped.[3] It inserts more medially and is responsible for 60% of the restraint to anterior and superior clavicular displacement and rotation.[1,2] The CC ligaments couple glenohumeral abduction and flexion to scapular rotation on the chest wall. Both ligaments must be disrupted to cause a complete AC joint dislocation. Data collected by Debski and colleagues in 2 separate studies revealed that after capsule transection, the conoid ligament provided the primary restraint to anterosuperior loading and the trapezoid ligament provided posterior restraint. They thus recommended that surgical reconstruction address both ligaments.[4,5]

Disruption of the AC ligaments alone does not significantly alter glenohumeral kinematics. However, combined sectioning of the AC and CC ligaments has been shown to result in significant alterations in glenohumeral kinematics during passive shoulder abduction.[46] The clinical significance of this is not known. Dynamic stabilization of the AC joint is provided by the trapezius, deltoid, capsule, and deltotrapezial fascia.[2]

Five primary biomechanical stages of throwing have been described: (1) windup, (2) cocking, (3) acceleration, (4) deceleration, and (5) follow-through.[6] Biomechanical studies have shown that the shoulder remains abducted approximately 100° throughout the arc of motion, with maximal external rotation of 175° seen directly before the acceleration phase. The shoulder additionally goes from 30° of abduction in late cocking to 10° of adduction at the completion of follow-through.[7] Peak shoulder torques of up to 52 Nm and arm speeds of greater than 7000°/s have been measured.[8] The stresses imparted across the AC joint during the throwing motion have not been fully evaluated.

MECHANISM OF INJURY

Traumatic injuries to the AC joint usually occur as a result of direct force on the adducted arm such as a hard fall onto the shoulder or with direct hits such as running into the outfield wall. The energy is transmitted to and disrupts the CC ligaments resulting in clavicle displacement. The acromion is then forced caudal, medial, and anterior. With sufficient energy, the trapezoid ligament ruptures; the scapula and acromion are forced medially, which ruptures the conoid. This disruption allows further medial translation of the acromion relative to the clavicle.[3] Less commonly, indirect force through a fall on an outstretched hand can cause AC joint injuries. The force is transmitted through the arm, into the humeral head, and then into the acromion process. The AC ligaments are the only ligaments disrupted in this setting because there is a decrease in the CC space secondary to the superior translation of the humeral head, protecting the CC ligaments.

THE PAINFUL AC JOINT

Osteolysis

Distal clavicle osteolysis is a relatively rare condition in the general population but more commonly affects male weight lifters or overhead athletes.[9] In a case series of 46 men with AC joint pain without antecedent trauma, Cahill reported that 45 lifted weights at least 3 times per week.[10] Patients with osteolysis typically present with an insidious onset of anterior distal clavicle pain exacerbated by weight lifting—particularly bench press, chest flies, power cleans, and push-ups.[11] Examination reveals tenderness to palpation of the AC joint and pain with cross-body adduction without other significant findings.

The first step in workup of AC joint pain is radiographic evaluation. Imaging of the AC joint is performed using the Zanca view, which involves angling the beam 15° cephalad in the anteroposterior plane, allowing AC joint visualization without scapular spine overlap.[12] Images may reveal widening of the AC joint, cystic changes or loss of subchondral bone, and distal clavicle osteopenia or tapering.[10,13]

Patient factors including age, activity level, level of impairment, and desire to return to competition influence the management of distal clavicle osteolysis.[9] Treatment ranges from conservative nonsurgical options to more invasive arthroscopic and open surgical operations. The most common initial approach to conservative management is activity modification, physical therapy, and nonsteroidal anti-inflammatory drugs (NSAIDs). Eliminating specific exercises, such as bench press and push-ups, and even minor adjustments such as changing bar grip distance may alleviate symptoms.[14] No high-quality evidence exists to support physical therapy in isolated cases of osteolysis; however, in instances of concomitant rotator cuff or impingement, formal physical therapy can be of benefit with goals of restoring flexibility and strength.[15]

Steroid injections may be considered as both a diagnostic and therapeutic intervention in patients with recalcitrant pain despite activity modification. Immediate pain relief with injection of both local anesthetic and steroid has been regarded as a reliable prognostic indicator of successful distal clavicle resection.[16] Accuracy of AC joint injections has been questioned, however. Borbas et al injected 40 patients without ultrasound guidance and 40 patients with ultrasound guidance. They reported 70% accuracy without ultrasound and 90% accuracy with ultrasound.[17]

Operative management is indicated when activity modification is unsuccessful in treating persistent pain. It is important to consider concomitant shoulder pathology, such as biceps tendinopathy and rotator cuff tears, which have been demonstrated to be present in 22% and 81%, respectively.[18] Therefore, obtaining an MRI (magnetic resonance imaging) is indicated to better evaluate the AC joint and possible concomitant shoulder pathology. MRI will demonstrate increased signal intensity of the AC joint on fat-suppressed T2-weighted and short-tau inversion recovery (STIR) images.[19] Distal clavicle bone marrow edema is also seen and has been shown to correlate with symptom severity.[19]

Determining between arthroscopic and open surgical techniques is based on individual surgeon preference and experience, secondary to a lack of level I or II studies comparing approaches.[20] Open distal clavicle excision has been reported to produce excellent results for various types of AC joint pathology including osteolysis. The largest case series of open clavicle resection for osteolysis was performed by Cahill, in which 21 patients underwent surgery and 25 underwent nonoperative management. Of the 21 operative patients, 19 reported symptom relief with a mean follow-up of 7 years.[10] Arthroscopic operations have also produced improved outcomes (Figure 21.1). Auge and Fischer reported on 10 weight lifters with unilateral distal clavicle osteolysis who underwent arthroscopic distal clavicle resection. All patients returned to his or her previous training program at an average of 9.1 days, with a mean follow-up of 18.7 months. The authors attributed the ability to continue training and improved cosmetic appearance to the arthroscopic approach.[21] Rabalais and McCarty performed a systematic review of open and arthroscopic distal clavicle resection and concluded both open and arthroscopic procedures improved symptoms in the presence of osteolysis and osteoarthritis. Open techniques attained good or excellent results in 76.3% of patients while arthroscopic procedures obtained good or excellent outcomes in 92.5%.[20] The review, however, was based mainly on level III and IV evidence, and the reviewed studies used several different systems of determining functional outcomes.

Osteoarthritis

AC joint arthritis presentation, diagnosis, and many aspects of management are similar to that of distal clavicle osteolysis. Radiographic differences include sclerotic changes in the AC joint seen in arthritis, which will be absent in osteolysis.[13] Management

similarly follows the same course with activity modification, physical therapy, and NSAIDs trialed first. If symptoms persist, operative management can be considered. Studies have documented that patients with traumatic and degenerative joint arthritis do worse than patients with distal clavicle osteolysis alone. Eskola et al performed distal clavicle resections in 73 patients: 32 with asymptomatic AC joint separation, 8 with distal clavicle fracture, and 33 with primary AC joint arthritis. A poor result, seen in 23 patients, was more common in patients with distal clavicle fracture. A good result, seen in 21 patients, was more common in patients in whom less than 10 mm of clavicle was resected.[22] The authors thus concluded that distal clavicle resection be performed with caution in patients with severe arthritis or after fracture and minimal resection be performed.

AC/CC Sprains and Dislocations

The spectrum of traumatic AC joint injury can range from minor sprains to complete dislocations. The true incidence of AC injuries seen by clinicians is likely underestimated, as many are not diagnosed or treated.[23] Rockwood developed a classification system on the basis of the number of ligaments involved, the severity of the injury, radiographic findings—including the position of the clavicle relative to the acromion—and reducibility of the AC joint with shoulder shrugging[24,25] (Table 21.1). As in most classification systems, Rockwood AC injury classification system arranges injuries to help guide treatment. Type I is a sprain of the AC ligaments without a complete tear. Type II is a tear of the AC ligament without a tear of the CC ligaments. Type III injuries tear both the AC and CC ligaments with 25% to 100% displacement as

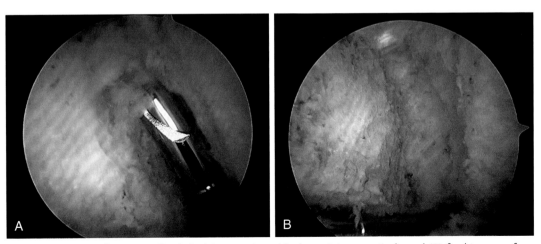

FIGURE 21.1 • (A) Arthroscopic distal clavicle resection with shaver intraoperatively, and (B) final images of distal clavicle resection with less than 1cm excision.

TABLE 21.1 Rockwood Classification of Acromioclavicular Injuries

Type	AC Ligaments	CC Ligaments	Deltopectoral Fascia	CC Interspace Distance	Radiographic Appearance
I	Sprained	Intact	Intact	Normal	Normal
II	Disrupted	Sprained	Intact	<25%	Widened
III	Disrupted	Disrupted	Disrupted	25%-100%	Widened
IV	Disrupted	Disrupted	Disrupted	Increased	Clavicle posterior
V	Disrupted	Disrupted	Disrupted	100%-300%	N/A
VI	Disrupted	Disrupted	Disrupted	Decreased	Clavicle inferior

AC, acromioclavicular; CC, coracoclavicular.

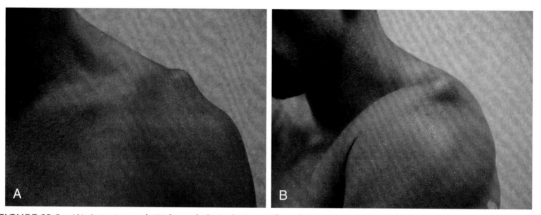

FIGURE 21.2 ● (A) Anterior and (B) lateral clinical views of grade III acromioclavicular (AC) joint separation.

compared with the contralateral, uninjured side. Type IV injuries involve complete AC dislocation with posterior displacement of the clavicle through or into the trapezius fascia. A type V injury is a complete AC dislocation with 100% to 300% superior displacement of the clavicle and also involves significant disruption of the deltotrapezial fascia. Type VI injuries are rare and involve inferior displacement of the clavicle into a subacromial or subcoracoid position.[24]

AC joint injury suspicion should be high in any athlete complaining of anterior and superior shoulder pain after a traumatic injury to the shoulder.[26] Most athletes will present with the injured upper extremity supported and adducted to alleviate pain.[27] Point tenderness, swelling, and localized pain can be expected in the acute posttraumatic period. The pain can also be emphasized with abduction and cross-body adduction of the arm, which load the AC joint.[28] To best assess the patient, they should be standing or seated with the arm hanging freely to increase any deformity due to the weight of the arm. Skin tenting may or may not be present and is seen more frequently in type III and V injuries (Figure 21.2). Sternoclavicular tenderness and pain may be present in type IV injuries due to the posterior displacement of the distal clavicle causing

concomitant anterior dislocation of the sternoclavicular joint.[27] Patients may also report neck or trapezius muscle pain, which occurs in type V and VI injuries as a result of deltotrapezial fascia injury.

The high incidence and favorable clinical course of AC separations has been well documented in contact sports. AC separations that occur during baseball are relatively rare.[28,43,44] As a result, treatment in this population is largely driven by anecdotal evidence and expert opinion. Kilcoyne et al[29] performed a study of Major League Baseball catchers' injuries resulting in disabled list (DL) placement and found the average time spent on the DL was 51 days. Interestingly, time lost was greater for noncollision injuries (53 days) compared with collision injuries (39 days). Only 1 AC injury was noted during the study period, which resulted in 17 missed days. Although significant AC injury is apparently rare, it is an important diagnosis to consider and treat accurately in overhead athletes.

Radiographs are the initial imaging modality of choice for diagnosis and classification of AC injuries. The Zanca view, as discussed above, is the most accurate radiograph for AC joint evaluation.[12] Stress views to help differentiate between type II and III injuries have been described; however, rarely is this difference

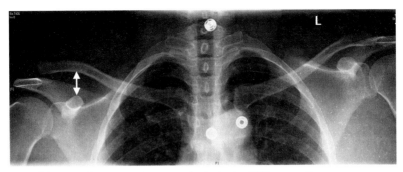

FIGURE 21.3 • X-ray with arrow demonstrating acromioclavicular (AC) separation.

clinically significant, and the provided information does not outweigh the added time, cost, and discomfort to the patient.[26] These views are accomplished by imaging the injured and noninjured sides. The normal extremity holds a 10 lb weight, and then comparison is made between the weighted and nonweighted images.[30] Additionally, an axillary view is essential in diagnosing type IV AC joint separations in which posterior displacement of the clavicle occurs. X-ray with both joints visualized can add further appreciation of the degree of separation (Figure 21.3).

Interest in utilizing MRI to diagnose AC injuries has increased owing to having the advantage of directly assessing ligamentous disruptions as opposed to inferring ligamentous injury based on osseous relationships.[27] MRIs have the added benefit of assessing for concomitant pathology.[31] In a study utilizing diagnostic arthroscopy to evaluate the incidence of associated injuries, Pauly et al[32] reported an incidence of 15% concomitant injuries requiring arthroscopic surgical management following type V injuries. Tischer et al[31] similarly found an incidence of 18.2% of patients with type III, IV, and V injuries also sustained intra-articular injuries requiring additional surgical intervention. Both sets of authors recommend obtaining preoperative MRI in patients with type V injuries.

Nonsurgical management is recommended and generally agreed upon for type I and type II AC joint injuries.[33-35] The affected extremity is typically immobilized in a simple sling for comfort as needed, usually 1 to 2 weeks. Routine modalities and athletic training room treatments are initiated early. Light shoulder strengthening and scapular control exercises begin once the athlete has regained a functional range of motion and is relatively pain free.[27] Position-specific rehabilitation (including return to hitting, return to throwing, and fielding drills) starts after motion and strength have fully returned to baseline. Time to return to play is variable and depends on a number of factors including playing position. In the senior authors' experience, the majority of athletes who experience

low-grade AC sprains return to play within 4 weeks of the injury. Pain in the AC joint may persist for as long as 6 months after the injury, with up to 33% of patients experiencing continued pain and AC instability at longer term (4-8 years) follow-up.[36] Bergfeld et al[37] found that up to 9% (9 of 97 patients with type I injuries) and 23% (7 of 31 patients with type II injuries) of patients in the United States Naval Academy reported severe pain with activity limitations at follow-up between 6 months and 3 years. Additionally, Mouhsine et al[36] retrospectively reviewed 33 patients with type I and II injuries and reported 50% of these patients were asymptomatic after 6.3 years follow-up with 9 patients (27%) symptomatic enough to undergo distal clavicle resection and AC ligament reconstruction.

Type III AC joint dislocation treatment is a matter of ongoing debate. Most published studies are case series with level IV evidence; there are very few reports of level II or III evidence available to guide treatment decisions.[27] Prospective and retrospective cohort analyses of untreated patients with type III injuries have helped form the basis of a treatment algorithm. Schlegel et al[38] prospectively evaluated a cohort of 25 patients with acute, untreated type III injuries. Objective assessment at 1 year postinjury revealed full painless range of motion in 80% of patients, a 17% loss of bench press strength compared with the contralateral side without significant strength loss during rotational motion testing.[38] In a critical analysis review of the literature, Virk et al[25] evaluated 14 studies comparing operative and nonoperative treatment. A cumulative total of 706 patients were included in the studies, and a favorable clinical outcome (defined as good or better symptom management) was reported in 88% of the operatively managed patients compared with 85% of the nonoperatively managed patients. Anatomic reduction was achieved in 59% of the operative group compared with 14.7% managed nonoperatively. Return to sport and work revealed a quicker recovery for the nonoperatively managed patients, who needed roughly half the time to return to the previous activity level.[25]

TABLE 21.2 Sample Rehabilitation Protocol for Grade III AC Joint Injury Recovery in an Overhead Athlete

Postinjury Day	Treatment
0	Sling, cryotherapy, oral methylprednisolone, passive rotation
5	Discontinue sling
7	Active motion and isometric exercises
14	Table-height push-ups, rotation with resistance bands
28	Two-handed swings
35	Interval throwing program
42	Batting practice on field
56	Medically clear

The scientific literature pertaining to the treatment of higher grade (type III and above) in the overhead athlete is even less robust. Bessette et al[28] reported a case of a Major League professional catcher who sustained a noncontact type III AC joint injury, which was treated nonoperatively. Despite having sustained a pisiform fracture in his rehabilitation program (Table 21.2), he returned to play at 77 days postinjury. The authors conclude that although baseball players place unique demands on their throwing shoulders making them vulnerable to AC injuries, high-level overhead athletes can still return to sport during the same season after a type III AC separation with nonoperative management. Successful return to play following nonoperative treatment of a type III AC sprain has also been reported in a collegiate pitcher.[46] There are no published studies comparing the results of nonoperative with operative management of Type III AC sprains in throwing athletes. McFarland surveyed 42 team orthopedists representing 28 Major League Baseball teams to ascertain their definitive treatment for a hypothetical starting rotation pitcher who had sustained a type III AC separation to his throwing arm 1 week before the season.[45] Twenty-nine (69%) of the physicians stated that they would treat the injury nonoperatively while 13 (31%) would operate immediately. Of the group surveyed, 25 (60%) had actually treated a pitcher or position baseball player with a type III AC separation in the throwing arm. Only 37% had been treated operatively. Of the remaining 67% treated without surgery, 80% regained normal function and achieved complete relief of pain while 18 (90%) had normal range of motion after treatment; of those treated operatively, 11 (92%) regained normal function, achieved complete relief of pain, and had normal range of motion after surgery.

Although patients have demonstrated good to excellent functional outcomes with nonsurgical management of their type III AC injuries,[39] some authors recommend surgical intervention in patients with higher functional demands.[34,40] Smith et al[41] performed a meta-analysis of 6 nonrandomized studies (380 patients) comparing nonoperative treatment with a sling and operative management by open reduction and fixation with a cancellous or malleolar screw and then pinning the AC joint with 2 Kirschner wires. The analysis found no difference in pain, throwing ability, strength, and AC joint arthritis incidence between the 2 groups ($P > .05$). The surgical group had significantly better cosmetic appearance ($P < .0001$), greater duration of sick leave ($P < .0001$), and significantly better Constant scores ($P = .03$). Additionally, complete anatomic reduction was not a requirement for optimal functional outcome in either nonoperatively or operatively treated groups.[41]

There is also a paucity of data to adequately answer the question of operative timing in type III AC injuries. A cumulative analysis of 5 retrospective comparative studies on early versus delayed operative treatment revealed 135 patients who underwent early operative management and 90 who underwent delayed operative management.[25] A favorable outcome, defined differently in each study, and a subjective measure was reported in 91% of the patients treated early compared with 73% of those in the delayed treatment group. On the basis of available literature, the current consensus is that no functional difference is demonstrated between operative and nonoperative management of type III injuries, and insufficient evidence exists to help guide timing.[25,27] With that in mind, it is generally recommended to treat the majority of uncomplicated type III injuries with nonsurgical management for 3 to 4 months. Surgical management should then be considered in patients with significant deformity, tenting of the skin, or persistent pain or in patients who place a higher functional demand on the injured shoulder.[27]

Considering the paucity of evidence-based studies on the outcomes of type III AC sprains in overhead athletes, it is the authors' opinion that the vast majority of these injuries can initially be treated nonoperatively with anticipated successful return to play. Failure to successfully complete a full return to throwing program owing to persistent symptoms referable to the AC joint would indicate a need for surgical intervention. As with other patients, overhead athletes who experience higher grade (IV and V) injuries should be strongly considered for early surgical stabilization.

It is generally agreed upon that type IV, V, and VI AC joint injuries should be treated operatively. As discussed previously, type IV and VI injuries are exceedingly rare, and most reported outcome data are presented as part of a case series or case reports.[42] Surgical management according to Li et al[27] includes 5 key elements: (1) anatomic and accurate reduction of the AC joint to correct superior displacement and anterior–posterior translation, (2) direct repair or reconstruction of the CC ligaments, (3) supplementation or protection of the CC ligament repair or reconstruction with synthetic material or rigid implant to maintain AC joint stability during the acute phases of healing, (4) repair of the deltoid and trapezial fascia, and (5) distal clavicular resection in patients with chronic AC injuries for which there is radiographic or clinical evidence of AC osteoarthritis. When considering surgery to treat symptomatic AC sprains in the overhead athlete, adherence to these key elements is paramount. However, given the heterogeneity among study populations and surgical techniques in the literature, it is difficult to recommend 1 particular repair or reconstruction technique over another.

MANAGER'S TIPS

- Traumatic injuries to the AC joint typically occur as a result of direct force on the adducted arm, such as running into the outfield wall, or indirect force through a fall on an outstretched hand
- Workup of the painful AC joint includes history and physical, radiographic evaluation including a Zanca view and occasionally MRI evaluation
- AC sprains and dislocations are treated based on the Rockwood classification (type I-VI)

- Nonsurgical management via simple sling for 1 to 2 weeks with position-specific rehabilitation starting after motion and strength have returned to baseline is indicated in players with type I and II injuries
- It is the authors' opinion that the vast majority of type III injuries can initially be treated nonoperatively with anticipated successful return to play. Failure to successfully complete a full return to throwing program would indicate a need for surgical intervention
- Surgical management via open repair of the AC joint ligaments is indicated in players with type IV, V, and VI injuries
- Rehabilitation for type III begins with active motion on postinjury day (PID) 7 and progresses to table-height push-ups on PID 14, then 2-handed swings on PID 28, interval throwing program on PID 35, batting practice on field on PID 42, and medically clear on PID 56

REFERENCES

1. Fukuda K, Craig EV, An KN, Cofield HR, Chao EY. Biomechanical study of the ligamentous system of the acromioclavicular joint. *J Bone Joint Surg Am.* 1986;68(3);434-440.

2. Renfree KJ, Wright TW. Anatomy and biomechanics of the acromioclavicular and sternoclavicular joints. *Clin Sports Med.* 2003,22(2):219-237.

3. Jones RB, Schickendantz MS. Acromioclavicular joint disorders. In: Krishnan S, ed. *The Shoulder and the Overhead Athlete.* New York: Lippincott-Williams Wilkins; 2004.

4. Costic RS, Labriola JE, Rodosky MW, Debski RE. Biomechanical rationale for development of anatomical reconstructions of coracoclavicular ligaments after complete acromioclavicular joint dislocations. *Am J Sports Med.* 2004;32(8):1929-1936.

5. Jari R, Costic RS, Rodosky MW, Debski RE. Biomechanical function of surgical procedures for acromioclavicular joint dislocations. *Arthroscopy.* 2004;20(3):237-245.

6. Ong BC, Skiya JK, Rodosky MW. Shoulder injuries in the athlete. *Curr Opin Rheumatol.* 2002(14):150-159.

7. Dillman CJ, Fleisig GS, Werner SL, et al. Biomechanics of the shoulder in sports: throwing activities. In: Matsen FA III, Fu FH, Hawkins RJ, eds. *The Shoulder: A Balance of Mobility and Stability.* Rosemont, IL: American Academy of Orthopaedic Surgeons; 1993:621.

8. Pappas ZM, Zawacki RM, Sullivan TJ. Biomechanics of baseball pitching: a preliminary report. *Am J Sports Med.* 1985;13:216.

9. DeFroda SF, Nacca C, Waryasz GR, Owens BD. Diagnosis and management of distal clavicle osteolysis. *Orthopaedics.* 2017;40(2):119-124.

10. Cahill BR. Osteolysis of the distal part of the clavicle in male athletes. *J Bone Joint Surg Am.* 1982;64(7): 1053-1058.

11. Haupt HA. Upper extremity injuries associated with strength training. *Clin Sports Med.* 2001;20(3):481-490.

12. Zanca P. Shoulder pain: involvement of the acromioclavicular joint: analysis of 1,000 cases. *Am J Roentgenol Radium Ther Nucl Med.* 1971;112(3):493-506.

13. Matthews LS, Simonson BG, Wolock BS. Osteolysis of the distal clavicle in a female boy builder: a case report. *Am J Sports Med.* 1993;21(1):150-152.

14. Shaffer BS. Painful conditions of the acromioclavicular joint. *J Am Acad Orthop Surg.* 1999;7(3):176-188.

15. Cibulka MT, Hunter HC. Acromioclavicular joint arthritis treated by mobilizing the glenohumeral joint: a case report. *Phys Ther.* 1985;65(10)1514-1516.

16. Worcester JN Jr, Green DP. Osteoarthritis of the acromioclavicular joint. *Clin Orthop Relat Res.* 1968;58:69-73.

17. Borbas P, Kraus T, Clement H, Grechenig S, Weinberg AM, Neidar N. The influence of ultrasound guidance in the rate of success of acromioclavicular joint injection: an experimental study on human cadavers. *J Shoulder Elbow Surg.* 2012;21(12):1694-1697.

18. Brown JN, Roberts SN, Hayes MG, Sales AD. Shoulder pathology associated with symptomatic acromioclavicular joint degeneration. *J Shoulder Elbow Surg.* 2000;9(30):173-176.

19. De la Puente R, Boutin RD, Theodorou DJ, Hooper A, Schewitzer M, Resnick D. Posttraumatic and stress-induced osteolysis of the distal clavicle: MR imaging findings in 17 patients. *Skeletal Radiol.* 1999; 28(4):202-208.

20. Rabalais RD, McCarty E. Surgical treatment of symptomatic acromioclavicular joint problems: a systematic review. *Clin Orthop Relat Res.* 2007;455:30-37.

21. Auge WK II, Fischer RA. Arthroscopic distal clavicle resection for isolated atraumatic osteolysis in weight lifters. *Am J Sports Med.* 1998;26(2):189-192.

22. Eskola A, Santavirta S, Viljakka HT, Wirta J, Partio TE, Hoikka V. The results of operative resection of the lateral end of the clavicle. *J Bone Joint Surg Am.* 1996;78(4):584-587.

23. Copeland S. *Shoulder Surgery.* London: WB Saunders; 1997.

24. Rockwood CA Jr. Injuries to the acromioclavicular joint. In: Rockwood CA Jr, Green DP, eds. *Fractures in Adults.* Vol 1, 2nd ed. Philadelphia: JB Lippincott; 1984:860-910.

25. Virk MS, Apostolakos J, Cote MP, Baker B, Beitzel K, Mazzocca AD. Operative and nonoperative treatment of acromioclavicular dislocation: a critical analysis review. *J Bone Joint Surg.* 2015;3(10):1-10.

26. Bishop JY, Kaeding C. Treatment of the acute traumatic acromioclavicular separation. *Sports Med Arthrosc Rev.* 2006;14(4):237-245.

27. Li X, Ma R, Bedi A, Dines DM, Altchek DW, Dines JS. Management of acromioclavicular joint injuries: current concepts review. *J Bone Joint Surg Am.* 2014;96:73-84.

28. Dragoo JL, Braun HF, Barlinski SE, Harris AH. Acromioclavicular joint injuries in National Collegiate Athletic Association football: data from the 2004-2005 through 2008-2009 National Collegiate Athletic Association Injury Surveillance System. *Am J Sports Med.* 2012;40:2066-2071.

29. Kilcoyne KG, Ebel BG, Bancells RL, Wilckens JH, McFarland EG. Epidemiology of injuries in major league baseball catchers. *Am J Sports Med.* 2015;43:2496-2500.

30. Chronopoulos E, Kim TK, Park HB, Ashenbrenner D, McFarland EG. Diagnostic value of physical tests for isolated chronic acromioclavicular lesions. *Am J Sports Med.* 2004;32(3):655-661.

31. Melenevsky Y, Yablon CM, Ramappa A, Hochman MG. Clavicle and acromioclavicular joint injuries: a review of imaging, treatment, and complications. *Skeletal Radiol.* 2011;40(7):831-842.

32. Pauly S, Gerhardt C, Haas NP, Scheibel M. Prevalence of concomitant intraarticular lesions in patients treated operatively for high-grade acromioclavicular joint separations. *Knee Surg Sports Traumatol Arthrosc.* 2009;17(5):513-517.

33. Tischer T, Salzmann GM, El-Azab H, Vogt S, Imhoff AB. Incidence of associated injuries with acute acromioclavicular joint dislocations type III through V. *Am J Sports Med.* 2009;37(1):136-139.

34. Toss JD, Mead NC, Sigmond HM. Acromioclavicular separations: useful and practical classification for treatment. *Clin Orthop Relat Res.* 1963:28:111-119.

35. Bannister GC, Wallace WA, Stableforth PG, Hutson MA. The management of acute acromioclavicular dislocation. A randomized prospective controlled trial. *J Bone Joint Surg Br.* 1989;71(5):848-850.

36. Cox JS. The fate of the acromioclavicular joint in athletic injuries. *Am J Sports Med.* 1981;9(1):50-53.

37. Mouhsine E, Garofalo R, Crevoisier X, Farron A. Grade I and II acromioclavicular dislocations: results of conservative treatment. *J Shoulder Elbow Surg.* 2003;12(6):599-602.

38. Bergfeld JA, Andrish JT, Clancy WG. Evaluation of the acromioclavicular joint following first and second degree sprains. *Am J Sports Med.* 1978;6(4):153-159.

39. Schlegel TF, Burks RT, Marcus RL, Dunn HK. A prospective evaluation of untreated acute grade III acromioclavicular separations. *Am J Sports Med.* 2001;29(6):699-703.

40. Bjerneld H, Hovelius L, Thorling J. Acromioclavicular separations treated conservatively: a five year follow up study. *Acta Orthop Scand.* 1983;54(5):743-745.

41. Dias JJ, Steingold RF, Richards RA, Tesfayohannes B, Gregg PJ. The conservative treatment of acromioclavicular dislocation: review after five years. *J Bone Joint Surg Br.* 1987;69(5):719-722.

42. Smit TO, Chester R, Pearse EO, Hing CB. Operative versus non-operative management following Rockwood grade III acromioclavicular separation: a meta-analysis of the current evidence base. *J Orthop Traumatol.* 2011;12(1):19-27.

43. Bessette M, Soloff L, Schickendantz M. Return to play after nonoperative treatment of type III acromioclavicular injury in a professional baseball player. *Ann Sports Med Res.* 2017;4(3).

44. Watson ST, Wyland DJ. Return to play after nonoperative management for a severe type III acromioclavicular separation in the throwing shoulder of a collegiate pitcher. *Phys Sportsmed.* 2015;43(1):99-103.

45. McFarland EG, Blivin SJ, Doehring CB, Curl LA, Silberstein C. Treatment of grade III acromioclavicular separations in professional throwing athletes: results of a survey. *Am J Orthop.* 1997;26(11):771-774.

46. Walley KC, Haghpanah B, Hingsammer A, et al. Influence of disruption of the acromioclavicular and coracoclavicular ligaments on glenohumeral motion: a kinematic evaluation. *BMC Musculoskelet Disord.* 2016;17(1):480.

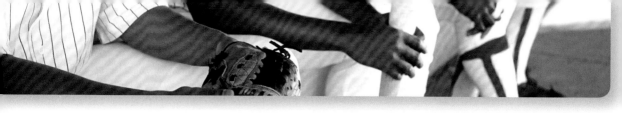

CHAPTER 22

Scapulothoracic Conditions and Baseball Players

W. Ben Kibler, MD | Stephen J. Thomas, PhD, ATC | Aaron Sciascia, PhD, ATC, PES

You could be a kid for as long as you want when you play baseball.

—*Cal Ripken Jr*

INTRODUCTION

The scapula serves many roles in shoulder function including (1) serving as a stable base for muscle activation, (2) dynamically moving in relation to the arm to create precise concavity-compression ball and socket kinematics throughout arm motion, (3) providing through its dynamic stability, optimal force and energy transfer from the core to the hand, and (4) moving to allow maximum arm abduction/external rotation (ABER). The most effective scapular position to achieve these goals is retraction, and the most effective motion is retraction and controlled protraction. Control of internal/external rotation (not allowing excessive internal rotation) and anterior/posterior tilting (not allowing anterior tilt) facilitates these goals.

SCAPULAR DYSKINESIS

Most scapular problems in throwing athletes can be traced to loss of control of normal resting scapular position and dynamic scapular motion, which will result in alterations in the position or motion that produce excessive protraction. This position and motion is considered an impairment, which in the face of functional demands of the overhead motion, can create inefficiencies and deficits in the kinematics of the shoulder, which can decrease performance and increase injury risk.[1]

Altered dynamic motion is termed scapular dyskinesis (dys—alteration of; kinesis—motion).[2] Dyskinesis has been found to be present in 67% to 100% of patients with shoulder injuries.[3,4] Dyskinesis results in scapular positions of increased anterior tilt, increased internal rotation, decreased upward rotation, and increased protraction. These positions have the effect of increasing the glenohumeral (GH) angle beyond the "safe zone," of increasing anterior shear, and of increasing tensile loads on the anterior band of the inferior GH ligament[5,6] and compression loads on the posterior labrum. Excessive scapular protraction also decreases maximum rotator cuff activation, decreasing the "compressor cuff" muscle function that establishes dynamic stability. In addition, the protraction diminishes dynamic subacromial clearance of the elevating humeral head and increases potential rotator cuff impingement on the glenoid.[7] It also diminishes the ability to move into maximal ABER, a position required for maximum performance.

Dyskinesis has multiple causes, which can be determined by appropriate history, examination, imaging, and special testing. Traumatic factors include clavicle fractures and high-grade acromioclavicular (AC) joint injuries.[8,9] Clavicle fractures may produce dyskinesis and protraction if the anatomy is not completely restored. High-grade (types III-VI) AC separations disrupt the strut function and allow a "third translation," in which the scapula translates inferior to the clavicle and medial on the thorax.

Intra-articular factors can produce dyskinesis by pain-derived muscle weakness, reflex-driven inhibition of coordinated muscle activation, or mechanical compensations to maintain GH concavity-compression when the static restraints are damaged. These factors include GH posttraumatic and multidirectional instability,[3,10-12] labral injuries,[13,14] biceps tendinopathy, and rotator cuff disease.[15]

The majority of scapular dyskinesis cases have root causes related to altered soft tissue and muscle function, ie, stiffness, inflexibility, decreased strength or strength imbalance, or altered muscle activation patterns. This would be expected, as scapular motion is largely dependent on coordinated muscle activation in force couples.

Stiffness/inflexibility may be due to muscle or joint causes.[16-19] The most common finding is coracoid-based inflexibility—pectoralis minor and biceps short head. Tightness of these muscles decreases scapular posterior tilt, upward rotation, and external rotation.[20] Upper trapezius tightness produces a shrug position, which can affect arm elevation. Pectoralis major and latissimus dorsi tightness can create dyskinesis through their action on the humerus.

Glenohumeral internal rotation deficit (GIRD), an altered joint motion, which is related to posterior muscle stiffness and capsular tightness, creates dyskinesis by producing a "windup" of the scapula into protraction as the arm rotates into follow-through.

Decreased strength is caused most commonly by fatigue or inhibition of activation. Fatigue that results in maladaptive patterns is commonly seen around the shoulder and in the lower trapezius,[21] posterior deltoid,[22] and supraspinatus.[11] It may occur in muscles that are deconditioned for the demands of the task or from exercise that is too strenuous for normally conditioned muscles. It occurs sooner in eccentric activities. Fatigue alters strength balance, joint motions, and joint loads.[23-25]

Inhibition of muscle activation is the most commonly encountered reason for muscle weakness. The neuromuscular axis is intact, but there is a decrease in the activation stimulus. Inhibition may be seen in GH joint internal derangements, such as labral injury or biceps tendinopathy, probably due to pain or capsular tension. Muscles such as the lower trapezius and serratus anterior appear to be more susceptible to this type of weakness, frequently being involved early in the injury and symptom process. Another effect of inhibition is alteration of the muscle activation patterns that involve the affected muscles. The lower trapezius has been shown to be delayed in muscle activation during arm elevation and descent in patients with impingement symptoms.[26]

Muscle imbalance can affect strength and force development, disrupt the coordinated sequencing of muscle activations in the kinetic chain, alter force couple activation, alter joint motion, and change joint loading patterns. Commonly observed alterations include stronger upper trapezius coupled with weaker lower trapezius/serratus anterior, stronger subscapularis coupled with weaker infraspinatus, stronger latissimus dorsi coupled with weaker lower trapezius, and stronger pectoralis minor coupled with weaker serratus anterior. Mechanisms creating the imbalances include inhibition of one muscle, acute or overload injury to one muscle, and hypertrophy of one muscle due to selective training or use.

Specific Problems in the Throwing Athlete

Scapular dyskinesis has been found in association with almost every pathologic injury in the shoulder and arm in the throwing athlete, including labral injury,[13,27] instability,[3] impingement,[28-30] rotator cuff disease,[4] clavicle fractures,[9,31-33] AC separations,[8] and elbow injury.[34] The incidence varies, but dyskinesis can be identified in between 50% and 100% of throwers with injuries.

Labral Injury

Scapular dyskinesis has a high association with labral injury with up to 94% of injured athletes demonstrating dyskinesis.[14,35] The altered position and motion of internal rotation and anterior tilt plus loss of upward rotation changes GH alignment, placing increased tensile strain on the anterior ligaments,[5] increases "peel-back" of the biceps/labral complex on the glenoid,[13] and creates pathologic internal impingement resulting in labral compression, tearing, and insubstance shearing.[35,36] Only a 10° loss of upward rotation increases the area and amount of compressive impingement, while a 10° increase in internal rotation increases the amount of compressive impingement.[37] These effects are magnified in the presence of GIRD, which creates increased protraction due to "windup" of the tight posterior structures in follow-through. Evaluation for dyskinesis in patients with suspected labral injury will be a key component in developing programs for nonoperative or postoperative rehabilitation. In addition, correction of the symptoms of pain found in the modified dynamic labral shear (M-DLS) test can be frequently demonstrated by the scapular retraction test (SRT). This indicates the presence of dyskinesis as part of the pathophysiology and the need for scapular rehabilitation to improve scapular retraction. A scapular-based rehabilitation program has been found to be successful to modify symptoms and improve performance so that surgery is not required in 41% of professional athletes[38] and 50% to 60% of nonprofessional but recreationally active athletes.[39]

Glenohumeral Instability

Many patients with instability demonstrate dyskinesis. The type of instability will usually determine how to address the dyskinesis. Traumatic anterior or posterior instability results in dyskinesis due to pain, muscle alteration(s), or altered joint mechanics, but dyskinesis can rarely be completely resolved in the presence of the anatomic lesion.

Symptoms in many other types of instability are more related to alterations of muscle function, which then create dyskinesis, and treatment of dyskinesis has been shown to have a more central effect on symptom resolution and functional restoration.[40-42] Because dyskinesis is so prevalent in patients with instability, evaluation for the presence or absence of scapular dyskinesis should be included as part of a comprehensive examination of the unstable shoulder.

Impingement

Impingement is frequently seen in throwing athletes but is rarely a primary or isolated diagnosis. Scapular dyskinesis is associated with impingement by altering scapular position at rest and on dynamic motion. Scapular dyskinesis in impingement is characterized by loss of acromial upward rotation, excessive scapular internal rotation, and excessive scapular anterior tilt.[28,30] These positions create scapular protraction, which may decrease the subacromial space,[43] increase contact on the glenoid,[7] and decrease demonstrated rotator cuff strength.[44,45]

Activation sequencing patterns and strength of the muscles that stabilize the scapula are altered in patients with impingement and scapular dyskinesis. Increased upper trapezius activity, imbalance of upper trapezius/lower trapezius activation, and decreased serratus anterior activation have been reported in patients with impingement.[26,30] Increased upper trapezius activity is clinically observed as a shrug maneuver, resulting in a type III dyskinesis pattern. This causes impingement owing to lack of acromial elevation. Frequently, lower trapezius activation is weak, inhibited, or delayed, and upper trapezius, pectoralis minor, and latissimus dorsi will be tight and painful to palpation. Serratus anterior activation has been shown to be decreased in patients with impingement, creating a lack of scapular external rotation and elevation with arm elevation.[26]

The pectoralis minor has been shown to be shortened in length in patients with impingement. This tight muscle creates a position of scapular protraction at rest and does not allow scapular posterior tilt or external rotation on arm motion, predisposing patients to impingement symptoms.[20] In this population of throwing athletes, even in the presence of positive impingement signs and impingement tests, most cases of impingement symptoms not associated with injury can be resolved by including restoration of scapular kinematics in the rehabilitation program.[46]

Rotator Cuff Injury

The rotator cuff is frequently clinically involved in throwers with shoulder symptoms, and symptoms can be exacerbated by dyskinesis. Upper trapezius spasm and tightness, pectoralis minor tightness, and lower trapezius and serratus anterior weakness are common findings. The dyskinetic protracted position that results in an internally rotated and anteriorly tilted glenoid increases the internal impingement on the posterior superior glenoid with arm external rotation and increases the torsional twisting of the rotator cuff, which may create the undersurface rotator cuff injuries seen in throwers.[13,47,48] In addition, scapular protraction creates superior compression loads on the rotator cuff. With continued activity, these loads result in histologic and mechanical changes in the tendon that are those seen in clinical tendinopathy.[15] Finally, positions of scapular protraction have been shown to be limiting to the development of maximal rotator cuff strength.

Rehabilitation programs that address restoration of scapular mechanics have been shown to decrease rotator cuff symptoms and decrease the requests for surgery, both in partial-thickness and full-thickness tears.[49] In both nonoperative and postoperative cases, early rehabilitation protocols should avoid exercises or arm positions that create protraction. These positions increase the compressive load on the tendon repair and can impair or delay optimum healing.[15,50]

Acromioclavicular Joint Injuries

AC joint injuries can create major 3-dimensional functional deficits owing to the disruption of the important AC linkage. High-grade AC separations alter the strut function of the clavicle on the scapula and change the biomechanical screw axis of scapulohumeral rhythm (SHR), allowing excessive scapular internal rotation and protraction and decreased dynamic acromial elevation when the arm is elevated.[51] The acromion will move inferiorly, anteriorly, and medially to the clavicle, resulting in the clinical deformity. The protracted scapular position creates many of the dysfunctional problems associated with chronic AC separations, including impingement and decreased demonstrated rotator cuff strength.

If dyskinesis is demonstrated on the clinical examination, this indicates the alteration of scapular kinematics that can affect shoulder function. In this case, increased attention should be directed toward correcting the biomechanical abnormality rather than just placing the arm in a sling. Treatment should include not only CC ligament reconstruction but also AC ligament reconstruction to completely restore the screw axis mechanism.[52]

Clavicle Fractures

Clavicle fractures have the capability, similar to high-grade AC joint injuries, of disrupting scapular kinematics and SHR. In midshaft clavicle fractures, the weight of the arm, the pull of the biceps and pectoralis muscles, and the torque transmitted to the clavicle through the CC ligaments by the protracted scapula all create a rotational displacement force, in addition to the amount of shortening and angulation that are also present. This 3-dimensional deficit yields a loss of strut efficiency for SHR and biomechanical problems including altered motion,[32,33,53] altered glenoid orientation,[54] and decreased strength.[31] Dyskinesis could be an important piece of information to identify patients who have altered anatomy that needs correction to restore normal shoulder function.

Scapula and the Elbow

Scapular function results in optimum position and force regulation throughout the entire arm. Dyskinesis can have several effects that can alter elbow motion, result in increased valgus load, and play a role in the etiology of elbow injuries, especially ulnar collateral ligament injuries.[23,25,55]

Fatigue of the scapular muscles, documented by muscle weakness and demonstrated by altered scapular internal/external rotation and anterior/posterior tilt, produces compensatory motions at the elbow and inability to reproduce elbow position,[21,23,25] both leading to increased loads.

A protracted scapula can result in altered GH angulation and potentiates the possibility of throwing out of the scapular plane, in a motion of relative humeral horizontal hyperabduction, a motion termed "slow arm" by pitching coaches. This motion increases the centripetal forces at the elbow.

Finally, dyskinesis can produce an altered arm position relative to the thorax, resulting in the "dropped elbow," a position in which the elbow is lower than the shoulder throughout a large part of the throwing motion and which has been termed by pitching coaches as "the kiss of death" of the elbow. In the dropped elbow, the elbow is in flexion for a longer time (increasing valgus stress) and the amount of time the medial ligaments experience these large loads is increased.

These scapular-based impairments interact with shoulder GIRD to affect the elbow. GIRD increases scapular protraction in follow-through, thereby increasing the scapular effects. GIRD also decreases the interactive moment that produces an elbow's varus acceleration, which counteracts the applied valgus load.[56-59]

PHYSICAL EXAMINATION

The goals of the physical examination of the scapula are to establish the presence or absence of scapular dyskinesis; to evaluate joint, muscle, and bone causative factors; and to employ dynamic corrective maneuvers to assess the effect of correction of dyskinesis on symptoms.

The scapular examination should largely be accomplished from the posterior aspect. The scapula should be exposed for complete visualization. The resting posture should be checked for side-to-side asymmetry but especially for evidence of a SICK position[60] or inferior medial or medial border prominence.

The SC joint and the AC joints should be evaluated for joint instability, and the clavicle should be evaluated for angulation, shortening, or malrotation. Anterior/posterior AC joint laxity can be evaluated by stabilizing the clavicle with one hand and grasping and mobilizing the acromion in an anterior/posterior direction with the other hand.

Identifying the physical impairment of scapular dyskinesis is best accomplished by observation of scapular motion using the scapular dyskinesis test.[61-63] The examination is conducted by having the patients raise the arms in forward flexion to maximum elevation and then lower them 3 to 5 times, with a 3- to 5-pound weight in each hand.[61,62] Prominence of any aspect of the medial scapular border on the symptomatic side is recorded as "yes" (prominence detected) or "no" (prominence not detected)[64] (Figure 22.1).

The scapular assistance test (SAT) and SRT are corrective maneuvers that can alter the injury symptoms and provide information about the role of scapular dyskinesis in the total picture of dysfunction that accompanies shoulder injury and needs to be restored.[63,65] In the SAT, the examiner applies gentle pressure to assist scapular upward rotation and posterior tilt as the patient elevates the arm (Figure 22.2). A positive result occurs when the painful arc of impingement symptoms

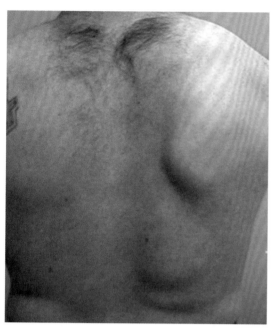

FIGURE 22.1 • Example of scapular dyskinesis showing medial border and inferior angle prominence.

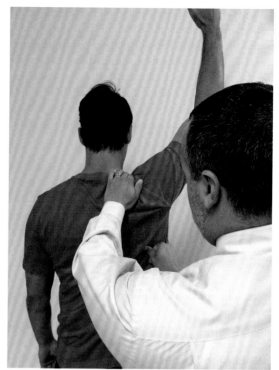

FIGURE 22.2 • Scapular assistance test.

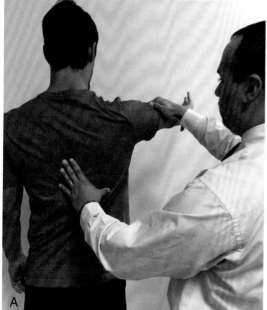

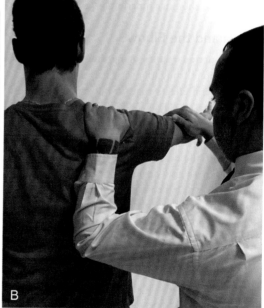

FIGURE 22.3 • Scapular retraction test. A, Standard manual muscle testing to assess flexion strength. B, Muscle testing of flexion with the scapula stabilized.

is relieved and the arc of motion is increased. In the SRT, the examiner first grades the strength in forward flexion following standard manual muscle testing procedures (Figure 22.3A) or evaluates the labrum by the M-DLS test[66] (Figure 22.4). The examiner then places and manually stabilizes the scapula in a retracted position (Figure 22.3B). A positive test occurs when the demonstrated strength is increased or the symptoms of internal impingement in the labral injury are relieved in the retracted position.

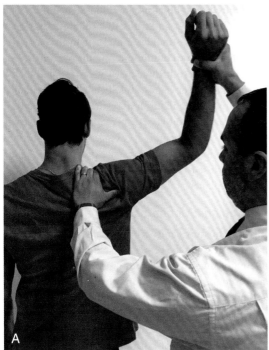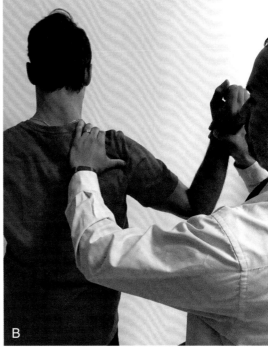

FIGURE 22.4 • The modified dynamic labral shear (M-DLS) for evaluating the presence of superior labral injury. A, Passive external rotation applied with the arm in 120 degrees of abduction. B, Manual shearing of the humeral head while maintaining the externally rotated position.

Coracoid-based inflexibility can be assessed by palpation of the pectoralis minor and the short head of the biceps brachii at their insertion in the coracoid tip. The muscles will usually be tender to palpation, even if they are not symptomatic in use, can be traced to their insertions on the ribs and arm as taut bands, and will create symptoms of soreness and stiffness when the scapulae are manually maximally retracted and the arm is slightly abducted to approximately 40° to 50°.

Standard GH examination techniques should be used to evaluate for internal derangement. Special attention should be paid to the examination for altered rotation, including internal, external, and total range of motion, and the evaluation of labral injuries, both of which are associated with dyskinesis. The methods of assessing shoulder rotation and motion include (1) internal rotation at 90° abduction[67] and (2) horizontal adduction with the arm at 90° flexion and the scapula restricted from moving into abduction.[68]

REHABILITATION

Three types of rehabilitation scenarios exist for throwing athletes: no activity with formal rehabilitation, limited/modified activity with supplemental rehabilitation, and full activity with supplemental conditioning. The key points for each level are described below.

No Activity With Formal Rehabilitation

Whether the athlete is experiencing general symptoms (soreness or pain with throwing, relative mild weakness, or a difficulty warming-up and/or getting loose) or specific symptoms that would suggest possible internal derangement, removing the high-load activity of throwing may help clinicians be more successful at reducing or alleviating impairments.

Many authors and clinicians have advocated for the identification of all potential culprits that could be affecting shoulder or scapular dysfunction in the overhead athlete and treating those culprits as part of shoulder rehabilitation.[14,69-71] It has been shown that the culprits can range from localized deficits at and around the shoulder to deficits distal to shoulder such as inflexibilities, weaknesses, and motor deficiencies at the trunk, pelvis, and lower extremity[72-74] (Figures 22.5 and 22.6). A full body assessment, or kinetic chain approach, appreciates the preference of the body to function as a unit to perform a multitude of tasks.[72]

A kinetic chain rehabilitation framework for shoulder dysfunction describes a rehabilitation approach that focuses on 3 critical characteristics.[75] First, patients are upright during exercise performance rather than be positioned supine or prone when possible to simulate functional demands.[75] Second, the lever arm on the shoulder and trunk is shortened to reduce the load on

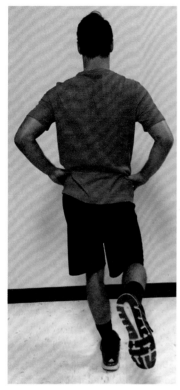

FIGURE 22.5 • Trendelenburg stance to detect gluteus medius weakness.

the injured arm. Finally, arm motions should be initiated using the legs and trunk to facilitate activation of the scapula and shoulder muscles, which is a typical neurologic pattern of motion.[76,77] This framework was later expanded to include a set of progressive goals[69]: (1) establish proper postural alignment; (2) establish proper motion at all involved segments; (3) facilitation of scapular motion via exaggeration of lower extremity/trunk movement; (4) exaggeration of scapular retraction in controlling excessive protraction; (5) utilize the closed-chain exercise early; and (6) work in multiple planes.

Posture and Motion

Proper posture and motion can be achieved by restoring skeletal segmental stability and mobility through muscle reeducation, soft tissue mobility, and spinal/rib mobilization. Muscle reeducation and strengthening of the core muscles should begin early in rehabilitation, targeting both local and global muscles.[70] In this first stage of the kinetic chain approach, soft tissue deficits of both upper and lower extremities should also be addressed. Segmental mobility of the thoracic spine and rib cage mobility is necessary for the scapula to synchronously move during arm motion.

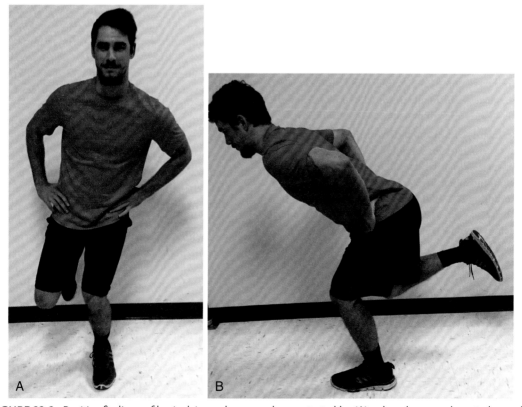

A   B

FIGURE 22.6 • Positive findings of leg/pelvis weakness as demonstrated by (A) valgus knee on decent phase of squat and (B) excessive trunk flexion as a compensation to align the knee during squatting.

Scapular Motion Facilitation

Primary stabilization and motion of the scapula on the thorax involves the coupling of the upper and lower fibers of the trapezius muscle with the serratus anterior and rhomboid muscles. Arm function overhead requires that the scapula obtains a position of posterior tilt and external rotation, which allows optimal shoulder muscle activation that is synergistic with trunk and hip musculature. This kinetic chain pattern of activation then facilitates maximal activation of the muscles attached to the scapula.[75] This integrated sequencing allows the retracted scapula to serve as a stable base for the origin of all the rotator cuff muscles, allowing optimal concavity-compression to occur.[78,79]

Controlling Protraction and Exaggerating Retraction

Although scapular protraction is a necessary kinematic translation, which occurs during the ball release through follow-through phases of the throwing motion, excessive scapular protraction does not allow optimal rotator cuff activation to occur.[44,45,80,81] The muscles responsible for performing scapular retraction can help control scapular protraction through eccentric control. When optimized, these muscles can properly maintain scapular stability, thus decreasing excessive protraction with arm movement. For this reason, the early phases of training should focus on scapular strengthening, especially in eccentric activation, in an attempt to restore normal scapular kinematics rather than placing an early emphasis on rotator cuff strengthening as performed in more traditional rehabilitation protocols. A basic exercise to utilize in this phase would be conscious correction of the scapula using visual feedback[82] (Figure 22.7).

Early Closed-Chain Implementation

Kinetic chain–based rehabilitation activities have been grouped into open and closed chain.[83-85] Typically, closed-chain exercises are implemented early in the rehabilitation process. These types of exercises are best suited for reestablishing the proximal stability and control in the links of the kinetic chain such as the pelvis and trunk. Open-chain exercises, which generate greater loads in comparison with closed-chain activities, should be utilized later in rehabilitation programs owing to the longer lever arm these exercises require, which causes increased demand on the soft tissue.

The rationale behind the closed-chain framework is to maximize the ability of the inhibited muscles to activate. This involves placing the extremity in a

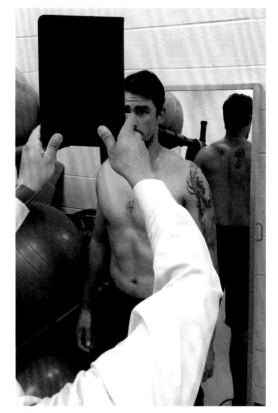

FIGURE 22.7 ⊛ Conscious correction of the scapula requires the patient to actively position the scapulae in retraction through the use of visual assistance.

closed-chain position, emphasizing normal activation patterns, and focusing on the muscle of interest by deemphasizing compensatory muscle activation. A closed-chain exercise such as the low row (Figure 22.8A and B) should be utilized because the short-lever positioning in conjunction with the pelvis and trunk acting as the driver facilitates lower trapezius and serratus anterior coactivation, which decreases the activation of the upper trapezius.[86] Once the normal activation pattern of retraction and depression has been restored, then more challenging exercises can be employed.

Working in Multiple Planes

During the functional phase in the later stages of the rehabilitation process, general GH strengthening would be introduced. Open-chain exercises attempt to isolate the rotator cuff muscles through long-lever arms performed in single-plane ranges of motion, which could potentially create shear force across the joint and cause muscular irritation. The patient should be positioned in standing positions to effectively use all segments within the kinetic chain.[87] This will simulate normal function and

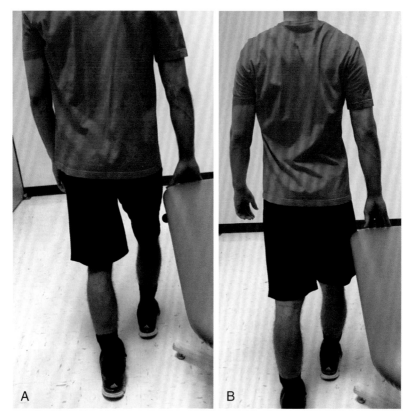

FIGURE 22.8 • Low row exercise: The patient is positioned standing with the hand of the involved arm against the side of a firm surface and legs slightly flexed (A). The patient should be instructed to extend the hips and trunk to facilitate scapular retraction and hold the contraction for 5 seconds (B).

limit attempts at trying to treat muscles in isolation.[87] The transverse plane should be exploited particularly in the early phases of rehabilitation, using diagonal and rotation exercises (Figures 22.9A, B and 22.10A, B), because most activities occur in the transverse plane.

Limited Activity With Supplemental Rehabilitation

At this level, the athlete would likely present similar to the athlete at the "no activity" level; however, the symptoms may be more general or vague suggesting something deleterious is beginning rather than fully existing. Additionally, chronic injury such as long-standing labral pathology or tendinopathy of the long head of the biceps brachii or rotator cuff may be detected but may not grossly affect function. Because of this less severe presentation, allowing the athlete to participate in some team activities is permissible and often tolerable. The activity modifications would include limited throwing volume and participation in field drills that only require gathering a ball and batting.

Supplemental rehabilitation involves supervised exercises and/or stretches that target specific muscles or tissues directly affecting scapular function, and the treatment plan would likely serve as an adjunct to strength training and conditioning. Similar to the exercise progression described for the "no activity with formal rehabilitation" level, the kinetic chain–based approach would be implemented to address scapular control and integration of all kinetic chain links. Examples would include reverse throwing (Figure 22.11A and B) and power position (Figure 22.12A and B). The strength training program would also be modified so that the athlete receives the training benefit but the injured or irritated tissue would not be overly stress or taxed. Examples would include modifying arm maneuvers to avoid hyperextension, horizontal abduction, or overhead positions. At this level, clinicians tend to address underlying kinetic chain concerns and inflexibilities of local muscles (ie, scapular stabilizers) while strength and conditioning specialists target muscle endurance of larger global muscles (ie, prime movers). It is important to note that communication between the clinician

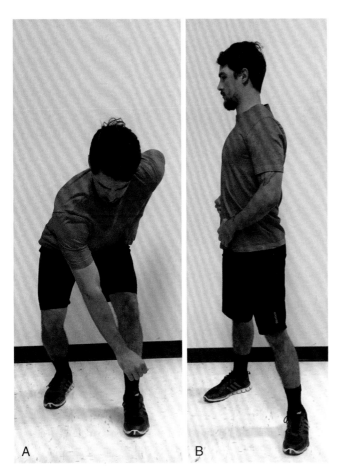

FIGURE 22.9 • Lawnmower exercise: The lawnmower begins with the hips and trunk flexed and the arm slightly forward elevated (A). The patient is instructed to extend the hips and trunk, followed by rotation of the trunk to facilitate scapular retraction (B).

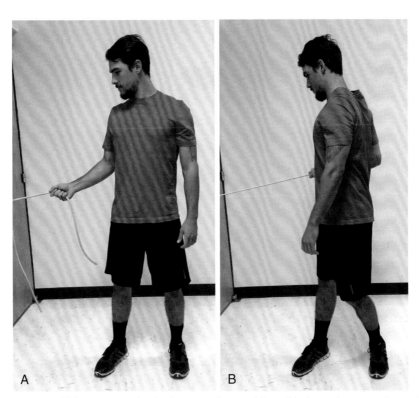

FIGURE 22.10 • Fencing: This maneuver begins in a standing position with the patient grasping resistance bands or tubing (A). It utilizes multiple kinetic chain segments to enhance proper muscle scapular muscle activation through activation of the legs, trunk, scapula, and arm (B).

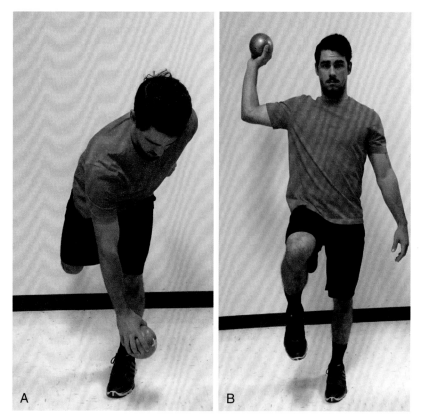

FIGURE 22.11 • Reverse throw: The patient begins with the trunk and hip flexed and standing on a single leg (A) and then actively extends the trunk and hip to bring the arm into a position of 90° abduction and 90° of elbow flexion (B).

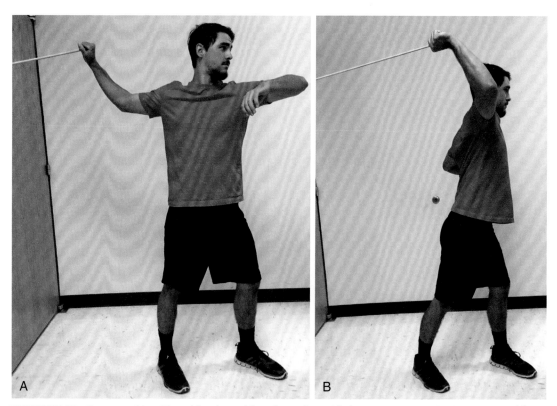

FIGURE 22.12 • Power position: The athlete is positioned standing with dominant arm in 90/90 position and forearm pronated (A). The athlete is instructed to rotate the trunk without moving the feet while maintaining the 90/90 position of the arm (B). The forearm should be allowed to supinate to imitate the act of the overhead throwing.

and strength specialist is important to avoid overlap in training programs that could be deleterious to recovery.

Full Activity With Supplemental Conditioning

In most cases, basic preexercise regimens and postexercise maintenance are effective at staving off soreness and injury. However, it is possible for baseball athletes to have 1 or 2 underlying deficiencies ranging from soft tissue inflexibility to muscle weakness or imbalance, all of which can contribute to habitual soreness. In these cases, clinicians should diligently assess all aspects of the athlete's regimen—mechanics during throwing, fielding, and hitting; technique during strength and conditioning maneuvers; volume and frequency of sporting drills; and off-season programming—to determine if an adjustment to current training should be employed. Furthermore, an assessment of the athlete's pre-throwing regimen should occur. The adjustments could be a modification of training interventions (more endurance-focused exercises rather than power-focused exercises), an addition of exercises not currently being performed, or a change in mechanics during drills or throwing. Pre- and postactivity measurements of GH rotation and scapular position should be obtained because a significant percentage of throwing athletes will demonstrate large changes that can have implications for shoulder and arm kinematics.[88-90]

MANAGER'S TIPS

- The scapula is a key component link in the kinetic chain that helps maximize function in throwing athletes
- Scapular roles in shoulder function include a stable base for muscle activation, providing dynamic to create precise concavity-compression, moving to allow maximum arm ABER, and facilitating force transfer
- Scapular dyskinesis is loss of control of resting position and dynamic motion. It should be considered an impairment of optimal scapular motion and has possible consequences to affect optimum scapular roles in throwing that can alter performance and increase injury risk. It may be seen as a limitation that increases injury risk in nonsymptomatic throwers, or it may be seen in association with overt injury and symptoms

- Dyskinesis has multiple causative factors. Traumatic factors include clavicle fractures and high-grade AC separations. Intra-articular factors include labral injury, rotator cuff disease, and GH joint instability. The most common factors include soft tissue alterations, including muscle and joint tightness, muscle weakness and imbalance, and altered muscle activation patterns. All these factors can be elucidated by dedicated and comprehensive evaluation of the history, physical examination, and imaging
- Dyskinesis has been associated with causation or exacerbation of virtually every shoulder and elbow injury, so the evaluation for dyskinesis should be included in the evaluation of all shoulder and elbow injuries
- Rehabilitation of scapular dyskinesis should be included as part of the overall treatment of all shoulder and elbow injuries. Three specific rehabilitation phases should be implemented depending on the capacity for throwing. They include no throwing activity with formal rehabilitation to restore the deficits discovered in the evaluation, limited/modified throwing activity with supplemental rehabilitation to optimize throwing capability, and full throwing activity with supplemental rehabilitation to maintain throwing capability in the face of continuing demands

ACKNOWLEDGMENT

The authors would like to sincerely thank Daniel Roberts, PT, ATC, Assistant Athletic Trainer, Houston Astros Baseball Organization, with reviewing and critiquing the rehabilitation section of this chapter. Without his expertise, the chapter would have been incomplete and limited in practicality.

REFERENCES

1. Hickey D, Solvig V, Cavalheri V, Harrold M, Mckenna L. Scapular dyskinesis increases the risk of future shoulder pain by 43% in asymptomatic athletes: a systematic review and meta-analysis. *Br J Sports Med.* 2018;52(2):102-110.

2. Kibler WB, Ludewig PM, McClure PW, Uhl TL, Sciascia AD. Scapula summit 2009. *J Orthop Sports Phys Ther.* 2009;39(11):A1-A13.

3. Warner JJP, Micheli LJ, Arslanian LE, Kennedy J, Kennedy R. Scapulothoracic motion in normal shoulders and shoulders with glenohumeral instability and impingement syndrome. *Clin Orthop Relat Res.* 1992;285(191):199.

4. Paletta GA, Warner JJP, Warren RF, Deutsch A, Altchek DW. Shoulder kinematics with two-plane x-ray evaluation in patients with anterior insta-bility or rotator cuff tears. *J Shoulder Elbow Surg.* 1997;6:516-527.

5. Weiser WM, Lee TQ, McQuade KJ. Effects of simu-lated scapular protraction on anterior glenohumeral sta-bility. *Am J Sports Med.* 1999;27:801-805.

6. Kibler WB, Uhl TL, Maddux JWQ, Brooks PV, Zeller B, McMullen J. Qualitative clinical evaluation of scapu-lar dysfunction: a reliability study. *J Shoulder Elbow Surg.* 2002;11:550-556.

7. Sarkar S, Seeley S, Beranek K, Blom K, Braman JP, Ludewig PM. Rotator cuff proximity to potential impinging structures during clinical impingement tests. In: *Paper Presented at: IXth Conference of the International Shoulder Group.* Wales, UK; 2012.

8. Gumina S, Carbone S, Postacchini F. Scapular dyskine-sis and SICK scapula syndrome in patients with chronic type III acromioclavicular dislocation. *Arthroscopy.* 2009;25(1):40-45.

9. Shields E, Behrend C, Beiswenger T, et al. Scapular dyskinesis following displaced fractures of the middle clavicle. *J Shoulder Elbow Surg.* 2015;24(12):e331-e336.

10. Barden JM, Balyk R, Raso VJ. Atypical shoulder muscle activation in multidirectional instability. *Clin Neurophysiol.* 2005;116:1846-1857.

11. Illyes A, Kiss RM. Kinematic and muscle activity char-acteristics of multidirectional shoulder joint instability during elevation. *Knee Surg Sports Traumatol Arthrosc.* 2006;14:673-685.

12. Ogston JB, Ludewig PM. Differences in 3-dimensional shoulder kinematics between persons with multidi-rectional instability and asymptomatic controls. *Am J Sports Med.* 2007;35:1361-1370.

13. Burkhart SS, Morgan CD, Kibler WB. The dis-abled throwing shoulder: spectrum of pathology. Part I: Pathoanatomy and biomechanics. *Arthroscopy.* 2003;19(4):404-420.

14. Kibler WB, Kuhn JE, Wilk KE, et al. The disabled throwing shoulder - spectrum of pathology: 10 year update. *Arthroscopy.* 2013;29(1):141-161.

15. Reuther KE, Thomas SJ, Tucker JJ, et al. Scapular dyskinesis is detrimental to shoulder tendon proper-ties and joint mechanics in a rat model. *J Orthop Res.* 2014;32(11):1436-1443.

16. Niederbracht Y, Shim AL, Sloniger MA, Paternostro-Bayles M, Short TH. Effects of a shoulder injury pre-vention strength training program on eccentric external rotation muscle strength and glenohumeral joint imbal-ance in female overhead activity athletes. *J Strength Cond Res.* 2008;22(1):140-145.

17. Butterfield TA. Eccentric exercise in vivo: strain-in-duced muscle damage and adaptation in a stable system. *Exerc Sport Sci Rev.* 2010;38(2):51-60.

18. Amin NH, Ryan J, Fening SD, Soloff L, Schickendantz MS, Jones M. The relationship between glenohumeral internal rotational deficits, total range of motion, and shoulder strength in professional baseball pitchers. *J Am Acad Orthop Surg.* 2015;23(12):789-796.

19. Myers N, Sciascia A, Westgate PM, Kibler WB, Uhl T. Increasing ball velocity in the overhead athlete: a meta-analysis of randomized controlled trials. *J Strength Cond Res.* 2015;29(10):2964-2979.

20. Borstad JD, Ludewig PM. The effect of long versus short pectoralis minor resting length on scapular kine-matics in healthy individuals. *J Orthop Sports Phys Ther.* 2005;35(4):227-238.

21. Ebaugh DD, McClure PW, Karduna AR. Effects of shoulder muscle fatigue caused by repetitive overhead activities on scapulothoracic and glenohumeral kine-matics. *J Electromyogr Kinesiol.* 2006;16:224-235.

22. Moore SD, Uhl TL, Kibler WB. Improvements in shoulder endurance following a baseball-specific strengthening program in high school baseball players. *Sports Health.* 2013;5(3):233-238.

23. Tripp BL, Boswell LL, Gansneder BM, Shultz SJ. Functional fatigue decreases three-dimensional multi-joint position reproduction acuity in the overhead throwing athlete. *J Athl Train.* 2004;39(4):316-320.

24. Forestier N, Nougier V. The effects of muscular fatigue on the coordination of a multijoint movement in human. *Neurosci Lett.* 1998;252(3):187-190.

25. Tripp B, Uhl TL, Mattacola CG, Srinivasan C, Shapiro R. Functional multijoint position reproduction acu-ity in overhead athletes. *J Athl Train.* 2006;41(2): 146-153.

26. Cools AM, Witvrouw EE, DeClercq GA, Danneels LA, Cambier DC. Scapular muscle recruitment pattern: tra-pezius muscle latency with and without impingement symptoms. *Am J Sports Med.* 2003;31:542-549.

27. Laudner KG, Stanek JM, Meister K. Differences in scapular upward rotation between baseball pitchers and position players. *Am J Sports Med.* 2007;35:2091-2095.

28. Kebaetse M, McClure PW, Pratt N. Thoracic posi-tion effect on shoulder range of motion, strength, and three-dimensional scapular kinematics. *Arch Phys Med Rehabil.* 1999;80:945-950.

29. Lukasiewicz AC, McClure P, Michener L, Pratt N, Sennett B. Comparison of 3-dimensional scapular posi-tion and orientation between subjects with and with-out shoulder impingement. *J Orthop Sports Phys Ther.* 1999;29(10):574-586.

30. Ludewig PM, Cook TM. Alterations in shoulder kinematics and associated muscle activity in people with symptoms of shoulder impingement. *Phys Ther.* 2000;80(3):276-291.

31. McKee MD, Pedersen EM, Jones C, et al. Deficits fol-lowing nonoperative treatment of displaced midshaft clavicular fractures. *J Bone Joint Surg Am.* 2006;88:35-40.

32. Matsumura N, Ikegami H, Nakamichi N, et al. Effect of shortening deformity of the clavicle on scapular kinematics: a cadaveric study. *Am J Sports Med.* 2010;38(5):1000-1006.

33. Hillen RJ, Burger BJ, Poll RG, van Dijk CN, Veeger DH. The effect of experimental shortening of the clavicle on shoulder kinematics. *Clin Biomech.* 2012;27(8):777-781.

34. Kibler WB, Sciascia AD. Kinetic chain contributions to elbow function and dysfunction in sports. *Clin Sports Med.* 2004;23(4):545-552.

35. Laudner KG, Myers JB, Pasquale MR, Bradley JP, Lephart SM. Scapular dysfunction in throwers with pathologic internal impingement. *J Orthop Sports Phys Ther.* 2006;36(7):485-494.

36. Myers JB, Laudner KG, Pasquale MR, Bradley JP, Lephart SM. Glenohumeral range of motion deficits and posterior shoulder tightness in throwers with pathologic internal impingement. *Am J Sports Med.* 2006;34:385-391.

37. Mihata T, Jun BJ, Bui CN, et al. Effect of scapular orientation on shoulder internal impingement in a cadaveric model of the cocking phase of throwing. *J Bone Joint Surg Am.* 2012;94(17):1576-1583.

38. Fedoriw WW, Ramkumar P, McCulloch PC, Lintner DM. Return to play after treatment of superior labral tears in professional baseball players. *Am J Sports Med.* 2014;42(5):1155-1160.

39. Edwards SL, Lee JA, Bell JE, et al. Nonoperative treatment of superior labrum anterior posterior tears: improvements in pain, function, and quality of life. *Am J Sports Med.* 2010;38(7):1456-1461.

40. Kibler WB. Management of the scapula in glenohumeral instability. *Tech Shoulder Elbow Surg.* 2003;4(3):89-98.

41. Burkhead WZ, Rockwood CA. Treatment of instability of the shoulder with an exercise program. *J Bone Joint Surg Am.* 1992;74-A(6):890-896.

42. Wilk KE, Macrina LC, Reinold MM. Non-operative rehabilitation for traumatic and atraumatic glenohumeral instability. *N Am J Sports Phys Ther.* 2006;1(1):16-31.

43. Ludewig PM, Reynolds JF. The association of scapular kinematics and glenohumeral joint pathologies. *J Orthop Sports Phys Ther.* 2009;39(2):90-104.

44. Kibler WB, Sciascia AD, Dome DC. Evaluation of apparent and absolute supraspinatus strength in patients with shoulder injury using the scapular retraction test. *Am J Sports Med.* 2006;34(10):1643-1647.

45. Tate AR, McClure P, Kareha S, Irwin D. Effect of the scapula reposition test on shoulder impingement symptoms and elevation strength in overhead athletes. *J Orthop Sports Phys Ther.* 2008;38(1):4-11.

46. Ellenbecker TS, Cools A. Rehabilitation of shoulder impingement syndrome and rotator cuff injuries: an evidence-based review. *Br J Sports Med.* 2010;44:319-327.

47. Mihata T, Gates J, McGarry MH, Lee JC, Kinoshita M, Lee TQ. Effect of rotator cuff muscle imbalance on forceful internal impingement and peel-back of the superior labrum: a cadaveric study. *Am J Sports Med.* 2009;37(11):2222-2227.

48. Mihata T, McGarry MH, Kinoshita M, Lee TQ. Excessive glenohumeral horizontal abduction as occurs during the late cocking phase of the throwing motion can be critical for internal impingement. *Am J Sports Med.* 2010;38(2):369-382.

49. Kuhn JE. Exercise in the treatment of rotator cuff impingement: a systematic review and a synthesized evidence-based rehabilitation protocol. *J Shoulder Elbow Surg.* 2009;18:138-160.

50. Sciascia A, Karolich D. A comprehensive approach for non-operative treatment of the rotator cuff. *Curr Phys Med Rehabil Rep.* 2013;1(1):29-37.

51. Sahara W, Sugamoto K, Murai M, Yoshikawa H. Three-dimensional clavicular and acromioclavicular rotations during arm abduction using vertically open MRI. *J Orthop Res.* 2007;25:1243-1249.

52. Kibler WB, Sciascia AD, Morris BJ, Dome DC. Treatment of symptomatic acromioclavicular joint instability by a docking technique: clinical indications, surgical technique, and outcomes. *Arthroscopy.* 2017;33(4):696-708.e2

53. Kibler WB, Sciascia AD, eds. *Disorders of the Scapula and Their Role in Shoulder Injury – a Clinical Guide to Evaluation and Management.* Switzerland: Springer; 2017.

54. Andermahr J, Jubel A, Elsner A, Prokop A, Tsikaras P, Jupiter J. Malunion of the clavicle causes significant glenoid malposition: a quantitative anatomic investigation. *Surg Radiol Anat.* 2006;28(5):447-456.

55. Wilk KE, Macrina LC, Fleisig GS, et al. Deficits in glenohumeral passive range of motion increase risk of shoulder injury in professional baseball pitchers: a prospective study. *Am J Sports Med.* 2015;43(10):2379-2385.

56. Fleisig GS, Barrentine SW, Escamilla RF, Andrews JR. Biomechanics of overhand throwing with implications for injuries. *Sports Med.* 1996;21:421-437.

57. Hirashima M, Kadota H, Sakurai S, Kudo K, Ohtsuki T. Sequential muscle activity and its functional role in the upper extremity and trunk during overarm throwing. *J Sports Sci.* 2002;20:301-310.

58. Hirashima M, Yamane K, Nakamura Y, Ohtsuki T. Kinetic chain of overarm throwing in terms of joint rotations revealed by induced acceleration analysis. *J Biomech.* 2008;41:2874-2883.

59. Putnam CA. Sequential motions of body segments in striking and throwing skills: description and explanations. *J Biomech.* 1993;26:125-135.

60. Burkhart SS, Morgan CD, Kibler WB. The disabled throwing shoulder: spectrum of pathology. Part III: The SICK scapula, scapular dyskinesis, the kinetic chain, and rehabilitation. *Arthroscopy.* 2003;19(6): 641-661.

61. McClure PW, Tate AR, Kareha S, Irwin D, Zlupko E. A clinical method for identifying scapular dyskinesis: Part 1: Reliability. *J Athl Train.* 2009;44(2):160-164.

62. Tate AR, McClure PW, Kareha S, Irwin D, Barbe MF. A clinical method for identifying scapular dyskinesis: Part 2: Validity. *J Athl Train.* 2009;44(2):165-173.

63. Kibler WB, Ludewig PM, McClure PW, Michener LA, Bak K, Sciascia AD. Clinical implications of scapular dyskinesis in shoulder injury: the 2013 consensus statement from the "scapula summit". *Br J Sports Med.* 2013;47:877-885.

64. Uhl TL, Kibler WB, Gecewich B, Tripp BL. Evaluation of clinical assessment methods for scapular dyskinesis. *Arthroscopy.* 2009;25(11):1240-1248.

65. Kibler WB. The role of the scapula in athletic function. *Am J Sports Med.* 1998;26:325-337.

66. Kibler WB, Sciascia AD, Dome DC, Hester PW, Jacobs C. Clinical utility of new and traditional exam tests for biceps and superior glenoid labral injuries. *Am J Sports Med.* 2009;37(9):1840-1847.

67. Wilk KE, Reinhold MM, Macrina LC, et al. Glenohumeral internal rotation measurements differ depending on stabilization techniques. *Sports Health.* 2009;1(2):131-136.

68. Laudner KG, Moline MT, Meister K. The relationship between forward scapular posture and posterior shoulder tightness among baseball players. *Am J Sports Med.* 2010;38:2106-2112.

69. Sciascia A, Cromwell R. Kinetic chain rehabilitation: a theoretical framework. *Rehabil Res Pract.* 2012;2012:1-9.

70. Kibler WB, Press J, Sciascia AD. The role of core stability in athletic function. *Sports Med.* 2006;36(3):189-198.

71. Sciascia A, Monaco M. When is the patient truly 'Ready to Return', a.k.a. kinetic chain homeostasis. In: Kelly IV JD, ed. *Elite Techniques in Shoulder Arthroscopy: New Frontiers in Shoulder Preservation.* Switzerland: Springer; 2016:317-327.

72. Sciascia AD, Thigpen CA, Namdari S, Baldwin K. Kinetic chain abnormalities in the athletic shoulder. *Sports Med Arthrosc Rev.* 2012;20(1):16-21.

73. Radwan A, Francis J, Green A, et al. Is there a relation between shoulder dysfunction and core instability? *Int J Sports Phys Ther.* 2014;9(1):8-13.

74. Reeser JC, Joy EA, Porucznik CA, Berg RL, Colliver EB, Willick SE. Risk factors for volleyball-related shoulder pain and dysfunction. *Phys Med Rehabil.* 2010;2(1):27-35.

75. McMullen J, Uhl TL. A kinetic chain approach for shoulder rehabilitation. *J Athl Train.* 2000;35(3):329-337.

76. Bouisset S, Zattara M. A sequence of postural movements precedes voluntary movement. *Neurosci Lett.* 1981;22:263-270.

77. Hodges PW, Richardson CA. Feedforward contraction of transversus abdominus is not influenced by the direction of arm movement. *Exp Brain Res.* 1997;114:362-370.

78. Lippitt S, Matsen Iii FA. Mechanisms of glenohumeral joint stability. *Clin Orthop Relat Res.* 1993(291):20-28.

79. Lippitt S, Vanderhooft JE, Harris SL, Sidles JA, Harryman II DT, Matsen III FA. Glenohumeral stability from concavity-compression: a quantitative analysis. *J Shoulder Elbow Surg.* 1993;2(1):27-35.

80. Smith J, Kotajarvi BR, Padgett DJ, Eischen JJ. Effect of scapular protraction and retraction on isometric shoulder elevation strength. *Arch Phys Med Rehabil.* 2002;83:367-370.

81. Smith J, Dietrich CT, Kotajarvi BR, Kaufman KR. The effect of scapular protraction on isometric shoulder rotation strength in normal subjects. *J Shoulder Elbow Surg.* 2006;15:339-343.

82. De May K, Danneels L, Cagnie B, Huyghe L, Seyns E, Cools AM. Conscious correction of scapular orientation in overhead athletes performing selected shoulder rehabilitation exercises: the effect on trapezius muscle activation measured by surface electromyography. *J Orthop Sports Phys Ther.* 2013;43(1):3-10.

83. Ellenbecker TS, Manske R, Davies GJ. Closed kinetic chain techniques of the upper extremities. *Orthop Phys Ther Clin N Am.* 2000;9(2):219-229.

84. Kibler WB, Livingston B. Closed-chain rehabilitation for upper and lower extremities. *J Am Acad Orthop Surg.* 2001;9(6):412-421.

85. Ellenbecker TS, Davies GJ. *Closed Kinetic Chain Exercise: A Comprehensive Guide to Multiple Joint Exercises.* Champaign: Human Kinetics; 2001.

86. Kibler WB, Sciascia AD, Uhl TL, Tambay N, Cunningham T. Electromyographic analysis of specific exercises for scapular control in early phases of shoulder rehabilitation. *Am J Sports Med.* 2008;36(9):1789-1798.

87. De May K, Danneels L, Cagnie B, Cools A. Are kinetic chain rowing exercises relevant in shoulder and trunk injury prevention training? *Br J Sports Med.* 2011;45(4):320.

88. Kibler WB, Sciascia AD, Moore SD. An acute throwing episode decreases shoulder internal rotation. *Clin Orthop Relat Res.* 2012;470:1545-1551.

89. Reinold MM, Wilk KE, Macrina LC, et al. Changes in shoulder and elbow passive range of motion after pitching in professional baseball players. *Am J Sports Med.* 2008;36(3):523-527.

90. Wilk KE, Macrina LC, Fleisig GS, et al. Loss of internal rotation and the correlation to shoulder injuries in professional baseball pitchers. *Am J Sports Med.* 2011;39(2):329-335.

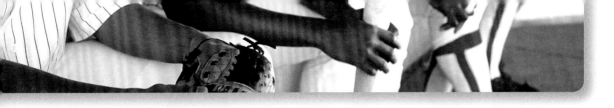

CHAPTER 23

Thoracic Outlet Syndrome and Neurovascular Conditions of the Shoulder in Baseball Players

Robert W. Thompson, MD

It was all I lived for, to play baseball.

—*Mickey Mantle*

INTRODUCTION

Major neurovascular conditions of the upper extremity are relatively rare and often difficult to recognize. These conditions are nonetheless quite important in baseball players and other overhead athletes, because they can seriously limit athletic performance and may even have limb-threatening consequences.[1] Some of the most significant upper extremity neurovascular disorders are related to compression of the brachial plexus nerves or the subclavian vessels and are therefore considered different forms of thoracic outlet syndrome (TOS).[2] In this chapter, current strategies for the diagnosis and treatment of these conditions are highlighted, both to avoid serious complications and to promote successful treatment outcomes. In most cases, early recognition, proper initial treatment, and comprehensive surgical care can allow the athlete to successfully return to previous levels of performance.

NEUROGENIC THORACIC OUTLET SYNDROME

Neurogenic TOS is caused by compression and irritation of the brachial plexus nerve roots within the scalene triangle at the base of the neck and/or the infraclavicular subcoracoid (pectoralis minor) space (Figure 23.1).[2,3] This condition is related to predisposing anatomical factors (such as cervical ribs, ligamentous bands, and scalene muscle abnormalities) combined with injury, fibrosis, hypertrophy, and chronic spasm of the scalene and pectoralis minor muscles.

Clinical Recognition

The symptoms of neurogenic TOS include pain, numbness, and paresthesia in the arm and/or hand.[3] These complaints do not correspond to the distribution of a single peripheral nerve or cervical nerve root and are often variable in intensity or duration, depending on the level of arm activity. Importantly, symptoms of neurogenic TOS are usually exacerbated by activities with the arm in an elevated position. Along with tenderness, muscle spasm, and reproduction of hand/arm symptoms upon palpation over the supraclavicular scalene triangle or subcoracoid pectoralis minor muscle tendon, positional complaints on physical examination can be useful in differentiating TOS from other conditions.[3] While diagnostic imaging and/or electrophysiological studies are usually negative, they help to exclude other (more common) conditions that might yield similar symptoms.[4] As outlined in Table 23.1, the recent publication of clinical diagnostic criteria for neurogenic TOS has helped provide more consistency in recognizing this condition.[5,6] In baseball players, the diagnosis of neurogenic TOS is often complicated by minimal symptoms at rest or with day-to-day activities but the presence of significant arm fatigue, heaviness, and other symptoms when throwing.[1] The use of exercise-enhanced anterior scalene and/or pectoralis minor muscle blocks with local anesthetic provides a

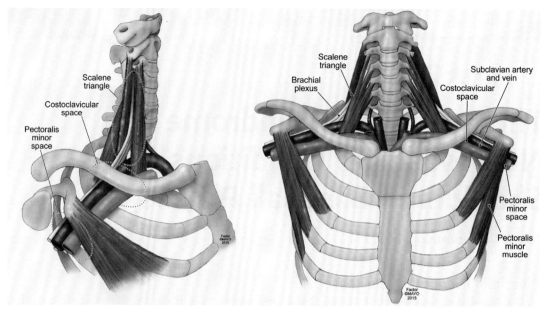

FIGURE 23.1 • **Anatomy of the thoracic outlet.** The 5 nerve roots comprising the brachial plexus (C5, C6, C7, C8, and T1) pass through the thoracic outlet within the base of the neck, including the scalene triangle (bordered by the anterior and middle scalene muscles and the first rib), the costoclavicular space, and the subcoracoid (pectoralis minor) space. The subclavian artery passes through the scalene triangle and over the first rib immediately anterior to the brachial plexus, while the subclavian vein crosses the first rib through the costoclavicular space, in front of the anterior scalene muscle and immediately behind the clavicle. (Adapted from Illig KA, Donahue D, Duncan A, et al. Reporting standards of the Society for Vascular Surgery for thoracic outlet syndrome: executive summary. *J Vasc Surg.* 2016;64(3):797-802. Copyright © 2016 by the Society for Vascular Surgery. With permission.)

useful adjunctive diagnostic test to help distinguish neurogenic TOS from other conditions and can also help predict the response to treatment.[7]

Treatment

Treatment for neurogenic TOS begins with rest of the affected extremity, physical therapy to relax and stretch the scalene and pectoralis minor muscles, and use of muscle relaxants and anti-inflammatory agents.[8-12] Botox injections to the scalene muscles have been explored for neurogenic TOS but have not been found to have a durable benefit compared with saline injections alone.[13] Surgical treatment is appropriate for those with substantial disability, when sufficient improvement has not been achieved with conservative approaches alone.[14-16] Thoracic outlet decompression for neurogenic TOS can be performed through either a transaxillary or supraclavicular approach, typically with removal of the first rib, resection of the anterior and middle scalene muscles, and brachial plexus neurolysis. In patients with physical examination findings related to the subcoracoid space, pectoralis minor tenotomy is also beneficial.[17] Some evidence suggests that the symptomatic recurrence rate is higher after transaxillary first rib resection compared with

supraclavicular decompression, particularly in long-term follow-up.[18] Other advantages of the supraclavicular approach include more complete anterior and middle scalenectomy, ease of identifying anatomic variations and anomalies, and ability to perform brachial plexus neurolysis with direct visual protection of the brachial plexus nerve roots.[19] In recent years, there has been some interest in video-assisted transpleural (thoracoscopic) first rib resection, but this remains an experimental approach with no proven advantages over standard surgical approaches.[20]

Rehabilitation

Initial care after thoracic outlet decompression revolves around control of postoperative pain, maintenance of shoulder range of motion, avoiding muscle spasm, and optimizing wound healing, although light conditioning activity is permitted (Table 23.2).[3,21] Regular physical therapy is started after the first 3 to 4 weeks, using a combination of passive and assisted exercises to emphasize shoulder range of motion; light upper extremity neural mobilization ("nerve glides"); gentle stretching of the levator, upper trapezius, and pectoral muscles; improving head, shoulder, and scapular posture; monitoring for scapular winging; increasing

TABLE 23.1 CORE-TOS Clinical Diagnostic Criteria for Neurogenic TOS

Upper extremity symptoms extending beyond the distribution of a single cervical nerve root or peripheral nerve present for at least 12 wk, not satisfactorily explained by another condition, **and** meeting at least 1 criterion in at least 4 of the following 5 categories:
Principal Symptoms
1A: Pain in the neck, upper back, shoulder, arm, and/or hand 1B: Numbness, paresthesia, and/or weakness in the arm, hand, or digits
Symptom Characteristics
2A: Pain/paresthesia/weakness exacerbated by elevated arm positions 2B: Pain/paresthesia/weakness exacerbated by prolonged or repetitive arm/hand use, including prolonged work on a keyboard or other repetitive strain tasks 2C: Pain/paresthesia radiate down the arm from the supraclavicular or infraclavicular spaces
Clinical History
3A: Symptoms began after occupational, recreational, or accidental injury of the head, neck, or upper extremity, including repetitive upper extremity strain or overuse 3B: Previous ipsilateral clavicle or first rib fracture, or known cervical rib 3C: Previous cervical spine or ipsilateral peripheral nerve surgery without sustained improvement in symptoms 3D: Previous conservative or surgical treatment for ipsilateral TOS
Physical Examination
4A: Local tenderness on palpation over the scalene triangle and/or subcoracoid space 4B: Arm/hand/digit paresthesia on palpation over the scalene triangle and/or subcoracoid space 4C: Objectively weak handgrip, intrinsic muscles, or digit 5, or thenar/hypothenar atrophy
Provocative Maneuvers
5A: Positive upper limb tension test (ULTT) 5B: Positive 3-minute elevated arm stress test (EAST)

Diagnostic criteria developed by the Consortium for Research and Education on Thoracic Outlet Syndrome (CORE-TOS).

(Reprinted from Balderman J, Holzem K, Field BJ, et al. Associations between clinical diagnostic criteria and pretreatment patient-reported outcomes measures in a prospective observational cohort of patients with neurogenic thoracic outlet syndrome. J Vasc Surg. 2017;66(2):533-544.e2. Copyright © 2017 Elsevier. With permission.)

movement of the scapula into upward rotation and elevation; improving diaphragm (vs chest) breathing patterns; and general conditioning (walking, bicycle, elliptical, treadmill). It is important at this stage to avoid vigorous use of involved upper limb, such as strengthening with weights or bands, manual therapies that may irritate sensitive healing tissue, or immersion in water, until after the incisions are fully healed. By 8 weeks after operation, the therapist may begin manual therapies and resisted strengthening exercises for the mid- and lower trapezius, serratus anterior, and rotator cuff muscles; continue to optimize range of motion of the upper limb, movement patterns, and the throwing motion; and introduce gentle throwing. Care may transition from the physical therapist to the athletic trainer at this stage, and a more formal gradual supervised throwing program may begin by 12 to 16 weeks after operation and progress over time as tolerated. It is important that the primary surgeon, TOS-specialist physical therapist, and athletic trainer work in concert during the rehabilitation process,

with patience and a highly individualized approach, and recognize the need to step back or move slower in the event that the athlete develops any worsening symptoms, to avoid excessive activity that might promote excessive muscle spasm, perineural scar tissue, or recurrent neurogenic TOS. From reported experience, it is expected that full rehabilitation to a return to competition will require 9 to 12 months after surgical treatment for neurogenic TOS.[22]

Outcomes

The outcomes of surgical treatment for neurogenic TOS are relatively well established, with substantial symptom improvement in 85% to 90% of patients, but for many years surgical treatment for neurogenic TOS in overhead throwing athletes has been relegated to case reports.[14-16] In the past decade, there has been increased awareness of this condition, particularly in professional and collegiate baseball, along with greater understanding that surgical treatment can allow many athletes to resume careers that might otherwise have

TABLE 23.2 Overview of Postoperative Rehabilitation for Neurogenic TOS

Stage I: Inpatient to Hospital Discharge
• Hospital length of stay 3-4 d • Patient self-exercises (cervical and shoulder ROM) • Surgeon office follow-up visit postoperative day 5-7, drain removal
Stage II: Postoperative Weeks 1-4
• Protection of surgical tissues to promote incisional healing and minimize muscle spasm (propping arm with pillows while sitting and sleeping, ice, medications) • Maintain cervical and glenohumeral range of motion (hospital self-exercises) • Light conditioning activity (walking, bicycle)
Stage III: Postoperative Weeks 4-8
• Physical therapist visits near home, 1-2 per week • Pain management (ice or heat to surgical area) • Scar hypersensitivity and local tissue edema • Posture (head, shoulders, and scapulae); monitor for scapular winging • Light neural mobilizations • Gentle stretching of levator, upper trapezius, and pectoral muscles • Movement of scapula into upward rotation and elevation • Breathing pattern (chest versus diaphragm) • Conditioning activity (walking, bicycle, elliptical, treadmill) but avoid vigorous use of the involved upper limb • Activities of daily living, ergonomics, work environment • Cautions: no strengthening including use of weights or bands; avoid manual therapies that may irritate sensitive healing tissue; no immersion in water until incisions fully healed
Stage IV: Postoperative Weeks 8-16
• Continue physical therapist visits near home, 1-2 per week • Symptom management, may introduce manual therapies • Continue conditioning activity (bicycling, walking, elliptical, treadmill) • Strengthening mid- and lower trapezius, serratus anterior, and rotator cuff muscles • Increasing range of motion of upper limb, throwing motion, optimize movement patterns • Introduce gentle throwing and progress as tolerated
Stage V: Postoperative Months 4-6

• Supervised throwing program, progressing as tolerated:
  • Step 1: 1 × 25 throws at 60 feet
  • Step 2: 2 × 25 throws at 60 feet
  • Step 3: 1 × 25 throws at 60 feet, 1 × 25 throws at 90 feet
  • Step 4: 1 × 30 throws at 60 feet, 1 × 25 throws at 90 feet
  • Step 5: 1 × 30 throws at 60 feet, 1 × 25 throws at 90 feet
  • Step 6: 1 × 30 throws at 90 feet, 1 × 25 throws at 120 feet
  • Step 7: 2 × 20 throws at 120 feet
  • Step 8: 1 × 20 throws at 120 feet, 1 × 20 feet at 150 feet
  • Step 9: 1 × 20 throws at 150 feet, 10 pitches from mound
  • Step 10: long toss, 35-pitch bullpen session
• Gradually increase activity toward unrestricted return to competition at 6-9 mo

come to an end. To better characterize the impact of surgical treatment on baseball pitching performance, we recently utilized objective metrics to assess the performance of Major League Baseball (MLB) pitchers before and after recovery from treatment for neurogenic TOS.[22] This study involved 10 pitchers who underwent operation between July 2001 and July 2014 and had achieved a sustained return to play in MLB, using traditional and advanced performance metrics acquired from public databases. The mean age was 30.2 ± 1.4 years at the time of surgery and the mean period of postoperative rehabilitation was 10.8 ± 1.5 months before the return to MLB. There were no significant differences comparing 3 years before and 3 years after surgery with regard to 15 traditional pitching metrics, including earned run average (ERA), fielding independent pitching (FIP), walks plus hits per inning pitched (WHIP), walks

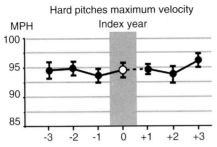
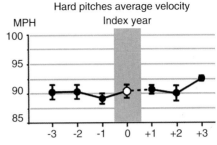

FIGURE 23.2 • **Performance metrics in MLB pitchers before and after surgical treatment for neurogenic TOS.** Pitch velocity metrics in the 3 years surrounding the index (surgical treatment) year for a series of MLB pitchers who underwent treatment for neurogenic TOS. Data shown illustrate the mean ± SEM for each year. There were no significant before-after differences for hard pitch maximum or average velocity. (Reprinted from Thompson RW, Dawkins C, Vemuri C, et al. Performance metrics in professional baseball pitchers before and after surgical treatment for neurogenic thoracic outlet syndrome. *Ann Vasc Surg.* 2017;39(1):216-227. Copyright © 2016 Elsevier. With permission.)

per 9 innings (BB/9), and strikeouts to walks ratio (SO/BB). There were also few differences observed in assessing 72 advanced metrics, even for maximal and average hard pitch velocity (Figure 23.2). This study thereby demonstrated that pitchers returning to MLB after surgery for neurogenic TOS have had capabilities equivalent to or better than before treatment and that when coupled with an ample period of postoperative rehabilitation, thoracic outlet decompression can provide effective treatment for professional baseball pitchers with this career-threatening condition.

More recently, Schutze et al surveyed a series of competitive athletes who had undergone surgical treatment for neurogenic TOS.[23] This included 67 athletes ranging from 14 to 48 years of age, an average of 3.9 years after surgery. The results demonstrated that 96% had an improvement in pain medication use, 75% would undergo surgical treatment on the contralateral side if recommended, 82% had experienced resolution of symptoms, and 94% were unlimited in performing activities of daily living. Moreover, 70% of these individuals had returned to the same or better level of athletic activity after surgical treatment, with 50% reaching this goal within 1 year of operation.

VENOUS THORACIC OUTLET SYNDROME

Venous TOS is characterized by axillary-subclavian vein effort thrombosis (Paget-Schroeter syndrome), and it represents the most frequently encountered vascular disorder in young competitive athletes.[24] Because delayed diagnosis or incomplete treatment can prevent further participation in sports, it is particularly important for sports medicine physicians to have a sound understanding of this condition. Fortunately, with proper initial treatment and definitive surgical

care, most athletes affected by venous TOS can return to previous levels of performance within several months.[25]

Pathophysiology

In the past, subclavian vein effort thrombosis was considered to be due to acute vein injury caused by compression of the subclavian vein between the clavicle and first rib, with superimposed thrombosis, or as a complication of a primary hypercoagulable disorder. It is now recognized that effort thrombosis is the acute clinical presentation of a more chronic condition, characterized by repetitive "mechanical" venous injury during arm elevation, associated with the anatomical constraints normally present at the level of the first rib (Figure 23.3).[25] During repetitive cycles of injury and repair over months to years, the site of subclavian vein compression becomes encased by constricting scar tissue. While this remains asymptomatic due to simultaneous expansion of venous collaterals, eventually thrombus formation within the narrowed subclavian vein can occlude the lumen and propagate peripherally to obstruct critical collaterals. The abrupt obstruction of pathways for venous flow results in the symptoms of "effort" thrombosis: marked arm swelling from the shoulder to the hand, cyanotic discoloration, heaviness, and pain or fatigue with use. Although pulmonary embolism may occur from thrombus formed within the proximal portion of the subclavian vein, this is much less frequent than in iliofemoral deep vein thrombosis and is usually of minor consequence.

Clinical Recognition

The presentation of any young, healthy, and active individual with sudden onset of arm swelling and cyanotic discoloration, as well as any young individual with otherwise unexplained pulmonary embolism, should

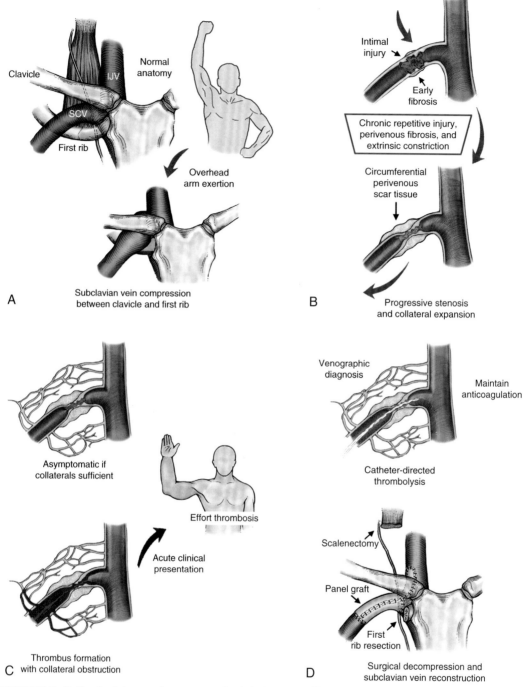

FIGURE 23.3 • **Pathophysiology and treatment of subclavian vein effort thrombosis.** A, Normal anatomy of the thoracic outlet with compression of the subclavian vein during arm elevation. B, Repetitive subclavian vein injury resulting in progressive stenosis. C, Collateral expansion may prevent symptoms of venous obstruction; however, eventual thrombus formation with obstruction of collaterals results in the acute clinical presentation of effort thrombosis. D, Catheter-directed venography and thrombolytic infusion improves venous flow and reveals underlying subclavian vein obstruction at the level of the first rib. Definitive treatment is achieved by thoracic outlet decompression with the first rib resection and subclavian vein reconstruction. SCV, subclavian vein; IJV, internal jugular vein. (Reprinted with permission from Thompson RW, Pearl GJ. Neurovascular injuries in the throwing shoulder. In: Dines JM, ElAttrache NS, Yocum LA, Altchek DW, Andrews J, Wilk KE, eds. *Sports Medicine of Baseball*. 1st ed. Philadelphia, PA: Lippincott Williams & Wilkins; 2012:180-193.)

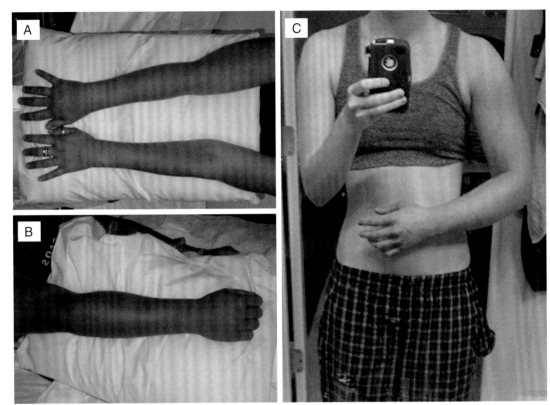

FIGURE 23.4 • **Clinical presentation of effort thrombosis.** Photographs depicting 3 otherwise healthy, active, young patients who had experienced the recent onset of upper extremity swelling and cyanotic discoloration, extending from the shoulder to the hand, due to SCV effort thrombosis. A, A 32-year-old woman with right SCV thrombosis. B, A 24-year-old man with right SCV thrombosis. C, A 17-year-old woman with right SCV thrombosis. (Reprinted from Vemuri C, Salehi P, Benarroch-Gampel J, McLaughlin LN, Thompson RW. Diagnosis and treatment of effort-induced thrombosis of the axillary subclavian vein due to venous thoracic outlet syndrome. *J Vasc Surg Venous Lymphat Disord.* 2016;4(4):485-500. Copyright © 2016 Elsevier. With permission.)

raise the suspicion of axillary-subclavian vein thrombosis (Figure 23.4).[24-26] This suspicion is strongly reinforced by a history of active use of the affected arm, especially in vigorous overhead activities or weight lifting. Physical examination typically reveals substantial arm swelling, up to twice the normal size, as well as cyanotic discoloration and distention of subcutaneous veins around the upper arm and shoulder. There may also be a sensation of heaviness with arm elevation and occasionally numbness and tingling in the hand with use. In contrast, there is usually no significant tenderness in the supraclavicular or infraclavicular space or other evidence of neurogenic TOS.

Upper extremity (ultrasound) Duplex imaging may be used in patients suspected to have axillary-subclavian vein effort thrombosis, but it is important to recognize that this testing approach has a substantial false-negative rate and cannot be used to exclude a diagnosis of venous TOS.[25,26] The possibility of effort thrombosis may also be assessed by contrast-enhanced

CT or MR venography, performed with the arm at rest and with the arm raised overhead, which avoids the limitations of ultrasound and can be used to exclude the diagnosis when negative.[4] More definitive diagnosis of venous TOS is obtained by traditional catheter-directed contrast venography. This approach provides the most complete anatomic information regarding the site and extent of thrombosis and evaluation of the status of the collateral veins. Because contrast venography is also required for catheter-based thrombolysis, the preferred initial step in treatment, this is often the initial diagnostic test of choice.

Anticoagulation and Thrombolysis

Initial treatment of patients suspected to have effort thrombosis should include anticoagulation with intravenous heparin to prevent the extension of thrombus. Following catheter-directed venography to verify the diagnosis, catheter-based mechanical thrombectomy combined with localized infusion of a small amount of

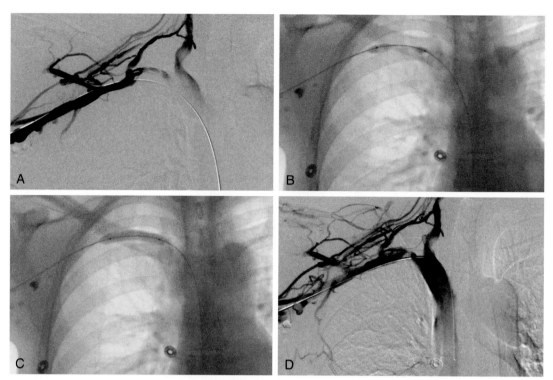

FIGURE 23.5 • **Venography and initial management of effort thrombosis.** Initial interventional management of a young woman with right-sided SCV effort thrombosis. A, Initial venogram confirming axillary-subclavian vein occlusion, with venous obstruction extending to the lateral chest wall and numerous enlarged collateral veins. B, Resolution of thrombus with catheter-directed thrombolytic therapy, clearing much of the axillary vein and SCV, with residual narrowing observed in the central SCV. C, Inflation of an angioplasty balloon across the area of residual SCV stenosis at the level of the first rib. D, Completion venogram demonstrating improved patency of the SCV. (Reprinted from Vemuri C, Salehi P, Benarroch-Gampel J, McLaughlin LN, Thompson RW. Diagnosis and treatment of effort-induced thrombosis of the axillary subclavian vein due to venous thoracic outlet syndrome. *J Vasc Surg Venous Lymphat Disord.* 2016;4(4):485-500. Copyright © 2016 Elsevier. With permission.)

a thrombolytic agent is used to clear any fresh or recent clot from the axillary-subclavian and collateral veins (Figure 23.5).[27] This usually results in an improvement in the venographic appearance and reveals focal high-grade stenosis or occlusion of the proximal subclavian vein at the level of the first rib. Residual subclavian vein stenosis may be treated by balloon angioplasty, but this is usually unsuccessful and does not represent definitive long-term treatment. It is also well established that placement of stents in the subclavian vein should be strongly avoided, owing to a predictably high rate of failure in the absence of venous decompression.[28]

Following thrombolysis, most patients experience a prompt reduction in symptoms of venous obstruction and should remain on systemic anticoagulation. Conservative treatment with long-term anticoagulation alone has been debated in the past, but this approach is associated with a substantial incidence of recurrent thrombosis, persistent symptoms, and residual limitations in arm activity. The proper

duration of anticoagulation for effort thrombosis is also unknown, given that venous TOS is caused by factors distinct from those underlying other forms of deep vein thrombosis, and lifelong anticoagulation with restrictions on use of the arm is recommended in the absence of surgical decompression. Such limitations are obviously unacceptable for young healthy athletes (and most patients with venous TOS), making surgical treatment the best recommendation. Thus, for almost all patients with venous TOS, prompt referral for definitive surgical management is recommended at the time of initial diagnosis or upon completion of thrombolytic therapy.

Surgical Management

Surgical protocols for the treatment of venous TOS are intended to decompress the axillary-subclavian vein and collateral venous pathways throughout the costoclavicular space and to restore and maintain normal blood flow through the subclavian vein.[24]

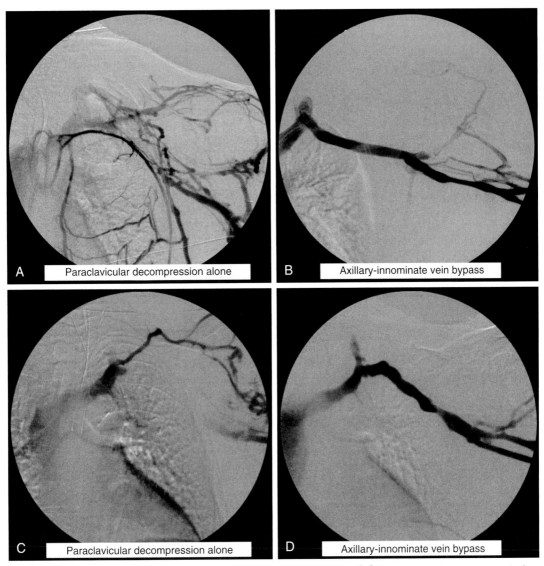

FIGURE 23.6 • Subclavian vein bypass graft reconstruction. Intraoperative left upper extremity venograms in 2 different patients depicting residual obstruction of the SCV immediately after paraclavicular decompression and external venolysis (A and C) and widely patent SCV bypass graft reconstructions with cryopreserved femoral vein conduits (B and D). (Reprinted from Vemuri C, Salehi P, Benarroch-Gampel J, McLaughlin LN, Thompson RW. Diagnosis and treatment of effort-induced thrombosis of the axillary subclavian vein due to venous thoracic outlet syndrome. *J Vasc Surg Venous Lymphat Disord.* 2016;4(4):485-500. Copyright © 2016 Elsevier. With permission.)

In all approaches, thoracic outlet decompression is accomplished by first rib resection along with division or removal of the anterior scalene and subclavius muscles, whether performed by transaxillary, supraclavicular, or infraclavicular (subclavicular) approaches, or combinations of these incisions. The transaxillary protocol typically involves partial resection of the first rib and simple division of its scalene muscle attachments. Because the subclavian vein cannot be completely exposed or controlled from this approach, these operations are usually coupled with a plan for intraoperative or postoperative venography and balloon angioplasty and/or stent placement to deal with any residual stenosis in the subclavian vein. In contrast, the infraclavicular and paraclavicular protocols permit complete first rib resection and more thorough resection of the anterior scalene and subclavius muscles, as well as direct subclavian vein reconstruction when necessary, during a single operative procedure (Figure 23.6).[25] Following surgical therapy by any of these protocols, interval anticoagulation and a comprehensive physical therapy and rehabilitation program are important in achieving a return to full function.

Outcomes

We have previously reviewed our results with operative treatment for venous TOS using the paraclavicular approach, in a series of 32 high-performance athletes with a median age of 20.3 years.[25] In this group, the mean interval between symptoms and definitive venographic diagnosis was 20.2 ± 5.6 days (range 1-120), and catheter-directed subclavian vein thrombolysis was performed in 26 (81%) with balloon angioplasty in 12. No patient in our experience required division of the clavicle, disruption of the sternoclavicular joint, or partial sternotomy. Patency of the axillary subclavian vein was restored by circumferential external venolysis alone in 56% or by direct axillary-subclavian vein reconstruction in 44%. All 32 athletes in this experience resumed unrestricted use of the upper extremity and returned to participate in sports, with a median interval of 3.5 months between operation and the return to competitive athletics (range 2-10 months). The overall duration of management (from symptoms to full athletic activity) was significantly correlated with the time interval from venographic diagnosis to operation and was longer in patients with persistent symptoms or rethrombosis before referral.

In a recent review, we also compared the published outcomes of treatment with 3 different surgical protocols for venous TOS.[26] In this study, protocols based on the transaxillary and infraclavicular approaches to surgical treatment resulted in successful outcomes in approximately 75% of patients, whereas 95% of patients had a successful outcome after treatment based on paraclavicular decompression. We have thereby concluded that successful outcomes for the management of venous TOS can be achieved using an aggressive multidisciplinary approach based on (1) early diagnostic venography, thrombolysis, and tertiary referral; (2) paraclavicular thoracic outlet decompression with external venolysis and frequent use of subclavian vein reconstruction; and (3) temporary postoperative anticoagulation. Optimal management of venous TOS is also dependent on early recognition by treating physicians, prompt referral for comprehensive surgical management, and well-integrated postoperative care in conjunction with a physical therapy team that has expertise in the management of all forms of TOS.

ARTERIAL THORACIC OUTLET SYNDROME

Arterial TOS is the least frequent form of TOS, representing only 1% to 3% of patients in most clinical series.[1,2] This condition is characterized by pathologic changes in the subclavian artery resulting in either thrombosis or aneurysm formation, in associated with a bony abnormality, such as a cervical rib.[29] Although positional compression of the subclavian artery is frequent on physical examination, vascular laboratory testing, or vascular imaging studies, this finding does not represent a source of clinical symptoms and is not considered to reflect arterial TOS. Indeed, positional compression of the subclavian artery is frequently misunderstood when encountered in a patient with upper extremity symptoms, which are usually attributable to neurogenic TOS.

Clinical Recognition

One of the most common presenting findings in patients with arterial TOS is unilateral digital ischemia, with symptoms including numbness, tingling, cold and painful sensations, cyanotic or pale discoloration, and delayed capillary refill in the fingers.[30] The brachial, radial, and/or ulnar pulses may be absent or decreased in the presence of a proximal arterial occlusion, with diminished blood pressure. Digital ischemia may also exist with normal radial and ulnar pulses if the site of obstruction is solely within the hand, which can occur with digital artery embolism from a more proximal site or with digital artery thrombosis secondary to local trauma. Digital ischemia usually coexists with and is exacerbated by local vasospasm, and in some circumstances, primary vasospasm can also result in digital ischemia in the absence of arterial thrombosis or embolism.

The presence of digital ischemia requires differentiation between proximal and distal arterial sources of thromboembolism, localized digital artery occlusion, and primary vasospasm (Table 23.3).[30] In most cases of upper extremity embolism, a proximal artery source must be considered, which is best evaluated by contrast-enhanced arteriography, with positional views of the neck and upper arm and high-resolution views of the hand. This may be accomplished with computed tomography or magnetic resonance imaging, but catheter-based (transfemoral) arteriography remains the most accurate and definitive approach.

Subclavian Artery Aneurysms

Subclavian artery aneurysms form as a result of sustained compression of the subclavian artery at the level of the first rib, almost always in association with a congenital cervical rib or anomalous first rib.[30] This type of aneurysm is caused by poststenotic dilatation with arterial wall degeneration, leading to ulceration, mural thrombus, and distal embolization. Anticoagulation

TABLE 23.3 Differential Diagnosis of Digital Ischemia

Thromboembolism from a cardiac source
Arrhythmia, valvular disease, septal defect (paradoxical)
Thromboembolism from a proximal arterial source
Aorta: endothelial erosion, ulceration, or penetrating ulcer
Subclavian or axillary arteries: aneurysm, occlusion, stenosis, or ulceration
Thromboembolism from a distal arterial source
Brachial, radial, or ulnar arteries: local trauma
Palmar arteries: hypothenar hammer syndrome
Systemic diseases associated with vasculitis
Scleroderma, rheumatoid arthritis, polyarteritis nodosa, Takayasu disease, Buerger disease
Local vascular diseases
Hemangioma, arteriovenous malformation, glomus tumor, synovitis
Primary digital artery thrombosis
Local repetitive trauma
Primary vasospasm
Raynaud disease, cold exposure, tobacco use, cocaine

and antiplatelet therapy should be started to limit the extent of arterial thrombosis, and contrast-enhanced arteriography is required to image the extent, location, and character of arterial occlusions and to detect the presence of subclavian artery compression and aneurysm formation (Figure 23.7). Although intra-arterial thrombolytic therapy may have a role in helping to resolve distal thromboembolism, this approach is better used in conjunction with or after definitive operative treatment.

Surgical treatment for subclavian artery aneurysms consists of supraclavicular thoracic outlet decompression with scalenectomy and removal of the cervical and first ribs, followed by excision of the aneurysmal segment of subclavian artery. In some cases, a second infraclavicular incision is needed to obtain distal arterial control at the level of the axillary artery. Interposition bypass graft reconstruction is then used to restore flow through the subclavian artery. After reconstruction of the subclavian artery, intraoperative contrast arteriography is performed to define the extent and distribution of any distal emboli, and thromboembolectomy is performed as necessary to clear the involved distal vessels to the extent feasible. When there is extensive digital artery embolism beyond the capabilities of surgical thrombectomy, adjunctive intra-arterial infusion of vasodilator and thrombolytic agents may help achieve optimal outcomes.

Outcomes

We recently reviewed our experience with patients undergoing primary or reoperative treatment for arterial TOS over an 8-year period.[29] This large single-institution series involved 40 patients with a mean age of 40.3 ± 2.2 years (range, 13-68 years), with over half presenting with upper extremity ischemia/emboli (n = 21) or posterior stroke (n = 2), including 8 who had required urgent brachial artery thromboembolectomy. There were also 17 (42%) patients with a nonvascular presentation, with 11 having neurogenic TOS and 6 having an asymptomatic neck mass or incidentally discovered subclavian artery dilatation. All 40 patients underwent thoracic outlet decompression, of which 75% had a cervical rib (24 complete, 6 partial), 5 had a first rib abnormality, and 4 had a clavicle fracture. Subclavian artery reconstruction was performed in 70%, but 30% had only mild arterial dilatation (<100%) that required no arterial reconstruction. Subclavian artery patency was 92% during mean follow-up of 4.5 ± 0.4 years; no patients had further dilatation or embolism, and chronic symptoms were present in 6 (4 postischemic/vasospasm and 2 neurogenic). Based on this review, we concluded that early thoracic outlet decompression and surgical treatment of subclavian artery aneurysms, with restoration of direct arterial flow to the hand and digits, can lead to excellent results and a full return to function over a period of several months. Unfortunately, owing to the insidious clinical presentation of subclavian aneurysms and delays in surgical treatment, many patients with this condition exhibit residual symptoms secondary to hand or digital thromboembolism that cannot be easily resolved.

LESIONS OF THE AXILLARY ARTERY AND ITS BRANCHES

There is a unique group of lesions that appear to occur almost exclusively in baseball pitchers and volleyball players, involving the third portion of the axillary artery

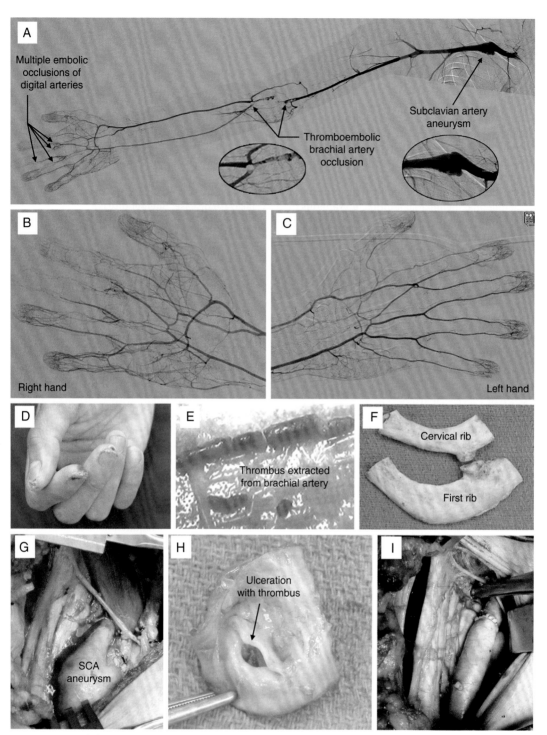

FIGURE 23.7 • **Subclavian artery (SCA) aneurysm causing digital ischemia.** Photographs depicting a 28-year-old right-handed man who presented with right hand ischemia. A, A right upper extremity arteriogram demonstrated a subclavian artery aneurysm, thromboembolic occlusion of the distal brachial artery, and multiple embolic digital artery occlusions. Magnified arteriographic views of the affected right hand (B) and normal left hand (C) illustrate the differences in perfusion. D, Ischemic fingertip lesions in the right hand. E, Brachial artery thromboembolectomy and patch angioplasty repair was initially performed. F, Operative specimens of the cervical and first ribs, removed during supraclavicular thoracic outlet decompression several days after thrombectomy. G, Subclavian artery aneurysm viewed from right supraclavicular exposure. H, The excised specimen of the subclavian artery aneurysm demonstrated intimal ulceration with thrombus. I, Subclavian artery repair with interposition bypass graft. (Reprinted by permission from Springer Thompson RW. Management of digital emboli, vasospasm, and ischemia in ATOS. In: Illig KA, Thompson RW, Freischlag JA, Donahue DM, Jordan SE, Edgelow PI, eds. *Thoracic Outlet Syndrome*. 1st ed. London: Springer; 2013:557-563.)

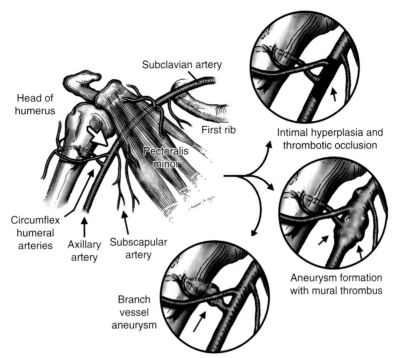

FIGURE 23.8 • **Pathogenesis of compressive axillary artery lesions.** Compression of the third portion of the axillary artery by anterior displacement of the humeral head during the overhead throwing motion, with the white arrow indicating the direction of force acting upon the artery. The axillary artery is relatively fixed in position at this site by the overlying fascia, branch vessel origins, and the pectoralis minor muscle. Repetitive compression can lead to intimal hyperplasia with stenosis, or aneurysm formation, with or without thrombotic occlusion. Similar lesions may also arise in the adjacent axillary artery branches (subscapular and circumflex humeral arteries). (Reprinted from Duwayri YM, Emery VB, Driskill MR, et al. Positional compression of the axillary artery causing upper extremity thrombosis and embolism in the elite overhead throwing athlete. *J Vasc Surg.* 2011;53(5):1329-1340. Copyright © 2011 Society for Vascular Surgery. With permission.)

and its branches (subscapular and circumflex humeral arteries).[31,32] In combination with anatomic fixation of the axillary artery underneath the pectoralis minor muscle and by the fascia at the location of the subscapular and circumflex humeral branch vessel origins, these lesions are caused by arterial compression and stretching by the head of the humerus as it moves forward during extremes of arm elevation and extension, as seen in the overhead pitching motion.[31] The response to repetitive axillary artery injury at this location can cause intimal hyperplasia and arterial stenosis, with subsequent thrombotic occlusion (Figure 23.8), or disruption and aneurysmal degeneration, with the formation of mural thrombus and distal thromboembolism. Axillary artery compression may also cause arterial dissection, which may extend proximally or distally to occlude additional segments of the circulation. Lastly, repetitive arterial injury affecting the first several centimeters of the branch vessels at this location, likely owing to stretch of the branch vessel origin from the axillary artery wall, typically leads to branch vessel aneurysm formation with thrombosis and distal embolism.

Clinical Recognition

Exertional arm fatigue, digital cutaneous microemboli, and/or acute hand/digital ischemia are the presenting symptoms typically caused by lesions of the axillary artery and its branches. Like subclavian artery aneurysms, initial treatment includes anticoagulation and diagnostic vascular laboratory tests to evaluate arterial flow to the arm, with imaging studies being required to visualize the site, extent, and character of the arterial lesion. This may be accomplished with either CT or MR angiography, but direct catheter-based arteriography is preferred.[4] If the artery is not completely occluded during arteriography at rest, elevation of the arm should be used to mimic the pitching motion, to determine if positional obstruction occurs at this location.

Treatment

Medical management with thrombolysis, anticoagulation, and/or antiplatelet therapy cannot assure against the recurrence of distal emboli from mural thrombus, and thrombolysis with balloon angioplasty and/

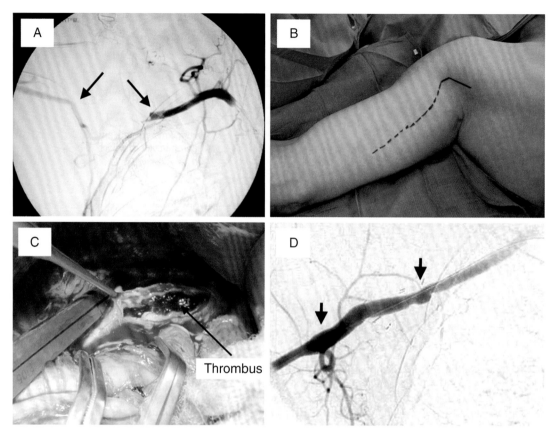

FIGURE 23.9 • **Axillary artery thrombosis.** Initial arteriogram demonstrating occlusion of the right axillary artery in a 29-year-old baseball pitcher, with the black arrows indicating the length of the occluded arterial segment (A). Surgical exploration through an upper arm incision (B), revealing acute thrombosis of the distal axillary artery (C), superimposed on an area of intimal thickening caused by focal intimal hyperplasia. The excised arterial segment was replaced by an interposition vein graft, illustrated on a completion arteriogram, with the black arrows indicating the length of the bypass graft (D). (Reprinted from Duwayri YM, Emery VB, Driskill MR, et al. Positional compression of the axillary artery causing upper extremity thrombosis and embolism in the elite overhead throwing athlete. *J Vasc Surg.* 2011;53(5):1329-1340. Copyright © 2011 Society for Vascular Surgery. With permission.)

or stent placement is unsatisfactory, as this does not correct the underlying cause and may introduce the potential for additional complications. Thus, surgical treatment is recommended for all lesions of the axillary artery and its branches.[31]

The preferred operative approach initially involves exposure through an upper medial arm incision and complete mobilization of the affected portion of the axillary artery to prevent future compression.[31] For lesions affecting the main axillary artery, the affected segment is usually excised and reconstructed with an interposition bypass, typically using a short reversed saphenous vein graft (Figure 23.9). It is preferable to include or reimplant at least one of the axillary artery branch vessels during construction of the distal anastomosis of the bypass graft (usually the posterior circumflex humeral artery), to maintain optimal perfusion to the humeral head and shoulder girdle musculature.

For aneurysms confined to the axillary artery branch vessels, ligation and excision of the affected branch is sufficient. Intraoperative completion arteriography should be performed to assess the distal circulation in the upper extremity, and localized thrombectomy may be needed in the brachial, radial, or ulnar arteries to reestablish direct arterial flow to the palmar arch of the hand. When there has been thrombosis within the palmar arch or digital arteries, intraoperative administration of thrombolytic agents and vasodilators may be valuable adjuncts.

Outcomes

Recovery from surgical treatment is typically complete within 6 to 12 weeks of operation, and a full return to previous levels of function can usually be expected. Nonetheless, it is recognized that in some patients a full functional recovery may remain limited by persistent digital ischemia owing to the existence of preexisting chronic thromboembolism, similar to that occasionally observed in patients with subclavian artery aneurysms.

We have recently reviewed our outcomes of surgical treatment in a series of 9 high-performance overhead athletes with axillary artery pathology, of whom 7 were elite baseball pitchers, with a mean age of 30.9 ± 2.9 years.[31] At angiography and surgical exploration at a mean of 2.5 ± 0.8 weeks after the onset of symptoms (range 1-8 weeks), 6 had occlusion of the distal axillary artery opposite the humeral head either at rest (3) or with arm elevation (3), 1 had axillary artery dissection with positional occlusion, and 2 had thrombosis of circumflex humeral artery aneurysms. Treatment included segmental axillary artery repair with saphenous vein (n = 7; 5 interposition bypass grafts and 2 patch angioplasties), ligation/excision of circumflex humeral artery aneurysms (n = 2), and distal artery thrombectomy/thrombolysis (n = 2). The mean postoperative hospital stay was 3.8 ± 0.5 days, and the time until resumption of unrestricted overhead throwing was 10.8 ± 2.7 weeks. At a median follow-up of 15 months, primary-assisted patency was 89% and secondary patency was 100%, and all 9 patients had continued careers in professional baseball. This led us to conclude that repetitive positional compression of the axillary artery can cause a spectrum of pathology in the overhead athlete, that prompt recognition of these rare lesions is crucial given their propensity toward thrombosis and distal embolism, and that full functional recovery can usually be anticipated within several months of surgical treatment.

MANAGER'S TIPS

- Neurogenic TOS is characterized by upper extremity pain, numbness, tingling, and fatigue and can be recognized with the help of recently published clinical diagnostic criteria and imaging-guided scalene muscle anesthetic blocks

- Surgical treatment for neurogenic TOS can provide effective treatment for professional baseball pitchers with this career-threatening condition, often to previous levels of athletic performance, at a median of 10 months after operation when coupled with an ample period of postoperative rehabilitation

- Subclavian vein "effort" thrombosis due to venous TOS is optimally treated by anticoagulation and catheter-directed thrombolysis, followed within several weeks by thoracic outlet decompression

- Athletes undergoing surgical treatment for venous TOS can usually expect a return to full activity within 3 to 4 months after operation, with an excellent prognosis for a return to sport

- Baseball players with arterial disease of the upper extremity often present with unilateral digital ischemia from emboli or vasospasm and may exhibit diminished upper extremity blood flow with arm elevation identified by contrast-enhanced imaging studies

- Arterial TOS is characterized by subclavian artery pathology (aneurysms or occlusive lesions) in association with a bony abnormality, such as a cervical rib

- Positional axillary artery compression associated with the baseball pitching motion can result in localized lesions that can cause thromboembolism and digital ischemia

- Prompt recognition and surgical treatment is required for all upper extremity arterial lesions, due to either arterial TOS or axillary artery compression, to optimize the potential for successful outcomes and a return to sport

ACKNOWLEDGMENTS

This work was supported by the Thoracic Outlet Syndrome Research and Education Fund of the Foundation for Barnes-Jewish Hospital, St. Louis, Missouri. We thank the referring physicians, team physicians, and athletic trainers who have allowed us to participate in the care of their patients.

REFERENCES

1. Thompson RW, Driskill MR. Neurovascular problems in the athlete's shoulder. *Clin Sports Med.* 2008;27:789-802 [PMID:19064156].
2. Illig KA, Thompson RW, Freischlag JA, Donahue DM, Jordan SE, Edgelow PI. *Thoracic Outlet Syndrome (TOS).* 1st ed. London: Springer-Verlag; 2013.
3. Thompson RW, Bartoli MA. Neurogenic thoracic outlet syndrome. In: Rutherford RB, ed. *Vascular Surgery.* 6th ed. Philadelphia: Elsevier Saunders; 2005:1347-1365.
4. Raptis CA, Sridhar S, Thompson RW, Fowler K, Bhalla S. Imaging of the patient with thoracic outlet syndrome. *Radiographics.* 2016;36(4):984-1000 [PMID:27257767].
5. Illig KA, Donahue D, Duncan A, et al. Reporting standards of the Society for Vascular Surgery for thoracic outlet syndrome: executive summary. *J Vasc Surg.* 2016;64(3):797-802 [PMID:27565596].
6. Balderman J, Holzem K, Field BJ, et al. Associations between clinical diagnostic criteria and pretreatment patient-reported outcomes measures in a prospective observational cohort of patients with neurogenic thoracic outlet syndrome. *J Vasc Surg.* 2017;66(2):533-544 [PMID:28735950].

7. Bottros MM, AuBuchon JD, McLaughlin LN, Altchek DW, Illig KA, Thompson RW. Exercise-enhanced, ultrasound-guided, local anesthetic anterior scalene/pectoralis minor muscle blocks can facilitate diagnosis of neurogenic thoracic outlet syndrome in the high-performance overhead athlete. *Am J Sports Med.* 2017;45(1):189-194 [PMID:27664077].

8. Totten PA, Hunter JM. Therapeutic techniques to enhance nerve gliding in thoracic outlet syndrome and carpal tunnel syndrome. *Hand Clin.* 1991;7(3):505-520 [PMID:1939356].

9. Aligne C, Barral X. Rehabilitation of patients with thoracic outlet syndrome. *Ann Vasc Surg.* 1992;6(4):381-389 [PMID:1390029].

10. Walsh MT. Therapist management of thoracic outlet syndrome. *J Hand Ther.* 1994;7(2):131-144 [PMID:8038876].

11. Wehbe MA, Schlegel JM. Nerve gliding exercises for thoracic outlet syndrome. *Hand Clin.* 2004;20(1):51-55 [PMID:15005384].

12. Watson LA, Pizzari T, Balster S. Thoracic outlet syndrome part 2: conservative management of thoracic outlet. *Man Ther.* 2010;15(4):305-314 [PMID:20382063].

13. Finlayson HC, O'Connor RJ, Brasher PM, Travlos A. Botulinum toxin injection for management of thoracic outlet syndrome: a double-blind, randomized, controlled trial. *Pain.* 2011;152(9):2023-2028 [PMID:21628084].

14. Caputo FJ, Wittenberg AM, Vemuri C, et al. Supraclavicular decompression for neurogenic thoracic outlet syndrome in adolescent and adult populations. *J Vasc Surg.* 2013;57(1):149-157 [PMID:23127984].

15. Peek J, Vos CG, Unlu C, van de Pavoordt HDWM, van den Akker PJ, de Vries JPM. Outcome of surgical treatment for thoracic outlet syndrome: systematic review and meta-analysis. *Ann Vasc Surg.* 2017;40:303-326 [PMID:27666803].

16. Rinehardt EK, Scarborough JE, Bennett KM. Current practice of thoracic outlet decompression surgery in the United States. *J Vasc Surg.* 2017;66(3):858-865 [PMID:28579292].

17. Sanders RJ, Annest SJ. Thoracic outlet and pectoralis minor syndromes. *Semin Vasc Surg.* 2014;27(2):86-117 [PMID:25868762].

18. Altobelli GG, Kudo T, Haas BT, et al. Thoracic outlet syndrome: pattern of clinical success after operative decompression. *J Vasc Surg.* 2005;42(1):122-128 [PMID:16012461].

19. Thompson RW, Vemuri C. Neurogenic thoracic outlet syndrome exposure and decompression: supraclavicular (chapter). In: Mulholland MW, Hawn MT, Hughes SJ, Albo D, Sabel MS, Dalman RL, eds. *Operative Techniques in Surgery.* Philadelphia: Wolters Kluwer Health; 2015:1848-1861.

20. Hwang J, Min BJ, Jo WM, Shin JS. Video-assisted thoracoscopic surgery for intrathoracic first rib resection in thoracic outlet syndrome. *J Thorac Dis.* 2017;9(7):2022-2028 [PMID:28840002].

21. Zajac JM, Angeline ME, Bohon TM, et al. Axillary artery thrombosis in a major league baseball pitcher: a case report and rehabilitation guide. *Sports Health.* 2013;5(5):402-406 [PMID:24427409].

22. Thompson RW, Dawkins C, Vemuri C, et al. Performance metrics in professional baseball pitchers before and after surgical treatment for neurogenic thoracic outlet syndrome. *Ann Vasc Surg.* 2017;39(1):216-227 [PMID:27522980].

23. Shutze W, Richardson B, Shutze R, et al. Midterm and long-term follow-up in competitive athletes undergoing thoracic outlet decompression for neurogenic thoracic outlet syndrome. *J Vasc Surg.* 2017;66(6):1798-1805 [PMID:28943009].

24. Illig KA, Doyle AJ. A comprehensive review of Paget-Schroetter syndrome. *J Vasc Surg.* 2010;51(6):1538-1547 [PMID:20304578].

25. Melby SJ, Vedantham S, Narra VR, et al. Comprehensive surgical management of the competitive athlete with effort thrombosis of the subclavian vein (Paget-Schroetter syndrome). *J Vasc Surg.* 2008;47(4):809-820 [PMID:18280096].

26. Vemuri C, Salehi P, Benarroch-Gampel J, McLaughlin LN, Thompson RW. Diagnosis and treatment of effort-induced thrombosis of the axillary subclavian vein due to venous thoracic outlet syndrome. *J Vasc Surg Venous Lymphat Disord.* 2016;4(4):485-500 [PMID:27639006].

27. Schneider DB, Curry TK, Eichler CM, et al. Percutaneous mechanical thrombectomy for the management of venous thoracic outlet syndrome. *J Endovasc Ther.* 2003;10(2):336-340 [PMID:12877619].

28. Urschel Jr HC, Patel AN. Paget-Schroetter syndrome therapy: failure of intravenous stents. *Ann Thorac Surg.* 2003;75(6):1693-1696 [PMID:12822601].

29. Vemuri C, McLaughlin LN, Abuirqeba AA, Thompson RW. Clinical presentation and management of arterial thoracic outlet syndrome. *J Vasc Surg.* 2017;65(5):1429-1439 [PMID:28189360].

30. Thompson RW. Management of digital emboli, vasospasm, and ischemia in arterial thoracic outlet syndrome (chapter). In: Illig KA, Thompson RW, Freischlag JA, Donahue DM, Jordan SE, Edgelow PI, eds. *Thoracic Outlet Syndrome (TOS).* 1st ed. London: Springer-Verlag; 2013:557-563.

31. Duwayri YM, Emery VB, Driskill MR, et al. Positional compression of the axillary artery causing upper extremity thrombosis and embolism in the elite overhead throwing athlete. *J Vasc Surg.* 2011;53(5):1329-1340 [PMID:21276687].

32. van de Pol D, Kuijer PPFM, Langenhorst T, Maas M. High prevalence of self-reported symptoms of digital ischemia in elite male volleyball players in The Netherlands: a cross-sectional national survey. *Am J Sports Med.* 2012;40(10):2296-2302 [PMID:22926747].

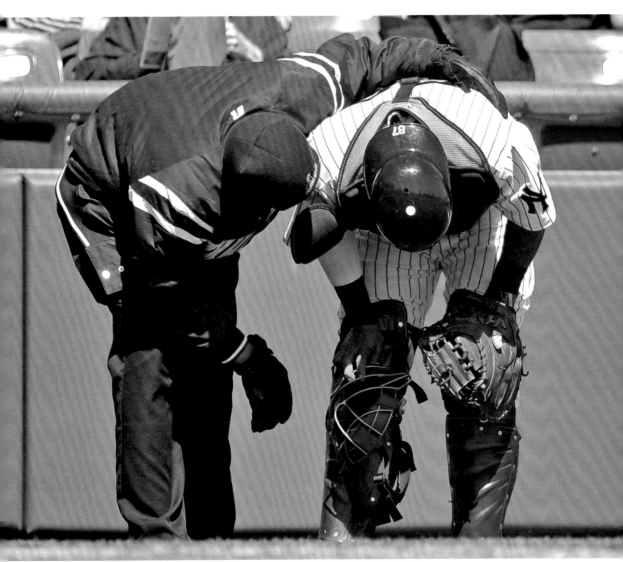

Aspen Photo / Shutterstock.com

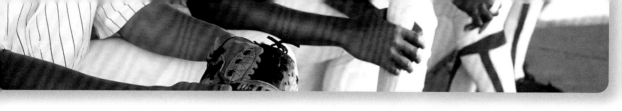

CHAPTER 24

Hip Injuries in Baseball Players

T. Sean Lynch, MD

During my 18 years I came to bat almost 10,000 times. I struck out about 1,700 times and walked maybe 1,800 times. You figure a ballplayer will average about 500 at bats a season. That means I played seven years without ever hitting the ball.

—*Mickey Mantle*

INTRODUCTION

The hip is a model of joint stability because it anchors the pelvis and lower appendicular skeleton. This anchoring is accomplished through the sacroiliac and femoroacetabular joints in combination with a complex arrangement of numerous muscles, tendons, and ligaments that cross these joints. Hip motion is controlled by not only the powerful thigh muscles but also the body's core (including the low lumbar musculature), with additional support from the adductors and gluteal muscles. The joint architecture allows the hip to withstand forces 6 to 8 times an individual's bodyweight during sporting activities. Significant force is necessary to injure the hip and its surrounding muscles. Baseball players, however, repetitively stress their hips and often have abnormal hip anatomy that makes the hip more vulnerable to injury.

Historically, athletic hip injuries were most commonly diagnosed as groin or hip flexor pulls. In some instances, this diagnosis would prematurely end an athlete's playing career. Over the last 10 to 15 years, specific diagnoses of hip injury have been refined through improved understanding of hip biomechanics, better physical examination skills, and imaging modalities.[1,2] Injury-specific treatment can now predictably return athletes to play. This chapter addresses the sports hip triad.[3] This injury pattern consists of intra-articular hip injuries, including femoroacetabular impingement (FAI) and labral injuries, with associated abnormalities to the adductor and rectus abdominis muscles, which share a common sheath and attachment, the pubic symphysis. The presence of motion-limiting FAI with a concomitant intra-articular injury can cause mechanical transfer of force to the pubis as well as the adductor and rectus abdominis muscles, which can lead to athletic pubalgia (refer to chapter 25) and osteitis pubis (Figure 24.1).

Recently, evidence and experience has created a good algorithm to approach this spectrum of injuries in high-level athletes. It is the goal of this chapter to familiarize the reader on these conditions while providing management pearls for the baseball player.

HIP INJURIES IN BASEBALL

Hip and groin injuries in baseball have a 5% to 6% incidence.[4,5] Although these are less than the more commonly discussed shoulder and elbow injuries, these athletic hip conditions can lead to long periods of disability, have a high rates of recurrence, and may even predispose to other injuries down the kinetic chain such as elbow injuries.[5-7] Hip injuries have been shown to cause an average of 23 days missed per athlete, which was similar to the more commonly highlighted elbow and knee injuries in the same study (23 and 27 days, respectively).[6]

Major League Baseball's (MLB's) Health and Injury Tracking System (HITS) database was recently used to analyze hip and groin injuries from 2011 to 2014.[4] Infield players sustained more hip injuries than outfielders, batters, or baserunners. The most frequent mechanism of injury was noncontact injuries during defensive fielding (74%), and infielders experienced the most hip and groin injuries (34%). This validates

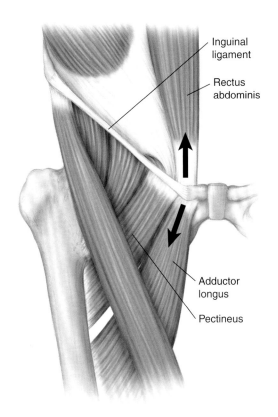

FIGURE 24.1 • Injury to the abdominal wall at the fascial attachments of the rectus and adductors onto the pubis is implicated in athletic pubalgia.

- Inguinal ligament
- Rectus abdominis
- Adductor longus
- Pectineus

the finding that muscle strains and contusions made up the majority of injuries in this series. Meanwhile, the pitcher's mound was the most common location for injuries, and these players had the longest time out from play.

Extra-articular hip injuries were most common, making up 95.4% of total injuries with almost all able to be treated nonoperatively. Many of these extra-articular injuries (79.1%) were strains or contusions of the adductor, iliopsoas, or gluteal muscles with a mean of 12.4 days missed. In contrast, in case of intra-articular injuries, 40.5% were treated surgically, and these players missed an average of 122.5 days; whereas players whose intra-articular injuries were treated nonsurgically missed a mean of 22.5 days.

ATHLETIC HIP INJURIES

Groin or pelvis pain in athletes can be challenging to diagnose because pain can be referred to or from several different anatomic locations, including the lower back/lumbar spine, abdominal and pelvic viscera,

genitourinary structures, and hip and knee joints. Hip and groin injuries in baseball players can be divided into 4 broad categories: adductor strains, osteitis pubis, athletic pubalgia (refer to chapter 25), and intra-articular hip pathology, such as FAI.

ADDUCTOR STRAINS

The adductor muscle complex includes the adductor longus, adductor magnus, and adductor brevis muscles, as well as the gracilis, obturator externus, and pectineus muscles. In MLB, adductor strains are the most common extra-articular groin injury accounting for 40.8% of all these injuries according to a recent review of all Minor League Baseball (MiLB) and MLB players.[4] In comparison, adductor strains in professional soccer players with these injuries represent 23% of all muscle injuries, resulting in a mean 2 weeks of lost playing time with a reinjury rate of 18%.[8] In athletes with reinjuries, return to play took considerably longer than the recovery time from their original injury. This stresses the importance of rehabilitation that emphasizes the correction of any predisposing factors that might put the athlete at risk for injury, including muscle tightness, weakness, or imbalances across the pelvis.[9]

These muscles are frequently susceptible to injuries during sporting activity from large mechanical loads placed onto the small tendon of the adductor longus during muscle contraction.[10] These injuries occur during eccentric contraction at the myotendinous unit or fibrocartilaginous insertion of the adductor tendon on the pubic bone, known as the adductor enthesis. Athletes report aching groin or medial thigh pain that is exacerbated with resisted adduction and passive stretching of the adductors. Athletes with an injury at the adductor enthesis have pain on palpation at or near the origin on the pubic bone (Figure 24.2). Myotendinous injuries present with pain that is further distal. Reduced adductor muscle strength, measured with the athlete lying on the side with the hip in neutral rotation, and the loss of hip range of motion (ROM) have been associated with an increased risk of subsequent strain injury.[9]

Management

Management of athletic hip injuries typically begins with nonsurgical care, consisting of cessation or modification of the offending sport, anti-inflammatory medications, and physical therapy. Rehabilitation should emphasize core strengthening and stabilization and postural retraining with normalization of the dynamic relationship between the hip and pelvic muscles. Local injections can be helpful in some cases to allow

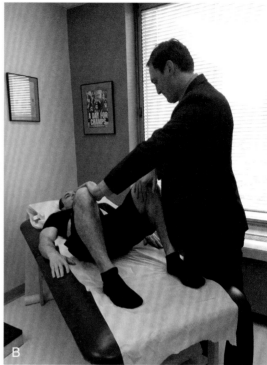

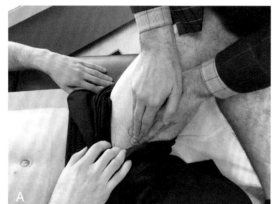

FIGURE 24.2 • A and B, Clinical photographs showing the evaluation of the athlete with adductor tendon/muscle injury. A, Tenderness is elicited at the origin of the adductors by palpation with resisted contraction. B, Pain with resisted hip adduction at 0°, 45°, and 90° of hip flexion, with the patient's feet on the table, can reproduce adductor pain and/or weakness.

continued participation of in-season athletes. Aggressive stretching to improve ROM should be avoided to prevent aggravation of hip pain in athletes with underlying FAI. Other exercises that should be avoided include deep hip flexion and low repetition and heavyweight strength training. After the athlete is pain free, a gradual return to play can be initiated (Figure 24.3).

In addition to first-line treatment strategies, adjuncts to the nonsurgical care of adductor injuries can include entheseal pubic cleft injections after a period of rest, anti-inflammatory medications, and physical therapy. For athletes with adductor tendinitis or tendinopathy, the injection is directed into the adductor enthesis (Figure 24.4).[11,12] In elite athletes, a study found that individuals with chronic adductor-related groin pain and normal magnetic resonance imaging (MRI) findings had no recurrence of pain at 1 year. However, athletes with evidence of enthesopathy on MRI did have recurrence of symptoms at a mean of 5 weeks after injection. This finding suggests that athletes with a chronic adductor injury but no evidence of enthesopathy on MRI have early, mild disease that could resolve with nonsurgical management, including corticosteroid injection. More advanced adductor disease seen on MRI appears to have poorer results after corticosteroid injection.

Other injection options include platelet-rich plasma (PRP), which has gained popularity within the last decade among the orthopedic community as a treatment modality to enhance tissue healing. The term "platelet-rich plasma" may be applied to any fraction of autologous blood that contains a higher concentration of platelets than baseline. In a retrospective case series, patients with adductor longus tendinopathy demonstrated significantly improved Western Ontario and Mc-Master Universities Osteoarthritis Index (WOMAC) scores at 6 weeks and a mean of 20.2 months after injection.[13] Ultrasound was also used to assess lesion size at baseline and 6 weeks postinjection, with adductor longus tendon lesion size decreasing from an average of 21.2 to 2.6 mm during this time.

Most adductor injuries are low-grade strains or partial tears that generally are amenable to nonsurgical care. In athletes who have sustained complete ruptures of the proximal adductor longus, surgical reattachment has allowed a return to play but with the added cost of extended time out for healing and recovery.[14,15] Schlegel et al demonstrated in National Football League players that nonsurgical management of complete ruptures resulted in a return to sport in half the time (an average of 6 weeks) of that of surgical reattachment

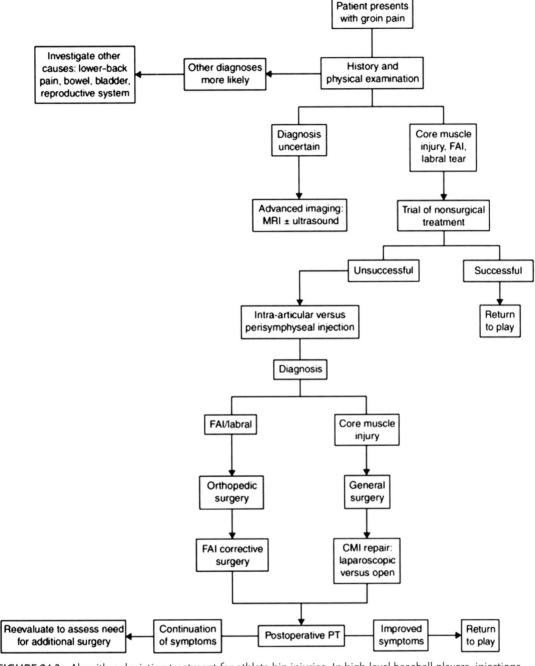

FIGURE 24.3 • Algorithm depicting treatment for athlete hip injuries. In high-level baseball players, injections can be done in conjunction with the initiation of nonsurgical management. FAI, femoroacetabular impingement, CMI, core muscle injury, PT, physical therapy.

(12 weeks).[16] For athletes with recalcitrant adductor enthesopathy, however, selective adductor release has been another option to be beneficial. Schilders et al concluded that selective partial adductor release in 43 professional athletes provided considerable pain relief.[12] All but one of the athletes were able to return to their preinjury level of sport at approximately 2 months.

OSTEITIS PUBIS

Osteitis pubis is a painful overuse stress injury of the pubic symphysis that can cause lower abdominal or groin pain secondary to excessive strain and motion of the joint. The pubic symphysis acts as a fulcrum for force generated at the anterior pelvis. The rectus

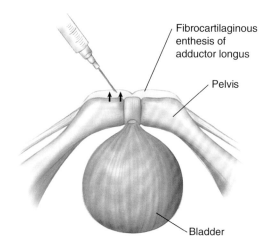

FIGURE 24.4 • Illustration demonstrating an entheseal injection, which is performed under image intensification or ultrasound guidance. A 21-gauge needle is inserted into the pubic cleft and moved a few millimeters into the fibrocartilaginous enthesis of the adductor longus. The injection contains triamcinolone acetonide (80 mg in 2 mL) mixed with bupivacaine hydrochloride (3 mL of a 0.5% solution). Reassessment is performed 5 minutes after the injection and consists of palpation over the adductor longus insertion site, passive stretching of the adductors, and active adduction against resistance.

abdominis tendon and the 3 adductor tendons attach to the fibrocartilage plate of the pubic symphysis to provide anterior pelvic stabilization. During core rotation and extension, these muscles act as antagonists; the rectus elevates the pelvis, and the adductors depress it. Injury to either tendon increases stress that can alter symphyseal biomechanics, ultimately causing a stress injury/reaction of the pubic bone. Later degeneration of the cartilage at the pubic symphysis can also result from these stresses.

An overlap of patient presentation and physical examination findings has been observed in athletic pubalgia, but a distinguishing feature is that pain can be elicited with palpation over the pubic symphysis and during a positive spring test (Figure 24.5). It is critical to ascertain whether the pain on palpation is truly a typical limiting pain for the athlete because tenderness in this region is common. In the setting of chronic osteitis pubis, characteristic radiographic findings include lytic changes at the pubic symphysis, sclerosis, and widening of the symphysis (Figure 24.6). MRI shows subchondral bone marrow edema with bilateral involvement that is more prominent on the affected side.[17] This finding can also be relatively frequent in asymptomatic athletes.

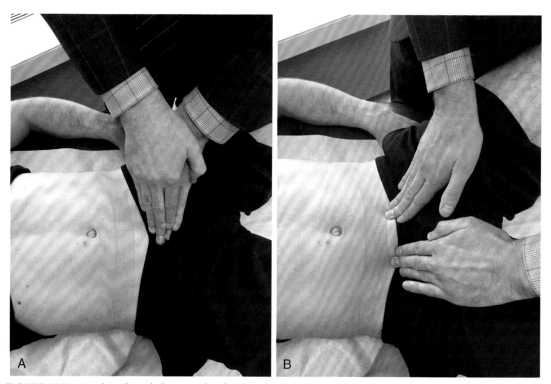

FIGURE 24.5 • A and B, Clinical photographs showing the evaluation of the athlete with osteitis pubis. A, Pain can often be elicited by manual palpation of the athlete's pubic symphysis. B, The most specific test for osteitis pubis is the direct pressure spring test in which the fingertips move laterally a few centimeters to the pubic symphysis and direct pressure is applied to the pubic rami. During application of pressure, the patient feels pain in the symphysis.

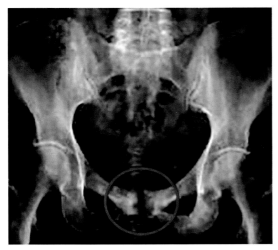

FIGURE 24.6 • AP radiograph demonstrating classic findings of osteitis pubis: cystic change, sclerosis, and widening of the pubic symphysis (circle).

Management

Corticosteroid injections also have been useful adjuncts in the treatment of osteitis pubis for pain relief and to accelerate an athlete's return to play.[18,19] Athletes who received corticosteroid injections into the symphyseal cleft and those who received injections within 2 weeks of diagnosis had the best results.[19] Nonsurgical care is generally successful from a symptom perspective; however, return to play can take time, and pain-free play can take even longer. In a series of professional Australian football players with pubic stress injuries, 89% of athletes were able to return to play by the next football season, 5 to 6 months after the diagnosis and initiation of treatment.[20]

Nonsurgical treatment fails in approximately 5% to 10% of athletes, who then require surgical treatment.[21] For the athletic population, surgical options include pubic symphyseal fusion, débridement of the pubic symphysis through open or endoscopic approaches, wedge resections, or surgical treatment of associated symptomatic FAI and/or athletic pubalgia[22-25] (Table 24.1). Surgical indications are not well defined, and considerable geographic differences in treatment and diagnosis exist. Some clinicians consider osteitis pubis to be an isolated entity, whereas others attribute the symptoms to be associated FAI and/or athletic pubalgia. Procedures directed at the pubic symphysis alone have been described in small series and can have important long-term complications, such as hemospermia, scrotal swelling, and stress fractures through the symphyseal arthrodesis.[22]

FEMOROACETABULAR IMPINGEMENT

FAI is the predominant cause of labral tears in nondysplastic hips and described it as a preosteoarthritic condition of the hip[26] (Figure 24.7). Cam-type impingement is due to an abnormal shear force between an aspherical femoral head and a normal acetabulum during hip flexion and internal rotation.[27] This abutment on the acetabular rim can displace the labrum toward the capsule, thus causing tears that are perpendicular to the articular surface in the labral transition zone between the fibrocartilage labrum and the articular hyaline cartilage.[28] Meanwhile, pincer-type impingement is secondary to acetabular overcoverage, which results in pathologic contact between the normal femoral head and this prominent portion of acetabulum. This causes crushing of the labrum between the femoral neck and acetabulum. The labrum fails first that causes eventual labral ossification, which further exacerbates this overcoverage.[26,29] Mixed FAI patterns are the predominant cause of hip pain among athletes with complaints of decreased hip ROM and impaired athletic performance.[30]

Athletes present with activity-related hip or groin pain that is exacerbated by hip flexion and internal rotation, with possible mechanical symptoms from labral tearing.[31] Pain location is variable, and in a study, 88% had groin pain, 67% had lateral hip pain, 35% had anterior thigh pain, 29% had buttock pain, 27% had knee pain, and 23% had low-back pain.[32] Patients with FAI will have limitations of hip ROM, as they can usually flex their hip to 90° to 110°, and in this position there is limited internal rotation and asymmetric external rotation relative to the contralateral leg.[33] The anterior impingement test is one of the most reliable tests for FAI (Figure 24.8A).[33] With the patient supine, the hip is dynamically flexed to 90°, adducted, and internally rotated. A positive test elicits deep anterior groin pain that generally replicates the patient's symptoms.[26] The posterior impingement test is also performed with the patient supine; the unaffected hip is flexed and held by the patient while the affected limb is extended and externally rotated by the examiner (Figure 24.8B). Buttock pain can result when the femoral head contacts the posterior acetabular cartilage and rim.[2,30]

Imaging traditionally begins with the use of radiographs, which should include an anteroposterior (AP) pelvic radiograph, a lateral (cross-table or Dunn view) radiograph, and a false-profile radiograph. Lateral imaging can help to evaluate cam-type impingement, femoral head asphericity, and insufficient head-neck offset. The false-profile view is also important to define coverage of

TABLE 24.1 Clinical Outcomes After Surgical Management of Osteitis Pubis

Study	Procedure	No. of Patients	Results
Williams[30]	Fusion with compression plating	7	All patients were able to RTP at approximately 6 mo
			All patients were pain free at final follow-up (52 mo)
Radic[33]	Curettage (no stabilization)	23	70% of patients able to RTP at 6 mo 39% remained asymptomatic
			26% had 1-time recurrence that improved with rest
			1 **patient** underwent late pubic symphyseal fusion
Hechtman[31]	Arthroscopically assisted curettage	4	Procedure preserved pubic ligament to reduce risk of instability
			RTP at 3 mo
			Pain free at final follow-up (50 mo)
Paajanen[32]	Mesh reinforcement	8	RTP within 8 wk for 7 of 8 patients
			All patients were pain free at final follow-up (2.7 y)

RTP, Return to play.

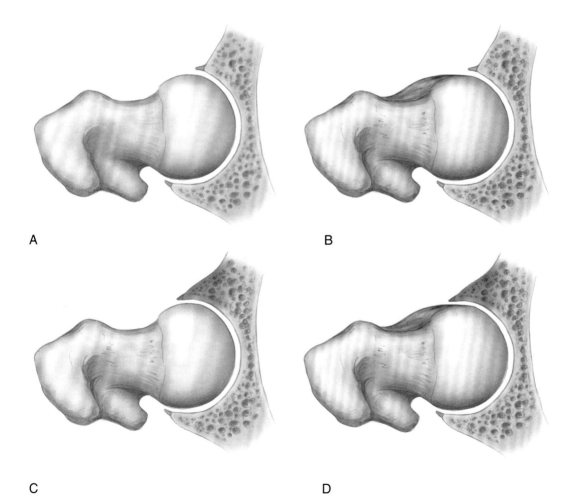

FIGURE 24.7 • Biomechanics of hip impingement as seen on the axial view of the hip joint. A, A normal hip. B, Reduced femoral head-neck offset (cam-type impingement). C, Excessive overcoverage of the femoral head (pincer-type impingement). D, Combination of cam and pincer types of impingement.

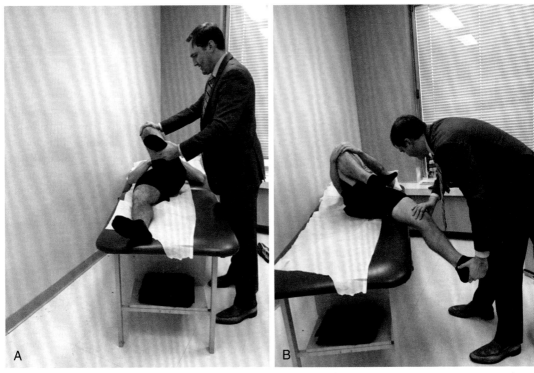

FIGURE 24.8 • Assessment for femoroacetabular impingement includes (A) anterior impingement test and (B) posterior impingement test.

the anterior aspect of the femoral head. MRI can help supplement radiographs to assess intra-articular lesions, particularly labral tears and chondral imaging. Protocols have been developed using noncontrast imaging that can identify these injuries noninvasively.[34]

Management

Hip arthroscopy can be successfully performed in both the supine and lateral decubitus positions. Portal positioning is critical to the success of the procedure. The standard portals are the anterior, anterolateral, midanterior, and posterolateral portals. The anterior portal is placed at the intersection of a line drawn down distally from the anterior superior iliac spine and a transverse line from the tip of the greater trochanter. This portal is at greatest risk of nerve injury with the lateral femoral cutaneous nerve in close proximity. Many surgeons have favored using a midanterior portal slightly distal and lateral to this location to afford greater protection to the lateral femoral cutaneous nerve. The anterolateral and posterolateral (optional) portals are placed at the superior border of the greater trochanter at its anterior and posterior borders, respectively. By respecting these landmarks, important neurovascular structures can be avoided (Figure 24.9).

Once appropriate portal placement and labral visualization have been accomplished by means of an

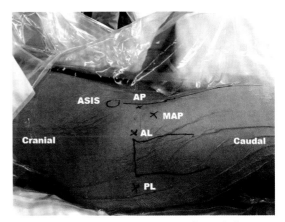

FIGURE 24.9 • Intraoperative setup of portal placement for intra-articular hip disorders of the right hip. ASIS, Anterior superior iliac spine; AP, anterior portal; AL, anterolateral portal; MAP, mid anterior portal; PL, posterolateral portal.

anterior capsulotomy, the labrum should be debrided of frayed, nonviable tissue. This can be performed with a variety of instruments, including radiofrequency ablation, motorized shavers, and biters. The preserved tissue should be probed to assess whether there is enough healthy tissue to merit repair. The acetabular rim should then be prepared to bleeding bone with a motorized burr with fluoroscopic assistance as needed.

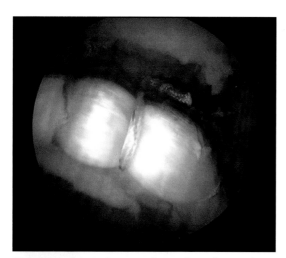

FIGURE 24.10 • Refixation is best achieved using a noneverting vertical mattress stitch that prevents labral deformity and preserves the suction-seal function of the reserved tissue.

Sutures are passed with the assistance of a suture penetrator or shuttle sutures (Figure 24.10).[35-38]

In patients with labral injuries, it is important to not only treat the labrum but also address the underlying osseous abnormalities. A failure to address these deformities is the most common cause for failure and revision FAI surgery.[39,40] Focal retroversion of the acetabulum ("pincer") at the cranial aspect of the acetabulum should be treated before labral refixation.

The cam lesion is then treated in the peripheral compartment to restore normal femoral offset and sphericity. A technical challenge is to address this deformity circumferentially but also proximodistally to assure a complete and thorough treatment of any source of mechanical impingement. Up to a 30% resection of the head-neck junction can be performed without compromising the safe load-bearing capacity for the femoral neck and increasing the risk of fracture.[41] Dunn or extended neck lateral fluoroscopic images can help to guide the intraoperative resection. However, a dynamic examination under direct arthroscopic visualization is essential to confirm elimination of the impingement and improvement in functional ROM.

Rehabilitation and Return to Play

When recommending rehabilitation protocols, hip arthroscopists must rely on a plethora of level IV evidence and informal expert opinion. As a result, significant variability exists between institutions and surgeons; however, there are 4 main phases of rehabilitation after hip arthroscopy: (1) maximum protection

and mobility, (2) controlled stability, (3) strengthening, and (4) return to sport.

Hip arthroscopy is a procedure that encourages athletes to get moving quickly after their surgery, as early rehabilitation on gluteal muscle groups, iliopsoas, and hip rotators are critical. Athletes can start using the stationary bike without resistance within 1 to 2 days after their procedure. This promotes muscle activation and prevents adhesions within the joint between the labrum and capsule. Elliptical and deep pool work focusing on aqua jogging, scissoring, and swimming while pulling can start after the first month. Antigravity treadmill or water running can be initiated at 8 weeks, with grass running and plyometric progression at 10 weeks. Functional baseball activities of batting and throwing can begin at 12 weeks. For batters, we recommend a 4-week interval hitting program to allow for a gradual progress back into the athlete's regular practice routine (Table 24.2). Meanwhile, for pitchers, we advise a 6-week throwing program to ensure return of appropriate throwing mechanics to prevent injury to the shoulder or elbow.

COMBINED ATHLETIC PUBALGIA AND FAI

There is often overlap between intra-articular and extra-articular pathology for patients presenting with lower abdominal, groin, or hip pain. Recently, using a cadaveric model, Birmingham and colleagues demonstrated that the presence of cam morphology places increased stresses and motion on the pubic symphysis. This was postulated to predispose patients to athletic pubalgia.[42] A subset of patients will present with combined FAI and core muscle injury/athletic pubalgia. Often, however, it remains difficult to determine the extent of the pain or disability that is attributable to each individual entity. In these cases, anesthetic intra-articular and extra-articular injections can assist in the diagnosis.

Treatment of only one of the symptomatic pathologies can lead to a suboptimal result. Pubalgia surgery alone has demonstrated a 25% return to the previous level of sport, whereas arthroscopic treatment of FAI alone resulted in a 50% return to the previous level in a study.[43] When both conditions were surgically managed either simultaneously or in a staged manner, 89% returned to sports without limitations. Similar results were noted in a series of professional athletes[44]; however, no patient within this series was able to return to sport after athletic pubalgia surgery alone. Therefore, it may be reasonable to counsel the athlete about FAI corrective surgery with later

TABLE 24.2 Four-Week Interval Hitting Program

Sunday	Monday	Tuesday	Wednesday	Thursday	Friday	Saturday
Rest	**Tee stand phase** Warm-up 15 swings at 50% effort Rest 5 min 15 swings at 50% effort	Thrower's 10/ physical therapy	Warm-up 20 swings at 50% effort Rest 5 min 20 swings at 60% effort	Rest Thrower's 10/physical therapy	Warm-up 15 swings at 75% effort Rest 5 min 15 swings at 75% effort	Rest Thrower's 10
Rest	Warm-up 25 swings at 75%-80% effort Rest 5 min 25 swings at 75%-80% effort	Rest Thrower's 10/ physical therapy	Warm-up 30 swings at 90% effort Rest 5 min 30 swings at 90% effort	Rest Thrower's 10/physical therapy	**Soft toss phase** Warm-up + 10-15 swings off tee 10 swings at 50% effort Rest 5 min 20 swings at 60% effort	Rest Thrower's 10
Rest	Warm-up + 10-15 swings off tee 15 swings at 75% effort Rest 5 min 15 swings at 75% effort Rest 5 min 15 swings at 75% effort	Rest Thrower's 10/ physical therapy	Warm-up + 10-15 swings off tee 15 swings at 90% effort Rest 5 min 15 swings at 90% effort Rest 5 min 15 swings at 90% effort	Rest Thrower's 10/physi-cal therapy	**Batting practice** Warm-up + 10-15 swings of soft toss 15 swings at 50% effort Rest 5 min 15 swings at 60% effort Rest 5 min 15 swings at 75% effort	Rest Thrower's 10
Rest	Warm-up + 10-15 swings of soft toss 15 swings at 75% effort Rest 5 min 15 swings at 80% effort Rest 5 min 15 swings at 80% effort	Rest Thrower's 10/ physical therapy	Warm-up + 10-15 swings of soft toss 15 swings at 80% effort Rest 5 min 15 swings at 90% effort Rest 5 min 15 swings at 100% effort	Rest Thrower's 10/physi-cal therapy	**Live pitching sequencing** See below for infor-mation on how to begin this phase*	Rest Thrower's 10

*Once you have finished your batting practice sequencing, you are ready to progress to **live pitching**. Start with a simulated game or gradually progress back into your regular practice routine.

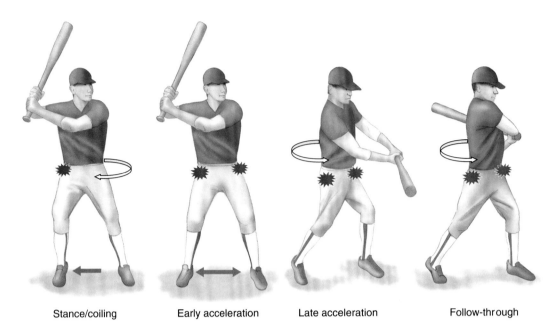

| Stance/coiling | Early acceleration | Late acceleration | Follow-through |

FIGURE 24.11 • Biomechanics of the hip joint during batting.

pubalgia surgery if symptoms do not fully resolve, given that half of the patients are able to return in this manner. However, when treating high-level athletes, surgical management of both the core muscle injury/athletic pubalgia and FAI in a staged or simultaneous manner may allow for a more predictable return to sport with minimal time lost.

LOWER EXTREMITY BODY MECHANICS OF THE BASEBALL ATHLETE

Understanding the relationship of hip and pelvic motion in relation to the batting and throwing athlete is important to understand the possible underlying causes of intra- and extra-articular hip injuries. This section will describe the biomechanics of common baseball specific skills of batting and throwing.

BATTING MOTION

The act of batting can be broken down into 3 distinct phases: preparatory, acceleration, and follow-through (Figure 24.11).

Preparatory

Each batter has a unique stance; however, there are certain characteristics that may describe this initiation position. Generally, athletes will have their shoulders, trunk, and pelvis perpendicular to the pitcher with their head rotated toward the pitcher's mound. The batters bodyweight will be over their back leg with the trunk erect and leaning slightly forward. The knees and hips will vary in the degree flexion based on individual preference (Figure 24.11A).

As the batter swings, there is a transition of weight away from the pitcher and onto the back leg, as gluteal muscles push into abduction with slight extension and external rotation. This is followed by a rotation of the upper torso and pelvis toward the dominant side. This helps to preload the trunk to store elastic energy that can be converted to power for the acceleration phase of batting.

Acceleration

This phase begins with lift off of the lead leg in a transfer of weight onto the dominant side. The lead leg then strides toward the target with an average stride length of 380% of the width of the hips, which places both hip joints toward the end range of abduction. As the lead leg makes contact with the dirt, it becomes a firm pillar, which helps to drive the lead pelvic ileum bone posterior to aid in the rapid acceleration of the pelvis, which rotates approximately 30° around the trunk's axis.[45] Rapid transfer of weight onto the lead leg follows. Powered by the gluteal muscles, the trailing hip abducts and externally rotates in a closed chain that is aided by knee extension of the lead leg. This creates a rigid lever and fulcrum

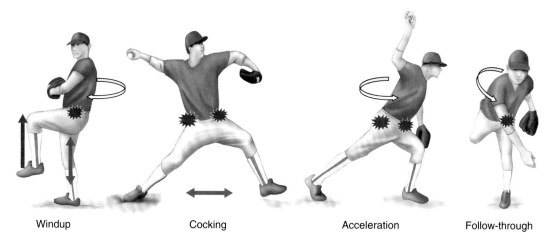

Windup   Cocking   Acceleration   Follow-through

FIGURE 24.12 • Biomechanics of the hip joint during throwing.

by which the pelvis rotates with pelvic acceleration estimated to be 714 °/second toward the pitcher. The upper extremity follows behind to bring the bat in contact with the ball (Figure 21.11C).

Follow-through

After the ball has been hit, the generated velocity continues to power the swing through the ball. The lead leg moves into maximal internal rotation as the pelvis rotates about axis of the trunk. Meanwhile, the trailing leg returns to a more neutral position but continues to remain in extension with slight internal rotation. When compared with the throwing motion, there is a more even distribution of weight through this phase that results in a more balanced finish position (Figure 24.11D).

THROWING MOTION

The phases of throwing can be divided into windup/cocking, acceleration, and follow-through (Figure 24.12).

Windup/Cocking

The initial phase of throwing starts from the lower extremity with the player creating forward momentum to propel the ball. This begins with a shuffle step as the thrower sets his feet and begins moving toward the target. The thrower faces perpendicular to home plate with his head, shoulders, and hips parallel to the direction of the intended target. The trailing leg accepts the majority of the weight as the thrower steps toward the target with the lead leg. This lead leg progresses through an open-chain adduction-internal rotation to abduction-external rotation through an arc of flexion

toward the target. The gluteal muscles of the trailing leg will power the dominant leg into abduction, external rotation, and extension (Figure 24.12B).

This creates separation of the feet in the form of stride length, which is a critical factor in determining ball velocity. As the hips and pelvis rotate, the trunk remains perpendicular to the target. This rotational movement stores elastic energy in preparation for propelling the ball forward.

Acceleration

Both feet are in contact with the ground to form a stable base that allows for the upper extremity to propel the ball toward home plate. Once the lead foot comes in contact with the ground, it accepts the weight and acts as a fulcrum by which the trunk and upper body rotate to accelerate the dominant arm through the throwing motion. Rotation of the pelvis causes extension of the trailing leg as the hip returns to neutral rotation and pivots toward the target. As the pelvis continues to rotate forward, the lead hip moves into internal rotation and adduction with hip flexion once the trunk bends forward and rotates as the ball is released (Figure 24.12C).

Follow-through

As the ball is released toward home plate, the momentum generated increases hip flexion, internal rotation, and adduction of the lead leg, as body weight is distributed onto the lead side. Meanwhile, the player lifts off the trail foot indicating that weight has shifted entirely onto the lead lower extremity. Hamstrings, gluteus maximus, external rotators of the hip, and the trunk extensors activate in an eccentric fashion to decelerate the trunk and conclude the sequence of throwing (Figure 24.12D).

THE ROLE OF HIP MOTION ON KINETIC CHAIN

Pitchers have been found to have reduced hip internal rotation ROM compared with position players,[46] with hip injuries, specifically FAI and labral tears,[47,48] being common among this population.[4] The deleterious effects of FAI exacerbating a pitcher's predisposition for reduced internal hip rotation likely places these throwers at a disadvantage for generating power from the lower extremities. As overhand throwing is a sequence of role-specific events in the kinetic chain coordinated to produce force on the ball,[49] a deficiency of the hips to generate power during the windup and early cocking phases may result in overcompensation of the upper extremities during the late cocking and early acceleration phases.[50] This phenomenon has been previously documented in the shoulder, wherein the majority of overhand throwers with superior labral tears from anterior to posterior (SLAP) were found to have significant deficits in internal rotation ROM of the hips.[51] If kinetic overcompensation instead manifests at the elbow, it may lead to repetitive microtrauma to the UCL. This can result in the gradual development of chronic changes, including heterotopic calcification and ligamentous attenuation, and ultimately rupture requiring reconstructive surgery.[52]

This stresses the importance of evaluating the whole batting or throwing athlete. Once the clinical evaluation of the overhead throwing motion and kinetic chain is completed, treatment of baseball injuries should focus on addressing any kinetic chain deficits or altered throwing/batting biomechanics, improving joint stability, and optimizing anatomy. Based on the specific node where the pathomechanics are identified, the rehabilitation may involve improving and optimizing hip ROM, hip and leg strength, core stability and strength, scapular control, shoulder ROM and strength, and restoration of glenohumeral rotation. Rehabilitation can help reduce injury risk and possible need for surgery.

MANAGER'S TIPS

- Athletic hip injuries in baseball players include adductor muscle strains, osteitis pubis, and FAI with acetabular labral tears
- Injuries can be treated with nonoperative care including rest, activity modifications, nonsteroidal anti-inflammatory drugs (NSAIDs), corticosteroid injections, and physical therapy focusing on core strengthening and stabilization, postural retraining, and reestablishing dynamic relationship between the hip and pelvic muscles

- Baseball players with hip labral tear miss the most time from play and often require surgical intervention in the form of a hip arthroscopy
- FAI can cause limitations of hip motion that can disrupt the transference of kinetic energy while throwing and subsequently lead to increased torque being placed on the throwing shoulder and/or elbow
- Deficits in hip ROM should be addressed in the prevention and rehabilitation of various shoulder and elbow pathologies that are common among baseball players

REFERENCES

1. Philippon MJ, Maxwell RB, Johnston TL, Schenker M, Briggs KK. Clinical presentation of femoroacetabular impingement. *Knee Surg Sports Traumatol Arthrosc.* 2007;15(8):1041-1047.
2. Lynch TS, Terry MA, Bedi A, Kelly BT. Hip arthroscopic surgery: patient evaluation, current indications, and outcomes. *Am J Sports Med.* 2013;41(5):1174-1189.
3. Feeley BT, Powell JW, Muller MS, Barnes RP, Warren RF, Kelly BT. Hip injuries and labral tears in the national football league. *Am J Sports Med.* 2008;36(11):2187-2195.
4. Coleman SH, Mayer SW, Tyson JJ, Pollack KM, Curriero FC. The epidemiology of hip and groin injuries in professional baseball players. *Am J Orthop (Belle Mead NJ).* 2016;45(3):168-175.
5. Posner M, Cameron KL, Wolf JM, Belmont PJ Jr, Owens BD. Epidemiology of major league baseball injuries. *Am J Sports Med.* 2011;39(8):1676-1680.
6. Li X, Zhou H, Williams P, et al. The epidemiology of single season musculoskeletal injuries in professional baseball. *Orthop Rev (Pavia).* 2013;5(1):e3.
7. Werner J, Hagglund M, Walden M, Ekstrand J. UEFA injury study: a prospective study of hip and groin injuries in professional football over seven consecutive seasons. *Br J Sports Med.* 2009;43(13):1036-1040.
8. Ekstrand J, Hagglund M, Walden M. Epidemiology of muscle injuries in professional football (soccer). *Am J Sports Med.* 2011;39(6):1226-1232.
9. Tyler TF, Nicholas SJ, Campbell RJ, McHugh MP. The association of hip strength and flexibility with the incidence of adductor muscle strains in professional ice hockey players. *Am J Sports Med.* 2001;29(2):124-128.
10. Renstrom P, Peterson L. Groin injuries in athletes. *Br J Sports Med.* 1980;14(1):30-36.
11. Schilders E, Bismil Q, Robinson P, O'Connor PJ, Gibbon WW, Talbot JC. Adductor-related groin pain in competitive athletes. Role of adductor enthesis, magnetic resonance imaging, and entheseal pubic cleft injections. *J Bone Joint Surg Am.* 2007;89(10):2173-2178.

12. Schilders E, Talbot JC, Robinson P, Dimitrakopoulou A, Gibbon WW, Bismil Q. Adductor-related groin pain in recreational athletes: role of the adductor enthesis, magnetic resonance imaging, and entheseal pubic cleft injections. *J Bone Joint Surg Am*. 2009;91(10):2455-2460.

13. Dallaudiere B, Pesquer L, Meyer P, et al. Intratendinous injection of platelet-rich plasma under US guidance to treat tendinopathy: a long-term pilot study. *J Vasc Interv Radiol*. 2014;25(5):717-723.

14. Dimitrakopoulou A, Schilders EM, Talbot JC, Bismil Q. Acute avulsion of the fibrocartilage origin of the adductor longus in professional soccer players: a report of two cases. *Clin J Sport Med*. 2008;18(2):167-169.

15. Rizio L III, Salvo JP, Schurhoff MR, Uribe JW. Adductor longus rupture in professional football players: acute repair with suture anchors: a report of two cases. *Am J Sports Med*. 2004;32(1):243-245.

16. Schlegel TF, Bushnell BD, Godfrey J, Boublik M. Success of nonoperative management of adductor longus tendon ruptures in National Football League athletes. *Am J Sports Med*. 2009;37(7):1394-1399.

17. Mullens FE, Zoga AC, Morrison WB, Meyers WC. Review of MRI technique and imaging findings in athletic pubalgia and the "sports hernia". *Eur J Radiol*. 2012;81(12):3780-3792.

18. O'Connell MJ, Powell T, McCaffrey NM, O'Connell D, Eustace SJ. Symphyseal cleft injection in the diagnosis and treatment of osteitis pubis in athletes. *AJR Am J Roentgenol*. 2002;179(4):955-959.

19. Holt MA, Keene JS, Graf BK, Helwig DC. Treatment of osteitis pubis in athletes. Results of corticosteroid injections. *Am J Sports Med*. 1995;23(5):601-606.

20. Verrall GM, Slavotinek JP, Fon GT, Barnes PG. Outcome of conservative management of athletic chronic groin injury diagnosed as pubic bone stress injury. *Am J Sports Med*. 2007;35(3):467-474.

21. Mehin R, Meek R, O'Brien P, Blachut P. Surgery for osteitis pubis. *Can J Surg*. 2006;49(3):170-176.

22. Williams PR, Thomas DP, Downes EM. Osteitis pubis and instability of the pubic symphysis. When nonoperative measures fail. *Am J Sports Med*. 2000;28(3):350-355.

23. Hechtman KS, Zvijac JE, Popkin CA, Zych GA, Botto-van Bemden A. A minimally disruptive surgical technique for the treatment of osteitis pubis in athletes. *Sports Health*. 2010;2(3):211-215.

24. Paajanen H, Hermunen H, Karonen J. Pubic magnetic resonance imaging findings in surgically and conservatively treated athletes with osteitis pubis compared to asymptomatic athletes during heavy training. *Am J Sports Med*. 2008;36(1):117-121.

25. Radic R, Annear P. Use of pubic symphysis curettage for treatment-resistant osteitis pubis in athletes. *Am J Sports Med*. 2008;36(1):122-128.

26. Ganz R, Parvizi J, Beck M, Leunig M, Notzli H, Siebenrock KA. Femoroacetabular impingement: a cause for osteoarthritis of the hip. *Clin Orthop Relat Res*. 2003(417):112-120.

27. Siebenrock KA, Wahab KH, Werlen S, Kalhor M, Leunig M, Ganz R. Abnormal extension of the femoral head epiphysis as a cause of cam impingement. *Clin Orthop Relat Res*. 2004(418):54-60.

28. Beck M, Kalhor M, Leunig M, Ganz R. Hip morphology influences the pattern of damage to the acetabular cartilage: femoroacetabular impingement as a cause of early osteoarthritis of the hip. *J Bone Joint Surg Br*. 2005;87(7):1012-1018.

29. Siebenrock KA, Schoeniger R, Ganz R. Anterior femoro-acetabular impingement due to acetabular retroversion. Treatment with periacetabular osteotomy. *J Bone Joint Surg Am*. 2003;85-A(2):278-286.

30. Philippon MJ, Schenker ML. Arthroscopy for the treatment of femoroacetabular impingement in the athlete. *Clin Sports Med*. 2006;25(2):299-308 [ix].

31. Redmond JM, Gupta A, Hammarstedt JE, Stake CE, Dunne KF, Domb BG. Labral injury: radiographic predictors at the time of hip arthroscopy. *Arthroscopy*. 2015;31(1):51-56.

32. Clohisy JC, Knaus ER, Hunt DM, Lesher JM, Harris-Hayes M, Prather H. Clinical presentation of patients with symptomatic anterior hip impingement. *Clin Orthop Relat Res*. 2009;467(3):638-644.

33. Klaue K, Durnin CW, Ganz R. The acetabular rim syndrome. A clinical presentation of dysplasia of the hip. *J Bone Joint Surg Br*. 1991;73(3):423-429.

34. Mintz DN, Hooper T, Connell D, Buly R, Padgett DE, Potter HG. Magnetic resonance imaging of the hip: detection of labral and chondral abnormalities using noncontrast imaging. *Arthroscopy*. 2005;21(4):385-393.

35. Shindle MK, Voos JE, Nho SJ, Heyworth BE, Kelly BT. Arthroscopic management of labral tears in the hip. *J Bone Joint Surg Am*. 2008;90(suppl 4):2-19.

36. Kelly BT, Weiland DE, Schenker ML, Philippon MJ. Arthroscopic labral repair in the hip: surgical technique and review of the literature. *Arthroscopy*. 2005;21(12):1496-1504.

37. Larson CM, Giveans MR. Arthroscopic debridement versus refixation of the acetabular labrum associated with femoroacetabular impingement. *Arthroscopy*. 2009;25(4):369-376.

38. Larson CM, Guanche CA, Kelly BT, Clohisy JC, Ranawat AS. Advanced techniques in hip arthroscopy. *Instr Course Lect*. 2009;58:423-436.

39. Philippon MJ, Schenker ML, Briggs KK, Kuppersmith DA, Maxwell RB, Stubbs AJ. Revision hip arthroscopy. *Am J Sports Med*. 2007;35(11):1918-1921.

40. Heyworth BE, Shindle MK, Voos JE, Rudzki JR, Kelly BT. Radiologic and intraoperative findings in revision hip arthroscopy. *Arthroscopy*. 2007;23(12):1295-1302.

41. Mardones RM, Gonzalez C, Chen Q, Zobitz M, Kaufman KR, Trousdale RT. Surgical treatment of femoroacetabular impingement: evaluation of the effect of the size of the resection. *J Bone Joint Surg Am.* 2005;87(2):273-279.

42. Birmingham PM, Kelly BT, Jacobs R, McGrady L, Wang M. The effect of dynamic femoroacetabular impingement on pubic symphysis motion: a cadaveric study. *Am J Sports Med.* 2012;40(5):1113-1118.

43. Larson CM, Pierce BR, Giveans MR. Treatment of athletes with symptomatic intra-articular hip pathology and athletic pubalgia/sports hernia: a case series. *Arthroscopy.* 2011;27(6):768-775.

44. Hammoud S, Bedi A, Magennis E, Meyers WC, Kelly BT. High incidence of athletic pubalgia symptoms in professional athletes with symptomatic femoroacetabular impingement. *Arthroscopy.* 2012;28(10):1388-1395.

45. Welch CM, Banks SA, Cook FF, Draovitch P. Hitting a baseball: a biomechanical description. *J Orthop Sports Phys Ther.* 1995;22(5):193-201.

46. Laudner KG, Moore SD, Sipes RC, Meister K. Functional hip characteristics of baseball pitchers and position players. *Am J Sports Med.* 2010;38(2):383-387.

47. Fukushima K, Takahira N, Imai S, et al. Prevalence of radiological findings related to femoroacetabular impingement in professional baseball players in Japan. *J Orthop Sci.* 2016;21(6):821-825.

48. Kelly BT, Bedi A, Robertson CM, Dela Torre K, Giveans MR, Larson CM. Alterations in internal rotation and alpha angles are associated with arthroscopic cam decompression in the hip. *Am J Sports Med.* 2012;40(5):1107-1112.

49. Putnam CA. Sequential motions of body segments in striking and throwing skills: descriptions and explanations. *J Biomech.* 1993;26(suppl 1):125-135.

50. Seroyer ST, Nho SJ, Bach BR, Bush-Joseph CA, Nicholson GP, Romeo AA. The kinetic chain in overhand pitching: its potential role for performance enhancement and injury prevention. *Sports Health.* 2010;2(2):135-146.

51. Ben Kibler W, Sciascia A. Kinetic chain contributions to elbow function and dysfunction in sports. *Clin Sports Med.* 2004;23(4):545-552 [viii].

52. Mulligan SA, Schwartz ML, Broussard MF, Andrews JR. Heterotopic calcification and tears of the ulnar collateral ligament: radiographic and MR imaging findings. *AJR Am J Roentgenol.* 2000;175(4):1099-1102.

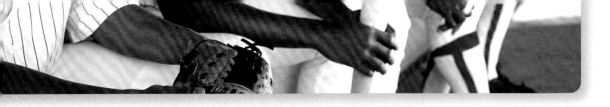

CHAPTER 25

Athletic Pubalgia and Oblique Injury and Prevention

T. Sean Lynch, MD

It's unbelievable how much you don't know about the game you've been playing all your life.

—*Mickey Mantle*

INTRODUCTION

Core muscles stabilize the spine and pelvis while generating and transferring energy from the center of the body to the extremities. This stability is critical for rotational movements involved in almost every sport and especially in baseball. Swinging a bat and throwing a ball require an athlete's body to shift and rotate weight and momentum smoothly with the legs generating power that is transferred through the torso and into the arms and hands. This is the essential mechanism that creates bat speed for hitters and arm momentum and ball velocity for pitchers. The core muscles that are important for the baseball athlete include internal and external oblique muscles, intercostal muscles, and rectus and transversus abdominis muscles.

Understanding the anatomic location and function of the core musculature helps skillful evaluation of these injuries. The external and internal oblique muscles are oriented in an oblique fashion and perpendicular to each other. They are responsible for flexion and rotation of the trunk, as well as providing trunk stabilization during complex movements. Meanwhile, the intercostal muscles are active in trunk stabilization and show side-specific activation during trunk rotation in electromyography (EMG) analysis.[1,2] Although, intercostals are thoracic muscles, they are part of the core musculature because of their continuity with the internal oblique muscles, and they have a similar injury presentation, treatment, and recovery.[3,4] Finally, the abdominal muscle attachments include the rectus abdominis and transversus abdominis, which provide posture and stabilize the lumbar spine and pelvis with lower extremity motion. The focus of this chapter is the 2 main abdominal core injuries that affect the baseball athlete: oblique muscle strains and athletic pubalgia.

OBLIQUE MUSCLE STRAINS

Abdominal oblique muscle strains, sometimes referred to as side strains, are common in baseball players. These injuries are characterized by an acute pain and localized tenderness over the lateral trunk near or directly over the rib cage after a throwing, swinging, or twisting.[5,6] It is most commonly reported in baseball players[4,6,7] and in cricket fast bowlers.[5,8-10] Other athletes affected include golfers, javelin throwers, rowers, rugby players, and tennis players.[5,10,11] The lateral trunk region affected by these oblique muscle injuries is composed of complex anatomical relationships between the external oblique, transversus abdominis, and intercostals, which can all be injured[8] (Figure 25.1).

The abdominal muscles mostly act synergistically for visceral support but also function separately to move and stabilize the trunk. As a consequence of their connection from the torso to the pelvis, the oblique abdominal muscles are particularly active during activities that require trunk stabilization with concomitant creation of side-specific axial torque, flexion and lateral flexion. These actions are required in sports that involve unilateral, asymmetrical, and explosive movements such as cricket and baseball,[6,11-13] and repetitive movement can result in asymmetrical changes in muscle size.[14]

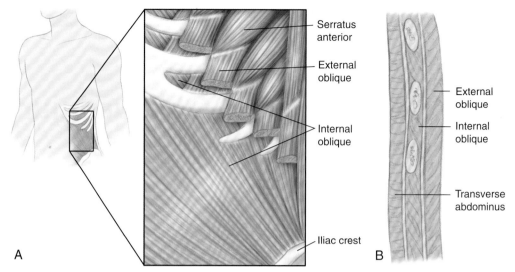

FIGURE 25.1 • Normal anatomy of the anterolateral abdominal wall. A, Internal oblique muscle originates from the iliac crest and inserts into the lowest 4 ribs beneath the external oblique. B, Coronal section through abdominal wall shows 3 flat muscles. Internal oblique muscle lies immediately underneath ribs.

Epidemiology

Conte et al. reviewed abdominal injuries from the Major League Baseball (MLB) disabled list over a 20-year season. There were 393 oblique injuries that made up 5% of all injuries.[6] The study also demonstrated an increasing incidence of oblique injuries. In terms of laterality, pitchers incurred 78% of injuries on the side contralateral to their throwing arm and position players sustained 70% of injuries contralateral to their dominant batting side.

Mechanisms of Injury

These injuries typically occur as an acute injury involving a single specific movement and resulting in acute pain that prevents further play.[7,8] In Conte's study, the mechanism of injury was not available; however, approximately half were sustained by pitchers, suggesting that throwing is the most common cause in baseball. The acute nature of the injury and the fact that it occurs during a specific sporting activity suggest that oblique injuries are precipitated by high-energy movements in asymmetrical motion. These actions typically require the trunk to act as a foundation from which sudden high forces and torques are produced to hit or throw an object such as a ball.

For baseball pitchers, the proposed moment of injury is the late cocking and early acceleration stages of throwing.[7] This involves the leading arm being "pulled down" (extended) from the position of maximal elevation with the trunk in contralateral side flexion placing the oblique muscles in a stretched position. Concomitantly, the trunk is rapidly flexed laterally away from the pitching arm. Fleisig et al. performed a kinematic study that concluded that the most demanding moment for the trunk during pitching was near the instant of front foot contact at which point there is maximum trunk rotation and high trunk axial acceleration where high torque is produced.[15] Meanwhile, swinging a baseball bat is another mechanism of injury in which the leading and trailing abdominal obliques demonstrate maximal activation through the swing, suggesting their role is more of trunk stabilization rather than power generation. This is evidenced by slight perturbations in balance while batting such as missing an off-speed pitch, which increases eccentric load on the abdominal obliques.

Diagnosis and Clinical Features

Clinical features include acute pain over the anterolateral or posterolateral thoracic wall over 1 or more of the lowest 4 ribs[4-8,10,11] (Figure 25.2). Deep inspiration may elicit pain,[4,5,11] and athletes are typically exquisitely tender to palpation at the injury site.[4-8,10,11] In the early stages, coughing and sneezing are painful while rolling over in bed, rising from sitting, and driving a car may also cause discomfort.

The athlete's pain is often reproduced by movements related to the initial mechanism of injury.[1] Lateral flexion range of motion (ROM) (Figure 25.3) and rotation both toward and away from the injured side are tested (Figure 25.4). Isometric resisted shoulder adduction at 90° abduction on the side of injury can also reproduce pain.

Advanced imaging such as ultrasound or magnetic resonance imaging (MRI) is routinely used in the acute setting in the assessment of high-level athletes. These imaging modalities determine the extent of injury, establish an accurate diagnosis, and have helped predict time to return to play.[4,6-8,11] Ultrasound can demonstrate

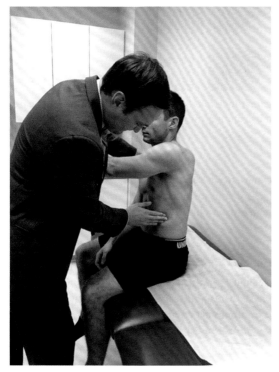

FIGURE 25.2 • Athletes present with pain to palpation over 1 or more of the 4 lowest ribs on the affected side.

internal oblique muscle tears that typically appear as a hypoechoic area with fibrillar disruption reflecting fluid collection, hematoma, and surrounding edema. On MRI, an acute side strain injury is characterized by high signal on short T1 Inversion Recovery and/or T2 images at the muscle, rib, or costal cartilage interface and typically categorized as either a complete or partial muscle tear (Figure 25.5). Imaging studies have shown that the internal oblique is the predominantly affected muscle with external oblique and transversus abdominis also being involved. Internal oblique muscle injury is most common at its 11th rib attachment, followed by the 10th, 9th, and 12th ribs. An important benefit of using MRI is that it demonstrates bone and cartilage pathology in addition to muscle strains.

Injury to the rib or costal cartilage may include osseous stress or avulsion fractures.[5,7,8] Additionally, periosteal stripping can occur when the muscular attachment is avulsed from the osseous or cartilaginous origin. This is an injury to the rib as well as the internal oblique muscle, which may result in hemorrhage and hematoma even with a low-grade muscle tear. Hematoma may track between the myofascial surfaces of the internal and external oblique muscles.

Risk and Associated Factors

Oblique injuries occur with higher incidence in the early part of the MLB season.[6] The first month of the season contributed over 25% of side strain injuries followed by a decrease in injury incidence during the second month of the season. The high early season incidence of side strains suggests that relative deconditioning in the off-season combined with a sharp increase in activity intensity when transitioning from preseason to competitive games may be a contributing factor.

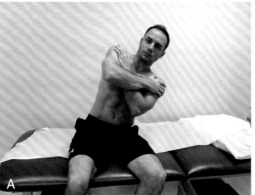
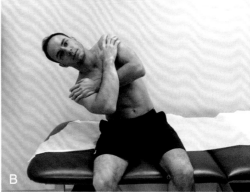

FIGURE 25.3 • Lateral flexion is typically reduced and limited by pain in both directions, particularly toward the injured side. This right hand dominant pitcher has limited flexion toward his left side compared with his right (A and B). The athlete will also report jamming or squashing symptoms when moving toward the injured side.

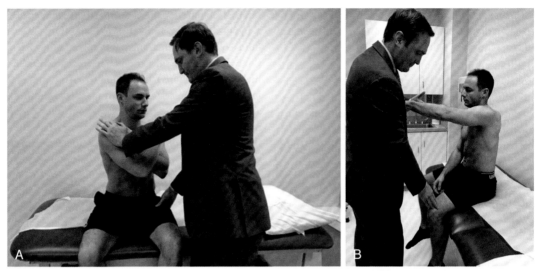

FIGURE 25.4 • Having the patient contract the muscle against resistance by rotating the torso can replicate the pain, assisting with diagnosis. This can be simulated by rotating the torso (A) or resisted shoulder adduction (B).

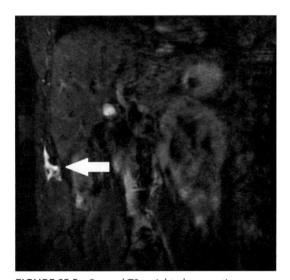

FIGURE 25.5 • Coronal T2-weighted magnetic resonance image of the abdomen showing internal oblique muscle tear with retraction (arrow) of the right 10th rib in a Major League Baseball (MLB) outfielder.

In cricket, an overhead throwing sport similar to baseball, age has been found to be a possible contributing factor, as cricket fast bowlers younger than 24 years are 3 times more likely to sustain a side strain injury than those older than 30 years. This same group of younger athletes is twice more likely to sustain the injury than those aged 25 to 29 years.[16] The reason for this increase in risk is unknown but could be related to being relatively unaccustomed to the demands of high-level competitive matches compared with their more experienced colleagues. This may also include a lack of musculoskeletal maturity to cope with the demands of elite sport.

Treatment and Recovery

Few studies outline the management of oblique muscle injuries in the baseball athlete. Treatment includes physiotherapy and surgery in rare recalcitrant cases. In the author's experience, manual therapy techniques to the area of injury may be beneficial to reduce muscle spasm and possibly encourage optimal soft tissue healing. Thoracic spine mobilization to restore extension, lateral flexion, and rotation ROM is also beneficial to expedite return to preinjury activities.

On resolution of pain on deep inspiration and coughing, the athlete will generally tolerate graded strengthening and cardiovascular exercise. This commences with isometric contractions that load the chest wall muscles in neutral trunk positions to minimize the effects of pain-inhibited muscle atrophy and provide a stimulus for muscle healing.[17] This can be progressed to concentric contractions in positions that load the area of injury such as trunk lateral flexion away from the injured side to further enhance the mechanotherapy effect on the healing muscle tissue. These exercises also have a functional role, as they mimic the windup components of baseball pitching and possibly retrain muscles for return to sport. The final stage of strengthening involves the transition from concentric to the eccentric and dynamic actions required for the propulsion phases of throwing. It is also important to consider the repetitive nature of pitching and hitting during the rehabilitation process so that high volumes of strengthening exercise are performed to cope with the demands of the sport. Functional retraining of the specific task with graded increases in quantity and intensity is paramount. The athlete may also need to initially return to a lower level of competition to complete his rehabilitation under game conditions and demonstrate his readiness to return to peak performance.

An extended return to play time of approximately 4 to 5 weeks has been reported for athletes following oblique injuries. It is imperative that the athlete has full asymptomatic lateral flexion ROM before return to sport. Recurrent side strain injuries have been reported with a recurrence rate of 12% with one-third of recurrences being sustained by pitchers.[6] These recurrences most commonly occurred in the same or following baseball season.

Time to return to able status in MLB has been affected by laterality of injury. Ipsilateral injuries took much longer to recover than contralateral injuries for pitchers whereas the opposite was true for position players.[6] It is possible that ipsilateral injury differs in severity or type of pathology (eg, periosteal stripping vs muscle injury) to contralateral injury and that this affects recovery time. Similarly, batting-induced injuries may have a different pathology to throwing injuries, thus affecting recovery time.

ATHLETIC PUBALGIA

Athletic pubalgia is another source of lower abdominal or groin pain that can be debilitating for a baseball player. This condition is commonly referred to as a sports hernia or core muscle injury; however, no hernia is seen with these injuries but rather a weakening or tearing of the abdominal wall is present. Athletes usually present with symptoms of gradually increasing activity-related lower abdominal and/or proximal hip adductor-related pain.[18,19] Trunk hyperextension and/or hip hyperabduction can also lead to increased tension in the pubic region and the development of acute pain if associated with partial or complete ruptures of the rectus abdominis/adductor aponeurosis.[20]

Diagnosis and Clinical Features

Affected athletes have unilateral or bilateral lower abdominal pain that can radiate toward the perineum and proximal adductors during sporting activities. Athletes participating in sports that require repetitive pivoting and cutting with quick starts are susceptible to these injuries.[21-23] In an epidemiologic study utilizing MLB's Health and Injury Tracking System (HITS), athletic pubalgia made up 1.8% (n = 32) of all hip and groin injuries over a 4-season period.[24]

A classic complaint is pain present with activity that prevents the athlete from playing at full potential but ceases with rest. Physical examination findings include pain with palpation over the pubis and the abdominal obliques and/or rectus abdominis insertion as well as occasional pain on palpation at the adductor longus tendon origin at or near the pubic symphysis. Pain also is exacerbated with resisted sit-ups at the inferolateral edge of the distal rectus abdominis and with resisted adduction[18] (Figure 25.6). MRI can show a cleft sign at the rectus abdominis/adductor aponeurosis about the anterior pelvis; however, it is important to note that these imaging findings are not infrequent in asymptomatic athletes[25] (Figure 25.7).

Treatment

Management of athletic pubalgia typically begins with nonsurgical care, consisting of cessation or modification of sporting activities, anti-inflammatory medications, and physical therapy. Rehabilitation should emphasize core strengthening and stabilization and postural retraining with normalization of the dynamic relationship between the hip and pelvic muscles. Local injections can be helpful in some cases to allow continued participation for an in-season athlete. After the athlete is pain free, a gradual return to play can be initiated.

Moderate to severe symptoms of athletic pubalgia rarely improve with nonsurgical care, and eventual surgical repair for the relief of symptoms is typically required to allow the athlete to return to play.[26,27] Some factors to remember regarding treatment include the level at which the athlete is competing and the timing of the baseball season. During the season, if the player can continue to function, then the previously described strategies can be used. A corticosteroid can also be employed for immediate pain relief to help the athlete get to the off-season, when surgical intervention can be considered without substantial time lost from sport. Surgery should be considered for the in-season athlete who cannot continue despite nonsurgical measures[28] (Figure 25.8).

Surgical options are numerous, and no consensus has been observed in the literature regarding a preferred surgical technique. Surgical procedures are divided into 3 general categories: open repair with or without mesh reinforcement, laparoscopic repair with mesh, and broad pelvic floor repair with possible adductor releases/repair and neurectomies. Primary repairs can be subdivided further into a modified

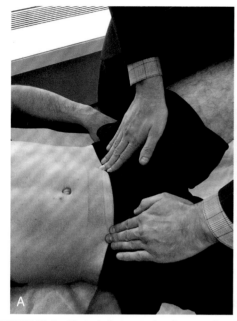
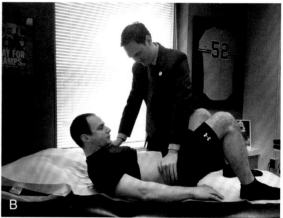

FIGURE 25.6 • Clinical photographs showing the physical examination for the diagnosis of athletic pubalgia. This condition can be challenging to diagnose, but the patient often presents with suprapubic pain, most commonly seen on the rectus abdominis origin or its lateral edge (A) and with resisted sit-ups (B).

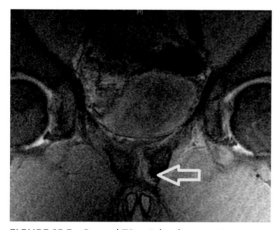

FIGURE 25.7 • Coronal T2-weighted magnetic resonance image of the pubic symphysis showing the secondary cleft sign in a 22-year-old outfielder with left-sided inguinal pain. A curvilinear area of hyperintense signal (arrow) that adjoins the high signal intensity of the medial pubic body can be seen near the rectus abdominis-adductor longus aponeurosis.

Bassini-type repair with or without adductor releases and a minimal repair with decompression of the genital branch of the genitofemoral nerve. Athletes are able to return to play at a rate of 80% to 100% regardless of the repair type and with considerable pain relief[18,19,26,27,29-35] (Table 25.1).

Meyers et al. described a primary repair in which the inferolateral border of the rectus abdominis is repaired to the pubis and the inguinal ligament to provide stability to the rectus.[18] For athletes with adductor pathology and pain, a repair or release also can be performed to help restore core muscle balance. In this series of high-performing athletes, approximately 88% were performing at or above their preinjury level within 3 months. This percentage increased to 96% at 6 months. The minimal repair technique of the transversalis fascia has been described by Muschaweck and Berger.[31,36] This technique focuses on the decompression of the genital branch of the genitofemoral nerve with tension-free repair of the posterior inguinal wall deficiency or defect (Figure 25.9). Athletes undergoing this minimal repair procedure can resume running and cycling on the postoperative day 2, can begin sports-specific training on postoperative day 3 or 4, and can train fully on postoperative day 5. This accelerated return to play is attributed to the tension-free repair that can enable athletes to return to play within 2 weeks.

Postoperative rehabilitation varies by the surgeon and the surgical technique, but programs should focus on a step-wise progression of exercise activity, with a focus on core and lower extremity strength, stability, flexibility, and balance. Emphasis should be placed on achieving proper muscle activation, and recruitment-pattern training is essential to proper recovery. Walking can be initiated early, and light jogging can be started by 3 to 4 weeks postoperatively. In our experience, athletes generally can return to baseball within 6 to 8 weeks of surgery.

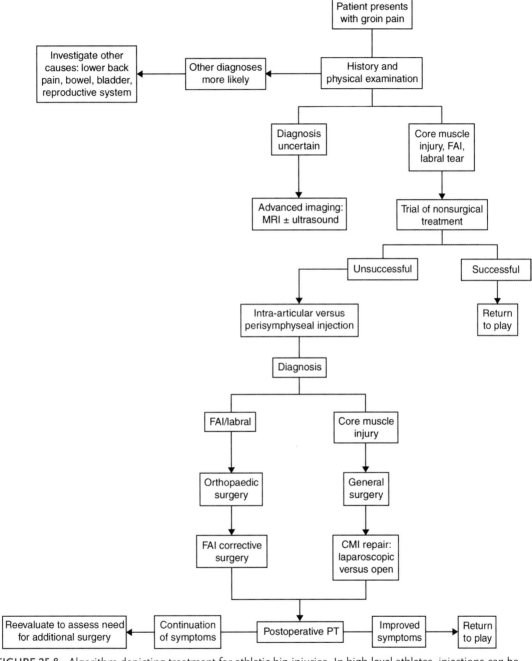

FIGURE 25.8 • Algorithm depicting treatment for athletic hip injuries. In high-level athletes, injections can be done in conjunction with the initiation of nonsurgical management. FAI, femoroacetabular impingement; CMI, core muscle injury; PT, physical therapy.

TRIP TO THE MOUND

The majority of abdominal baseball injuries are related to overuse or maximal exertion of the musculature. These injuries should not be written off as an isolated event, and correcting the root cause of the injury may be more important than treating the injury itself. There is a growing evidence that suggests that core stabilization is an important component of gross motor activities and that core strengthening has a role in injury prevention. The role of core musculature in batting and pitching has been assessed in electromyographic studies. Hip and trunk muscles play an important role in stabilizing the core while limb movements are carried out. Core muscles are also activated in a side-specific manner to generate torque, especially in pitching. Kinetic chain research demonstrates the importance of core muscle activated before carrying out athletic limb movement. These studies suggest that developing core stability may reduce overall injury rates and should be incorporated into players' workouts and rehabilitations.

There is often overlap between intra-articular and extra-articular pathology for patients presenting with lower abdominal, groin, or hip pain. The presence of cam morphology on the femoral head places increased stress and motion on the pubic symphysis; thus, causing a subset of patients to present with combined femoroacetabular impingement (FAI) and core muscle injury/athletic pubalgia. This is important to note, as treatment of only 1 of the symptomatic pathologies can lead to suboptimal results. Therefore, when treating high-level baseball player, surgical management of both the core muscle injury/athletic pubalgia and FAI in a staged or simultaneous manner may allow for a more predictable return to sport with minimal time lost.

TABLE 25.1 Clinical Outcomes After Surgical Management of Athletic Pubalgia

Study	Level of Evidence	No. of Athletes (Hips)	Follow-up (%)	Mean Age in Year (Range)	Surgical Approach	Return to Play
Brannigan[27]	Prospective, IV	85 (100)	100%	24 (18-50)	Open, no mesh	96% within 15 wk
Hackney[35]	Retrospective, IV	15	100%	NR (18-38)	Open, no mesh	87%
Brown[30]	Retrospective, IV	98 (107)	100%	NA (19-40)	Open, mesh	99%
Kluin[29]	Prospective, IV	14 (17)	100%	32.7 (12-56)	Lap mesh	93% within 3 mo
Genitsaris[33]	Retrospective, IV	131	100%	23.5 (18-36)	Lap mesh	100% within 2-3 wk
Muschaweck and Berger [31]	Prospective, IV	129 (132)	97%	25 (21-29)	Open, minimal repair	84% within 4 wk
Meyers[18]	Retrospective, IV	175	100%	NA	Open broad pelvic floor repair	95% within 3 mo
Meyers[19]	Retrospective, III	5218 (5460)	NA	NA (11-77)	Open broad pelvic floor repair	95% within 3 mo
Jakoi[32]	Case cohort, III	43	100%	NA	Various	80% for at least 2 seasons

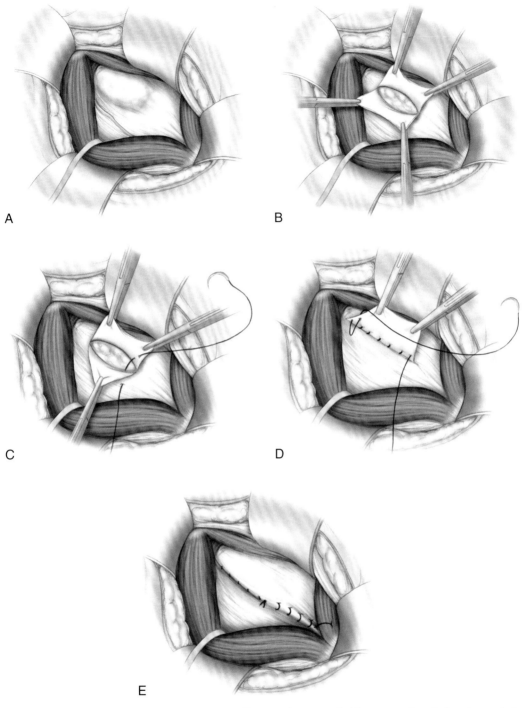

A

B

C

D

E

FIGURE 25.9 • Minimal repair technique: (A) A small tear in the external oblique was identified and extended to expose the posterior wall of the inguinal canal. B, The weakness in the posterior floor of the inguinal canal was identified and opened. C-E, The defect in the posterior wall was repaired in a running fashion.

MANAGER'S TIPS

- Oblique injuries are injuries of many names: internal/external oblique, intercostal oblique, abdominal muscle, rib muscle, or rectus abdominus strains
- Majority of these injuries are sustained while batting or pitching with high incidence of injuries occurring early in the season
- These injuries must be treated properly to avoid reinjury
- Athletic pubalgia is another core muscle injury sustained by baseball players and frequently requires surgical management
- Athletic pubalgia frequently seen in conjunction with FAI with labral tear. Athlete should also be assessed for FAI if concerned about core muscle injury

REFERENCES

1. Rimmer KP, Ford GT, Whitelaw WA. Interaction between postural and respiratory control of human intercostal muscles. *J Appl Physiol (1985)*. 1995;79(5):1556-1561.
2. Whitelaw WA, Ford GT, Rimmer KP, De Troyer A. Intercostal muscles are used during rotation of the thorax in humans. *J Appl Physiol (1985)*. 1992;72(5):1940-1944.
3. Gregory PL, Biswas AC, Batt ME. Musculoskeletal problems of the chest wall in athletes. *Sports Med*. 2002;32(4):235-250.
4. O'Neal ML, McCown K, Poulis GC. Complex strain injury involving an intercostal hematoma in a professional baseball player. *Clin J Sport Med*. 2008;18(4):372-373.
5. Connell DA, Jhamb A, James T. Side strain: a tear of internal oblique musculature. *AJR Am J Roentgenol*. 2003;181(6):1511-1517.
6. Conte SA, Thompson MM, Marks MA, Dines JS. Abdominal muscle strains in professional baseball: 1991-2010. *Am J Sports Med*. 2012;40(3):650-656.
7. Stevens KJ, Crain JM, Akizuki KH, Beaulieu CF. Imaging and ultrasound-guided steroid injection of internal oblique muscle strains in baseball pitchers. *Am J Sports Med*. 2010;38(3):581-585.
8. Humphries D, Jamison M. Clinical and magnetic resonance imaging features of cricket bowler's side strain. *Br J Sports Med*. 2004;38(5):E21.
9. Boyce Cam NJ, Muthukumar N, Boyle S, Lawton JO, Stretch R. Rib impingement in first class cricketers: case reports of two patients who underwent rib resection. *Br J Sports Med*. 2006;40(8):732-733 [discussion 733].
10. Obaid H, Nealon A, Connell D. Sonographic appearance of side strain injury. *AJR Am J Roentgenol*. 2008;191(6):W264-W267.
11. Maquirriain J, Ghisi JP. Uncommon abdominal muscle injury in a tennis player: internal oblique strain. *Br J Sports Med*. 2006;40(5):462-463.
12. Shaffer B, Jobe FW, Pink M, Perry J. Baseball batting. An electromyographic study. *Clin Orthop Relat Res*. 1993(292):285-293.
13. Watkins RG, Dennis S, Dillin WH, et al. Dynamic EMG analysis of torque transfer in professional baseball pitchers. *Spine (Phila Pa 1976)*. 1989;14(4):404-408.
14. Hides J, Stanton W, Freke M, Wilson S, McMahon S, Richardson C. MRI study of the size, symmetry and function of the trunk muscles among elite cricketers with and without low back pain. *Br J Sports Med*. 2008;42(10):809-813.
15. Fleisig GS, Hsu WK, Fortenbaugh D, Cordover A, Press JM. Trunk axial rotation in baseball pitching and batting. *Sports Biomech*. 2013;12(4):324-333.
16. Humphries D, Orchard J, Kontouris A. Abdominal wall injuries at the elite level in Australian male professional cricketers. *J Postgrad Med Educ Res*. 2015;49(4):155-158.
17. Khan KM, Scott A. Mechanotherapy: how physical therapists' prescription of exercise promotes tissue repair. *Br J Sports Med*. 2009;43(4):247-252.
18. Meyers WC, Foley DP, Garrett WE, Lohnes JH, Mandlebaum BR. Management of severe lower abdominal or inguinal pain in high-performance athletes. PAIN (performing athletes with abdominal or inguinal neuromuscular pain study group). *Am J Sports Med*. 2000;28(1):2-8.
19. Meyers WC, McKechnie A, Philippon MJ, Horner MA, Zoga AC, Devon ON. Experience with "sports hernia" spanning two decades. *Ann Surg*. 2008;248(4):656-665.
20. Palisch A, Zoga AC, Meyers WC. Imaging of athletic pubalgia and core muscle injuries: clinical and therapeutic correlations. *Clin Sports Med*. 2013;32(3):427-447.
21. Anderson K, Strickland SM, Warren R. Hip and groin injuries in athletes. *Am J Sports Med*. 2001;29(4):521-533.
22. Susmallian S, Ezri T, Elis M, Warters R, Charuzi I, Muggia-Sullam M. Laparoscopic repair of "sportsman's hernia" in soccer players as treatment of chronic inguinal pain. *Med Sci Monit*. 2004;10(2):CR52-CR54.
23. Irshad K, Feldman LS, Lavoie C, Lacroix VJ, Mulder DS, Brown RA. Operative management of "hockey groin syndrome": 12 years of experience in National Hockey League players. *Surgery*. 2001;130(4):759-764 [discussion 764-756].
24. Coleman SH, Mayer SW, Tyson JJ, Pollack KM, Curriero FC. The epidemiology of hip and groin injuries in professional baseball players. *Am J Orthop (Belle Mead NJ)*. 2016;45(3):168-175.
25. Zoga AC, Kavanagh EC, Omar IM, et al. Athletic pubalgia and the "sports hernia": MR imaging findings. *Radiology*. 2008;247(3):797-807.

26. LeBlanc KE, LeBlanc KA. Groin pain in athletes. *Hernia*. 2003;7(2):68-71.

27. Brannigan AE, Kerin MJ, McEntee GP. Gilmore's groin repair in athletes. *J Orthop Sports Phys Ther*. 2000;30(6):329-332.

28. Lynch TS, Bedi A, Larson CM. Athletic hip injuries. *J Am Acad Orthop Surg*. 2017;25(4):269-279.

29. Kluin J, den Hoed PT, van Linschoten R, IJzerman JC, van Steensel CJ. Endoscopic evaluation and treatment of groin pain in the athlete. *Am J Sports Med*. 2004;32(4):944-949.

30. Brown RA, Mascia A, Kinnear DG, Lacroix V, Feldman L, Mulder DS. An 18-year review of sports groin injuries in the elite hockey player: clinical presentation, new diagnostic imaging, treatment, and results. *Clin J Sport Med*. 2008;18(3):221-226.

31. Muschaweck U, Berger L. Minimal Repair technique of sportsmen's groin: an innovative open-suture repair to treat chronic inguinal pain. *Hernia*. 2010;14(1):27-33.

32. Jakoi A, O'Neill C, Damsgaard C, Fehring K, Tom J. Sports hernia in National Hockey League players: does surgery affect performance? *Am J Sports Med*. 2013;41(1):107-110.

33. Genitsaris M, Goulimaris I, Sikas N. Laparoscopic repair of groin pain in athletes. *Am J Sports Med*. 2004;32(5):1238-1242.

34. Radic R, Annear P. Use of pubic symphysis curettage for treatment-resistant osteitis pubis in athletes. *Am J Sports Med*. 2008;36(1):122-128.

35. Hackney RG. The sports hernia: a cause of chronic groin pain. *Br J Sports Med*. 1993;27(1):58-62.

36. Muschaweck U, Berger LM. Sportsmen's groin-diagnostic approach and treatment with the minimal repair technique: a single-center uncontrolled clinical review. *Sports Health*. 2010;2(3):216-221.

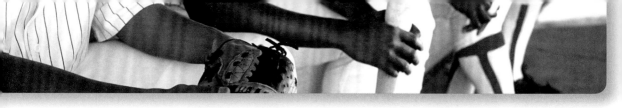

CHAPTER 26

Knee Injuries in Baseball Players

Charles A. Bush-Joseph, MD | Nathan Krebs, DO | Brandon J. Erickson, MD

I never give up. If you beat me, you have to beat me one, three, four, five times, and I still don't give up.

—*Mariano Rivera*

INTRODUCTION

Baseball is one of the most popular sports in the United States and is played by millions of people each year.[1] The majority of the literature involving baseball-related injuries is focused on the upper extremity, although recent attention has been brought to the morbidity associated with lower extremity injuries. Epidemiologic studies have shown that knee injuries represent 3.5% to 6.5% of all injuries in baseball but are the fifth most common cause of missed time with an average of 16.2 days missed.[1-5] As would be expected, lower extremity injuries are much more prevalent in position players and base runners than in pitchers.[6,7] Nearly half of all knee injuries have been found to occur by noncontact mechanisms. Contusions are the most prevalent type of knee injury, comprising nearly one-third of all knee injuries, and are associated with the fastest return to play at 7 days.[2] At this time there is a paucity of literature on baseball-specific knee injuries and outcomes. This chapter will review knee injuries involving the meniscus, ligaments, and cartilage along with semitendinosus avulsions and patellar tendinopathy.

MENISCAL INJURIES

Clinical Evaluation

The menisci are fibrocartilaginous structures that function as shock absorbers for the articular surfaces of the femur and tibia. They also provide proprioception and stability to the knee joint. Meniscal injuries represent approximately 10% to 13% of all knee injuries in baseball players, with medial meniscus injuries more common than lateral.[2,8,9] Tears can be broken down into acute injuries and chronic, degenerative tears. Medial meniscal tears are more commonly chronic in nature when compared with the lateral meniscus, which is most commonly injured in a traumatic event.[10]

History

Athletes presenting with a meniscal injury typically complain of localized joint line pain, often with associated locking, catching, and pain with rotational movements of the knee. They may complain of intermittent swelling of the knee. The pain is often localized to the area of the meniscal tear.

Physical Examination

Clinically, there is usually a knee effusion appreciated on examination. Joint line tenderness is a common clinical finding for a meniscus tear.[11] The McMurray and Apley compression tests may also be used to reproduce symptoms and localize the area of injury, although the most sensitive and specific examination is the Thessaly test. The Thessaly test when performed with 20° of knee flexion has a sensitivity of 89% and specificity of 97% for medial meniscus tears and a sensitivity of 92% and specificity of 96% for lateral meniscal tears.[11]

Imaging

Provided initial radiographs of the knee (anteroposterior, lateral, sunrise, and Merchant views) do not show any other osseous abnormalities, a magnetic resonance imaging (MRI) test is commonly ordered. An MRI is the imaging study of choice to diagnose a meniscal tear and commonly demonstrates increased signal within the meniscus extending to the articular surface.[11] Occasionally, there can be a bucket-handle

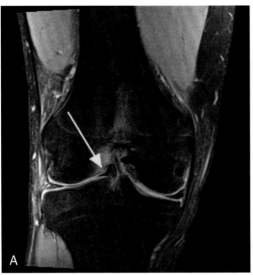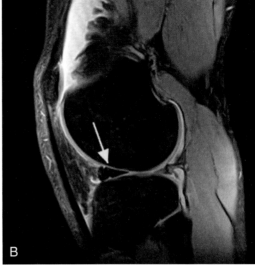

FIGURE 26.1 • Anteroposterior (A) and sagittal (B) MRI demonstrating an isolated bucket-handle lateral meniscal tear (yellow arrows).

tear of the meniscus where part of the meniscus flips into the notch (Figure 26.1A and B). This particular tear pattern can block motion of the knee.

Treatment

Nonoperative

Meniscal injuries may be treated initially with rest, cryotherapy, and elevation in addition to non–weight bearing on the involved extremity. Weight bearing may be advanced as tolerated, and the patient may benefit from physical therapy. Nonsteroidal anti-inflammatory drugs are typically used as first-line treatment for pain control; intra-articular steroid injections may also be used. Biologics, such as platelet-rich plasma (PRP) or bone marrow aspirate concentrate (BMAC), are another option that can be used to help optimize the anti-inflammatory environment of the knee to allow the athlete to return to play.[12,13]

Operative

Although nonsurgical treatment modalities can be offered, most meniscal injuries in athletes require surgical intervention. Mitchell et al found that 75% of meniscal injuries sustained during baseball required surgical intervention.[9] Surgical treatment options for meniscal injuries include debridement or repair. There are many factors that come into play when deciding between a repair and a meniscectomy including the location and type of tear, age of the athlete, and timing of the injury. A discussion between the athlete and treating surgeon is paramount to explain the differences in short- and long-term outcomes of a repair versus a debridement as well as the amount of time that will be missed for each. A meniscal repair can be performed all inside, outside in, or inside out with vertical mattress suture configuration, which is the current gold standard (Figure 26.2A-D).

Authors' Preferred Surgical Technique

A partial meniscectomy is performed with the patient in the supine position with the use of a lateral post to allow for valgus stress on the knee to give access to the medial compartment. If there is a possibility of performing a meniscal repair, the patient's leg should be placed in a leg holder and the foot of the bed dropped to allow easier access to the knee. Following standard prepping and draping, an inferolateral arthroscopy portal is created off the lateral edge of the patellar tendon at the level of the inferior pole of the patella. A complete diagnostic arthroscopy is performed, and the meniscal tear is assessed. An 18-g spinal needle is used to localize the inferomedial portal to allow access to the meniscal tear. If a partial meniscectomy is the best treatment option, a combination of an arthroscopic shaver and arthroscopic biter are used to debride the tear back to a stable rim. Great care is taken to avoid damage to the chondral surfaces of the knee.

If the tear pattern is amenable to a meniscal repair, the surgeon must assess if the tear can be repaired using the all-inside technique or if an inside out technique is required. If an all-inside technique is utilized, a sled is introduced into the knee to protect the chondral surfaces, followed by the meniscal repair device. The device is deployed in a vertical mattress configuration, taking care to ensure the device

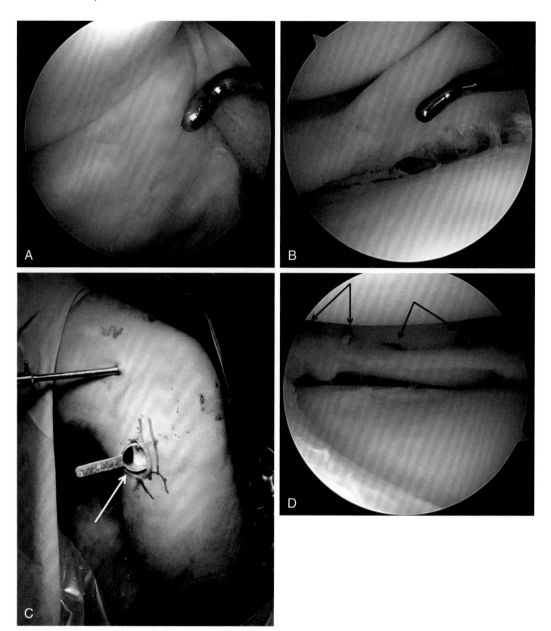

FIGURE 26.2 • A, Arthroscopic image demonstrating a locked bucket-handle tear of the lateral meniscus with the meniscus flipped into the notch. B, Arthroscopic image demonstrating a bucket-handle tear of the lateral meniscus following reduction of the meniscus back into the lateral compartment of the knee. C, The lateral aspect of the knee is exposed for a lateral meniscal repair with a retractor in place (arrow) to allow the surgeon to catch the needles as they are passed. D, Arthroscopic image demonstrating the final product of an inside out lateral meniscal repair utilizing high-tensile suture (arrow). A superolateral outflow cannula is also in place.

has deployed properly. The tail of the repair device is cut after cinching it down completely. If an inside out repair is required, an incision is made on either the medial (for a medial meniscal repair) or lateral (for a lateral meniscal repair) side of the knee, taking care to avoid neurovascular structures. The plane in between the gastrocnemius and capsule is developed, and a Henning retractor is placed behind the capsule to catch the needles as they are passed to avoid damaged to the surrounding structures. High-tensile suture is then passed through the tear in a vertical mattress configuration using long, sharp needles that are retrieved out of the skin incision. Great care is taken to avoid tissue bridges in between the sutures. Once all the sutures have been passed, these are tied down sequentially over the capsule.

Following a partial meniscectomy, patients are made weight bearing as tolerated (WBAT) and have no restrictions on knee range of motion (ROM) or activities. They begin rehabilitation during the first postoperative week to work on strengthening and ROM. Plyometric exercises and progression to return to sport (RTS) begin once they have full strength and ROM back and have a "dry" knee (no evidence of swelling). Patient who underwent a meniscal repair are placed into a hinged knee brace and are made WBAT in full extension. They are allowed to unlock the brace from 0° to 90° for ROM exercises. At 2 weeks, they are allowed to be WBAT with the braces unlocked from 0° to 90° and, at 4 to 6 weeks, can discontinue the use of the brace. They then progress through physical therapy and work on RTS when they have full ROM and strength and restore their proprioception. Patients are instructed to take a baby aspirin once a day for 3 weeks to minimize the risk of a blood clot.

Results

Kim et al found that athletes requiring meniscectomies had significantly shorter return to play times if they were younger than 30 years of age or were of higher activity level. The return to play was faster in athletes requiring lateral meniscectomy at 61 days compared with return to play in 79 days after medial meniscectomy. Additionally, it was found that almost half of the lateral meniscectomy patients experienced recurrent pain and/or effusion at return to play.[14] Postoperatively, athletes who undergo a meniscectomy are allowed to fully weight bear and begin training when they feel comfortable, whereas those who undergo a meniscal repair require a period of protected weight bearing and several months of rehabilitation.

Complications

Complications following a partial meniscectomy are infrequent with some patients reporting continued pain. Patients who undergo a meniscal repair are at risk of the repair failing. If this happens, the patient often requires a second surgery to remove the damaged meniscus, as a second attempt at a repair is often unsuccessful.

LIGAMENT INJURIES

Anterior Cruciate Ligament

Anterior cruciate ligament (ACL) tears are infrequent in baseball but responsible for the greatest mean days missed of all knee injuries.[2] ACL tears are most commonly sustained during a noncontact cutting or pivoting movement. The most common mechanism of ACL injury is seen when fielding, followed by base running.[15] There is a high association between ACL ruptures and other intra-articular injuries, such as meniscal tears.[9]

Clinical Evaluation

History

Athletes presenting with an ACL tear will often state they felt a "pop" in their knee, followed by a significant effusion. This pop is often the result of a noncontact pivoting injury to the knee. They may also complain of instability of the knee, but this will vary from person to person.

Physical Examination

A complete physical examination of the knee should be performed, including assessing ROM, varus/valgus laxity, etc. ACL-specific examinations include the Lachman, anterior drawer, and pivot shift tests. The Lachman test, performed with the knee in 30° of flexion, is positive when the examiner can anteriorly translate the tibia while holding the femur stable, more than 5 to 10 mm with a soft endpoint. This test is the gold standard for diagnosing an ACL tear. The pivot shift test is commonly performed in the operating room after the patient is sedated, as this test is not typically tolerated well in office.

Imaging

Standard knee radiographs mentioned previously are performed and, although often normal, can sometimes demonstrate an avulsion of the lateral capsule off of the tibia (Segond fracture), which is pathognomonic for an ACL tear. An MRI is commonly performed to confirm the diagnosis of a suspected ACL tear as well as to rule out any concomitant pathology (meniscal, chondral, etc) (Figure 26.3A and B).[16]

Treatment

Nonoperative

Nonoperative treatment is generally unsuccessful in patients participating in competitive athletics, as many will complain of persistent instability and will not be able to RTS at the same level as before their injury.[17]

Operative

The gold standard for treatment of an ACL tear in an athlete who wishes to RTS is an anterior cruciate ligament reconstruction (ACLR). There are multiple surgical techniques (accessory anteromedial, transtibial) and graft choices (bone-patellar tendon-bone [BTB] autograft, hamstring autograft, quadriceps tendon autograft, and BTB allograft) for performing an

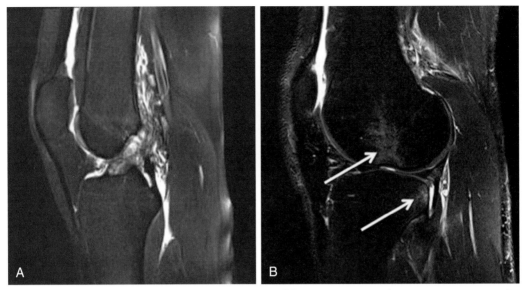

FIGURE 26.3 • A, Sagittal MRI image demonstrating a tear of the anterior cruciate ligament (ACL). Notice the fibers are not in complete continuity and have significant edema within them. B, Sagittal MRI of a patient who sustained an isolated ACL tear demonstrating significant bone marrow edema in the lateral femoral condyle and posterolateral tibial plateau (arrows). This bone bruise pattern is pathognomonic for an ACL tear.

ACLR. Autograft is preferred for competitive athletes, with BTB commonly referred to as the current gold standard and the most common graft choice by collegiate and professional football team physicians.[18-20] The surgical technique should focus on recreating the orientation of the native anatomy, either using the transtibial or anteromedial portal methods for drilling the femoral tunnel (Figure 26.4A-D).[21]

Authors' Preferred Surgical Technique

In our opinion, the patient age and position dictates the graft choice. A BTB autograft is the graft of choice in most professional baseball players, while a hamstring autograft should be used in catchers because of the nature of their position with kneeling, bending, etc. An ACLR is performed with the patient supine on the operating room table, the operative leg in a leg holder, the nonoperative leg in lithotomy position, the foot of the bed completely dropped, and the bed reflexed approximately 15°. An examination under anesthesia, including a pivot shift, is performed to confirm the ACL tear. If the pivot shift is positive, the graft can be harvested before inserting the arthroscope. A tourniquet is inflated and a paramedian incision is made, and dissection is sharply taken down to the paratenon of the patellar tendon. The paratenon is incised, and scissors are used to elevate this off of the patellar tendon. Once the tendon is exposed, a 10 mm graft is harvested from the central third of the patellar tendon, taking great care to remain parallel to the tendon fibers when harvesting the graft to avoid convergence. Tibial

(10 by 25 mm) and patellar (20 by 10 mm) bone plugs are then harvested using an oscillating saw, making sure not to go too deep with the saw on the patella to violate the cartilage or increase the risk for fracture. The graft is taken to the back table and prepped by the assistant to ensure it will pass through 10 mm tunnels. High-tensile sutures are placed in via drill holes into both bone plugs.

Once the graft is harvested, the arthroscope is introduced into the knee via an inferolateral portal. A diagnostic arthroscopy is performed. The inferomedial portal is created under direct visualization. Any other intra-articular pathology is addressed at this point. The old ACL stump is completely debrided, and a notchplasty is performed if needed to see around the back of the lateral femoral condyle. Once the femoral and tibial footprints have been exposed, a femoral drilling guide is inserted via the inferomedial portal, and the pin is placed at the center of the anatomic footprint of the ACL on the lateral femoral condyle. Great care is taken to ensure that there is 7 mm between where the pin is placed and the back wall to minimize the chance of back wall blowout. The knee is hyperflexed, and the pin is advanced out the lateral thigh. The pin should exit in the middle of the iliotibial band. The knee is kept in the hyperflexed position while the 10-mm reamer is introduced (making sure to avoid the cartilage on the medial femoral condyle) and reamed to but not through the second cortex. The reamer is removed, and a passing stitch is placed through the

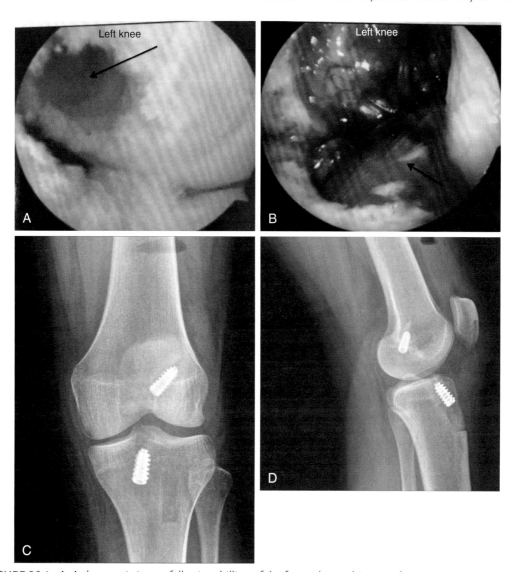

FIGURE 26.4 • A, Arthroscopic image following drilling of the femoral tunnel (arrow) during an anterior cruciate ligament reconstruction of the left knee. B, Arthroscopic image following passage of the new anterior cruciate ligament (ACL) graft (arrow) during an anterior cruciate ligament reconstruction of the left knee. Postoperative anteroposterior (C) and lateral (D) radiographs demonstrating 2 metal interference screws used to fix the reconstructed anterior cruciate ligament (ACL) (in this patient a bone-patellar tendon-bone graft was used).

beath pin and pulled out the lateral thigh. This is clamped proximally. The tibial drilling guide is then set to 55° (in most cases unless the graft is excessively long or short) and placed in the knee via the inferomedial portal. Once the tip of the guide is in the center of the anatomic ACL tibial footprint, a guide pin is advanced into the joint. Once the position is good, a 10-mm reamer is used to create the tibial tunnel. Bone is collected during this reaming process to graft the patellar and tibial harvest sites at the end of the case. A shaver and electrocautery device are used to clean the orifices of the tunnels and to remove any bone dust from the knee.

The passing stitch is then retrieved out of the tibial tunnel, and the graft is passed. Once the femoral plug is in place, a notcher is used to create a path for the metal interference screw. The superior and anterior portion should be notched, as this is where the screw should go to prevent blowing out the back wall. A guidewire is placed, and then the 7 × 20 mm cannulated screw is placed. Tension is held on both ends of the graft during screw placement to ensure the graft does not continue to advance into the tunnel. The knee is taken through a ROM to ensure the graft does not impinge. The arthroscope is then removed, and the tibial bone plug is fixed with a 9 × 20 mm metal interference screw. A Lachman and pivot shift are checked to ensure the knee is stable. The incisions are closed in layered fashion, and postoperative hinged knee brace (HKB) is applied.

Following ACLR, the patient is WBAT with the HKB locked in extension for 1 week. They can unlock the brace to work on ROM. At 1 week, the brace can be unlocked for ambulation. Patients begin physical therapy to regain ROM followed by strength immediately. If they are progressing well, they can begin an elliptical and jog at 8 weeks, run/sprint at 10 to 12 weeks, and cut/pivot at 12 weeks. RTS is dictated by return of ROM, strength, and proprioception. If there is any question, patients undergo a functional sports assessment to look at their mechanics for an added data point for understanding when they can RTS.

Results

RTS ranges from 81% to 94% in baseball players following ACLR.[15,22,23] Mei et al found that the average time to return to play was 418 days in Major League Baseball (MLB) players, demonstrating the significant loss of time from sport with these injuries.[23] In a study of MLB players by Fabricant el al, 88% were able to return to play following ACLR. Additionally, it was found that there was a significant reduction in number of games played postoperatively and that there was a decreased batting average after return if the rear leg was the operative extremity.[22]

Complications

Although many players are able to RTS following ACLR, some do have continued pain or loss of motion in the knee. Anterior knee pain and difficulty kneeling is a common problem affecting patients who underwent ACLR using a BTB autograft, while hamstring weakness can affect those who underwent ACLR with a hamstring autograft. Loss of terminal knee extension can impede RTS in these athletes, as failure to fully extend the knee can result in altered running and walking mechanics, quadriceps fatigue, etc. One of the most dreaded complications following ACLR is rerupture. Reruptures are less common on baseball players given the nature of the sport but are still a concern. For this reason, autograft is commonly used as the graft of choice to minimize this risk.

OTHER LIGAMENT INJURIES

Medial Collateral Ligament

Medial collateral ligament (MCL) sprains are relatively common, representing approximately 5.5% of all knee injuries in baseball players.[2] These injuries commonly occur from a valgus stress to the knee and result in a grade 1 sprain. A grade 1 sprain is defined as tenderness localized over the superficial MCL, but no abnormal laxity appreciated on examination.[24] They are described as tension injuries to the medial ligaments of the knee and usually are the result of a direct blow to the lateral knee.[24]

Athletes with MCL sprains often present with localized tenderness and swelling along the medial aspect of the knee. Valgus stress testing of the knee is performed at 30° of knee flexion to isolate the MCL and at 0° of flexion to test for concomitant cruciate ligament injury.[25] Grading the severity of the sprain is based on physical examination findings, with grade 1 sprains having less than 5 mm of medial knee opening with a valgus stress applied at 30° of knee flexion.[26] Radiographs should routinely be performed to rule out fracture, and an MRI may be performed if clinical examination suggests multiligamentous injury.[24]

The majority of athletes who sustain an MCL injury will achieve their preinjury activity level with nonoperative treatment alone.[25] Nonoperative treatment consists of 72 hours of protected weight bearing with rest, ice, and elevation. Following this, the athletes may progress to be WBAT in a hinged knee brace with physical therapy. Players with grade 1 injuries can expect to return to play in 1 to 2 weeks, while it takes a significantly longer period of time to return to play for those with grade 2 and 3 injuries.[26] Although the vast majority of MCL injuries can be treated conservatively, acute repair is indicated in complete tibial-sided avulsion or bony avulsion of the MCL (Figure 26.5).[25] Some athletes will experience concomitant MCL/ACL tears, but nonoperative management even in the setting of concomitant ACL injury has comparable results in terms of stability, without surgical morbidity and with an earlier RTS.[27]

Lateral Collateral Ligament

Grade 1 lateral collateral ligament (LCL) sprains account for 2.1% of all knee injuries in professional baseball players.[2] Isolated high-grade injury to the LCL is very rare, and the high-energy force required typically involves the other additional structures comprising the posterolateral corner of the knee, which include the popliteus tendon, popliteofibular ligament, lateral capsule, and biceps femoris.[28] Most injuries occur by a varus stress to an extended knee, usually resulting from a direct blow to the medial knee.

Athletes with LCL sprains will present with localized pain and swelling to the lateral aspect of the knee. Isolated LCL injuries will have laxity with a varus stress at 30° of flexion and normal findings with varus stress in a fully extended knee, unless the posterolateral corner of knee capsule was injured as well. Radiographs should be performed to rule out fracture. MRI may be performed with high-grade sprains and clinical findings suggestive of multiligamentous injury (Figure 26.6A and B).

Grade 1 and 2 LCL sprains may be treated successfully without surgery.[29] Treatment involves a short period of protected weight bearing with rest, ice, and elevation. Next, the athlete may progress to WBAT with a hinged knee brace and begin physical therapy.

High-grade injuries of the LCL typically involve damage to the cruciate ligaments along with the other structures of the posterolateral corner. These injuries commonly require surgical intervention, which consists of a posterolateral corner reconstruction. This is associated with an extensive recovery period. Methods used for posterolateral corner reconstructions include the anatomic LaPrade and modified Larson techniques.[30]

Chondral Injuries

The incidence and prevalence of symptomatic focal chondral defects in the athletic population is unknown. These lesions are associated with acute traumatic injury and chronic repetitive damage.[31] Chondral defects are found concomitantly in up to 50% of ACL tears.[32] Most commonly, symptomatic focal chondral lesions are associated with a specific traumatic event that resulted in osteochondral fracture.[33] Athletes who sustain a chondral injury will present with a knee effusion and may or may not have examination findings of localized tenderness over the area of the chondral defect. MRI is the imaging study of choice to diagnose chondral injuries of the knee.

Cartilage has little inherent capacity to heal. It is known that a significant decline in function and ability is seen over time in athletes with cartilage injury secondary to the significant repetitive mechanical stresses placed on the joint during sports activity.[31,34] Steroid injections and hyaluronic acid injections are options that can be used for symptom control. Further nonoperative treatment

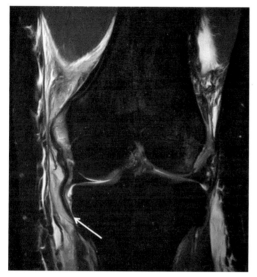

FIGURE 26.5 • Coronal MRI demonstrating a tibial-sided avulsion of the medial collateral ligament (MCL) (arrow).

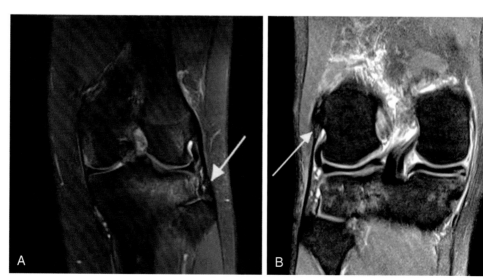

FIGURE 26.6 • Coronal MRI images demonstrating isolated distal (A) and proximal (B) lateral collateral ligament (LCL) injuries (arrows) that were both treated nonoperatively.

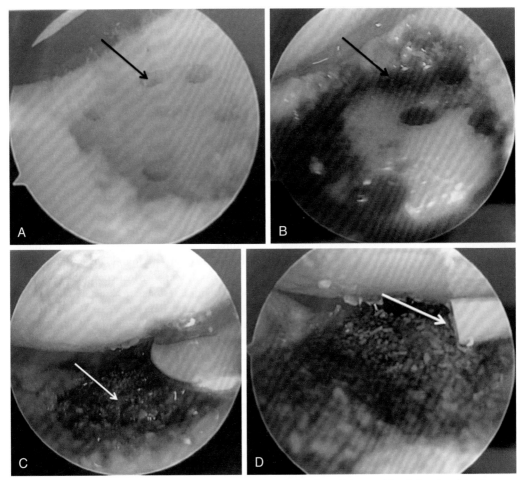

FIGURE 26.7 • A, Arthroscopic image demonstrating a chondral defect of the trochlea following debridement and microfracture. Notice the multiple perforations in the bone (arrow) site. B, Arthroscopic image after the fluid was turned off, which confirms good bleeding from the microfracture sites (arrow). C, Arthroscopic image after the biocartilage was placed and was spread out evenly with the use of a freer (arrow). D, Arthroscopic image demonstrating fibrin glue being inserted over the biocartilage to hold it in place (arrow).

options include PRP and BMAC, which may help return the athlete to sport by decreasing inflammation about the knee and easing the symptoms of the defect.[12,35,36]

The majority of athletes with persistently symptomatic chondral defects will elect for surgical treatment. Approximately 75% of athletes who undergo cartilage restoration surgery return to sport.[32,34] Treatment options include debridement, reparative (microfracture), and restorative procedures. Restorative procedures include biocartilage (Figure 26.7A-D), osteochondral autograft transplantation, osteochondral allograft transplantation (OAT), and matrix autologous chondrocyte implantation (MACI).[33] The particular type of procedure chosen is often dictated by the size and location of the lesion, with lesions on the patella presenting a particularly difficult treatment dilemma. In athletes, the

OAT procedure has been found to be associated with better outcomes and faster return to play when compared with other cartilage interventions.[31,32,34,37] The average RTS for athletes after a cartilage procedure is 9 months. Improved outcomes are seen with smaller defects in younger patients, with a shorter preoperative duration of symptoms, and no prior surgical intervention.[31]

MISCELLANEOUS

Distal Semitendinosus Avulsions

Distal hamstring avulsion injuries are uncommon in baseball players, and most occur in the setting of knee dislocation or multiligament injuries.[38] Distal semitendinosus avulsion injuries, in particular, appear to be associated with elite-level athletes. The mechanism of injury is usually from sprinting or during an extended stride. These injuries are known to cause significant morbidity, and there is scant literature regarding the appropriate treatment.[39]

Athletes will describe feeling a "pop" and having a sharp pain during the act of running. Commonly, there will be pain, difficulty fully straightening the leg, and ambulating. Clinically, there will be swelling and ecchymosis over the medial popliteal region and possibly a tender mass appreciated. Knee flexion will exacerbate symptoms, and resisted knee flexion will demonstrate weakness compared with the contralateral extremity.[39] MRI is used to confirm the diagnosis.

Nonoperative treatment consists of rest and physical therapy. Athletes are allowed to progress to running and sport-specific activities as tolerated. In a study by Cooper et al, it was found that 42% of athletes do not recover after nonoperative treatment. In athletes that did respond to conservative treatment, the average return to play was at 10.4 weeks.[40] The current literature recommends surgical treatment for distal semitendinosus avulsions. As it is known that athletes have little morbidity after harvesting of medial hamstring tendons for ligament reconstructions, treatment involves resection of the avulsed tendon. Some of the complications seen with the harvesting of medial hamstring tendons include residual hamstring weakness, anterior knee pain, and, less commonly, anterior knee numbness.[19] After operative treatment, the average time to return to play for professional baseball players is 6.8 weeks.[40]

Patellar Tendinopathy

Patellar tendinopathy is a prevalent knee condition and was found to have an incidence of approximately 10% when evaluating professional baseball players.[2] This condition is generally referred to as an overuse type of injury and can be a cause of significant morbidity and time lost from play. The diagnosis is made by clinical examination with localized pain at the distal pole of the patella and pain with extension of the knee. Ultrasonography or MRI may be used to aid in diagnosis (Figure 26.8). MRI is preferred secondary to greater sensitivity and the ability to rule out concomitant pathology.[41]

Eccentric quadriceps therapy is effective in most athletes for conservative management. The minimum duration of treatment should be 6 weeks. PRP or shockwave treatment may also be considered as first-line treatment or in cases refractory to physical therapy.[42]

Surgical treatment is only considered if there is no improvement of symptoms after 6 months of therapy.

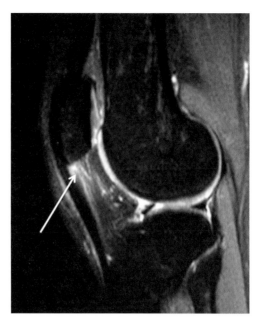

FIGURE 26.8 • Sagittal MRI of a patient with patellar tendonitis demonstrating increased signal at the inferior pole of his patella (arrow).

Options include arthroscopic or open distal patellar debridement. Both interventions have been found to have satisfactory results with arthroscopic debridement resulting in a faster recovery time.[42,43]

REFERENCES

1. Conte S, Requa R, Garrick JG. Disability days in major league baseball. *Am J Sports Med.* 2001;29(4):431-436.
2. Dahm DL, Mayer SW, Tyson JJ, et al. The epidemiology and impact of knee injuries in major and minor league baseball players. *Am J Orthop.* 2016;45(3):E54-E62.
3. Dick R, Sauers EL, Agel J, et al. Descriptive epidemiology of collegiate men's baseball injuries: National Collegiate Athletic Association Injury Surveillance System, 1988-1989 through 2003-2004. *J Athl Train.* 2007;42(2):183-193.
4. Ingram JG, Field SK, Yard EE, et al. Epidemiology of knee injuries among boys and girls in us high school athletics. *Am J Sports Med.* 2008;36(6):1116-1122.
5. McFarland EG, Wasik M. Epidemiology of collegiate baseball injuries. *Clin J Sport Med.* 1998;8(1):10-13.
6. Posner M, Cameron KL, Wolf JM, et al. Epidemiology of major league baseball injuries. *Am J Sports Med.* 2011;39(8):1676-1680.
7. Erickson BJ, Chalmers PN, Bush-Joseph CA, et al. Predicting and preventing injury in major league baseball. *Am J Orthop.* 2016;45(3):152-156.
8. Baker BE, Peckham AC, Pupparo F, et al. Review of meniscal injury and associated sports. *Am J Sports Med.* 1985;13(1):1-4.

9. Mitchell J, Graham W, Best TM, et al. Epidemiology of meniscal injuries in US high school athletes between 2007 and 2013. *Knee Surg Sports Traumatol Arthrosc.* 2016;24(3):715-722.

10. Doherty DB, Lowe WR. Meniscal root tears: identification and repair. *Am J Orthop.* 2016;45(3):183-187.

11. Karachalios T, Hantes M, Zibis AH, et al. Diagnostic accuracy of a new clinical test (the Thessaly test) for early detection of meniscal tears. *J Bone Joint Surg Am.* 2005;87(5):955-962.

12. Hsu WK, Mishra A, Rodeo SR, et al. Platelet-rich plasma in orthopaedic applications: evidence-based recommendations for treatment. *J Am Acad Orthop Surg.* 2013;21:739-748.

13. Greis PE, Holmstrem MC, Bardana DD, et al. Meniscal injury: II. Management. *J Am Acad Orthop Surg.* 2002;10:177-187.

14. Kim SG, Nagao M, Kamata K, et al. Return to sport after arthroscopic meniscectomy on stable knees. *BMC Sports Sci Med Rehabil.* 2013;5(1):23.

15. Dugas JR, Bedford BB, Andrachuk JS, et al. Anterior cruciate ligament injuries in baseball players. *Arthroscopy.* 2016;32(11):2278-2284.

16. Bronstein RD, Schaffer JC. Physical examination of knee ligament injuries. *J Am Acad Orthop Surg.* 2017;25:280-287.

17. Strehl A, Eggli S. The value of conservative treatment in ruptures of the anterior cruciate ligament (ACL). *J Trauma.* 2007;62:1159-1162.

18. Erickson BJ, Harris JD, Fillingham YA, et al. Anterior cruciate ligament reconstruction patterns by NFL and NCAA football team physicians. *Arthroscopy.* 2014;30(6):731-738.

19. Shelton WR, Fagan BC. Autografts commonly used in anterior cruciate ligament reconstruction. *J Am Acad Orthop Surg.* 2011;19:259-264.

20. West RV, Harner CD. Graft selection in anterior cruciate ligament reconstruction. *J Am Acad Orthop Surg.* 2005;13:197-207.

21. Dhawan A, Gallo RA, Lynch SA. Anatomic tunnel placement in anterior cruciate ligament reconstruction. *J Am Acad Orthop Surg.* 2016;24:443-454.

22. Fabricant PD, Chin SC, Conte S, et al. Return to play after anterior cruciate ligament reconstruction in major league baseball athletes. *Arthroscopy.* 2015;31(5):896-900.

23. Mai HT, Chun DS, Schneider AD, et al. Performance-based outcomes after anterior cruciate ligament reconstruction in professional athletes differ between sports. *Am J Sports Med.* 2017;1:363546517704834.

24. Reider B. Medial collateral ligament injuries in athletes. *Sports Med.* 1996;21(2):147-156.

25. Chen L, Kim PD, Ahmad CS, et al. Medial collateral ligament injuries of the knee: current treatment concepts. *Curr Rev Musculoskelet Med.* 2008;1(2):108-113.

26. Roach CJ, Haley CA, Cameron KL, et al. The epidemiology of medial collateral ligament sprains in young athletes. *Am J Sports Med.* 2014;42(5):1103-1109.

27. Scuderi GR, McCann PD. *Sports Medicine: A Comprehensive Approach.* 2nd ed. Philadelphia: Mosby; 2005:346-387.

28. Bushnell BD, Bitting SS, Crain JM, et al. Treatment of magnetic resonance imaging-documented isolated grade III lateral collateral ligament injuries in National Football League athletes. *Am J Sports Med.* 2010;38(1):86-91.

29. Kannus P. Nonoperative treatment of grade II and III sprains of the lateral collateral ligament compartment of the knee. *Am J Sports Med.* 1989;17(1):83-88.

30. Crespo B, James EW, Metsavaht L. Injuries to posterolateral corner of the knee: a comprehensive review from anatomy to surgical treatment. *Rev Bras Ortop.* 2014;50(4):363-370.

31. Harris JD, Brophy RH, Siston RA, et al. Treatment of chondral defects in the athlete's knee. *Arthroscopy.* 2010;26(6):841-852.

32. Krych AJ, Pareek A, King AH, Johnson NR, Stuart MJ, Williams RJ III. Return to sport after the surgical management of articular cartilage lesions in the knee: a meta-analysis. *Knee Surg Sports Traumatol Arthrosc.* 2017;25(10):3186-3196.

33. Alford JW, Cole BJ. Cartilage restoration, part 2: techniques, outcomes, and future directions. *Am J Sports Med.* 2005;33(3):443-460.

34. Mithoefer K, Hambly K, Della Villa S, et al. Return to sports participation after articular cartilage repair in the knee: scientific evidence. *Am J Sports Med.* 2009;37(suppl 1):167S-176S.

35. Chahla J, Dean CS, Moatshe G, et al. Concentrated bone marrow aspirate for the treatment of chondral injuries and osteoarthritis of the knee: a systematic review of outcomes. *Orthop J Sports Med.* 2016;4(1):2325967115625481.

36. Dold AP, Zywiel MG, Taylor DW, et al. Platelet-rich plasma in the management of articular cartilage pathology: a systematic review. *Clin J Sport Med.* 2014;24(1):31-43.

37. Gudas R, Stankevicius E, Monastyreckiene E, et al. Osteochondral autologous transplantation versus microfracture for the treatment of articular cartilage defects in the knee joint in athletes. *Knee Surg Sports Traumatol Arthrosc.* 2006;14:834-842.

38. Sivasundaram L, Matcuk GR, White EA, et al. Partial semitendinosus tendon tear in a young athlete: a case report and review of the distal semitendinosus anatomy. *Skeletal Radiol.* 2015;44:1051-1056.

39. Lempainen L, Sarimo J, Mattila K, et al. Distal tears of the hamstring muscles: review of the literature and our results of surgical treatment. *Br J Sports Med.* 2007;41(2):80-83.

40. Cooper DE, Conway JE. Distal semitendinosus ruptures in elite-level athletes: low success rates of nonoperative treatment. *Am J Sports Med*. 2010;38(6):1174-1178.

41. Figueroa D, Figueroa F, Calvo R. Patellar tendinopathy: diagnosis and treatment. *J Am Acad Orthop Surg*. 2016;24:e184-e192.

42. Everhart JS, Cole D, Sojka JH, et al. Treatment options for patellar tendinopathy: a systematic review. *Arthroscopy*. 2017;33(4):861-872.

43. Pascarella A, Alam M, Pascarella F, Latte C, Di Salvatore MG, Maffulli N. Arthroscopic management of chronic patellar tendinopathy. *Am J Sports Med*. 2011;39(9):1975-1983.

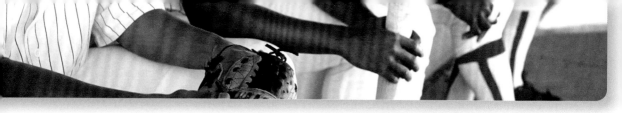

CHAPTER 27

Leg Injuries in Baseball Players

James Irvine, MD | T. Sean Lynch, MD

Control is what kept me in the big leagues for twenty-two years.

—*Cy Young*

INTRODUCTION

Our appreciation of lower extremity injuries in collegiate and professional baseball players has greatly evolved in recent years. Early data published on this topic was compiled from the National Collegiate Athletic Association (NCAA) Injury Surveillance System, which reviewed 17 seasons from 1988 through 2004.[16] The authors showed that 35.2% of game day injuries involved the lower extremity.[16] While the incidence of lower leg injuries were behind the upper extremity, these lower extremity injuries were found to be more severe with a higher prevalence of 10+ days (19.7%) out from play when compared with shoulder and elbow injuries (14.3%). McFarland and Wasik analyzed injury data from 3 collegiate baseball seasons and reported a similar incidence of lower extremity injuries at 31%.[43]

At the professional baseball level, limited epidemiologic studies were available before 2010. In collaboration with MLB (Major League Baseball) and its Players Association (MLBPA) as well as Minor League Baseball (MiLB), MLB Injury Surveillance System and Health and Injury Tracking System (HITS) was implemented. HITS keeps track of all MLB and MiLB players medical history and injuries with the goal of optimizing treatment algorithms, which may aid in safe return to play and the development of injury prevention programs. Dahm et al reviewed HITS data from 2011 to 2014 with a focus on knee injuries and reported that 44% of knee injuries were noncontact, with injuries occurring in the infield causing the most time away from sport.[15] Base runners were at greatest risk for sustaining a knee injury.

MLB Baseball rule 7.13 is a prime example of how injury data from the HITS database were used to change rules in the name of injury prevention. This particular rule focuses on reducing collisions at home plate between the base runner and catcher by not allowing the base runner to run into the catcher if he has an avoidable path to home plate, or else the runner is called out. The rule also states that the catcher cannot block the path to home plate if they do not have possession of the ball. In 2011, analysis of HITS data on these specific collisions revealed that 23 knee injuries occurred from collisions at home plate, and these injuries reduced to a total of 2 injuries in 2014 when rule 7.13 went into effect. As more data become available, additional changes to the game are likely to occur in an effort to maximize player safety.

MUSCLE INJURIES OVERVIEW

Muscle injuries to the lower leg of baseball players are composed of direct trauma as in the case of a contusion, as well as muscular strain, which may occur through an indirect mechanism. Within this injury spectrum, there are also muscle tears, ruptures, and cramps. Muscle injuries are incredibly common with contusion/hematoma recently reported as the most frequent knee-related injury at 30.5%, which resulted in an average of 6 days missed. When analyzing HITS data, muscle strain, tear, rupture, and cramps were lumped as a common diagnosis and accounted for 1.1% of all knee-related injuries with an average of 9.9 days missed.[15]

Contusions or hematomas may result from being hit by a pitch, collision with another player, base pad, or any structure surrounding the perimeter of the field. These traumatic impacts result in significant muscle damage, so prompt diagnosis and management is critical for both pain control and minimizing time

TABLE 27.1 Grade of Muscle Strain With Associated MRI Findings

Grade of Muscle Strain	Muscle Fiber Injury	MRI Findings
1	Few fibers torn	Edema but no architectural disruption
2	Moderate number of fibers torn	Edema and architectural disruption
3	Complete tear	Total muscle or tendon rupture

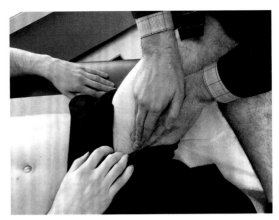

FIGURE 27.1 • An examiner palpates the adductor muscles to assess for strains along the muscle or tendon

away from sport. A major sequela of these injuries is the development of myositis ossificans, which can be present if the player is not getting better within 7 to 10 days or if pain increases in subsequent weeks. Myositis ossificans has been reported in 9% to 17% of contusions.[7]

Strains and tears may occur when a sudden burst of energy is needed to make a play such as leaping on the wall to prevent a home run, running after a fly ball, or trying to steal a base (Table 27.1).[17] Injury may also occur from a noncontact mechanism such as when trying to avoid collisions and inadvertently placing muscles and tendons under maximal strain, which results in muscle tearing or even tendon avulsions. Biarticular (span 2 joints) fast twitch muscles such as the rectus femoris and gastrocnemius are at the greatest risk when undergoing an eccentric contraction, and these muscle injuries occur most commonly at the musculotendinous junction.[32,55]

Contusions and strains regardless of their size cause trauma to underlying blood vessels, resulting in bleeding in the surrounding muscles. This is the basis for rest, ice, compression, and elevation (RICE), which is aimed at minimizing hematoma formation and fluid accumulation to optimize the healing environment and avoid further trauma to the soft tissues. An ideal period of rest is approximately 1 week to allow for early healing, but range of motion should promptly follow to optimize muscle regeneration and avoid scar formation.[1,35,36]

UPPER LEG STRAINS AND CONTUSIONS

Adductor Strain

Adductor strain is the most common extra-articular groin injury accounting for 40.8% of all extra-articular hip and groin injuries according to a recent review of all MiLB and MLB players.[12] The function of the adductor muscle complex is to help stabilize the pelvis while walking and running. It works in coordination with the abdominal muscles, which attach to the anterior ring of the pelvis.[42] These injuries are classically associated with soccer owing to the cutting and pivoting maneuvers required during a match, but the HITS data revealed that they are also a common cause of injury among professional baseball players. Coleman et al reported that infielders more commonly sustained hip and groin injuries compared with other positions and that the pitcher's mound was the single most common location for these injuries.[12] This finding highlights the importance of a pitcher's core strength and surrounding hip and groin musculature for stabilizing his pelvis while pitching.

Adductor strains result in acute medial groin pain. Clinical examination may reveal pain to palpation over the pubis at the adductor insertion and along the muscle belly as well as painful resisted adduction (Figure 27.1). Passive range of motion of the hip in the acute setting can be very painful. A thorough examination is critical because athletic pubalgia/sports hernias and femoroacetabular impingement can have overlapping symptoms in players who may be suffering from a combination of underlying pathology. One radiographic study evaluating athletes with chronic adductor pain noticed underlying FAI findings in 94% of patients.[60] FAI has been associated with decreased hip range of motion, which puts the adductor and hamstring muscles at risk, as the body tries to compensate for underlying mechanical blockage.[28] Further workup includes X-ray and magnetic resonance imaging (MRI) to help make an accurate diagnosis.

Nonoperative management consists of rest, ice, compression, and anti-inflammatory medications followed by range of motion exercise to avoid stiffness.

As the pain begins to abate, the player may begin a multimodal approach to rehabilitation with the initial priority on regaining full range of motion, followed by a strengthening program, and finally functional activities.[5] Coleman et al reported an average of 12.4 days missed from play when compared with 66.6 days in the rare instance that surgery was required.[12]

Quadriceps Strain

Quadriceps strain in professional baseball players accounts for less than 1% of knee-related injuries according to HITS data.[12] They may result from a sudden change in body position requiring knee flexion and hip extension coupled with an eccentric muscle contraction.[38] These injuries can occur anywhere along the group of quadriceps muscles but has a predilection for the rectus femoris because it is the only biarticular muscle of the quadriceps. The most common site of injury is the musculotendinous junction of the rectus femoris in the distal thigh.[32] In addition to injuries during a baseball game, quadriceps strains may also occur from excessive passive stretching during warm-ups.[38]

Players are likely to complain of pain in their anterior thigh, which is reproducible with palpation. A more indolent presentation may not bring it to player's attention until the end of the game or practice. Meanwhile, high-grade strains or an avulsion may leave the player on the ground without the ability to ambulate unassisted.[29] Clinical examination is usually sufficient with the athlete having tenderness over the site of the muscle strain and possibly a palpable defect with high-grade strains or avulsion/tendon rupture. Advanced imaging such as MRI would be indicated in the acute setting if the athlete has a palpable defect or there is concern for complete or near-complete tear of the quadriceps.[38] This may also be extended to the player with chronic thigh pain that has failed to resolve with conservative management.

Quadriceps strains at the musculotendinous junction are treated nonsurgically with RICE in the active phase, which is generally the first 24 to 72 hours. Avulsion injuries at the anterior inferior iliac spice (AIIS) with less than 2 cm of retraction may also be treated conservatively, whereas greater tendon retraction is less likely to heal without surgical intervention.[25] Strains and minimally avulsed tendons may undergo a graduated physical therapy program. Once the pain is under control, they can begin stretching, range of motion, and a sequential strengthening program that advances through isometric, isotonic, isokinetic, and then functional activities. A pain-free range of motion should be maintained throughout the player's rehabilitation. Injury-specific

rehabilitation should be accompanied by aerobic fitness such as swimming to aid in recovery and health. Case series of both acute surgical repair and nonoperative management of avulsion injuries have been studied in professional soccer and football players, respectively with good results in both groups; however, larger studies comparing these 2 options are still needed.[25,33]

Following rehabilitation, players should have full and pain-free knee range of motion, nearly equal side-to-side strength testing, and be able to perform all functional requirements of their position before return to game play. The study by Dahm et al listed muscle strains, tears, ruptures, and cramps around the knee as a single diagnosis and determined an average of 9.9 days missed for players with these injuries.[15]

Quadriceps Contusion

Contusion around the knee is the most common knee-related injury among professional baseball players.[15] They accounted for 30.5% of all knee-related injuries, but the specific percentage involving the quadriceps was not specified by the HITS data. Quadriceps contusions may result from being hit by a pitch, collision with another player or any object surrounding the field. The trauma results in muscle injury and is accompanied by hematoma formation.[36] The mechanism is important in these injuries because it has been shown that active quadriceps contraction at the time of injury has the ability to absorb more of the blunt force and result in a less severe injury.[7]

Players are usually able to recall the traumatic event associated with a quadriceps contusion and may complain of localized pain, swelling, and decreased range of motion. They are also likely to have pain to palpation of the surrounding area, but the amount of active knee flexion that the player can perform is more diagnostic of injury severity. Mild injuries are associated with knee flexion greater than 90° and normal gait, while severe injuries are associated with less than 45 degrees of knee flexion and an antalgic gait.[34]

These injuries need to be managed actively during the first 24 hours with the affected knee placed into 120 degrees of knee flexion, which may be achieved with a locked hinged knee brace or an elastic compression wrap (Figure 27.2).[3,37,54] Standard ice and compression will also aid in minimizing hematoma formation and pain control. Immobilization should be discontinued after 24 hours and proceed with active pain-free range of motion plus quadriceps stretching and isometric strengthening. Functional rehabilitation should be held until 120 degrees of knee flexion can be accomplished without pain.

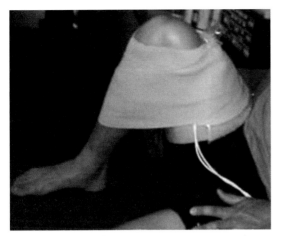

FIGURE 27.2 • An elastic compression wrap can be used to maintain 120 degrees of knee flexion for the first 24 hours after a quadriceps contusion, which aims to minimize hematoma formation as well as pain.

Studies have shown that the addition of NSAIDs may help prevent myositis ossificans following severe muscle contusion (Figure 27.3).[7,57] This sequela should be considered if pain is not improving after a week or if the player experiences a relatively pain-free period followed by an atraumatic increase in pain around the original site of trauma.[13]

In warrior athletes from West Point, cadets were able to return to play within 13 to 21 days.[54] HITS data on knee contusion and hematoma have shown that professional baseball players had an average of 6.0 days missed; however, a limitation of this system was that there is no specific category for quadriceps.[15] Regardless of severity, they should have at least 120° of pain-free flexion and be able to perform all functional activities related to their position before return to play.

Hamstring Strain

Ahmad et al reported that hamstring strains are the most common injury among MLB and MiLB players, which result in significant time loss from the game.[2] In-depth analysis of HITS data revealed that two-thirds of hamstring strains occurred during base running with a majority happening while running to first base. The detailed mechanism is an ongoing area of study, but research on the biomechanics of sprinting has shown that the hamstrings are at risk during the end of swing phase, as this position places the muscle under maximal stretch coupled with an eccentric contraction before heel strike.[30,64]

In mild presentations, the player may recall a "pull" and feel pain in the back of his mid-thigh. A stiff-legged gait is associated with a more severe strain or possibly

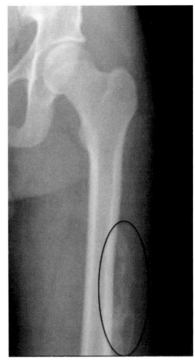

FIGURE 27.3 • An AP radiograph of the left proximal femur taken 6 weeks after injury shows myositis ossificans (black oval) along the lateral aspect of the thigh.

avulsion, as he is trying to avoid flexing his hip. Severe strains may also develop swelling and ecchymosis and have reproducible pain to palpation over the involved posterior thigh (Figure 27.4).[11] Additionally, active range of knee motion with the hip flexed and in the supine position can be utilized to diagnose a hamstring injury (Figures 27.5 and 27.6).[58] Avulsions are important to recognize, and if there is any uncertainty, X-rays may be obtained to assess for bony avulsion off of the ischium, but more commonly an MRI should be performed to diagnose strain severity as well as for presence of tendon avulsion (Figures 27.7 and 27.8A, B).[52]

Fortunately, strains of the musculotendinous junction account for about 90% of proximal hamstring injuries and have better outcomes compared with multiple tendon avulsion injuries, which generally require surgery.[39] Treatment protocols for nonoperative management begin with RICE in the acute phase to minimize hemorrhage and swelling. Stretching and passive range of motion is utilized to avoid stiffness, and isometric strengthening allows for minimal to pain-free muscle contraction to help avoid atrophy. This is followed by full active range of motion as well as isotonic and isokinetic strengthening. During this process, the muscle continues to remodel and strengthen to allow for eccentric loading of the muscle before introduction of functional activities.

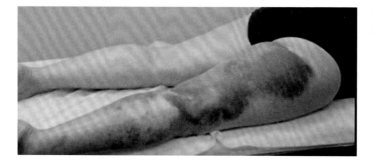

FIGURE 27.4 • Posterior thigh ecchymosis from hamstrings avulsion injury.

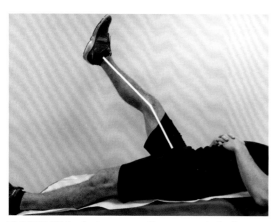

FIGURE 27.5 • Active range of motion with the hip flexed to 90° and the knee extended. This represents normal hamstring function.

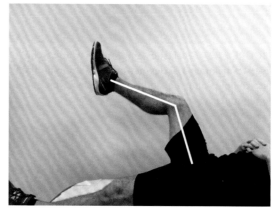

FIGURE 27.6 • Active range of motion with the hip flexed to 90° and the knee extended. The patient is unable to fully extend the knee as a result of a proximal hamstring injury.

Surgical repair is typically warranted in cases of 2 or 3 tendons involved with more than 2 cm of retraction; meanwhile, single tendon injuries can usually avoid surgical intervention.[11] Earlier surgical intervention is favored to aid surgical repair and to optimize the chance of healing and minimize scar tissue formation between tendon and sciatic nerve. After surgery, athletes are braced for approximately 6 weeks to avoid hip flexion and knee extension that will stress the repair. Strengthening can be implemented around 3 weeks with return to play at 6 to 9 months.

Utilizing HITS data, Ahmad et al found that professional baseball players missed 24 to 27 days for these injuries, which is almost twice the number of days of an National Football League (NFL) player (13.2 days).[2,18] It is important to keep this 24- to 27-day range in mind when considering the timing of return to play in baseball players, especially since the data have shown a 20% recurrence rate when comparing the 2010 and 2011 seasons. Rushing the player back too soon will most likely increase his chances of reinjury, which usually requires a longer period of recovery than the initial injury. Baseball players should be able to perform all functional activities of their position as well as run the bases pain free before their return to play.

LOWER LEG STRAINS

Gastrocnemius, Plantaris, and Soleus Strains

The calf muscles are composed of the gastrocnemius, plantaris, and soleus muscles and are collectively known as the *triceps surae*. Their aponeuroses unite to form the Achilles tendon, which attaches distally onto the calcaneus. Strains of the calf most commonly involve the medial head of the gastrocnemius muscle. The anatomical origins and insertion of the gastrocnemius are biarthrodial (crosses the knee and ankle joints), which places players at increased risk for these injuries when the knee is fully extended and the foot is dorsiflexed due to maximal stretch of the muscle.[9] Similarly, the plantaris muscle also spans the knee and ankle joints but is a rare injury and has been grouped along with calf strains. The soleus muscle is the other remaining calf muscle and is different in that it only crosses the ankle joint but, like the plantaris, is exceedingly rare compared with strains of the gastrocnemius.[10] The incidence of lower leg strains is seemingly low in professional baseball players, given their lack

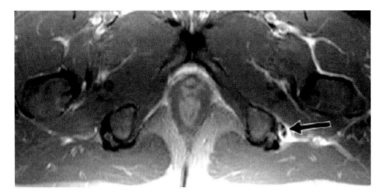

FIGURE 27.7 • Transverse fat-suppressed T2-weighted image at the level of the ischial tuberosity in a 23-year-old outfielder with a high-grade strain of the semimembranosus but no evidence of tendon avulsion. Arrow demonstrates a high grade strain at the origin of the semimembranosus.

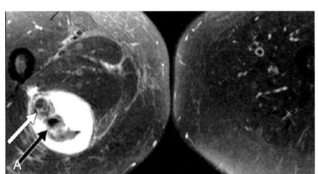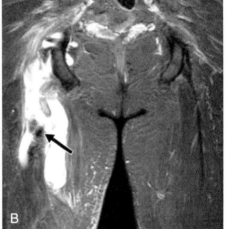

FIGURE 27.8 • A, Transverse fat-suppressed T2-weighted image through the proximal thigh in a 26-year-old pitcher with acute proximal hamstrings avulsion. Imaging demonstrates a large hematoma around the retracted semimembranosus tendon (black arrow) and sciatic nerve (white arrow). B, Coronal STIR image shows distal retraction of torn hamstring tendon (black arrow), with large surrounding hematoma.

of discussion in the published epidemiologic works regarding MLB injuries.

Players will complain of a pop in their calf while running and may be able to localize the area of injury by palpation. Given the small size of the plantaris, it is often difficult to isolate it as the source of injury without advanced imaging such as MRI or ultrasound. Meanwhile, a player's history coupled with examination findings should help distinguish between gastrocnemius and soleus strains.[10] Painful palpation of the medial head of the gastrocnemius is fairly diagnostic while pain about the lateral aspect of the calf is more commonly associated with soleus strains (Figure 27.9).[9,19] Stressing the calf with specific motor strength testing can also help determine the diagnosis. Testing the foot in plantarflexion under maximal knee flexion isolates the soleus muscle; full knee extension allows for more focused testing of the gastrocnemius (Figures 27.10 and 27.11).[10]

RICE is an important early intervention to help minimize bleeding, swelling, and pain. Passive stretching and isometric strengthening can be introduced as the pain is resolving in the acute period. The subacute phase introduces isotonic and isokinetic exercises to allow for continued muscle healing as well as gradual strengthening.[10] Eventually, functional activities are introduced with the timeline dependent on the severity of the injury and the athlete's progression with therapy.

THE USE OF PLATELET-RICH PLASMA FOR LOWER EXTREMITY INJURIES

Platelet-rich plasma (PRP) is a form of growth factor therapy, which is composed of autologous blood cells with a high concentration of platelets. Platelets contain multiple growth factors including

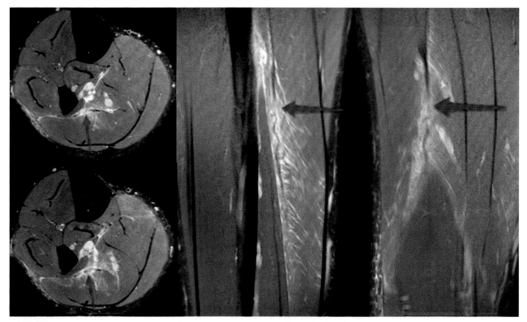

FIGURE 27.9 • Transverse and coronal fat-suppressed T2-weighted images through the lower leg with high-grade strain of the soleus. Edema and collagen fiber disruption within the lateral portion of the soleus muscle (red arrows).

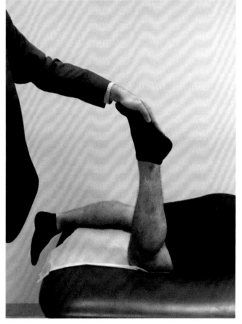

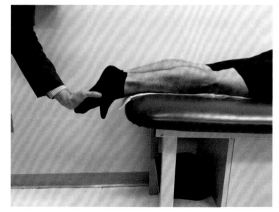

FIGURE 27.11 • Strength testing of the gastrocnemius is performed with knee extension and in the prone position.

FIGURE 27.10 • Isolated strength testing of the soleus muscle is performed with knee flexion and in the prone position.

platelet-derived growth factor (PDGF), fibroblast growth factor (FGF), epidermal growth factor, insulinlike growth factor 1 (IGF-1), vascular endothelial growth factor (VEGF), and transforming growth factor β1 (TGF-β1).[22] These growth factors are known to play critical roles in the healing process of musculoskeletal tissues. For example, in the case of tendon healing, FGF helps promote collagen production to aid in repair while VEGF is able to stimulate angiogenesis, which helps bring in additional nutrients necessary for matrix production. Histamine and serotonin are also released from the platelets, which increase local capillary permeability and thus further aid in local tissue repair.[22] In addition to the growth factor–rich platelets, PRP also contains leukocytes, neutrophils, and red blood cells. From the bench to the bedside, there is still a lot of work to be done to

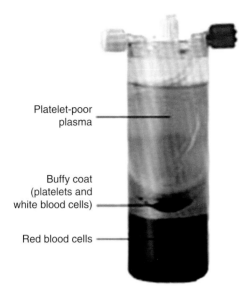

Platelet-poor plasma

Buffy coat (platelets and white blood cells)

Red blood cells

FIGURE 27.12 • Platelet-rich plasma in GPS kit after centrifugation. (GPS III is a product of Biomet Orthopedics Warsaw, IN.)

unlock the full potential of PRP. Research is currently underway to better understand the clinical impact of these additional components in an effort to optimize the healing response.[27]

A recent review of commercially available PRP extraction kits analyzed platelet and white blood cell composition to better characterize the final end product.[21] At the time of the study, there were only 4 commercially available products in the testing country and they included GPS III (Biomet Biologics), SmartPrep2 (Terumo Harvest), Magellan (Arteriocyte Medical Systems), and ACP (Device Technologies, Arthrex). The plasma-based system (ACP) is unique among these products in that it increased platelets by approximately 1.5-fold and decreased white blood cell count by 5 to 22 times. In comparison, the other extraction products are known to take from the "buffy layer," which is more cellular and not only increases platelets by 3 to 6 times but also increases white blood cells 3 to 5 times the baseline. These differences in the relatively acellular plasma layer versus buffy coat after centrifugation can be appreciated in the sample shown in Figure 27.12.

The effect of white blood cells in the sample is an active area of investigation, as they may aid in signal modulation and tissue repair. The leukocyte-rich PRP (LR-PRP) kits are most effective for tendinopathy treatment according to a recent meta-analysis, while early reports have demonstrated that leukocyte-poor PRP (LP PRP) may benefit those with osteoarthritis.[20,44,50] Additional studies are

needed to provide optimal patient-specific treatments based on diagnosis.

Studies looking at the impact of PRP on NFL player return to play after incomplete hamstring injury have yielded inconsistent results.[45,49] Mejia and Bradley found a 1-game difference in return to play after PRP injections for MRI grade 1 or 2 injuries in their sample size of 12 players.[45] In contrast, a small case-control study of 10 NFL players with acute hamstring injuries compared PRP plus rehabilitation program with a rehabilitation program alone and found a median return to play of 20 days for the PRP group and 17 days in the non-PRP group.[49] Larger, randomized controlled trials are warranted for hamstring injuries as well as other tendinopathies given the limited availability of high-level studies.

LOWER LEG PAIN DISORDERS

Medial Tibial Stress Syndrome (Shin Splints)

Stress-related disorders of the tibia fall into a spectrum of overuse injuries. Medial tibial stress syndrome (MTSS), commonly referred to as shin splints, can be grouped with tibial stress reaction and tibial stress fractures. It is a common source of exertional-related leg pain in athletes with an incidence ranging from 20% to 44% in active populations.[31,61,62] The exact etiology is still a topic of debate, but some believe it to arise as a response to traction from lower leg muscles and resulting in enthesopathy and periostitis. Meanwhile, a radiographic study using CT scans revealed a relative osteopenia of the anterior tibial cortex (Figure 27.13).[41] Clinically, it is associated with pain along the posteromedial border of the tibia that manifests from prolonged running.

Initial treatment strategies for MTSS are based on prospective studies from the military.[61,62] Treatment consists of rest with rehabilitation emphasizing calf stretching and strengthening and then gradual return of running. A recent prospective investigation of runners demonstrated that 37 of 38 participants had an average recovery period of 72 days before cessation of symptoms.[46] In chronic cases of more than 6 months in duration, extracorporeal shock wave therapy has shown to be beneficial over home therapies with an underlying theory that it induces microfractures in the trabecular bone, which induces a healing response.[51] Players should be able to fully participate in all functional

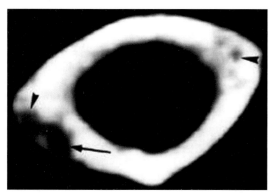

FIGURE 27.13 • CT scan image of a 23-year-old male runner with an 18-day history of worsening pain in the left tibia. A transverse 2-mm-thick high-spatial resolution CT scan through the mid-tibia demonstrates areas of osteopenia within the anterior and posterior cortices (arrowheads). Some areas have greater than 50% cortical thickness involvement (arrow).

TABLE 27.2 Fredericson MRI Classification Table of Tibial Stress Injuries

Grade of Stress Injury	MRI Findings
0	No abnormality
1	Periosteal edema with no associated bone marrow signal abnormalities
2	Periosteal edema and bone marrow edema visible only on T2-weighted images
3	Periosteal edema and bone marrow edema visible on both T1-weighted and T2-weighted images
4a	Multiple focal areas of intracortical signal abnormality and bone marrow edema visible on both T1-weighted and T2-weighted images
4b	Linear areas of intracortical signal abnormality and bone marrow edema visible on both T1-weighted and T2-weighted images

activities of their fielding position and run the base pads without reproduction of their pain before return to play.

Tibial Stress Reaction

Further along this spectrum of tibial disorders has been described as a tibial stress reaction. While shin splints are classically symptomatic during intense activity, tibial stress reactions may be painful with walking and activities of daily living. MRI studies have shown it to go beyond the anterior tibial cortex to include the underlying bone marrow. Fredericson et al graded tibial stress disorders based on review of MRI, with grades 1, 2, and 3 representing progressive tibial stress reactions and grade 4 being a stress fracture (Table 27.2).[23]

Surprisingly enough, athletes may not always complain of pain in the setting of tibial stress reactions. In a study of collegiate long-distance runners, MRIs were obtained of asymptomatic athletes and 9 of the 21 subjects (43%) had MRI changes, which demonstrated increased edema in the periosteum and bone marrow changes.[8] Thus, players with this condition may or may not present with pain over the medial aspect of the tibia, but tibial stress disorders should be in the differential diagnosis of a baseball player with atraumatic tibial pain. Symptomatic athletes will also have reproduction of their symptoms with palpation over the involved area. Low-grade tibial stress reactions may be missed because they are often asymptomatic, but for those who present with pain, they may need to refrain from sport for 4 to 6 weeks or until symptoms resolve. During this time, they may remain weight bearing as tolerated. For higher grade stress reactions, they should be treated similarly to a stress fracture, which includes non–weight bearing with possible need for surgical intervention. Similarly to MTSS, players should be able to perform all of their functional activities pain free before return to play.

Tibial Stress Fracture

In its most severe form, stress injuries of the tibia may advance to stress fractures. These overuse injuries are more likely to surface in baseball players during spring training when these athletes are returning from a period of relative inactivity and engaging in intense strengthening and conditioning. In an evaluation of runners with these stress fractures, athletes typically demonstrate Achilles tendon stiffness, decreased Achilles tendon elongation with maximal isometric contraction, and plantar-flexor stiffness, which impair normal gait mechanics and impart increased levels of stress to the tibia.[47]

Players will complain of increasing pain about their posteromedial tibia that is worse with intense activity and can cause discomfort with normal ambulation. Plain radiographs, MRI, and CT scan may provide the diagnosis (Figure 27.14).[56] Routine blood work should be evaluated to assess calcium and vitamin D, and parathyroid hormone levels assess for underlying deficiencies or metabolic disorders that may be either correctable risk factors or modifiable conditions. Baseball players should consume a minimum of 1000 mg of

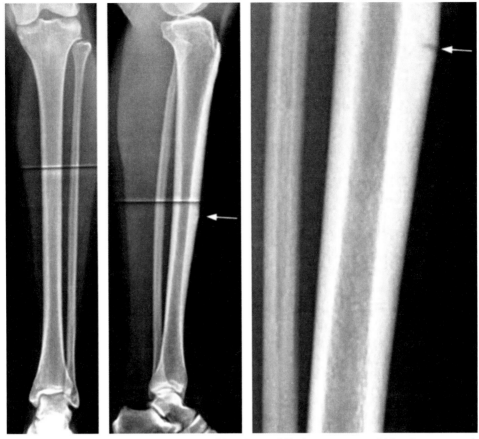

FIGURE 27.14 • Plain AP and lateral radiographs of the tibia and fibula in a 23-year-old first baseman with an anterior tibial stress fracture (white arrows).

calcium and 600 IU of vitamin D a day; however, higher doses might be necessary, as recent prospective studies have shown a 20% decrease in the incidence of stress fractures in those who consumed 2000 mg of calcium and 1000 IU of vitamin D daily.[24,40]

In addition to proper nutrition, rest and restricted weight bearing is beneficial. Both pulsed ultrasound and electronic shock wave therapy have been studied in the treatment of these injuries, but neither has proven to be beneficial in the acute setting.[6,53] The time to heal and return to play can be dictated by stress fracture location with ones involving the anterior tibial cortex more at risk for nonunion than those of the posteromedial cortex. Those involving the anterior cortex of the tibia have a reported nonunion rate as high as 60% and may take upward of 12 months to heal. Therefore, it is important to diagnose these injuries to have a discussion with the player and team regarding the risks of delayed healing as well as introduce the idea of surgical treatment. The player is typically out for 10 to 12 weeks after surgery with options including intramedullary

nail as well as anterior-tension band plating (Figure 27.15).[14,63] Return to play should be avoided until the player has pain-free functional activity.

Chronic Exertional Compartment Syndrome

Chronic exertional compartment syndrome (CECS) is a unique cause of lower leg pain. Different theories have been proposed as to the underlying pathophysiological mechanism. It is commonly believed to be an exercise-induced increase in intracompartmental pressure that hinders adequate perfusion resulting in pain, but nuclear medicine studies have failed to demonstrate consistent ischemic changes in these patients following exercise.[4,26] Regardless of the mechanism, it commonly causes bilateral lower leg pain, which differentiates it from tibial stress–related disorders. Athletes will also describe a fullness in their calves with possible paresthesias with activity. It should be considered in any baseball player presenting with chronic anterior or lateral lower leg pain that is worse with exercise and goes away following cessation of activity.

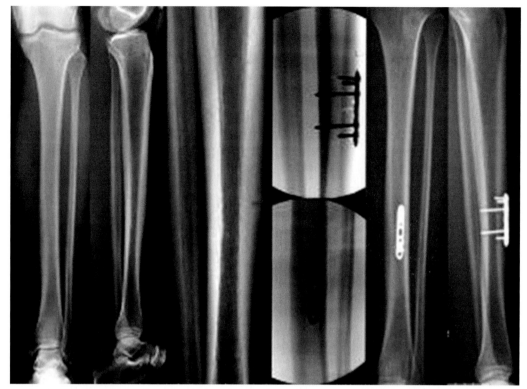

FIGURE 27.15 • A Division I College Baseball outfielder who failed 1 year of nonoperative treatment of an anterior tibial stress fracture. The images to the left demonstrate the stress fracture whereas the ones on the right are following open reduction and internal fixation with a 2.7-mm plate and screws in tension band mode.

The clinical objective assessment for CECS most commonly involves an invasive intracompartmental pressure measurement with a Stryker needle (Figure 27.16). The criteria for the diagnosis of CECS are based on compartment pressure monitoring as described by Pedowitz.[48] In the presence of appropriate clinical findings, the presence of 1 or more of the following intramuscular pressure criteria is considered diagnostic: (1) a pre-exercise pressure greater than or equal to 15 mm Hg, (2) a 1-minute postexercise pressure of greater than or equal to 30 mm Hg, or (3) a 5-minute postexercise pressure greater than or equal to 20 mm Hg. Although the Pedowitz criteria are considered the "gold standard," recent studies have shown that continuous measurements during simulated activities are even more beneficial.[48]

Once a baseball player has been diagnosed with CECS, it is important to gauge the impact on his ability to play the game. Truly debilitating cases may warrant surgical fasciotomies to help alleviate their symptoms, but the player should understand that this approach does not always cure the problem. Research on a military population comprising 611 patients with CECS reported that 44.7% had recurrence after fasciotomy and 27.7% could not get back to their previous activity

level.[59] Nonoperative management includes participating in less intense activities and, in some instances, changing sport or activity to avoid the impact levels that provoke their symptoms. Avoidance of excessive high-impact activities and supplementing with lower impact exercise such as the stationary bike is a way of augmenting training to maintain health and avoid recurrence of CECS. A baseball player's return to play from CECS is driven by his ability to participate in full functional activities without debilitating pain.

In conclusion, lower extremity injuries are common among professional baseball players, with hamstring strains representing the most frequent event requiring time away from the game. Fortunately, these injuries rarely require surgical intervention, but it is vital to treat all injuries appropriately to allow the athlete to return to play expeditiously, but without the risk of recurrence. Additionally, changes on the field, such as rule 7.13, has reduced collision-associated injuries at home plate, while ongoing research into PRP off the field is geared toward aiding player recovery and reducing time away from the game. The combination of data analysis and advances in therapeutic treatments will continue to evolve the game by increasing player safety and optimizing rehabilitation protocols.

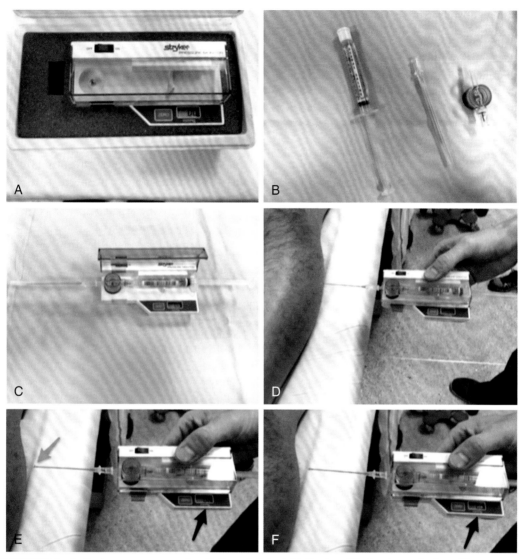

FIGURE 27.16 • A, Stryker pressure monitor. B, From left to right: 3-ml prefilled syringe of saline, 18-gauge needle and diaphragm chamber. C, Assembled pressure monitor. D, Hold monitor parallel to the floor. E, Purge all air in the system until drops of saline are seen at the end of the needle (blue arrow). Please notice that the monitor no longer reads 00 mm Hg (black arrow). F, Zero the monitor and confirm the reading is back to "00 mm Hg" (black arrow) in preparation for compartment pressure measurement.

REFERENCES

1. Aarimaa V, Rantanen J, Best T, Schultz E, Corr D, Kalimo H. Mild eccentric stretch injury in skeletal muscle causes transient effects on tensile load and cell proliferation. *Scand J Med Sci Sports*. 2004;14(6): 367-372.

2. Ahmad CS, Dick RW, Snell E, et al. Major and minor league baseball hamstring injuries: epidemiologic findings from the major league baseball injury surveillance system. *Am J Sports Med*. 2014;42(6):1464-1470.

3. Almekinders LC, Gilbert JA. Healing of experimental muscle strains and the effects of nonsteroidal antiinflammatory medication. *Am J Sports Med*. 1986;14(4):303-308.

4. Amendola A, Rorabeck CH, Vellett D, Vezina W, Rutt B, Nott L. The use of magnetic resonance imaging in exertional compartment syndromes. *Am J Sports Med*. 1990;18(1):29-34.

5. Anderson K, Strickland SM, Warren R. Hip and groin injuries in athletes. *Am J Sports Med*. 2001;29(4):521-533.

6. Beck BR, Matheson GO, Bergman G, et al. Do capacitively coupled electric fields accelerate tibial stress fracture healing? A randomized controlled trial. *Am J Sports Med*. 2008;36(3):545-553.

7. Beiner JM, Jokl P. Muscle contusion injuries: current treatment options. *J Am Acad Orthop Surg*. 2001;9(4):227-237.

8. Bergman AG, Fredericson M, Ho C, Matheson GO. Asymptomatic tibial stress reactions: MRI detection and clinical follow-up in distance runners. *AJR Am J Roentgenol.* 2004;183(3):635-638.

9. Brukner P, Khan K. *Clinical Sports Medicine.* 2nd ed. Sydney, New York: McGraw-Hill; 2001.

10. Bryan Dixon J. Gastrocnemius vs. soleus strain: how to differentiate and deal with calf muscle injuries. *Curr Rev Musculoskelet Med.* 2009;2(2):74-77.

11. Cohen S, Bradley J. Acute proximal hamstring rupture. *J Am Acad Orthop Surg.* 2007;15(6):350-355.

12. Coleman SH, Mayer SW, Tyson JJ, Pollack KM, Curriero FC. The epidemiology of hip and groin injuries in professional baseball players. *Am J Orthop (Belle Mead NJ).* 2016;45(3):168-175.

13. Cross MJ, Vandersluis R, Wood D, Banff M. Surgical repair of chronic complete hamstring tendon rupture in the adult patient. *Am J Sports Med.* 1998;26(6):785-788.

14. Cruz AS, de Hollanda JP, Duarte A Jr, Hungria Neto JS. Anterior tibial stress fractures treated with anterior tension band plating in high-performance athletes. *Knee Surg Sports Traumatol Arthrosc.* 2013;21(6):1447-1450.

15. Dahm DL, Curriero FC, Camp CL, et al. Epidemiology and impact of knee injuries in major and minor league baseball players. *Am J Orthop (Belle Mead NJ).* 2016;45(3):E54-E62.

16. Dick R, Sauers EL, Agel J, et al. Descriptive epidemiology of collegiate men's baseball injuries: National Collegiate Athletic Association Injury Surveillance System, 1988-1989 through 2003-2004. *J Athl Train.* 2007;42(2):183-193.

17. Ekstrand J, Lee JC, Healy JC. MRI findings and return to play in football: a prospective analysis of 255 hamstring injuries in the UEFA Elite Club Injury Study. *Br J Sports Med.* 2016;50(12):738-743.

18. Elliott MC, Zarins B, Powell JW, Kenyon CD. Hamstring muscle strains in professional football players: a 10-year review. *Am J Sports Med.* 2011;39(4):843-850.

19. Entwisle T. Lateral Soleus Intramuscular Aponeurosis Tear.

20. Fitzpatrick J, Bulsara M, Zheng MH. The effectiveness of platelet-rich plasma in the treatment of tendinopathy: a meta-analysis of randomized controlled clinical trials. *Am J Sports Med.* 2017;45(1):226-233.

21. Fitzpatrick J, Bulsara MK, McCrory PR, Richardson MD, Zheng MH. Analysis of platelet-rich plasma extraction: variations in platelet and blood components between 4 common commercial kits. *Orthop J Sports Med.* 2017;5(1):2325967116675272.

22. Foster TE, Puskas BL, Mandelbaum BR, Gerhardt MB, Rodeo SA. Platelet-rich plasma: from basic science to clinical applications. *Am J Sports Med.* 2009;37(11):2259-2272.

23. Fredericson M, Bergman AG, Hoffman KL, Dillingham MS. Tibial stress reaction in runners. Correlation of clinical symptoms and scintigraphy with a new magnetic resonance imaging grading system. *Am J Sports Med.* 1995;23(4):472-481.

24. Gaffney-Stomberg E, Lutz LJ, Rood JC, et al. Calcium and vitamin D supplementation maintains parathyroid hormone and improves bone density during initial military training: a randomized, double-blind, placebo controlled trial. *Bone.* 2014;68:46-56.

25. Gamradt SC, Brophy RH, Barnes R, Warren RF, Thomas Byrd JW, Kelly BT. Nonoperative treatment for proximal avulsion of the rectus femoris in professional American football. *Am J Sports Med.* 2009;37(7):1370-1374.

26. Goldfarb SJ, Kaeding CC. Bilateral acute-on-chronic exertional lateral compartment syndrome of the leg: a case report and review of the literature. *Clin J Sport Med.* 1997;7(1):59-61; discussion 62.

27. Hall MP, Band PA, Meislin RJ, Jazrawi LM, Cardone DA. Platelet-rich plasma: current concepts and application in sports medicine. *J Am Acad Orthop Surg.* 2009;17(10):602-608.

28. Hammoud S, Bedi A, Voos JE, Mauro CS, Kelly BT. The recognition and evaluation of patterns of compensatory injury in patients with mechanical hip pain. *Sports Health.* 2014;6(2):108-118.

29. Hasselman CT, Best TM, Hughes CT, Martinez S, Garrett WE Jr. An explanation for various rectus femoris strain injuries using previously undescribed muscle architecture. *Am J Sports Med.* 1995;23(4):493-499.

30. Heiderscheit BC, Hoerth DM, Chumanov ES, Swanson SC, Thelen BJ, Thelen DG. Identifying the time of occurrence of a hamstring strain injury during treadmill running: a case study. *Clin Biomech.* 2005;20(10):1072-1078.

31. Hubbard TJ, Carpenter EM, Cordova ML. Contributing factors to medial tibial stress syndrome: a prospective investigation. *Med Sci Sports Exerc.* 2009;41(3):490-496.

32. Hughes CT, Hasselman CT, Best TM, Martinez S, Garrett WE Jr. Incomplete, intrasubstance strain injuries of the rectus femoris muscle. *Am J Sports Med.* 1995;23(4):500-506.

33. Irmola T, Heikkila JT, Orava S, Sarimo J. Total proximal tendon avulsion of the rectus femoris muscle. *Scand J Med Sci Sports.* 2007;17(4):378-382.

34. Jackson DW, Feagin JA. Quadriceps contusions in young athletes. Relation of severity of injury to treatment and prognosis. *J Bone Joint Surg Am.* 1973;55(1):95-105.

35. Jarvinen M. Immobilization effect on the tensile properties of striated muscle: an experimental study in the rat. *Arch Phys Med Rehabil.* 1977;58(3):123-127.

36. Jarvinen TA, Jarvinen M, Kalimo H. Regeneration of injured skeletal muscle after the injury. *Muscles Ligaments Tendons J.* 2013;3(4):337-345.

37. Kannus P, Parkkari J, Jarvinen TL, Jarvinen TA, Jarvinen M. Basic science and clinical studies coincide: active treatment approach is needed after a sports injury. *Scand J Med Sci Sports.* 2003;13(3):150-154.

38. Kary JM. Diagnosis and management of quadriceps strains and contusions. *Curr Rev Musculoskelet Med.* 2010;3(1-4):26-31.

39. Koulouris G, Connell D. Evaluation of the hamstring muscle complex following acute injury. *Skeletal Radiol.* 2003;32(10):582-589.

40. Lappe J, Cullen D, Haynatzki G, Recker R, Ahlf R, Thompson K. Calcium and vitamin d supplementation decreases incidence of stress fractures in female navy recruits. *J Bone Miner Res.* 2008;23(5):741-749.

41. Magnusson HI, Westlin NE, Nyqvist F, Gardsell P, Seeman E, Karlsson MK. Abnormally decreased regional bone density in athletes with medial tibial stress syndrome. *Am J Sports Med.* 2001;29(6):712-715.

42. Mann RA, Moran GT, Dougherty SE. Comparative electromyography of the lower extremity in jogging, running, and sprinting. *Am J Sports Med.* 1986;14(6):501-510.

43. McFarland EG, Wasik M. Epidemiology of collegiate baseball injuries. *Clin J Sport Med.* 1998;8(1):10-13.

44. Meheux CJ, McCulloch PC, Lintner DM, Varner KE, Harris JD. Efficacy of intra-articular platelet-rich plasma injections in knee osteoarthritis: a systematic review. *Arthroscopy.* 2016;32(3):495-505.

45. Mejia HA BJ. The effects of platelet-rich plasma on muscle: basic science and clinical application. *Operat Tech Sports Med.* 2011;19(3):149-153.

46. Nielsen RO, Ronnow L, Rasmussen S, Lind M. A prospective study on time to recovery in 254 injured novice runners. *PLoS One.* 2014;9(6):e99877.

47. Pamukoff DN, Blackburn JT. Comparison of plantar flexor musculotendinous stiffness, geometry, and architecture in male runners with and without a history of tibial stress fracture. *J Appl Biomech.* 2015;31(1):41-47.

48. Pedowitz RA, Hargens AR, Mubarak SJ, Gershuni DH. Modified criteria for the objective diagnosis of chronic compartment syndrome of the leg. *Am J Sports Med.* 1990;18(1):35-40.

49. Rettig AC, Meyer S, Bhadra AK. Platelet-rich plasma in addition to rehabilitation for acute hamstring injuries in NFL players: clinical effects and time to return to play. *Orthop J Sports Med.* 2013;1(1):2325967113494354.

50. Riboh JC, Saltzman BM, Yanke AB, Fortier L, Cole BJ. Effect of leukocyte concentration on the efficacy of platelet-rich plasma in the treatment of knee osteoarthritis. *Am J Sports Med.* 2016;44(3):792-800.

51. Rompe JD, Cacchio A, Furia JP, Maffulli N. Low-energy extracorporeal shock wave therapy as a treatment for medial tibial stress syndrome. *Am J Sports Med.* 2010;38(1):125-132.

52. Rubin DA. Imaging diagnosis and prognostication of hamstring injuries. *AJR Am J Roentgenol.* 2012;199(3):525-533.

53. Rue JP, Armstrong DW III, Frassica FJ, Deafenbaugh M, Wilckens JH. The effect of pulsed ultrasound in the treatment of tibial stress fractures. *Orthopedics.* 2004;27(11):1192-1195.

54. Ryan JB, Wheeler JH, Hopkinson WJ, Arciero RA, Kolakowski KR. Quadriceps contusions. West Point update. *Am J Sports Med.* 1991;19(3):299-304.

55. Safran MR, Garrett WE Jr, Seaber AV, Glisson RR, Ribbeck BM. The role of warmup in muscular injury prevention. *Am J Sports Med.* 1988;16(2):123-129.

56. Shindle MK, Endo Y, Warren RF, et al. Stress fractures about the tibia, foot, and ankle. *J Am Acad Orthop Surg.* 2012;20(3):167-176.

57. Sodl JF, Bassora R, Huffman GR, Keenan MA. Traumatic myositis ossificans as a result of college fraternity hazing. *Clin Orthop Relat Res.* 2008;466(1):225-230.

58. Verrall G. Clinical and imaging diagnosis and grading of hamstring injuries. *Sports Radiology.* 2013;2.

59. Waterman BR, Laughlin M, Kilcoyne K, Cameron KL, Owens BD. Surgical treatment of chronic exertional compartment syndrome of the leg: failure rates and postoperative disability in an active patient population. *J Bone Joint Surg Am.* 2013;95(7):592-596.

60. Weir A, de Vos RJ, Moen M, Holmich P, Tol JL. Prevalence of radiological signs of femoroacetabular impingement in patients presenting with long-standing adductor-related groin pain. *Br J Sports Med.* 2011;45(1):6-9.

61. Yagi S, Muneta T, Sekiya I. Incidence and risk factors for medial tibial stress syndrome and tibial stress fracture in high school runners. *Knee Surg Sports Traumatol Arthrosc.* 2013;21(3):556-563.

62. Yates B, White S. The incidence and risk factors in the development of medial tibial stress syndrome among naval recruits. *Am J Sports Med.* 2004;32(3):772-780.

63. Young AJ, McAllister DR. Evaluation and treatment of tibial stress fractures. *Clin Sports Med.* 2006;25(1):117-128, x.

64. Yu B, Queen RM, Abbey AN, Liu Y, Moorman CT, Garrett WE. Hamstring muscle kinematics and activation during overground sprinting. *J Biomech.* 2008;41(15):3121-3126.

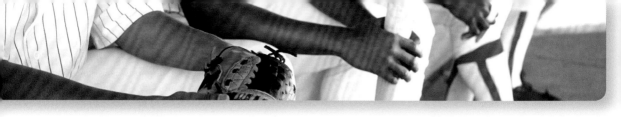

CHAPTER 28

Foot and Ankle Injuries in Baseball Players

Stephen White, MD | Robert B. Anderson, MD

You play the game to win the game and not worry about what's on the back of the baseball.

—*Paul O'Neil*

INTRODUCTION

Injuries to the foot and ankle are common in the baseball athlete. There is a broad scale of severity from nagging ailments to devastating injuries. Regardless of the baseball player's position, an injury to the foot and ankle, whether acute or chronic, can certainly affect the athlete's performance. This chapter will discuss some of the common disorders, as well as some of the more concerning foot and ankle injuries seen in baseball players.

ANKLE SPRAINS

Just like many other sports, ankle sprains are relatively common injury in baseball players. There are many types of ankle sprains with different mechanisms of injury. One must be aware of the different injury patterns to properly treat these injuries accordingly.

CLINICAL EVALUATION

History

The "classic" lateral ankle sprain has an inversion/plantarflexion mechanism of injury. This can occur in a number of ways, often from sliding into a base. This often results in injury to the lateral ligament complex, including the anterior talofibular ligament (ATFL) and the calcaneofibular ligament (CFL) (Figure 28.1). These patients often present with lateral ankle pain and swelling. There is also a medial ankle sprain that can occur with an eversion-type injury, although this is

less common. This usually results in disruption of the deltoid ligament complex. These patients will present with pain and often swelling over the medial aspect of ankle. Lastly, there is the "high ankle sprain," which is a syndesmosis injury often occurring from an external rotation mechanism of injury. This type of injury has seen an increase in incidence over the last several years, which could be due to increased awareness by clinicians. It occurs in approximately 17% of ankle sprains,[1] although this percentage has varied. These patients often have anterior lateral ankle pain and can often have medial-sided pain as well. These variants more commonly have difficulty weight bearing on the injured extremity.

Physical Examination

In athletes with a lateral or medial ankle sprain, patients will have tenderness to palpation over the involved ligaments. They could also have a range of swelling from mild to severe depending on how acute the injury is and how severe the ankle sprain was. Most "low" ankle sprains will be able to bear weight; however, there are a smaller percentage of higher severity "low" ankle sprains that have difficulty weight bearing initially, as well as inability to perform a single-limb heel rise on the effected extremity. In the classic lateral ankle sprain, patients may have a positive anterior drawer test, which is anterior talar translation compared with the uninjured side, which indicates injury to the lateral ligament complex.[2] A positive anterior drawer test should also be performed on the eversion injury as well, which includes external rotation to help assess the integrity of the superficial deltoid ligament.

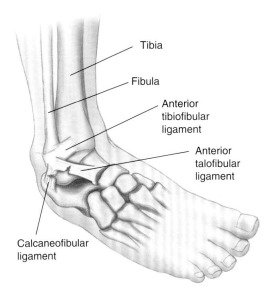

Tibia

Fibula

Anterior tibiofibular ligament

Anterior talofibular ligament

Calcaneofibular ligament

FIGURE 28.1 • Diagram showing injury of calcaneofibular and anterior talofibular ligament.

In patients with a high ankle sprain, as stated earlier, the patient may have difficulty with weight bearing, particularly if told to stand or hop on the injured extremity. They will often have a positive "squeeze test," in which compression of the tibia and fibula at the mid-calf will cause pain at the syndesmosis. The patient can have increased pain and/or translation of the fibula at the level of the syndesmosis with an anterior and posterior drawer force placed on the fibula. They can also have a positive external rotation stress test, which is performed with the knee flexed to 90° and external rotation/dorsiflexion of the foot. A positive test elicits pain at the level of the syndesmosis.

Imaging

Indications for radiographs with an ankle sprain follow the Ottawa ankle rules.[3] These include inability to bear weight, medial/lateral malleolus point tenderness, fifth metatarsal base tenderness, or navicular tenderness. If any of these is present, it is best to obtain appropriate X-rays. As a good rule of thumb, if there is any clinical suspicion of fracture or if something does not seem consistent to the history or examination, it is always best to side on caution and perform the X-rays. Three views of the ankle including anteroposterior (AP), lateral, and mortise are standard. If foot pathology is suspected, obtain 3 X-rays of the foot including AP, lateral, and oblique views.

If a high ankle sprain is suspected, it is reasonable to obtain an X-ray of the entire tibia/fibula in addition to the images stated earlier. This may detect a proximal fibula fracture, which could be indicative of a Maisonneuve-type injury. Also, an external rotation stress X-ray or a gravity stress X-ray could also be utilized to potentially show a syndesmotic injury. Lastly, standing AP ankle radiographs in comparison with the uninjured side may highlight areas of subtle diastasis and instability. An increased "medial clear space" is one such finding to be aware of.

Magnetic resonance imaging (MRI) can also be utilized to help detect suspected syndesmosis injuries with normal radiographs, as well as to assess for intra-articular lesions. This modality should also be utilized if patients have symptoms from a seemingly benign ankle sprain that persist beyond 8 weeks.

TREATMENT

Nonoperative

With "low" ankle sprains, rest, ice, compression, and elevation (RICE) are generally the first line of treatment. Some patients with more severe ankle sprains (those who are unable to bear weight or complete a single-limb heel rise) may require a short period of immobilization (3-6 days) in a walking boot or cast. The additional injection of cortisone or platelet-rich plasma (PRP) into the area of soft tissue injury remains controversial and without scientific validity. Following the acute phase after the initial inflammation has subsided, physical therapy is often utilized. This usually includes neuromuscular training. Proprioception and peroneal muscle strengthening are key components of therapy.

In treatment of "stable" high ankle sprains, patients are often placed in a non–weight bearing boot or cast for approximately 1 to 2 weeks. Once pain free, they can begin weight bearing and a physical therapy protocol.

Operative

Indications

Low ankle sprains with persistent pain and instability after failing conservative management will likely require surgical stabilization of the injured side, whether that is the lateral ligament complex (classic lateral sprain) or the deltoid ligament (medial sprain). Also, consider the alternative that there could be a "missed" high ankle sprain with persistent subtle instability if pain and dysfunction persist.

For any high ankle sprain with documented instability and/or diastasis on stress radiographs, operative fixation is indicated.

Surgical Options

In the classic lateral ankle sprain, reconstruction of the lateral ligament complex can be performed in a number of ways. The Brostrom anatomic reconstruction with the Gould modification is one of the more common procedures performed and is also the author's preferred method of treatment. This involves an anatomic shortening and reinsertion of the ATFL and CFL to essentially tighten the lateral ligament complex and thus increase stability. There are also various techniques that include tendon transfer and tenodesis to reconstruct the lateral ligament complex.

For deltoid ligament injuries, this is usually repaired with nonabsorbable sutures to reapproximate and tighten the ligament fibers. Anchors into the medial malleolus are often used when there are avulsion-type tears.

For syndesmosis injuries requiring operative treatment, syndesmosis stabilization and fixation is accomplished using either screw fixation, suture button fixation, or combination thereof. With screw fixation, generally 2 screws are placed from the fibula into the tibia approximately 1.5 to 5 cm above the tibial plafond. The same is true for suture button fixation, placing 2 devices in divergent fashion that are tensioned around the syndesmosis. This is the authors' preferred method of treatment as seen in Figures 28.2 and 28.3.

Postsurgical Rehabilitation

After lateral ligament repair, the patient is placed in a short leg splint with the foot in neutral dorsiflexion and slight eversion. The repair is generally protected for approximately 4 to 6 weeks. Light physical therapy is begun at that point and then progressed with the same therapy protocol as stated earlier for nonoperative ankle sprains.

For postoperative care of deltoid reconstruction, the ankle is splinted in dorsiflexion and the patient is kept non–weight bearing for approximately 2 weeks. The patient is then placed in a dorsiflexed cast and allowed to partially bear weight for an additional 2 to 3 weeks. At that point, the patient can progress to full weight bearing in a walking boot.

For high ankle sprains undergoing stabilization, the patient is typically non–weight bearing in a splint for 2 weeks. At that point, they are placed into a neutral cast and are continued non–weight bearing for 2 weeks. At 4 weeks postoperative, they are progressed to partial weight bearing in a boot for another 2 weeks and then full weight bearing in a boot for an additional 4 weeks. They will begin progressive strengthening at 10 weeks.

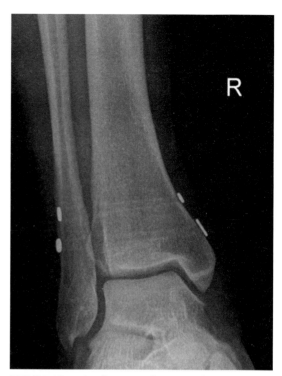

FIGURE 28.2 • Syndesmosis fixation with 2 suture buttons (mortise view). (Reprinted from Tanaka H, Mason L. Chronic ankle instability. *Orthop Trauma*. 2011;25(4):269-278. with permission from Elsevier.)

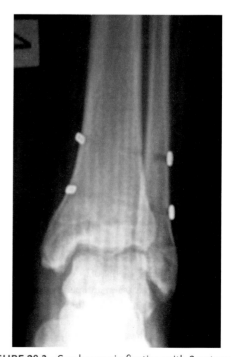

FIGURE 28.3 • Syndesmosis fixation with 2 suture buttons (AP view). (Reprinted from Tanaka H, Mason L. Chronic ankle instability. *Orthop Trauma*. 2011;254:269-278. Copyright © 2011 Elsevier. With permission.)

RESULTS

After a lateral ligament repair (Brostrom with Gould modification), there is an 85% to 95% success rate.[4] Medial ankle sprains have also shown promising results after repair and imbrication of the medial ligaments.[5] In high ankle sprain treatment, studies have shown favorable outcomes with syndesmosis stabilization; the type of fixation, whether screw or suture button, has been shown by some studies to make little difference.[6]

COMPLICATIONS

Patients can often have continued pain and instability after treatment of an ankle sprain. Most often this is due to a concomitant injury, which could include osteochondral lesions, peroneal tendon injuries, ankle impingement, tarsal coalitions, or missed fractures. Thus, it is important to look for concomitant injuries.

SCOUTING REPORT

- Have a high suspicion of a high ankle sprain if the patient is unable to bear weight or perform a single-limb heel rise
- Most "lateral" ankle sprains do well with nonoperative treatment but require comprehensive rehab (peroneals)
- If a player is not improving, suspect for subtle instability (deltoid/syndesmotic) and be aware of concomitant injuries to the joint itself

---

FOUL BALL INJURIES

The foul ball injury is another common injury among baseball players. The ball, as it comes off the bat, usually strikes the foot or ankle at high speeds and in areas with little soft tissue padding. The anterior tibia, malleoli, talus, navicular, and first metatarsal are common symptomatic sites that are struck.

CLINICAL EVALUATION

History

The patient will describe pain and perhaps note swelling and bruising at the site of impact of a foul ball.

They most commonly occur in the batter, but occasionally the catcher (or umpire) can be struck by a foul ball as well. These injuries can often be acutely painful, but most players return to play immediately and will seek treatment after the game.

Physical Examination

The patient will often have ecchymosis and possibly swelling at the site of impact. There will be point tenderness over the area. Depending on severity and location, the patient may have trouble with weight bearing and athletic performance.

Imaging

X-rays are usually recommended to assess the area of impact to rule out any fractures, unless the patient reports only minor pain and minimal functional loss and shows no evidence of a limp, etc. Given normal X-rays, if the patient is unable to bear weight, then an MRI is warranted.[7] If MRI shows bone edema (Figure 28.4), a computed tomography (CT) scan should be ordered to further evaluate for an occult fracture.

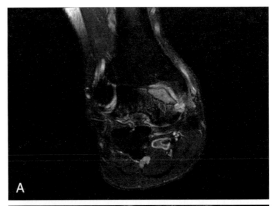

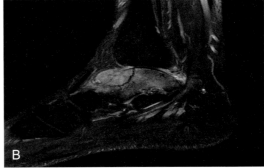

FIGURE 28.4 • MRI showing bone edema in the talus. A, Coronal view. B, Sagittal view. (Reprinted from Naqvi G, Shafqat A, Awan N. Tightrope fixation of ankle syndesmosis injuries: Clinical outcome, complications and technique modification. *Injury*. 2011;43(6):838-842. Copyright © 2011 Elsevier. With permission.)

TREATMENT

Nonoperative

Most of the cases of foul ball injuries are bone contusions and can be treated nonoperatively. This includes ice/nonsteroidal anti-inflammatory drugs (NSAIDs), weight bearing boot to protect the injury, and occasionally a bone stimulator for nondisplaced fractures. Indomethacin is a preferred choice of an NSAID, as it can also prevent the heterotopic ossification that occasionally occurs at the sites of these injuries. Patients can return to play when they can hop on the injured extremity 30 times (in 3 series) or do a minimum of 20 single-leg heel rise maneuvers.

Operative Indications

The only indication for operative fixation of these injuries is the rare case of a displaced fracture or a nonunion of a fracture after failure of conservative treatment.

Surgical Options

The surgery performed would vary depending on the site of the displaced fracture or nonhealing fracture.

RESULTS

Most players return to full level of play with little sequelae.

COMPLICATIONS

Patients can occasionally develop heterotopic ossification at the site of impact, which can sometimes be symptomatic. It is usually treated on a symptomatic basis and will rarely have to be excised when limiting performance.

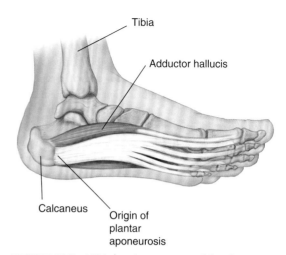

FIGURE 28.5 ● MRI showing anatomy of the plantar fascia. (Reprinted from Elsayed H, Puttaraju A, Crib G, et al. Osteoblastoma of the Talus: A case report and review of the literature. *Foot*. 2017;30:59-62. Copyright © 2017 Elsevier. With permission.)

PLANTAR FASCIA RUPTURE

Plantar fascia rupture occurs on a spectrum of disease that includes plantar fasciitis. Plantar fasciitis is a common complaint seen by orthopedic surgeons who treat the foot and ankle. It is caused by inflammation of the plantar aponeurosis at its origin on the calcaneus (Figure 28.5). It is usually from chronic overuse, which leads to microtears at this origin of the plantar fascia. It is commonly seen in athletes, including baseball players, and causes plantar-medial heel pain, which can be debilitating. Complications of this condition include plantar fascia rupture, which is more common in athletes and even more so in those who have had greater than 1 corticosteroid injection to treat the plantar fasciitis.

CLINICAL EVALUATION

History

Ruptures present with acute sharp tearing pain in the arch, plantar ecchymosis, and swelling usually after a forced planting maneuver. The foot is often difficult to walk on after the rupture.

Physical Examination

Examination will show acute tenderness in the involved foot. The foot, as noted earlier, will have plantar ecchymosis and swelling. There may be loss of arch height. The clinician can often palpate the loss of tension in the medial band of the plantar fascia when comparing with the uninjured foot.

SCOUTING REPORT

- Most of these injuries are contusions and can be treated nonoperatively. There is little risk of continuing athletic participation if pain and function allow
- Workup should include X-rays and an MRI if the player is unable to bear weight
- Obtain CT if MRI notes bone edema

Imaging

X-rays of the foot will generally be normal. Rarely, and typically in the chronic situation, they may show loss of arch height on a lateral weight bearing X-ray. MRI will identify the ruptured plantar fascia, whether partial or complete. There will be significant edema surrounding the area of rupture. It can also show surrounding soft tissue inflammation and hypertrophy in late presentation.

TREATMENT

Nonoperative

It is extremely important to diagnose plantar fascia rupture early so as to begin treatment as soon as possible. Most cases can be treated nonoperatively. Treatment includes placing into a short leg cast with a well-molded arch and weight bearing as tolerated. Patient will follow up weekly for serial examinations. If they are still tender on examination, then continue casting. The average time of casting is 2½ to 3½ weeks. After casting, therapy is begun, which includes night splints (Figure 28.6), plantar fascial stretching, Achilles stretching, and toe flexor strengthening. Patients are allowed to return to play when pain allows, which is usually at 4 to 6 weeks. They need to use an orthotic device for arch support (Figure 28.7), a full-length turf toe plate, and taping as needed.

RESULTS

Most patients achieve favorable results and return to preinjury level of play if treated with the abovementioned protocol. The key is treating ruptures early to maintain arch height and prevent late sequelae. Saxena et al in 2004 studied 18 athletes treated with nonoperative management that all returned to play at an average of 9 weeks.[8] In the author's experience, most athletes returned to play at an average of 4 to 5 weeks with this protocol.

COMPLICATIONS

The main complications that occur are due to late sequelae of improperly treated plantar fascia ruptures. This includes loss of arch height leading to a pronation deformity of the foot. Patients can develop lateral column foot pain, which can be caused by calcaneal-cuboid joint synovitis or cuboid stress reaction

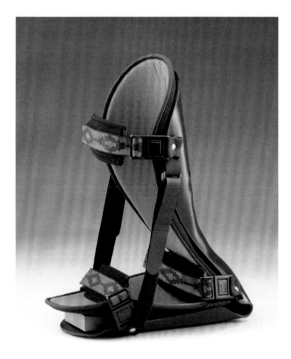

FIGURE 28.6 • Night splint. (Reprinted from Attard J, Singh D. A comparison of two night ankle-foot orthoses used in the treatment of inferior heel pain: a preliminary investigation. *Foot Ankle Surg.* 2012;18(2):108-110. Copyright © 2011 European Foot and Ankle Society. With permission.)

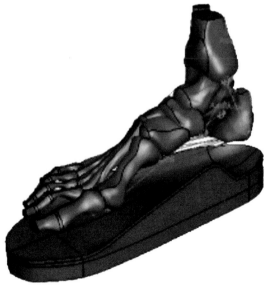

FIGURE 28.7 • Orthotic with arch support. (Reprinted from Cheung J, Zhang M. Parametric design of pressure-relieving foot orthosis using statistics-based finite element method. *Med Eng Phys.* 2008;18(2):269-277. Copyright © 2007 IPEM. With permission.)

(Figures 28.8 and 28.9). Patients can also develop metatarsal stress fractures (Figures 28.10 and 28.11) due to these biomechanical changes.

SCOUTING REPORT

- Early diagnosis is the key!
- For acute injuries, place foot directly into short leg cast with a well-molded arch
- Focus of treatment should be on maintaining and protecting the arch

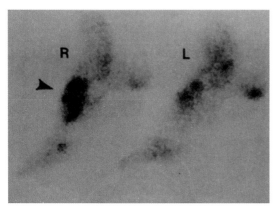

FIGURE 28.8 • Bone scan showing cuboid stress reaction (arrowhead).

SESAMOID DISORDERS

The sesamoids of the hallux have many functions. They modify pressure by absorbing the majority of the weight of the first metatarsal, and they help protect the flexor hallucis longus tendon. They also increase the mechanical leverage of the musculature of the first metatarsal, improving push-off. There are 2 sesamoids: the fibular (lateral) and the tibial (medial) (Figure 28.12). They are joined by an intersesamoid ligament and suspended by metatarsal-sesamoid ligaments. There is a delicate balance between the 2 to function appropriately. Injury to this complex can throw off this delicate balance, thus affecting function, which in turn can affect a player's performance.

CLINICAL EVALUATION

History

Pitchers are at risk for this disorder, given the pressure placed on the forefoot through the throwing sequence. Patients will typically present with sharp plantar pain under the first metatarsophalangeal (MTP) joint, which worsens with activity. It can be severe, and the discomfort can restrict performance. Patients may even have a limp. They can sometimes feel an acute pop in the area during activity. Patients often have pain with positions or maneuvers that cause extension of the first MTP joint, such as base running or a catcher's squatting position.

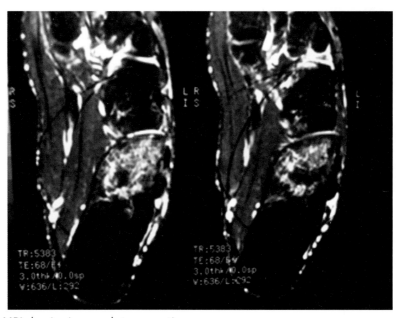

FIGURE 28.9 • MRI showing increased stress reaction.

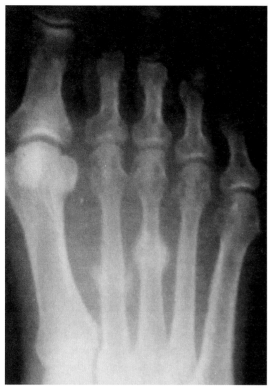

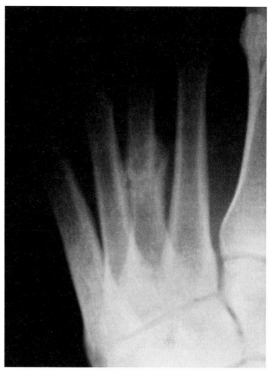

FIGURE 28.11 • X-ray showing metatarsal stress fracture.

FIGURE 28.10 • X-ray showing metatarsal stress fractures.

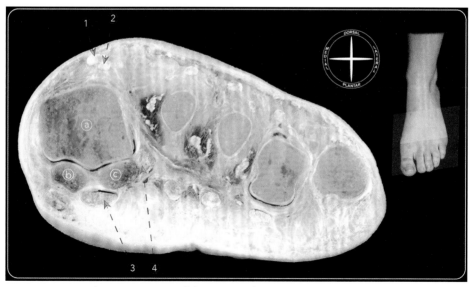

FIGURE 28.12 • Diagram showing anatomy of the sesamoids. a, 1st metatarsal. b, Tibial sesamoid. c, Fibular sesamoid. 1, Extensor hallucis longus tendon. 2, Extensor hallucis brevis tendon. 3, Flexor hallucis longus tendon. 4, Adductor hallucis tendon. (Reprinted from Malagelada F, Dalmau-Pastor M, Fargues B, Manzanares-Céspedes MC, Peña F, Vega J. Increasing the safety of minimally invasive hallux surgery – an anatomical study introducing the clock method. *Foot Ankle Surg.* 2018;24(1):40-44. Copyright © 2016 European Foot and Ankle Society. With permission.)

Physical Examination

Patients will typically have point tenderness directly underneath one of the sesamoids. Patients also have pain on passive extension (dorsiflexion) of the first MTP joint. However, they will often exhibit normal range of motion of the first MTP joint. Some of these patients will have high arched (cavus) feet, which predisposes them to these types of injuries.

Imaging

Plain X-rays of the foot can often be very helpful in diagnosing sesamoid disorders. An axial sesamoid view can also be helpful. It is good practice to view the contralateral foot for comparison, particularly in cases of subluxation or proximal migration of the sesamoids. Fractures, osteochondrosis, avascular necrosis, and bipartite sesamoids can also be noted on X-rays.

If the diagnosis cannot be determined on X-ray or if proximal migration of the sesamoid is noted, MRI is recommended as a next step. This can often help identify areas of inflammation, articular surface damage, soft tissue injuries, and avascular necrosis. It is also helpful for identifying stress fractures.

TREATMENT

Nonoperative

Nonoperative treatment for acute sesamoid complex injuries includes NSAIDs, cast/boot/sandal, and physical therapy. For more chronic-type injuries, an orthosis to offload the injured area is often helpful. A shoe with rigid sole/cushion is another option. Although there are different schools of thought on the topic, corticosteroid injections are occasionally performed to decrease inflammation.

Operative Indications

Operative indications generally include failure of conservative treatment for greater than 6 months. If a patient has pain or tenderness localized to 1 sesamoid and diagnostic studies identify an abnormality that obviously needs surgical intervention, then surgery is indicated at that point. There is always discussion in the professional athlete as to when to proceed with surgery, as many do not have the luxury of a 6-month trial of conservative treatment; thus, an operation may be performed sooner in this population, given significant sesamoid pathology.

Surgical Options

Owing to the various pathologies that occur to or around the sesamoid complex, there are a variety of surgeries and techniques that can be performed, which are too detailed for the purpose of this chapter. A few of the more common procedures performed are the total and partial sesamoidectomy, plantar shaving to decrease pressure on the problem sesamoid, bone grafting and/or fixation of fractures or nonunions, and soft tissue reconstruction for the turf toe injury.

AUTHORS' PREFERRED SURGICAL TECHNIQUE

Sesamoidectomy is the most commonly preferred technique, and it is of note that it is not a career-ending surgery. Many athletes return to the same level of play after this procedure. There are several important points to note while performing this procedure. A medial-plantar approach is performed for the tibial sesamoid, and plantar approach is performed for the fibular sesamoid. The surgeon must identify and protect the digital nerves throughout the procedure. After the sesamoid is removed, the surgeon must repair the resulting defect that will include repair of the flexor hallucis brevis and the volar plate. In the instance of a tibial sesamoidectomy, a tendon transfer of the abductor hallucis may be performed to reinforce the repair, provide flexion power, and improve long-term function. A concomitant release of the adductor hallucis tendon is recommended to remove subsequent unbalanced forces on the hallux.

Postsurgical Rehabilitation

Patients are typically kept non–weight bearing in a splint for 2 weeks. It is important to maintain hallux alignment and to protect in boot for 6 to 8 weeks total. Patients should not begin running until 3 months. An orthosis (turf toe plate) is used to protect the repair for 6 months postoperative.

RESULTS

Many patients' symptoms resolve with conservative treatment. As noted earlier, of the athletes that require surgical treatment, the vast majority return to the previous level of play with few complications.[9]

COMPLICATIONS

A cock-up toe deformity can occur if both the sesamoids are removed and with loss of push-off strength. This situation can also occur if the flexor hallucis brevis is weakened and not repaired appropriately. Hallux valgus may occur after tibial sesamoid excision, and similarly hallux varus can result from a fibular sesamoid excision in which the resulting soft tissue defect is not repaired and protected.[10]

STRESS FRACTURES (NAVICULAR)

Stress fractures are not exclusive to baseball—they occur in all sports. While many etiologies have been described, these fractures are basically caused by excessive repetitive forces that eventually exceed the bone's ability to withstand. Stress fractures begin as microfractures in the bone, and these stresses on the bone continue to overpower the body's healing response. They are often difficult to diagnose; thus, one has to have a high suspicion, as there is always a possibility in any running athlete with unexplained or vague pain. Navicular stress fractures are the most concerning and for whatever reasons are not uncommon in baseball players.

CLINICAL EVALUATION

History

The patient will often present with vague anterior ankle or foot pain without any noticeable pathology. The patient may even have a cramping in the area. Onset is usually insidious. They may report a recent history of increased activity level or even a position change. The pain may be worsened in an airline flight due to pressure changes.

Physical Examination

Patients may have swelling of the midfoot on occasion. They will also have tenderness to palpation of the midfoot, particularly over the "N-spot" (Figure 28.13).[11] Patients usually have full range of motion of the ankle

and subtalar joint. Hopping on a plantarflexed foot has also been shown to illicit pain in this area.[12]

Imaging

X-rays are often negative at initial presentation. MRI or bone scan must be utilized early if there is any suspicion of a stress fracture (Figures 28.14 and 28.15).

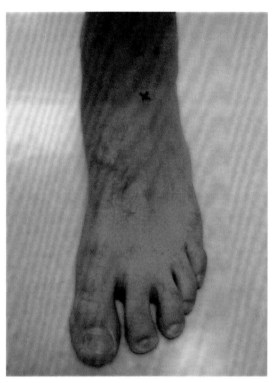

FIGURE 28.13 • Mark on skin shows location of "N-spot."

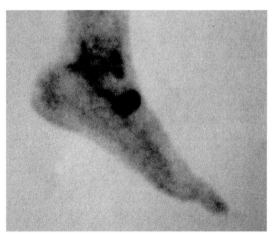

FIGURE 28.14 • Bone scan showing increased signal in navicular. (Reprinted from Lee S, Anderson R. Stress fracture of the tarsal navicular. *Foot Ankle Clin.* 2004;9:(1):85-104. Copyright © 2004 Elsevier. With permission.)

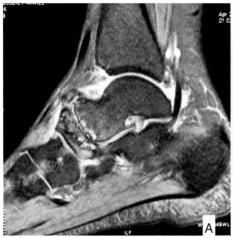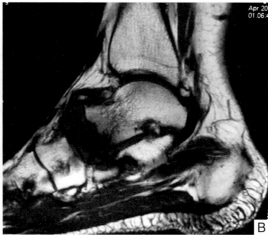

FIGURE 28.15 • A, Fluid sensitive MRI showing increased signal in navicular. B, T1 MRI showing decreased signal in navicular. (Reprinted from Vijay V, Gupta N, Vaishya R, et al. Tuberculosis around the tarsal navicular: a rare entity. *Foot.* 2016;28:20-25. Copyright © 2016 Elsevier. With permission.)

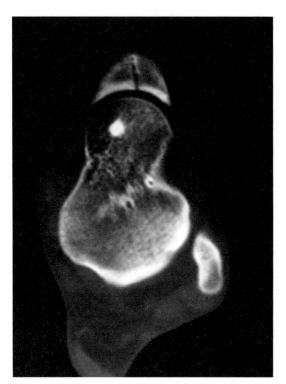

FIGURE 28.16 • CT scan showing stress fracture across navicular. (Reprinted from Reid J, Pinney S. Midfoot injuries in athletes: fundamentals of examination and treatment. *Oper Tech Sports Med.* 2010;18(1):46-49. Copyright © 2010 Elsevier. With permission.)

CT scan is mandatory if the MRI is abnormal (Figure 28.16). CT will help differentiate a stress reaction versus fracture versus nonunion, as well as its exact location and extent.

TREATMENT

Nonoperative

Many of these patients with an early presentation and incomplete fracture can be treated nonoperatively with a high success rate. Treatment protocol includes non–weight bearing in a cast for 6 to 8 weeks.[13] The use of a bone stimulator can also be used to stimulate a healing response.

Operative

Indications

In patients who have failed the nonoperative protocol or in certain professional athletes where timing of treatment is an issue, operative treatment is appropriate.[12] Any displaced fracture is an operative indication. Beware of "incomplete" stress fractures, as they can have a tendency to progress to complete fractures or nonunion (Figures 28.17 and 28.18). Thus, they need to be followed with a CT scan every 6 weeks. Early aggressive operative treatment may be utilized in these progressive cases.

Surgical Options

Most navicular stress fractures are treated operatively with 2 screws, plus or minus bone grafting. This can be performed in an open or percutaneous fashion. If a nonunion is present, some form of bone grafting, preferably autograft, is mandatory along with internal fixation. In these cases, it is important to delineate the orientation of the fracture line on CT scan, and try to orient the screw perpendicular to the fracture line.

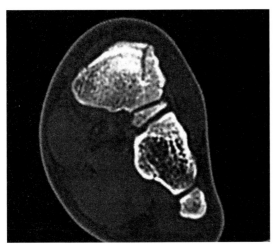

FIGURE 28.17 • CT scan showing "incomplete" stress fracture of navicular. (Reprinted from Jones M, Amendola A. Navicular stress fractures. *Sports Med Clin.* 2006;25(1):151-158. Copyright © 2005 Elsevier. With permission.)

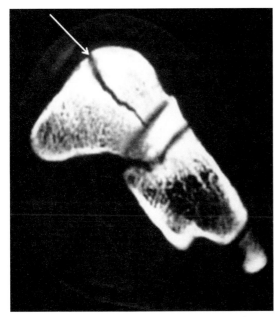

FIGURE 28.18 • CT scan showing progression of navicular fracture to complete (arrow). (Reprinted from Newman JS, Newberg AH. Basketball injuries. *Radiol Clin North Am.* 2010;48(6):1095-1111. Copyright © 2010 Elsevier. With permission.)

AUTHORS' PREFERRED SURGICAL TECHNIQUE

The author prefers to use two 4.0-mm partially threaded cannulated screws that are placed perpendicular across the fracture site with fluoroscopic guidance. The screws are often placed in a dorsolateral to plantar-medial orientation to cross perpendicular to the oblique fracture site. This is usually performed in a percutaneous fashion unless there is significant sclerosis, displacement, or presence of nonunion in which an open approach and bone grafting is preferable.

POSTSURGICAL REHABILITATION

Patients are kept non–weight bearing in a splint/boot for 6 weeks initially. They then proceed with weight bearing in a boot for 6 weeks. CT scan is performed at 12 weeks. Most athletes are running at 3 to 5 months, depending on initial fracture severity and healing progression.

RESULTS

Patients have a success rate of over 80% with nonoperative and operative treatment. According to a study, the average return to activity was 3.8 months with operative treatment versus 5.6 months with conservative treatment.[14] These numbers do vary according to the severity of the fracture and the timing of treatment.

COMPLICATIONS

Delayed union or nonunion is the most common complication of navicular stress fractures. These occurrences are confirmed by CT scan. Once diagnosed, those patients who were initially treated nonoperatively will undergo operative fixation, often with bone grafting. In the revision setting after failed screw fixation, the fracture site must be opened and sclerotic bone is removed, followed by bone grafting and internal fixation. A bone stimulator is typically recommended for these cases. An osteotomy of the calcaneus and/or first metatarsal may be required in the revision situation. The most concerning complication with the navicular stress fracture is that of avascular necrosis of the bone itself. There are very few options to manage this potentially devastating situation, and it can be career ending.

SCOUTING REPORT

- Stress fractures are difficult to diagnose
- Clinician must have a high suspicion, as an early diagnosis and appropriate treatment improves outcome
- Remember, stress fractures are always a possibility in the running athlete!
- If vague anterior ankle pain is present without obvious pathology, obtain an MRI

REFERENCES

1. Gerber JP, Williams GN, Scoville CR, Arciero RA, Taylor DC. Persistent disability associated with ankle sprains: a prospective examination of an athletic population. *Foot Ankle Int.* 1998;19(10):653-660.

2. Maffulli N, Ferran NA. Management of acute and chronic ankle instability. *J Am Acad Orthop Surg.* 2008;16(10):608-615.

3. Stiell IG, Greenberg GH, McKnight RD, Nair RC, McDowell I, Worthington JR. A study to develop clinical decision rules for the use of radiography in acute ankle injuries. *Ann Emerg Med.* 1992;21(4):384-390.

4. Baumhauer JF, O'Brien T. Surgical considerations in the treatment of ankle instability. *J Athl Train.* 2002;37(4):458-462.

5. Hintermann B, Valderrabano V, Boss A, Trouillier HH, Dick W. Medial ankle instability: an exploratory, prospective study of fifty-two cases. *Am J Sports Med.* 2004;32(1):183-190.

6. Cottom JM, Hyer CF, Philbin TM, Berlet GC. Transosseous fixation of the distal tibiofibular syndesmosis: comparison of an interosseous suture and endobutton to traditional screw fixation in 50 cases. *J Foot Ankle Surg.* 2009;48(6):620-630.

7. Baker JC, Hoover EG, Hillen TJ, Smith MV, Wright RW, Rubin DA. Subradiographic foot and ankle fractures and bone contusions detected by MRI in elite ice hockey players. *Am J Sports Med.* 2016;44(5):1317-1323.

8. Saxena A, Fullem B. Plantar fascia ruptures in athletes. *Am J Sports Med.* 2004;32(3):662-665.

9. Saxena A, Krisdakumtorn T. Return to activity after sesamoidectomy in athletically active individuals. *Foot Ankle Int.* 2003;24(5):415-419.

10. Mann RA, Coughlin MJ. Hallux valgus–etiology, anatomy, treatment and surgical considerations. *Clin Orthop Relat Res.* 1981(157):31-41.

11. Khan KM, Fuller PJ, Brukner PD, Kearney C, Burry HC. Outcome of conservative and surgical management of navicular stress fracture in athletes. Eighty-six cases proven with computerized tomography. *Am J Sports Med.* 1992;20(6):657-666.

12. Fitch KD, Blackwell JB, Gilmour WN. Operation for non-union of stress fracture of the tarsal navicular. *J Bone Joint Surg Br.* 1989;71(1):105-110.

13. Khan KM, Brukner PD, Kearney C, Fuller PJ, Bradshaw CJ, Kiss ZS. Tarsal navicular stress fracture in athletes. *Sports Med.* 1994;17(1):65-76.

14. Saxena A, Fullem B, Hannaford D. Results of treatment of 22 navicular stress fractures and a new proposed radiographic classification system. *J Foot Ankle Surg.* 2000;39(2):96-103.

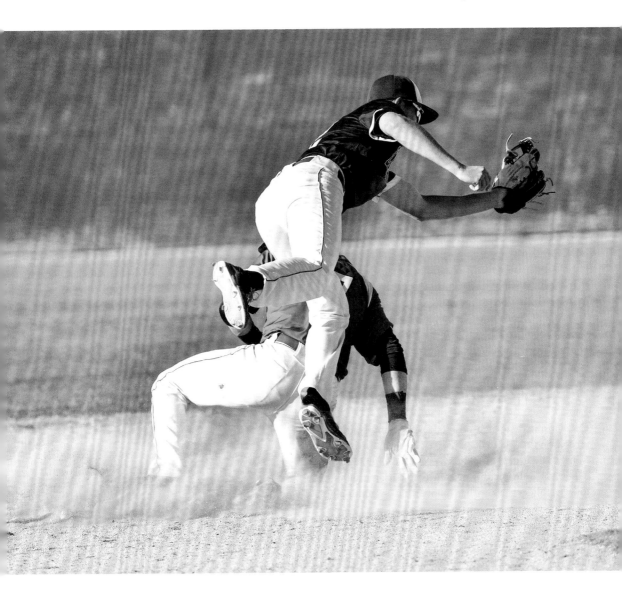

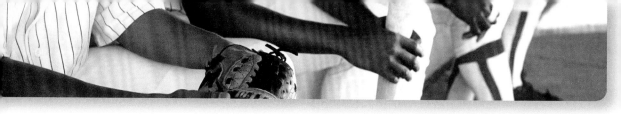

CHAPTER 29

Concussion and Brain Injury in Baseball Players

Steven Wakeman, MD | Gary Green, MD | Alex Valadka, MD

Whoever wants to know the heart and mind of America had better learn baseball.

—Jacques Barzun

INTRODUCTION

Popular interest in concussion has grown dramatically in recent years. Endless media reports create the impression that concussions occur everywhere and that they inevitably lead to severe neurologic disability. Much of this recent interest grew from recognition of the effects of traumatic brain injury (TBI) on military personnel in Iraq and Afghanistan. The National Football League's handling of concussions has also kept this issue high in public consciousness.

DEFINITION

Often lost in these high-profile conversations is proper recognition of what concussion is, and what it is not. Many definitions have been proposed. In a 2004 review, 41 different sets of concussion-related guidelines were identified.[1] That number has undoubtedly increased during the intervening years.

The American Association of Neurological Surgeons website defines concussion as "a clinical syndrome characterized by immediate and transient alteration in brain function, including alteration of mental status and level of consciousness, resulting from mechanical force or trauma."[2] Key points: (1) occurrence immediately after trauma, even though recognition may be delayed; (2) almost always transient; (3) caused by mechanical force; and (4) disturbance of function but not structure. The definition adopted by the expert panel at the 5th International Conference on Concussion in Sport, held in Berlin in October 2016, adds that sports-related concussion "may be caused either by a direct blow to the head, face, neck or elsewhere on the body with an impulsive force transmitted to the head" and that "clinical signs and symptoms cannot be explained by drug, alcohol, or medication use, other injuries (such as cervical injuries, peripheral vestibular dysfunction, etc) or other comorbidities (eg, psychological factors or coexisting medical conditions)."[3]

Simply put, concussion is a subtype of mild TBI in which brain imaging studies are normal. Recent investigations suggest that magnetic resonance imaging (MRI) in some patients with concussion may detect abnormalities not seen on computed tomography (CT) scans.[4] The implications of these findings for patient management as well as for defining concussion remain topics of ongoing debate.

Unfortunately, popular usage often eliminates the distinction between concussion and more severe forms of brain injury, such as news media reporting that surgery was needed to treat a "severe" concussion.[5]

EPIDEMIOLOGY

Fortunately, concussions occur less frequently in baseball than in most other sports. Combined data from the major and minor leagues from the 2011 to 2012 seasons revealed a game rate of concussions of 0.42 per 1000 athlete-exposures, representing 1% of all injuries that resulted in time lost from competition.[6] Subsequent changes to the rules of competition may have lowered this rate even further.[7] Despite these improvements, however, concussions continue to occur during routine baseball activities, such as base running and fielding.

Catchers account for a disproportionately large share of concussions sustained by players on defense.[6] Collisions with other players and contact with batted balls (foul tips to the facemask) cause most concussions among catchers. Similarly, umpires also can sustain concussions from foul tips to the face mask.

Many authors report that a patient's risk for future concussions increases after he or she sustains a first concussion.[8] However, this raises a chicken-and-egg question: did a greater susceptibility to concussions predispose to the first and subsequent concussions, or did an initial concussion really lower the threshold for suffering subsequent concussions?

ASSESSMENT

As always, assessment begins with a careful history and examination. A useful approach (even in patients whose concussion was not sustained during athletic events) is outlined in the SCAT5, or Sport Concussion Assessment Tool 5th Edition, which was produced by the panelists at the Berlin conference in 2016.[3]

The SCAT5 begins with an immediate, on-field assessment for the presence of "red flags" or indicators of potentially severe neurologic injury. *Neurologic deterioration or any other evidence of brain injury more significant than concussion requires that concussion protocols be abandoned and that the patient be treated as having a more severe brain injury.*

The SCAT5 then moves to an assessment of memory via Maddocks questions, followed by assessment of the Glasgow Coma Scale (GCS) score. However, the Major League Baseball (MLB) adaptation of the SCAT5 omits the GCS because significant abnormalities on the GCS would have been detected during the screen for red flags.

For off-field or office assessment, the SCAT5 scores 22 common symptoms of concussion. A brief cognitive assessment (the Standardized Assessment of Concussion) and tests of memory and concentration are performed. Balance testing (Modified Balance Error Scoring System) is also conducted.

MLB incorporates the most recent version of the SCAT in its rigorous protocol for player evaluation for possible concussion. The athletic trainer or team physician includes the SCAT results in the information that is sent to the MLB Medical Director.

Some clinicians group symptoms of concussion into certain categories, such as cognitive (eg, confusion, memory problems, impaired concentration), affective (eg, depression, anxiety, irritability), somatic (eg, headache, sleepiness, nausea, insomnia, fatigue), and vestibular (eg, dizziness, balance problems). Abnormalities with vision, and especially with extraocular movements, represent another common set of signs and symptoms that form the basis for many commercially available products that attempt to diagnose concussions.

Several important points must be kept in mind when evaluating these patients:

1. Concussion may occur without loss of consciousness. Some data suggest that as many as 90% of all concussions take place without loss of consciousness

2. Grading schemes for concussion are no longer used. Several schemes were popular in the past, but they were abandoned after it became clear that the assigned grades did not correlate with natural history or outcome. In other words, there is little meaning to saying someone has a "grade 1, grade 2, or grade 3" concussion

3. The SCAT5 is only a tool to aid a clinician's decision-making. It should not be used as a stand-alone test for diagnosing concussion, measuring recovery, or evaluating readiness to return to play

Should a CT scan be obtained as part of the evaluation of a patient with concussion? Medical literature and widespread clinical experience suggest that the answer is no.[9,10] Most concussion patients demonstrate neurologic improvement soon after injury, and the rest remain neurologically stable. The most worrisome red flags suggesting that immediate CT scanning is needed are progressive sleepiness and loss of consciousness. Other warning signs may include progressively worsening headache or repeated episodes of vomiting.

Concussion is a clinical diagnosis. Neuropsychological testing may be helpful in certain cases, such as in patients who fail to recover as quickly as expected. In athletes or other patients who will return to an activity that poses a risk of repeat concussion, such testing can provide extra assurance that concussive symptoms have resolved before clearance is given to return. Because formal neuropsychological testing is time-consuming and expensive, computerized evaluations have become popular in sports medicine. These are most useful when a preseason baseline has been obtained to facilitate comparisons to postinjury assessments. MLB requires that all Major and Minor League players undergo a baseline computerized neuropsychological assessment. MLB does not specify which particular test should be used. Such computerized assessment tools are only an aid to clinical decision-making; their results should not be followed blindly.

MANAGEMENT

There exists no effective treatment for the early period (the first few days or weeks) after a concussion. Fortunately, the vast majority of these injuries resolve spontaneously. Several days, and sometimes 7 to 10 days or more, may have to pass before athletes can return to competition. Several years ago, MLB created a 7-day disabled list (DL) only for patients with concussion. Before that time, the shortest DL was 15 days. Managers had to decide whether to place a player on the 15-day DL even though he might be recovered from his concussion in a week or less versus letting a concussed player take up a slot on the roster even though he might not be able to play or even practice for a week or longer. The 7-day DL has proven to be useful for management of concussed players. Longer periods on a DL are used when needed.

One of the areas of strongest agreement among clinicians who work in the concussion field is that a patient must be protected from sustaining a second concussion while he or she is still symptomatic from an earlier concussion. Of note, the first concussion may have been sustained in activities not related to sports and thus may be unknown to the team's medical personnel. A subsequent concussion may exacerbate symptoms and prolong recovery from a still-unresolved earlier one. Of much greater concern is the potential for second-impact syndrome, or massive and often fatal brain swelling produced by the second hit.[11] It is thought that the initial injury may impair the cerebral vasculature's ability to autoregulate cerebral blood flow. When this crippled vasculature sustains a second hit, it cannot adequately regulate the large amount of blood that normally flows to the brain, resulting in massive hyperemia, edema, and often herniation. Death or severe disability is frequent. This syndrome affects teenagers and younger players. Fortunately, such cases are rare, but their catastrophic outcomes make second-impact syndrome a much-feared and often much-publicized occurrence.

Complete "brain rest" had been a popular treatment, but the theoretical basis for this practice has always been thin. Experimental and clinical data about brain metabolism after severe TBI are often applied inappropriately to the much milder type of injury seen in concussions. Fortunately, encouraging these patients to be more active during their recoveries is gaining increasing acceptance.

Numerous products are touted as helping recovery from concussion, including memory or concentration games, extraocular movement exercises, balance and posture devices, and many others. Solid clinical evidence to support such products is lacking.

Pharmacologic intervention other than acetaminophen or other nonsteroidal anti-inflammatory agents for headache is probably best avoided by practitioners who lack experience in managing these patients. When symptoms of concussion persist for several weeks, some practitioners have begun trying various medications, but targeting specific drugs to specific types of symptoms is still a highly empirical process.

When an athlete's symptoms have resolved, he or she can gradually resume activity according to a graduated scheme, such as the 6-step strategy proposed by the 2016 Berlin conference panelists.[3] The first stage consists of routine daily activities. This is followed by light aerobic exercise, such as walking or stationary cycling at a slow pace. The third stage is sport-specific activity such as running, but with no head impacts. Next come harder training drills, and resistance training may also commence. The fifth stage is full-contact practice, followed by the sixth and final stage, which is return to play. Recurrence of symptoms at a specific level of activity suggests that the player's recovery should be paused at just below the symptom-inducing level for a short time, with a repeat attempt at the problematic level often being made on the next day.

Before a player can return to competition, MLB requires that players be asymptomatic and fully recovered from the effects of the concussion. Players must also achieve baseline or near-baseline results on repeat computerized neuropsychological testing. The team physician submits this documentation to the league office, and the MLB Medical Director and the MLB Players' Union jointly agree on when return to play is appropriate.

A minority of concussion patients will go on to have long-term problems, in what is often described as postconcussion syndrome (PCS). Our understanding of this condition is frustratingly sparse. It has been suggested that trauma-induced axonal injury, which normally resolves, may become permanent or even lead to formation of dysfunctional new neural pathways. There is a pressing need to identify why these patients have a postinjury course that differs so much from that of most concussion patients. Treatment may include time, activity-based interventions, medications, and counseling. Cognitive behavioral therapy may be helpful,[12] perhaps because risk of developing PCS may be associated with a personal or family history of mood disorders or other psychiatric illness.[13] Depending on a patient's specific symptomatology, vestibular or cervical rehabilitation may be helpful. Rarely, mild TBI can be season-ending or even career-ending.

LONG-TERM EFFECTS

The possibility that numerous concussions could have cumulative long-term deleterious effects has been recognized for perhaps a century or longer. Affected boxers were sometimes described as "punch drunk[14]" and subsequently as suffering from "dementia pugilistica.[15]" The term "chronic traumatic encephalopathy" (CTE) was described in 1949[16] and subsequently modified in 1973.[17] CTE has been used to describe certain neuropathologic findings seen on autopsied brains of former football players and other athletes. A prominent histologic finding is accumulation of phosphorylated tau protein that can form dense neurofibrillary tangles, but unlike Alzheimer disease, beta-amyloid protein deposition occurs minimally or not at all. Retrospective "psychological autopsies" of these cases have been interpreted as suggesting the existence of behavioral problems that the investigators attributed to the neuropathologic findings, which in turn were attributed to a history of numerous sports-related concussions or even to frequent subconcussive blows.

Unfortunately, media sensationalism and numerous legal actions have made it difficult to conduct a scientifically valid assessment of these findings and their potential significance. Only a small number of cases have been described. Many former athletes go on to have highly productive lives and careers after their playing days are over, raising questions about what might have been different in those who reportedly developed CTE. Carefully conducted prospective longitudinal studies are needed, but the expense, long time horizon, and sustained commitment required to complete such studies will always be formidable obstacles to their initiation, much less completion.

PREVENTION

Preventing concussions is much more effective than treating them. An obvious place to start in baseball players is improved head protection. Various modifications to batting helmets have been tried, but none has added much to the protection provided by existing helmet designs. Protection for pitchers against hard line drives to the head has evolved from a bulky cushion around the forehead, temples, and occiput to a sleeker visor-type helmet, but few pitchers have chosen to wear these. Of interest, a survey of professional catchers found that hockey-style masks were felt to provide better overall safety and protection, yet many catchers preferred conventional masks because of such perceived advantages as lightweight, ease of removability, and better visualization of the field of play (manuscript under review).

MLB has implemented several changes to the rules of competition that remove players from the risk of concussion. These include prohibitions against collisions between base runners and position players at home plate and the other bases. Preliminary data demonstrate that this rule change was highly effective in reducing the incidence of concussions.[7] Minimizing the risk of concussion in catchers and umpires is another important area of focus.

MANAGER'S TIPS

- Concussion is a clinical diagnosis characterized by alteration in brain function
- The vast majority of players who suffer a concussion never lose consciousness
- Various diagnostic tools are just that—tools. They should not be used in isolation to diagnose or manage concussion. Clinical judgment is always most important
- Players should not be cleared to return to competition if they are still symptomatic after a concussion
- Catchers have especially high rates of concussion
- Most concussions resolve on their own

REFERENCES

1. Peloso P, Carroll L, Cassidy JD, et al. Critical evaluation of the existing guidelines on mild traumatic brain injury. *J Rehabil Med*. 2004;36:106-112.
2. Concussion [Internet]. Rolling Meadows, IL: American Association of Neurological Surgeons. Available at http://www.aans.org/patient%20information/conditions%20and%20treatments/concussion.aspx.
3. McCrory P, Meeuwisse W, Dvorak J, et al. Consensus statement on concussion in sport—the 5th international conference on concussion in sport held in Berlin, 2016. *Br J Sports Med*. 2017;51:838-847.
4. Yuh EL, Mukherjee P, Lingsma HF, et al. Magnetic resonance imaging improves 3-month outcome prediction in mild traumatic brain injury: MRI in MTBI. *Ann Neurol*. 2013;73:224-235.
5. Safety questioned after Southern California high school football player's severe concussion [Internet]. San Francisco: ABC Inc, KGO-TV San Francisco; © 2017. Available at abc7news.com. http://abc7news.com/sports/safety-questioned-after-football-players-severe-concussion/1055792/.
6. Green GA, Pollack KM, D'Angelo J, et al. Mild traumatic brain injury in major and minor league baseball players. *Am J Sports Med*. 2015;43:1118-1126.
7. Green G, D'Angelo J, Coyles J, Valadka A. Effect of a rule change on concussions and other injuries in professional baseball. In: *Presented at the 5th International Consensus Conference on Concussion in Sport, Berlin*. October 2016.

8. Giza CC, Kutcher JS, Ashwal S, et al. Summary of evidence-based guideline update: evaluation and management of concussion in sports. Report of the Guideline Development Subcommittee of the American Academy of Neurology. *Neurology*. 2013;80:2250-2257.

9. Haydel MJ, Preston CA, Mills TJ, et al. Indications for computed tomography in patients with minor head injury. *N Engl J Med*. 2000;343:100-105.

10. Stiell IG, Wells GA, Vandernheen K, et al. The Canadian CT Head Rule for patients with minor head injury. *Lancet*. 2001;357:1391-1396.

11. Weinstein E, Turner M, Kuzma BB, Feuer H. Second impact syndrome in football: new imaging and insights into a rare and devastating condition: case report. *J Neurosurg Pediatr*. 2013;11:331-334.

12. Al Sayegh A, Sandford D, Carson AJ. Psychological approaches to treatment of postconcussion syndrome: a systematic review. *J Neurol Neurosurg Psychiatry*. 2010;81:1128-1134.

13. Morgan CD, Zuckerman SL, Lee YM, et al. Predictors of postconcussion syndrome after sports-related concussion in young athletes: a matched case-control study. *J Neurosurg Pediatr*. 2015;15:589-598.

14. Martland HS. Punch drunk. *J Am Med Assoc*. 1928;91:1103-1107.

15. Millspaugh JA. Dementia pugilistica. *US Nav Med Bull*. 1937;35:297-303.

16. Critchley M. Medical aspects of boxing, particularly from a neurological standpoint. *Br Med J*. 1957;1(5015):357-362.

17. Corsellis JA, Bruton CJ, Freeman-Browne D. The aftermath of boxing. *Psychol Med*. 1973;3:270-303.

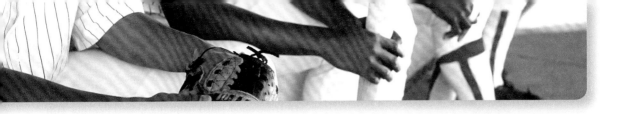

CHAPTER 30

Cervical Spine Injuries in Baseball Players

James D. Lin, MD | J. Alex Sielatycki, MD | Jamal N. Shillingford, MD | Ronald A. Lehman, Jr, MD

The greatest manager has a knack for making ballplayers think they are better than they think they are.

—*Reggie Jackson*

INTRODUCTION

Cervical spine injuries in baseball players can range from relatively common paraspinal muscular strains and herniated disks to rare but serious cervical spine fracture dislocations.[1] The frequency of common upper extremity conditions affecting throwing athletes such as rotator cuff tears, scapulothoracic conditions, and neurovascular conditions such as cubital tunnel syndrome may complicate the timely diagnosis of cervical spine pathology, which often manifests as periscapular pain, upper extremity radiculopathy, and/or weakness. A heightened awareness by the medical personnel can help achieve accurate diagnosis, appropriate treatment, and timely return to play. Unlike contact sports such as football, catastrophic cervical spinal injuries occur relatively infrequently with an estimated frequency of 0.08/100,000 injuries, approximately 10 times less than in football.[2] However, serious spinal injuries do occur, commonly in the setting of player-player collisions or ball-related injuries.[3] Team physicians, trainers, and managers should be prepared to recognize cervical spine injuries and spinal cord injury, perform appropriate sideline management, and refer to trauma or spinal cord injury center when indicated. The purpose of this chapter is to review the common cervical spine injuries encountered in baseball players with a focus on diagnosis, initial management, and treatment options.

CLINICAL EVALUATION

History

Effective communication between the patient, athletic trainer, and physician will help rule out serious diagnoses, while leading toward a definitive diagnosis. The intensity and location of pain should be described by the patient as well as circumstances that both exacerbate or alleviate the pain. Patients should be asked about the development of additional symptoms including numbness and/or paresthesias in specific dermatomal distributions.

Physical Examination

The on-field examination should focus initially on the presence of any obvious deformity, pain, or neurologic dysfunction that can confirm the information elicited from the patient's history. The examiner should palpate the spine to note any areas of malalignment, tenderness, or step-offs that could suggest more serious injuries such as a posterior ligamentous complex injury, fracture, or dislocation. A full sensory and motor neurologic examination should be conducted from head to toe, identifying any areas of weakness or abnormal sensation. The head and cervical spine must be stabilized by an assistant while log-roll maneuvers are utilized during physical examination to avoid movements that may exacerbate any existing injury. If there are no red flags or concerning signs, then range of motion in

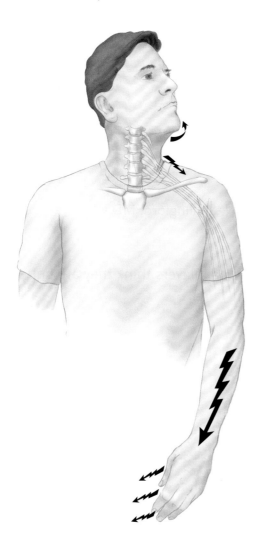

FIGURE 30.1 • Spurling maneuver.

flexion, extension, and rotation should be performed to assess for painful movement and symmetry. Provocative testing may include the Spurling maneuver with maximal neck extension, lateral flexion, and rotation toward the painful side, with axial compression applied, which may identify areas of foraminal neural compression or brachial plexus injury while shoulder abduction may provide relief[4] (Figure 30.1). If the player fails any portion of the on-field examination, they are immobilized in a cervical collar and removed from competition.

Two diagnostic dilemmas are often encountered when evaluating the throwing athlete with possible cervical spine pathology.

C8-T1 Radiculopathy Versus Cubital Tunnel Syndrome

It is important to distinguish between C8-T1 radiculopathy and peripheral ulnar nerve compression (cubital tunnel syndrome) because these 2 entities may have overlapping symptoms. In both cases, patient may experience ulnar-sided hand numbness. Patients with C8-T1 radiculopathy may experience ulnar forearm numbness/paresthesias secondary to the effect on the medial antebrachial cutaneous nerve along with weakness in the finger flexors. Patients with cubital tunnel syndrome do not have forearm sensory disturbance or finger flexor weakness and generally do not have weakness in the thenar muscles innervated by the median nerve.

C5 Radiculopathy Versus Rotator Cuff Tears

Both C5 radiculopathy and rotator cuff disorders can result in arm abduction weakness and pain in the shoulder area. These entities can typically be differentiated with provocative tests for shoulder impingement (Neer test, Hawkins test) as well as a detailed neurologic exam. Patients with rotator cuff disorders generally do not have neurologic findings such as paresthesias in a dermatomal distribution or biceps weakness, which can be present in C5 radiculopathy.

Sideline Management

The existence of a cervical spine injury must be assumed in the unconscious player, which then requires removal of any face masks and immediate neck immobilization before being moved. Prevention of catastrophic cervical spine injuries is key, and having a well-prepared and efficient plan can lead to successful transportation of the injured player. The tools necessary for successful immobilization and transportation include instruments necessary for face mask removal, a cervical collar, a hard backboard, and an equipped ambulance.[5] The effective transfer of a player to the backboard requires a minimum of 6 individuals and a well-rehearsed routine. The team leader controls the head and neck, while 2 people are on each side of the torso, and one at the feet. This allows the team to lift the player high enough to quickly shift the backboard underneath. A well-fitting cervical collar should be placed, and the head should be immobilized in a neutral position that restricts movement on the spine board. If no cervical collar is available, sandbags can be placed adjacent to the head to prevent cervical motion, which can exacerbate the damage to the spinal cord and nerve roots in the unstable spine.[6]

Imaging

Spine-related pain commonly resolves within 2 to 12 weeks with appropriate conservative management;

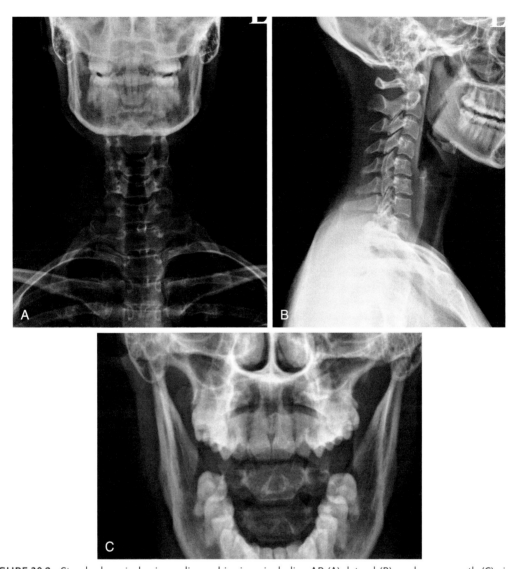

FIGURE 30.2 • Standard cervical spine radiographic views including AP (A), lateral (B), and open-mouth (C) views.

therefore, advanced imaging is often unnecessary. Players with severe persistent neck or radicular pain, neurologic impairment, altered mental status, a high-energy mechanism of injury, significant signs of trauma on physical examination, distracting injuries, or cardiorespiratory compromise should obtain a radiologic evaluation. Radiologic evaluation should include an anteroposterior, lateral, and open-mouth odontoid views, allowing visualization from the base of the skull down to the cervicothoracic junction (Figure 30.2). For patients with severe neurologic symptoms, advanced imaging with a computed tomography (CT) scan and/or magnetic resonance imaging (MRI) is necessary to better visualize the neural anatomy and areas of cord or root compression (Figure 30.3). For detection and evaluation of ligamentous injuries, MRI is more sensitive than X-ray and CT scan.[7,8]

A known risk factor for injuries of the cervical spine is congenital cervical stenosis. The Torg ratio is calculated by the width of the spinal canal compared with the width of the vertebral body at that same level. High-risk players at risk of cervical spine injuries are those with Torg ratios <0.8. Meyer and colleagues showed that football players with a Torg ratio less than 0.8 had a 3-fold risk of incurring a stinger.[9,10] Additionally, Castro et al showed that a Torg ratio of 0.7 or less may place college football players at increased risk of experiencing recurrent stingers.[11] Torg and colleagues also reported that cervical central stenosis placed athletes at risk for neuropraxia of the cervical spinal cord with transient quadriplegia.[12]

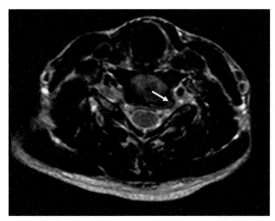

FIGURE 30.3 • Axial MRI showing herniated disk (arrow) in left neuroforamen.

HERNIATED DISK

Overview

Herniated nucleus pulposus (HNP) in the cervical spine, commonly referred to as a herniated or "ruptured" disk, may result in compression and/or irritation of the nearby cervical nerve root. Disk material may mechanically impinge on the nerve root, as it takes off from the spinal cord or as the nerve traverses the neuroforamen. In addition, herniated material from the nucleus pulposus can incite a localized inflammatory response, which itself may cause nerve root irritation. Sharp or electric-like pain may radiate from the neck into the arm, and there may be associated neurologic deficits such as numbness, paresthesias, or muscle weakness along the affected dermatome or myotome. A history of trauma precedes cervical radiculopathy in only 15% of cases in the general population.[13] In the general population, the most common cause of cervical radiculopathy is chronic changes from decreased foraminal height, osteophytes, and calcified disks. Acute soft disk herniation is responsible for only 25% of cases. Specifically in baseball players, the time course and onset has not been reported in the literature; however, one may suppose that disk ruptures occurring in this generally younger, active population are more often acute and related to an inciting event.

Nonoperative Treatment

There is a wide range of nonoperative treatment strategies in the setting of an acute disk herniation. It has been well demonstrated that the majority of acute HNP resolve over time without any intervention.[14] However, baseball players anxious to return to play warrant symptomatic treatment. Immobilization in a cervical collar is thought to decrease irritation and

inflammation about a nerve root by decreasing motion in the neck. Some patients find that a soft collar worn backward may alleviate symptoms by promoting a relatively flexed neck posture, which increases the space in the neuroforamen. It is generally not recommended that collars be used for longer than 2 to 3 weeks as a nonoperative treatment modality to avoid associated cervical muscular deconditioning and atrophy.

Nonsteroidal anti-inflammatory drugs (NSAIDs) are very commonly prescribed for treatment of musculoskeletal pain and may often provide significant symptom relief while a patient awaits further treatment and full recovery. Patients with renal dysfunction, hypertension, bleeding disorders, or peptic ulcer disease should consult with their primary physician before utilizing NSAIDs. Short courses of oral glucocorticoid steroids may provide significant pain relief in the acute setting of painful HNP. Patients with diabetes should be cautioned that systemic corticosteroids are likely to alter blood glucose levels, and careful attention should be paid to glycemic control during their use.

The use of epidural and transforaminal steroid injections for cervical HNP is widespread and has been shown to have both diagnostic and therapeutic benefits.[15] Unlike systemic corticosteroids, locally delivered steroids can mitigate the systemic side effects and theoretically deliver a high concentration of medication to the site needed. Unlike other nonsurgical modalities, spinal steroid injections are a more invasive procedure that does carry some inherent risk including rare cases of brainstem infarcts and death. Such complications are exceedingly rare among the many patients receiving injections every day in the United States.

Physical therapy (PT) is another nonsurgical modality with widespread use and often great clinical success. Many patients report significant symptom relief after participating in organized PT; however, it is unclear whether improvement is a direct result of therapy or in line with the natural course of the disease.[16,17] PT should be used with great care in patients with myelopathy or progressive weakness, and excessive manipulation of the neck should be avoided in this setting.

Surgical Options

Surgical intervention in the setting of cervical HNP with radiculopathy is occasionally indicated. Because the natural history of cervical HNP tends to favor resolution, surgical management is typically reserved as a second or third line of treatment. The patient's symptoms, physical examination findings, and correlative imaging should correlate to explain the patient's condition. If the diagnosis is in question, further studies or investigation are essential. Common indications for operative intervention in the setting of cervical HNP include the following:

1. Persistent, debilitating pain that is refractory to nonsurgical treatment
2. Progressive weakness along the myotome of the affected nerve root
3. Progressive or constant numbness along the affected dermatome
4. Numbness or weakness that has persisted for 6 to 12 weeks and that would be bothersome to the patient if the deficits were to become permanent
5. Spinal cord dysfunction/myelopathy

Unlike the general population, professional baseball players may have a greater stake in rapid recovery from a cervical radiculopathy. Surgical indications in elite athletes with severe pain or significant weakness related to cervical HNP may differ from those for an elderly patient with the same condition. For example, subtle bicep weakness may be largely insignificant for a sedentary patient and can thus be observed, while the same degree of weakness may inhibit top athletic performance. In such cases, it is important for the surgeon to discuss all treatment options with the athlete so that a reasonable, mutual decision can be made.

There are generally 3 primary surgical options in treating cervical HNP with radiculopathy: (1) anterior diskectomy and fusion; (2) posterior foraminotomy; (3) anterior diskectomy and arthroplasty.

Anterior Cervical Diskectomy and Fusion

Anterior cervical diskectomy and fusion (ACDF) is a surgical procedure performed to remove the diseased disk and promote fusion between the adjacent vertebral segments. It allows direct removal of compressive lesions without retraction of neural structures. In most settings of HNP, the offending pathology is ventral to the nerve root, and thus an anterior approach is the simplest means to obtain access to remove the lesion. The surgical exposure for ACDF utilizes a true intermuscular plane between the strap muscles of the neck and sternocleidomastoid, thus is largely a muscle-sparing procedure with generally minimal postsurgical pain. Once the intervertebral disk has been removed, a variety of graft options exist to fill this space, restore disk height, and induce fusion across the operative level. Historically, the gold standard graft choice has been autogenous bone graft harvested from the patient's iliac crest. In recent years, a large variety

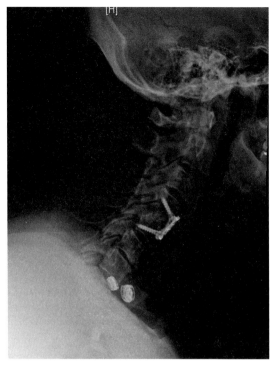

FIGURE 30.4 • Lateral radiograph of a patient after C4-5 anterior cervical diskectomy and fusion (ACDF).

of premachined allografts, synthetic cages, titanium implants, and bone substitutes are now available for use. In addition, locked anterior cervical plating has been introduced and shown to decrease nonunion rates and improve outcomes in ACDF; as such, most surgeons now utilize anterior plating techniques[4] (Figure 30.4).

The postoperative recovery from ACDF is generally well tolerated, with little pain or disability experienced by most patients. As with any surgical procedure, there are risks that must be considered. Devastating complications such as spinal cord injury, paralysis, blindness, stroke, esophageal perforation, vocal cord paralysis, asphyxiation, and infection are fortunately very rare.[4]

Nonunion (pseudarthrosis) at the site of intended fusion is a primary risk of any fusion operation. In general, fusion rates are very high in plated anterior cervical fusion, with rates reported at 95% or above.[18-20] Factors that may contribute to decreased fusion include tobacco use, osteoporosis, malnourishment, increased number of levels operated on, and poor surgical technique.[21,22] Importantly, the occurrence of a pseudarthrosis is not always associated with the need for further surgery. A significant number of patients without successful radiographic fusion may remain asymptomatic and thus would not require further surgical intervention.[21] When a nonunion is symptomatic, revision fusion from a posterior approach has a high success rate in achieving solid fusion, approaching 100% in most reports.[21]

Speech and swallowing difficulties are another important complication that can be associated with anterior cervical approaches. In general, mostly all patients undergoing this operation will experience some amount of mild transient dysphagia postoperatively. It is estimated that 2% to 5% of patients undergoing and anterior cervical operation may experience more severe, long-lasting dysphagia.

Adjacent segment degeneration (ASD) after ACDF is defined as disk degeneration at levels above and below the site of a prior fusion. There remains some controversy over whether ASD is a result of additional stresses placed at mobile segments above or below fusion constructs or whether ASD simply represents the natural history of disk degeneration in a patient with such genetic propensity. ASD is reported to occur in roughly 3% of patients per year or 25% of patients in the first 10 years after ACDF.[23]

The question of return to play is likely to be at the forefront in treating athletes with ACDF. There are no longitudinal studies to define the optimal time required before return to play is allowed. Most surgeons are likely to hold players out from competition for a minimum of 2 to 3 months after the procedure. In a study of 15 professional athletes (various sports), 13 of the 15 players returned to their sport between 2 and 12 months after surgery. In Hsu's review of baseball pitchers with cervical HNP, 7 of 8 pitchers undergoing ACDF were able to return to play the following season.[24] Ultimately, the decision on when an athlete should be allowed to return to the field will be up to the discretion of the treating surgeon. Our preferred postoperative protocol is a soft collar for 1 week, running at 8 weeks, and light throwing at 8 to 12 weeks with progression to full throwing based on radiographic assessment of fusion.

Posterior Cervical Foraminotomy

If a fusion is not desired, posterior cervical foraminotomy may be a reasonable alternative to preserve motion while achieving adequate neural decompression. This procedure is performed by making a posterior approach to the level in question and removing the dorsal portion of the neuroforamen to allow indirect decompression of the nerve root (Figure 30.5). Ideally, this operation is indicated when the compressive lesion is situated such that unroofing the neuroforamen posteriorly will afford sufficient decompression of the nerve.

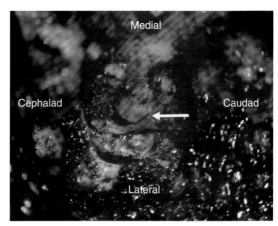

FIGURE 30.5 ● Intraoperative image from a posterior cervical foraminotomy. Removal of the medial aspect of the superior and inferior articular facets decompresses the underlying cervical nerve root (white arrow).

The primary advantage of PCF is the avoidance of fusion and thus theoretical decreased risk of ASD. However, there are also drawbacks associated with the foraminotomy procedure. In particular, recurrence of symptoms at the same level is reported at rates of roughly 5%.[25] Additionally, some studies have even reported ASD at rates of 6.7% after foraminotomy; thus ASD is not completely averted using this approach.[25] Nerve root palsy is also reported after this procedure owing to the need for neural retraction, with a reported incidence around 1.2% to 3.2%.[26]

Foraminotomy has a reported success rate of roughly 90% in the short term and thus may be a reasonable consideration for many patients with cervical HNP.[27] Specifically for baseball athletes, foraminotomy may be an attractive option in that there is no need for prolonged activity restriction, as there is no fusion that must occur. Once the incision has healed from this operation, players should in theory be allowed to return to play as their symptoms allow. The surgeon must be cautious, however, and carefully assess whether the impinging lesion will be accessible through this approach. Our preferred postoperative protocol is a soft collar for several days for patient comfort and progression of activities as symptoms subside with no restrictions.

Cervical Disk Arthroplasty

Cervical disk arthroplasty (CDA) (also known as disk replacement) was developed to mitigate the limitations of ACDF by allowing anterior decompression without the need for fusion. Rather than fusing the motion segment, a prosthetic disk is inserted in its place (Figure 30.6). The goal of this method is to

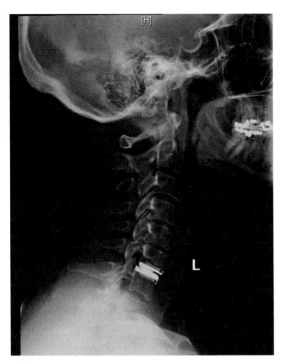

FIGURE 30.6 • Lateral radiograph of a patient after C6-7 cervical disk arthroplasty.

preserve motion at that level and theoretically mitigate the need for immobilization and activity restrictions and potentially decrease the development of ASD.

CDA has now been widely studied in several rigorous randomized-controlled trials of CDA versus ACDF, with promising results. In a multicenter randomized trial of single-level ACDF versus single-level CDA, Heller et al reported that both groups showed significant improvement in neck-related disability (NDI) at 12 and 24 months. In this study, the CDA group showed overall greater improvement in NDI from baseline, as well as fewer implant-related adverse events (1.7% vs 3.2%). In addition, patients receiving the artificial disk returned to work 2 weeks sooner on average compared with ACDF.[28] Sasso et al reported greater improvement in NDI and overall success rate with CDA at 4 years, with CDA patients showing overall success of 85.1% compared with 72.5% in the ACDF group at 4 years.[29]

Despite the theoretical advantage of protecting adjacent motion segments, the efficacy of CDA in preventing ASD has yet to be rigorously proven. In a 2013 meta-analysis of 6 prospective trials with pooled data on 777 ACDF patients and 809 CDA patients, the rate of reoperation for adjacent segment disease in CDA was 5.1% versus 6.9% in ACDF at 2 to 5 years, with no statistically significant difference.[30] Future studies with longer follow-up are needed to answer this question.

The surgical approach for CDA is the same as for ACDF, and thus many of the surgical risks between these 2 operations are similar. Compared with ACDF, there are, however, some risks unique to CDA. Spontaneous fusion, or heterotopic ossification, of the diskectomy level has been reported in CDA patients at a rate of 9% to 11%.[31,32] In such cases, recurrence of neck pain and radiculopathy may require revision of the arthroplasty to a fusion. Biomechanical testing of arthroplasty implants has shown good evidence to suggest that the devices are durable; however, the long-term durability of CDA implants remains unknown in clinical practice.

Finally, while CDA has been shown to have at least equivalent or slightly improved outcomes at 4 years compared with ACDF in the general population, the use of CDA in high-level athletes has not been specifically studied. In Hsu's review of major league pitchers, there was only 1 patient who had CDA, and he was able to return to play.[24] Anecdotally, the senior author (RAL) has had personal patients return to high-level military maneuvers and athletic activity relatively quickly after CDA, with 1 patient returning to skydiving just 4 weeks after CDA without untoward results.

Because CDA is not a fusion procedure, it is similar to a posterior foraminotomy in that prolonged immobilization is not necessary. Our preferred postoperative protocol is a soft collar for several days for patient comfort. Athletes are encouraged to return to running and throwing activities as soon as symptoms dissipate, with no restrictions to activities.

The available data and anecdotal experience provide good reason to believe that CDA is a good option for athletes that may both provide lasting symptom relief and more rapid return to play; however, more rigorous prospective studies are needed to confirm the efficacy and durability of CDA in high-level athletes.

Choosing the Best Operation

There are few absolute indications for one surgical approach over another in treating cervical radiculopathy. Appropriate decompression of the symptomatic nerve roots has a high overall success rate regardless of which approach is used.

CERVICAL STRAINS AND SPRAINS

Overview

Cervical sprains and strains are common cervical spine injury in athletes. By definition, muscle strains are partial tearing of the musculature or myotendinous junction, whereas sprains are ligamentous injuries.[33] Both can result in pain, spasm, and dysfunction. In practice, the diagnosis is often made when no objective signs of injury to the spine are apparent and neurovascular structures are intact.

Cervical sprains and strains can be caused by any force to the neck, which can include sudden flexion or extension as seen in whiplash-type injuries.[34,35] The resulting injury results in muscle spasm and pain. The athlete often reports neck pain and stiffness and may present with limited and painful range of motion.[36] Radiographic examination is normal and should show no signs of subluxation or instability.[37] Flexion and extension radiographs are useful to exclude occult ligamentous injuries.[34]

On examination, the athlete is typically tender to palpation over the paraspinal musculature. Flexion, extension, and rotation may exacerbate and help identify the source of pain. It is important to palpate the spinous processes, as direct midline pain suggests more serious bony injury. With isolated cervical sprains and strains, neurologic examination is generally normal. Neurologic deficits should prompt the examiner to search a more serious diagnosis.

Treatment

The key to treatment for paraspinal muscle strain and associated spasm are rest, ice, NSAIDs, muscle relaxants, and PT. Early mobilization leads to faster recovery than prolonged immobilization.[38] Any presumed sprain/strain associated with neurologic dysfunction or fails to improve with a short period of rest may warrant an MRI.

CERVICAL SPINE FRACTURES

Overview

There is a large spectrum of cervical spine fractures that vary by anatomic location (upper cervical vs lower cervical), fracture pattern, and presence or absence of concomitant spinal cord injury. In the setting of baseball injuries, these injuries often occur during player collisions or ball injuries and can occur during games or during practice settings.[3] Upper cervical spine injuries, including fractures and dislocations involving the atlanto-occipital joint, C1, or C2, are rare in athletes.[1] Moreover, given the relatively larger amount of space in the spinal canal in the upper cervical region, these injuries are less likely to be associated with spinal cord injury.

Subaxial cervical spine injuries are defined as injuries involving C3 and below and make up for over 70% of cervical spine fractures.[39] Several different methods have been described to classify cervical spine fractures, including the historical Allen Ferguson mechanistic classification, the algorithm-based subaxial injury classification, and most recently the AOSpine classification system.[40-42] However, a single classification has yet to be universally adopted.[43] Treatment decisions regarding cervical spine fractures and dislocations are ultimately based on a combination of fracture pattern, predicted spinal stability, presence of neurologic injury, and alignment.[41,43]

Key to understanding treatment of cervical spine fractures is understanding various anatomic elements that are prone to injury, including the vertebral bodies, intervertebral disk, anterior and posterior longitudinal ligaments, facet joint capsules, interspinous ligaments, supraspinous ligaments, and neurovascular structures including the spinal cord, nerve roots, and vertebral arteries. The particular combination of structures injured determines the injury classification and informs the treating physician about the likely stability of the spine and the need for surgery.

In the setting of baseball injuries, injury types more likely encountered are compression/burst fractures and injuries to the posterior tension band.[1] Discussion will be limited to management of these 2 types of injuries. In general, stable injury patterns without neurologic injury, such as compression fractures and most burst fractures, can be treated nonoperatively with a hard cervical orthosis. Unstable injury patterns likely to result in posttraumatic deformity or neurologic sequelae, such as those with posterior ligamentous complex disruption, are treated surgically.

Compression and Burst Fractures

Compression fractures occur in the setting of an axial force with the neck in a neutral or slightly flexed position.[1] This results in compression of the anterior vertebral body (compression fracture), without involvement of the posterior wall of the vertebral body (burst fracture). These are generally considered stable injuries.

Burst fractures occur in the setting of an axial force with the neck in the neutral position. This results in compression of the vertebral body with retropulsion of vertebral body fragments into the spinal canal. Because the posterior elements are loaded in compression, theoretically posterior ligamentous complex is intact.

In the absence of neurologic injury, compression and burst fractures injuries can often be treated nonoperatively with a hard cervical collar.[1] Other treatment options include skull traction or halo vest.[44]

Operative indications for burst fractures include neurologic injury and progressive deformity indicating spinal instability. Some authors have defined 1 cm height loss and substantial kyphosis as operative indications. When surgical treatment is chosen, burst fractures are generally treated with anterior vertebral body resection and fusion, to allow for decompression of the retropulsed fragments.[45,46] When anterior decompression is not necessary, posterior fusion with lateral mass screws is an option as well.[47]

Posterior Tension Band Injuries

Injuries to the posterior tension band can vary widely and range from unilateral or bilateral facet subluxations to unilateral or bilateral facet fracture dislocations. These injuries typically occur with a hyperflexion mechanism and are often associated with compression of neural elements. Definitive management of facet dislocations involves reduction to realign the spine, followed by definitive stabilization. Closed reduction can be achieved using skull tongs with traction to realign the spine under a monitored setting. Controversy remains regarding the need for an MRI before reduction, to identify a herniated disk that could be forced into the spinal canal during the reduction maneuver.[47,48]

If closed reduction fails, open reduction and definitive surgical stabilization of the injury can be performed from either an anterior or posterior approach.[45,49] If a disk herniation is identified on preoperative MRI, an anterior approach is recommended to decompress the spinal canal. If there is no disk herniation, either an anterior or posterior approach can be done, based on surgeon and patient preference.[45]

Brodke et al reported on results of 52 patients with cervical spine injuries and associated spinal cord injury randomized to anterior versus posterior surgical approaches. There were no differences in fusion rates, alignment, or neurologic recovery.[50] Kwon et al reported on a prospective randomized trial of anterior versus posterior surgery for unilateral facet injuries. Patients treated with anterior surgery had less pain, lower injection rates, and better alignment, but had increased swallowing difficulty.[51]

MANAGER'S TIPS

- Cervical spine injuries are common and include disk herniations, paraspinal muscle strains, and fractures or dislocations
- The natural history of cervical disk herniation tends to favor resolution, and surgical management is typically reserved as a second or third line of treatment

- Cervical sprains and strains are typically treated with rest, NSAIDs, and early mobilization
- Suspected spinal cord injury (SCI) should be managed with immobilization with hard cervical collar, rigid backboard, and urgent referral to SCI or trauma center

REFERENCES

1. Schroeder GD, Vaccaro AR. Cervical spine injuries in the athlete. *J Am Acad Orthop Surg.* 2016;24(9):e122-e133. doi:10.5435/JAAOS-D-15-00716.
2. Carll KE, Park AE, Tortolani PJ. Epidemiology of catastrophic spine injuries in high school, college, and professional sports. *Semin Spine Surg.* 2010;22(4):168-172. doi:10.1053/j.semss.2010.06.007.
3. Boden BP, Tacchetti R, Mueller FO. Catastrophic injuries in high school and college baseball players. *Am J Sports Med.* 2004;32(5):1189-1196. doi:10.1177/0363546503262161.
4. Rhee JM, Yoon T, Riew KD. Cervical radiculopathy. *J Am Acad Orthop Surg.* 2007;15(8):486-494.
5. Herkowitz HN, Garfin SR, Eismont FJ, Bell GR, Balderston RA. *Rothman-Simeone the Spine.* Philadelphia, PA: Elsevier; 2011.
6. Waninger KN. Management of the helmeted athlete with suspected cervical spine injury. *Am J Sports Med.* 2004;32(5):1331-1350. doi:10.1177/0363546504264580.
7. Ajani AE, Cooper DJ, Scheinkestel CD, Laidlaw J, Tuxen D V. Optimal assessment of cervical spine trauma in critically ill patients: a prospective evaluation. *Anaesth Intensive Care.* 1998;26(5):487-491.
8. Diaz JJJ, Aulino JM, Collier B, et al. The early work-up for isolated ligamentous injury of the cervical spine: does computed tomography scan have a role? *J Trauma.* 2005;59(4):897-903 [discussion 903-904]. doi:10.1097/01.ta.0000188012.84356.dc.
9. Meyer SA, Schulte KR, Callaghan JJ, et al. Cervical spinal stenosis and stingers in collegiate football players. *Am J Sports Med.* 1994;22(2):158-166. doi:10.1177/036354659402200202.
10. Eismont FJ, Clifford S, Goldberg M, Green B. Cervical sagittal spinal canal size in spine injury. *Spine (Phila Pa 1976).* 1984;9:663-666. doi:10.1097/00007632-198410000-00001.
11. Castro FP Jr, Ricciardi J, Brunet ME, Busch MT, Whitecloud TS III. Stingers, the Torg ratio, and the cervical spine. *Am J Sports Med.* 1997;25(5):603-608. doi:10.1177/036354659702500503.
12. Torg JS, Pavlov H, Genuario SE, et al. Neurapraxia of the cervical spinal cord with transient quadriplegia. *J Bone Joint Surg Am.* 1986;68(9):1354-1370. http://www.ncbi.nlm.nih.gov/pubmed/3782207.

13. Carette S, Fehlings MG. Clinical practice. Cervical radiculopathy. *N Engl J Med*. 2005;353(4):392-399. doi:10.1056/NEJMcp043887.

14. Lees F, Turner JW. Natural history and prognosis of cervical spondylosis. *Br Med J*. 1963;2(5373):1607-1610. doi:10.1136/bmj.2.5373.1607.

15. Sasso RC, Macadaeg K, Nordmann D, Smith M. Selective nerve root injections can predict surgical outcome for lumbar and cervical radiculopathy: comparison to magnetic resonance imaging. *J Spinal Disord Tech*. 2005;18(6):471-478. doi:00024720-200512000-00001 [pii].

16. Levine M, Albert T, Smith M. Cervical radiculopathy: diagnosis and nonoperative management. *J Am Acad Orthop Surg*. 1996;4(6):305-316. doi:10.1016/0003-9993(94)90040-X.

17. Hurwitz EL, Aker PD, Adams AH, Meeker WC, Shekelle PG. Manipulation and mobilization of the cervical spine. A systematic review of the literature. *Spine (Phila Pa 1976)*. 1996;21(15):1746-1759 [discussion 1759-1760]. doi:10.1097/00007632-199608010-00007.

18. Fraser JF, Härtl R. Anterior approaches to fusion of the cervical spine: a metaanalysis of fusion rates. *J Neurosurg Spine*. 2007;6(4):298-303. doi:10.3171/spi.2007.6.4.2.

19. Wang JC, McDonough PW, Endow KK, Delamarter RB. Increased fusion rates with cervical plating for two-level anterior cervical discectomy and fusion. *Spine (Phila Pa 1976)*. 2000;25(1):41-45. doi:10.1097/00007632-200001010-00009.

20. Yue W-M, Brodner W, Highland T. Long-term results after anterior cervical discectomy and fusion with allograft and plating: a 5- to 11-year radiologic and clinical follow-up study. *Spine (Phila Pa 1976)*. 2005;30(19):2138-2144. doi:00007632-200510010-00004 [pii].

21. Phillips FM, Carlson G, Emery SE, Bohlman HH. Anterior cervical pseudarthrosis. Natural history and treatment. *Spine (Phila Pa 1976)*. 1997;22(14):1585-1589. doi:10.1097/00007632-199707150-00012.

22. Mummaneni PV, Burkus JK, Haid RW, Traynelis VC, Zdeblick TA. Clinical and radiographic analysis of cervical disc arthroplasty compared with allograft fusion: a randomized controlled clinical trial. *J Neurosurg Spine*. 2007;6(3):198-209. doi:10.3171/spi.2007.6.3.198.

23. Cho SK, Riew KD. Adjacent segment disease following cervical spine surgery. *J Am Acad Orthop Surg*. 2013;21(1):3-11. doi:10.5435/jaaos-21-01-3.

24. Roberts DW, Roc GJ, Hsu WK. Outcomes of cervical and lumbar disk herniations in major league baseball pitchers. *Orthopedics*. 2011;34(8):602-609. doi:10.3928/01477447-20110627-23.

25. Clark JG, Abdullah KG, Steinmetz MP, Benzel EC, Mroz TE. Minimally invasive versus open cervical foraminotomy: a systematic review. *Global Spine J*. 2011;1(1):9-14. doi:10.1055/s-0031-1296050.

26. Choi KC, Ahn Y, Kang BU, Ahn ST, Lee SH. Motor palsy after posterior cervical foraminotomy: anatomical consideration. *World Neurosurg*. 2013;79(2). doi:10.1016/j.wneu.2011.03.043.

27. Henderson CM, Hennessy RG, Shuey HM, Shackelford EG. Posterior-lateral foraminotomy as an exclusive operative technique for cervical radiculopathy: a review of 846 consecutively operated cases. *Neurosurgery*. 1983;13(5):504-512. doi:10.1227/00006123-198311000-00004.

28. Heller JG, Sasso RC, Papadopoulos SM, et al. Comparison of BRYAN cervical disc arthroplasty with anterior cervical decompression and fusion: clinical and radiographic results of a randomized, controlled, clinical trial. *Spine (Phila Pa 1976)*. 2009;34(2):101-107. doi:10.1097/BRS.0b013e31818ee263.

29. Sasso RC, Anderson PA, Riew KD, Heller JG. Results of cervical arthroplasty compared with anterior discectomy and fusion: four-year clinical outcomes in a prospective, randomized controlled trial. *J Bone Joint Surg Am*. 2011;93(18):1684-1692. doi:10.2106/JBJS.J.00476.

30. Verma K, Gandhi SD, Maltenfort M, et al. The rate of adjacent segment disease in cervical disc arthoplasty versus single level fusion: a meta-analysis of of prospective studies. *Spine (Phila Pa 1976)*. 2013;38(26):2253-2257. doi:10.1097/BRS.0000000000000052.

31. Mehren C, Suchomel P, Grochulla F, et al. Heterotopic ossification in total cervical artificial disc replacement. *Spine (Phila Pa 1976)*. 2006;31(24):2802-2806. doi:10.1097/01.brs.0000245852.70594.d5.

32. Leung C, Casey AT, Goffin J, et al. Clinical significance of heterotopic ossification in cervical disc replacement: a prospective multicenter clinical trial. *Neurosurgery*. 2005:759-763. doi:10.1227/01.NEU.0000175856.31210.58.

33. Krabak BJ, Kanarek SL. Cervical spine pain in the competitive athlete. *Phys Med Rehabil Clin N Am*. 2011;22(3):459-471. doi:10.1016/j.pmr.2011.02.007.

34. Boden BP, Jarvis CG. Spinal injuries in sports. *Neurol Clin*. 2008;26(1):63-78. doi:10.1016/j.ncl.2007.12.005.

35. Swartz EE, Boden BP, Courson RW, et al. National athletic trainers' association position statement: acute management of the cervical spine–injured athlete. *J Athl Train*. 2009;44(3):306-331. doi:10.4085/1062-6050-44.3.306.

36. Zmurko MG, Tannoury TY, Tannoury CA, Anderson DG. Cervical sprains, disc herniations, minor fractures, and other cervical injuries in the athlete. *Clin Sports Med*. 2003;22(3):513-521. doi:10.1016/S0278-5919(03)00003-6.

37. Cantu RC. Cervical spine injuries in the athlete. *Semin Neurol*. 2000;20(2):173-178. doi:10.1055/s-2000-9825.

38. Borchgrevink I, Lereim G, Kaasa A, McDonagh D, Stiles T, Haraldseth O. Acute treatment of whiplash neck sprain injuries. A randomized trial of treatment during the first 14 days after a car accident. *Spine (Phila Pa 1976)*. 1998;23(1):25-31. doi:10.1097/00007632-199801010-00006.

39. Goldberg W, Mueller C, Panacek E, Tigges S, Hoffman JR, Mower WR. Distribution and patterns of blunt traumatic cervical spine injury. *Ann Emerg Med.* 2001;38(1):17-21. doi:10.1067/mem.2001.116150.

40. Allen BL, Ferguson RL, Lehmann TR, O'brien RP. A mechanistic classification of closed, indirect fractures and dislocations of the lower cervical spine. *Spine (Phila Pa 1976).* 1982;7(1):1-27. doi:10.1097/00007632-198200710-00001.

41. Vaccaro AR, Koerner JD, Radcliff KE, et al. AOSpine subaxial cervical spine injury classification system. *Eur Spine J.* 2016;25(7):2173-2184. doi:10.1007/s00586-015-3831-3.

42. Vaccaro AR, Hulbert RJ, Patel AA, et al. The subaxial cervical spine injury classification system: a novel approach to recognize the importance of morphology, neurology, and integrity of the disco-ligamentous complex. *Spine (Phila Pa 1976).* 2007;32(21):2365. doi:10.1097/BRS.0b013e3181557b92.

43. Patel AA, Hurlbert RJ, Bono CM, Bessey JT, Yang N, Vaccaro AR. Classification and surgical decision making in acute subaxial cervical spine trauma. *Spine (Phila Pa 1976).* 2010;35(21). doi:10.1097/BRS.0b013e3181f330ae.

44. Koivikko MP, Myllynen P, Karjalainen M, Vornanen M, Santavirta S. Conservative and operative treatment in cervical burst fractures. *Arch Orthop Trauma Surg.* 2000;120:448-451.

45. Dvorak M, Fisher C, Fehlings M, et al. The surgical approach to subaxial cervical spine injuries: an evidence-based algorithm based on the SLIC classification system. *Spine (Phila Pa 1976).* 2007;32(23):2620-2629. doi:10.1097/BRS.0b013e318158ce16.

46. Ripa DR, Kowall MG, Meyer PR Jr, Rusin JJ. Series of ninety-two traumatic cervical spine injuries stabilized with anterior ASIF plate fusion technique. *Spine (Phila Pa 1976).* 1991;16(0362-2436):S46-S55.

47. Kwon BK, Vaccaro AR, Grauer JN, Fisher CG, Dvorak MF. Subaxial cervical spine trauma. *J Am Acad Orthop Surg.* 2006;14(2):78-89.

48. Grauer JN, Vaccaro AR, Lee JY, et al. The timing and influence of MRI on the management of patients with cervical facet dislocations remains highly variable: a survey of members of the Spine Trauma Study Group. *J Spinal Disord Tech.* 2009;22(2):96-99. doi:10.1097/BSD.0b013e31816a9ebd.

49. Del Curto D, Tamaoki MJ, Martins DE, Puertas EB, Belloti JC. Surgical approaches for cervical spine facet dislocations in adults. *Cochrane Database Syst Rev.* 2014;10:CD008129. doi:10.1002/14651858.CD008129.pub2.

50. Brodke DS, Anderson PA, Newell DW, Grady MS, Chapman JR. Comparison of anterior and posterior approaches in cervical spinal cord injuries. *J Spinal Disord Tech.* 2003;16(3):229-235. doi:10.1097/00024720-200306000-00001.

51. Kwon BK, Fisher CG, Boyd MC, et al. A prospective randomized controlled trial of anterior compared with posterior stabilization for unilateral facet injuries of the cervical spine. *J Neurosurg Spine.* 2007;7(1):1-12. doi:10.3171/SPI-07/07/001.

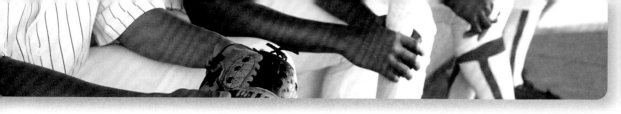

CHAPTER 31

Lumbar Spine Injuries in Baseball Players

Ronald A. Lehman, Jr, MD | Joseph M. Lombardi, MD | Melvin C. Makhni, MD | David P. Trofa, MD

Winning is the most important thing in my life, after breathing. Breathing first, winning next.

—*George Steinbrenner*

INTRODUCTION

Overuse injuries of the athlete are becoming increasingly prevalent owing to an active population and a societal emphasis on excessive training often associated with inadequate recovery time after activity.[1-5] Additionally, poor mechanics, improper exercise regimens, and unhealthy training environments can contribute to musculoskeletal injuries.[6,7] The lumbar spine is a common source of pain secondary to overuse injuries in the athlete, with some studies reporting up to 30% incidence of lower back pain in this demographic.[8] Those sports, which subject the athlete's lumbar spine to repetitive flexion or explosive extension moments, have a greater prevalence of lower back pain. Wrestlers, elite gymnasts, and football linemen have been shown to have increased rates of lower back pain versus age-matched controls.[9,10] Such injuries include muscular back pain, spondylolysis, acute herniation of nucleus pulposus, and sacroiliac joint pain, as well as mimickers of lumbar disease including hip labral and greater trochanteric pathologies. When performing a physical examination of an athlete with lower back pain, a clinician should have a high suspicion for these various conditions. Correct diagnosis will often require use of specific provocative maneuvers, in addition to a routine neurologic examination of the spine. In this review, we aim to guide clinicians on the proper physical examination of the lumbar spine with a focus on the athlete.

GENERAL EVALUATION

Casual observation of a patient presenting with lumbar spine discomfort is essential to guide the clinician as to the source and degree of pain. This should begin with observing the patient's walk into the examination room, making note of wincing or limping.[11] An examination of the patient's overall global alignment including posture and sagittal balance should be noted. This will require removal of all garments except underwear and use of a gown allowing for exposure of the patient's back. Evaluate for the presence of a normal lumbar and cervical lordosis as well as thoracic kyphosis (Figure 31.1A and B). Alignment of the head with respect to the center of the pelvis, shoulder heights, and pelvic tilt are important indicators of truncal shift[12] (Figure 31.2A and B). Other abnormalities including erythema, muscular atrophy, and skin pigmentation may be indicative of underlying infection or congenital pathologies.

Gait analysis is vital for identifying underlying spinal cord disease states. Antalgic or shortened stance phase gait is typical for musculoskeletal injury to a unilateral lower extremity. A spastic or scissored gait can be indicative of upper motor neuron injury including cord compression, trauma, or a tumor. Inability to perform a tandem gait (heel-to-toe) is often seen in patients with underlying ataxia. Identification of these gait patterns will aid the clinician in understanding pain patterns as well as neurologic dysfunction. Additionally, they may help to identify extraspinal pathologies such as leg length discrepancy or contractures.

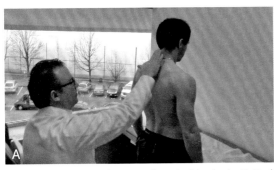
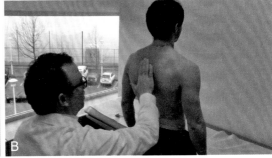

FIGURE 31.1 • A, Evaluation of cervical lordosis. B, Evaluation of thoracic kyphosis.

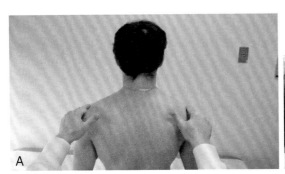
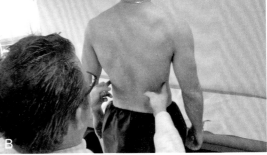

FIGURE 31.2 • A, Evaluation of shoulder height. B, Evaluation of waist symmetry.

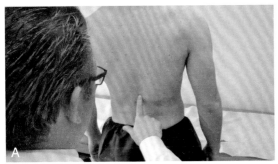
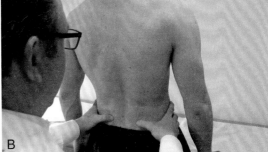

FIGURE 31.3 • A, Palpation of spinous processes. B, Palpation of posterior superior iliac spine.

PALPATION

The examiner should position himself behind the patient placing his hands on the patient's hips while palpating the spinous processes with his thumbs. Palpation should extend along the iliac crest (L4-L5) interspace as well as the sacroiliac joint and posterior superior iliac spine, which lies closest to the S2 vertebral level (Figure 31.3A and B). Palpation should be performed noting for any tenderness or step-off suggestive of spondylolisthesis. Absence of posterior bony structures with or without the presence of a hair tuft or skin pigmentation may be indicative of a congenital neural tube defect. Pain emanating from the lateral aspect of the spine on palpation may point to transverse process pathology. It is important to rule out muscular etiologies of pain, as these are among the most common generators of lumbar symptoms. The paraspinal musculature should be palpated carefully along the entire course of the spine. Tenderness to the sciatic notch is suggestive of sciatic nerve irritation. Likewise, pain with palpation to the greater trochanter points to greater trochanteric bursitis, which can often mimic an L5 radiculopathy (Figure 31.4).

SENSORY EXAMINATION

An understanding of dermatomal distribution can aid the clinician in localizing spinal pathology (Figure 31.5). A sensory examination may be elicited by use of light touch, pinprick, light and/or deep pressure, temperature, and vibration. Dermatomes corresponding to pathologic nerve roots have significant more sensory dysfunction than unaffected nerve roots.[13] Suri et al demonstrated 20% sensitivity and 93% specificity for the pinprick test in diagnosing lumbar radiculopathy.[14] Interestingly,

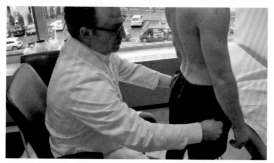

FIGURE 31.4 • Palpation of greater trochanter to evaluate for bursitis commonly seen in L5 radiculopathy.

these values increased to 36% and 92%, respectively, when the examiner knew the results of the patient MRI, demonstrating an inherent bias. Despite this, Bradley et al showed that compressed nerve roots may manifest in sensory deficits in only one-half of instances.[15]

The L1 dermatome runs from the medial aspect of the thigh, along the inguinal crease toward the groin. The L2 dermatome takes a similar path over a more distal and anterior area while the L3 dermatome encompasses the region just medial to the patella, traveling inferiorly down the medial aspect of the leg (Figure 31.6). The L4 dermatome crosses the anterior aspect of the knee, moving caudally down the anteromedial aspect of the lower leg (Figure 31.7). The L5 dermatome includes the lateral leg, the first dorsal web space, and the dorsal aspect of the middle toe, whereas the S1 most commonly includes the lateral aspect of the foot and the fifth digit (Figure 31.8A and B).

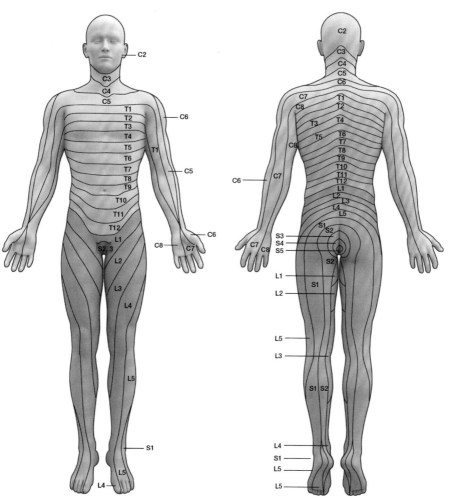

FIGURE 31.5 • Dermatome map.

MOTOR EXAMINATION

Motor testing serves to grade muscle strength on a scale from 0 to 5 (Table 31.1). Strength impairment on physical examination has been shown to correlate with high likelihood of associated anatomical abnormalities on MRI, with a predictive odds ratio of 5.2.[16]

L1-L3

The iliopsoas serves as the primary flexor of the hip. It has a collective innervation from the L1-L3 nerve roots, and therefore testing of hip flexion strength serves to evaluate the motor innervation for L1-L3. This is best evaluated by asking the patient to move

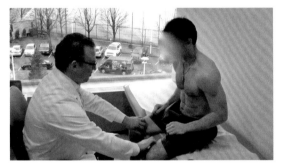

FIGURE 31.6 • Evaluation of the L3 sensory distribution.

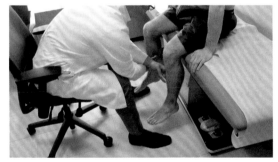

FIGURE 31.7 • Evaluation of the L4 sensory distribution.

to the edge of the table with his legs dangling off the end. The patient is then asked to lift his knee toward the ceiling while the examiner provides a resistive force just proximal to the knee. This method of motor testing was found to have a sensitivity between 39% and 48% and a specificity of 86% and 89%[14] (Figure 31.9).

L2-L4

The quadriceps and hip adductors have a collective innervation from the L2-L4 nerve roots. Quadriceps strength should be evaluated by allowing the patient to sit comfortably with his knees bent while his feet are relaxed and dangling. The examiner should stabilize the leg by placing one hand on the thigh and the other on the anterior surface of the tibia and ask the patient to extend his leg against resistance. Standing, single-leg squats can also be utilized to evaluate for quadriceps strength (Figure 31.10).

Hip adductors can be tested in the supine patient starting with the patient's knees extended and hips abducted so that the feet are just beyond shoulder width. The examiner should place the hands on the medial aspects of the knees and ask the patient to bring both legs together while leaving his heels on the examination table.

L4-L5

The superior gluteal nerve (originating from L5) provides innervation to the gluteus medius, which is the major abductor of the hip. Assessing hip abduction strength is an important tool, as it may be the only means of testing for L5 compromise in the setting of a great toe metatarsophalangeal and/or ankle arthrodesis. Hip abduction can be tested by asking the supine patient to place his legs together with the knees extended. The examiner then provides a resistive force to the patient's thigh while asking him to abduct his leg.

The most common method of testing for L4 and L5 nerve root function is by evaluation of tibialis anterior and extensor hallucis longus (EHL) strength,

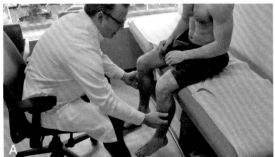
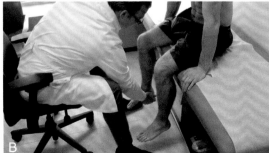

FIGURE 31.8 • A, Evaluation of L5 sensory distribution. B, Evaluation of S1 sensory distribution.

TABLE 31.1 Manual Muscle Strength Grading Chart

Grade	Percentage	Description
5 (normal)	100	Complete range of motion against gravity with full resistance
4 (good)	75	Complete range of motion against gravity with some resistance
3 (fair)	50	Complete range of motion against gravity with no resistance
2 (poor)	25	Complete range of motion with gravity eliminated
1 (trace)	10	Evidence of slight contractility with no evidence of joint motion even with gravity eliminated
0 (zero)	0	No evidence of muscle contractility

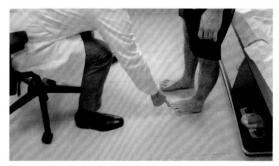

FIGURE 31.11 • Strength testing of the extensor hallucis longus.

dorsiflex his ankle with slight inversion. The examiner will then provide a plantarflexion force against the dorsum of the foot. Similarly, the examiner should then place a stabilizing force on the calcaneus and ask the patient to dorsiflex his great toe while applying a downward pressure on the first toe interphalangeal joint, assessing for weakness. Patients can also demonstrate L4-L5 integrity by performing heel-walks, which require contraction of tibialis anterior and EHL. It is our preferred technique to have the patient perform dorsiflexion exercises of the tibialis anterior and EHL 20 times before motor testing, as fatigue of the muscles can more clearly elucidate motor deficits (Figure 31.11).

S1

The S1 nerve root provides innervation to the gastrocnemius-soleus complex, which is the primary plantarflexor of the foot. Testing can be performed by asking the patient to plantarflex his foot either supine or with legs hanging off the side of the table. Resistance is placed on the sole of the foot by the examiner. Alternatively, the patient can be asked to toe-walk to isolate the gastrocnemius-soleus complex. Likewise, it is our preferred method to fatigue this muscle group before formal testing. This can be achieved by asking the patient to perform 20 single-leg heel rises while supporting himself against a wall or rail (Figure 31.12).

REFLEXES

Abnormal deep tendon reflexes can be harbingers for nerve root or spinal cord injury. It is vital to ensure that the muscle group of interest is completely relaxed before testing tendon reflexes. Oftentimes, it may help to distract the patient by asking them to engage other muscle groups. For example, when testing the knee jerk reflex, ask patients having difficulty relaxing to clasp their hands together and pull apart until reflex testing is completed. Always evaluate for any asymmetry between the sides.

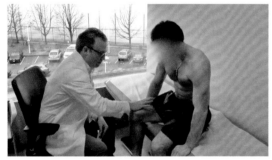

FIGURE 31.9 • Strength testing of the iliopsoas muscle group.

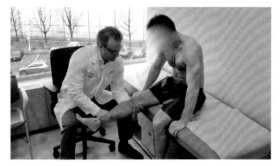

FIGURE 31.10 • Strength testing of the quadriceps group.

respectively. The patient should sit on the examination table with his knees flexed off the side, allowing their ankles to rest in neutral dorsiflexion. To isolate the tibialis anterior, the patient will be instructed to maximally

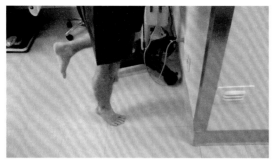

FIGURE 31.12 • Strength testing of gastrocsoleus complex.

TABLE 31.2 Reflex Grading Chart

• Deep tendon reflexes • Reflexes should be graded on a 0-4 "plus" scale:	
Tendon Reflex Trading Scale	
Grade	Description
0	Absent
1+ or +	Hypoactive
2+ or ++	"Normal"
3+ or +++	Hyperactive without clonus
4+ or ++++	Hyperactive with clonus

Reflexes are graded from absent (0) to hyperactive (4+) as seen in Table 31.2. These relative values should be assigned keeping patient age in perspective, as "normal" reflex response may deteriorate with age. Hyperreflexia and/or clonus suggest involvement of upper motor neurons. Hyporeflexia could indicate damage to the nerve roots, peripheral nerves, neuromuscular junctions, or muscles themselves. However, hyporeflexia is more commonly the natural consequence of aging and degeneration.

LUMBAR SPINE INJURIES IN THE ATHLETE

Spondylolysis

Lower back pain is a significant cause of loss of play in the young athlete, with up to 30% of athletes reporting such pain in a study by Videman et al[17] Spondylolysis and spondylolisthesis together account for nearly 50% of lower back pain in this population.[18] Spondylolysis is defined as a defect in the pars interarticularis, which is multifactorial in etiology across the general population. However, in the elite athlete, this pathology is believed to be the result of repetitive hyperextension of the lumbar spine with 71% to 95% of cases occurring at the L5 vertebra compared with 5% to 23% at

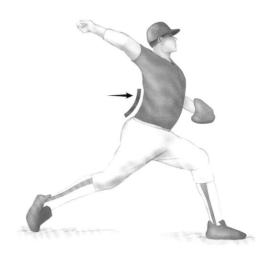

FIGURE 31.13 • Lumbar hyperlordosis as experienced by pitchers during the late cocking and early acceleration phase of overhead throwing.

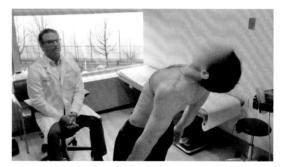

FIGURE 31.14 • Hyperextension of the lumbar spine often exacerbating symptoms of spondylolysis.

L4[19,20] (Figure 31.13). Shah et al demonstrated a high propensity for adolescent soccer players to develop this condition, postulating that the first phase of kicking demands a hyperextension of the lumbar spine to generate force.[21] An early recognition of this condition is vital, as it can often be treated nonoperatively after a period of restricted activity.

Athletes will typically present with an insidious onset of axial lower back pain. This may be associated with radicular pain to the buttock or down to posterior thigh. Symptoms are often exacerbated by activity, particularly hyperextension of the lumbar spine (Figure 31.14). The classic "stiff-legged" gait seen in these patients is the result of a shortened stride length due to hamstring spasm and increased limitation in forward flexion. Physical examination should begin with observation of the athlete's posture and gait. On occasion, these patients may exhibit a lumbar hyperlordosis due to compensatory measures

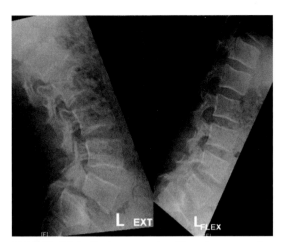

FIGURE 31.15 • Flexion-extension films demonstrating a fixed instability in a 15-year-old pitcher with grade 3 spondylolisthesis.

by unaffected levels above the spondylolisthesis. Palpation is vital, as it often elicits local axial back pain. Paraspinal pain may also be present due to muscular spasm. Additionally, in cases of severe spondylolisthesis, a palpable step-off can be appreciated. Commonly, these patients will also exhibit hamstring tightness. Spondylolysis and more often spondylolisthesis can cause a radiculopathy at the exiting nerve root. This is typically at the L5 level causing a radiating pain down the buttock and rarely motor weakness through the L5 distribution.

Initial workup should include plain standing anteroposterior (AP) and lateral radiographs (Figure 31.15). Flexion and extension films are useful for the diagnosis of spondylolisthesis with dynamic instability. Single-photon emission computed tomography scans may play an important role in prognosis. A positive scan reveals an active healing process in the fractured pars, whereas a normal or cold scan may be indicative of a healed injury or nonunion.[22] MRI plays a role in the diagnosis of atypical spondylolysis, particularly those that involve soft tissue neural impingement such as disk, ligamentum flavum, or pars fibrocartilage.[23]

The majority of athletes with symptomatic spondylolisthesis can be managed nonoperatively through restricted activity, aggressive rehabilitation, and bracing.[24] Research has demonstrated that even in the presence of nonunion, 91% of athletes report good to excellent outcomes with all returning to play.[25] The period of immobilization is controversial and can vary from 4 to 12 weeks depending on the provider. Despite this, the patient should always be symptom free before returning to play.[26,27] Surgical treatment with stabilization with or without decompression is typically reserved for patients who remain symptomatic after 9 to 12 months despite conservative therapy, spondylolisthesis greater than 50% of vertebral body, and unremitting radiculopathy or stenosis.[28,29]

Herniated Nucleus Pulposus

Herniation of the nucleus pulposus or more commonly referred to as a herniated disk is the result of a tear in the annulus of the disk complex, resulting in the escape of nuclear material into the surrounding epidural space. The presence of disk herniation in the setting of acute trauma and degenerative disease has been well documented in the literature. However, recent literature has shed more light on the association between degenerative disk disease (DDD) and the elite athlete. Sward et al demonstrated the prevalence of DDD in athletes (75%) versus their nonathlete counterparts (31%).[30] Likewise, Ong et al showed an increased loss of disk height and signal intensity and higher prevalence of disk displacement in Olympic athletes presenting with lower back pain.[31] However, these findings have been shown to vary by sport as demonstrated by Capel et al who demonstrated a lower incidence of degenerative disk changes in flamenco and ballet dancers when compared with a nonathlete control.[32] It has been postulated that this pathology is more closely related to impact sports as shown by an increased incidence of disk disease in professional volleyball players when compared with professional swimmers.[33] It has been demonstrated that professional weight lifters who perform half squats with 1.6 times their bodyweight put a compressive load across the L3-L4 segment roughly 10 times their bodyweight. These compressive loads can surpass 17,000 N in this population.

Disk herniations will classically present with radicular symptoms, which correlate to extruded nucleus pulposus upon the traversing or rarely exiting nerve root. Pain is usually exacerbated by lumbar flexion or performance of the Valsalva maneuver and alleviated by lying flat.[34,35] Radicular symptoms may manifest as dermatomal paresthesia or less commonly weakness. While adults can present with neurologic weakness, it is less common in the adolescent athletic population.[36] One study that evaluated herniated disks in elite tennis players noted their occurrence almost exclusively in the L4-L5 and L5-S1 levels.[37] Herniations at the L4-L5 level will typically result in a L5 radiculopathy manifesting in paresthesias in the L5 dermatome as well as weakness in great toe and less commonly ankle dorsiflexion. Likewise, disk herniations at the

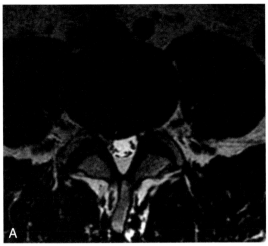
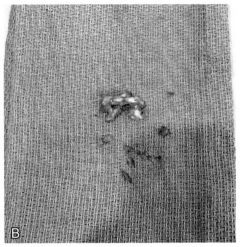

FIGURE 31.16 • A 30-year-old man presenting with 8 weeks of right leg radicular pain with progressive weakness along the L5 distribution. An MRI demonstrates a right-sided paracentral disk herniation (A). Clinical photo (B) demonstrates the extruded disk removed following diskectomy.

L5-S1 level may present as an S1 paresthesia and/or weakness with ankle eversion and plantarflexion strength. Decreases in the Achilles tendon reflex may also be observed.

Specific physical examination maneuvers are vital to assist the examining clinician in making the diagnosis of a herniated disk. The most specific tests are maneuvers, which reproduce the radicular symptoms the patient is experiencing, often referred to as "dural tension" signs. The classic example is the straight leg test, which serves to reproduce radicular pain by bringing the nerve root into contact with the extruded disk material. Xin et al demonstrated an 88.5% ability to accurately pinpoint the location of a disk herniation based on the symptoms elicited from a straight leg examination[38] (Figure 31.16).

Straight Leg Raise

The straight leg raise (SLR) is performed by placing the patient supine on the examination table and then raising the leg with the knee fully extended to reproduce radicular symptoms between 30° and 70° of elevation.[39] The sensitivities and specificities of this maneuver for lumbar disk herniation are 36% to 97% and 11% to 84%, respectively.[40-43] Part of the inconsistency with the examination relates to the variability in defining a positive result, such as the degree of elevation at which symptoms occur or the type of symptom produced. When comparing mid-lumbar (L2-L4) with low lumbar (L5-S1) regions, the SLR test is much more sensitive and specific for low lumbar root impingement.[44] Cecin sign is a variation of this tension examination in which a Valsalva maneuver is incorporated as well. The standing patient is

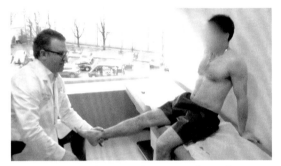

FIGURE 31.17 • The "tripod sign" resulting after a provocative straight leg raise.

asked to flex the lumbar spine forward to the point where pain is experienced and then asked to cough to simulate the Valsalva maneuver. Worsening radicular pain is considered a positive Cecin sign, which has a sensitivity of 73% and a specificity of 95% in patients with lumbar disk herniation proven on MRI.[45] Often, patients who exhibit a positive SLR will lean back on the examination table to alleviate the nerve root irritation. This compensatory action, in which the patient will place both hands behind him in support, is often referred to as the tripod sign (Figure 31.17).

Lasègue Sign, Bowstring Sign

Several other variations on the SLR test exist including the Lasègue and the Bowstring signs. As a specific maneuver was never described by Lasègue himself,[46] the sign attributed to him has variable descriptions in the literature. One version of the positive Lasègue sign refers to radicular pain elicited when the foot is dorsiflexed after the leg had been raised to the point of symptom reproduction and then slightly lowered. Foot dorsiflexion adds further tension to the irritated lumbosacral nerve root such that the leg symptoms are reproduced.[47,48] A second description involves raising the leg with the knee semiflexed and then extending the knee until symptoms are reproduced.

The Bowstring sign elicits pain during a leg raise with a semiflexed knee followed by application of manual pressure within the popliteal fossa to tension the tibial nerve.[49] In contrast, placing tension on the medial and lateral hamstring tendons instead should not re-create pain in a patient with organic spinal pathology.[50] When correlated with intraoperative pathologic findings, the Lasègue and bowstring signs had 71% and 69% specificity for lumbar disk herniation but did not assist with preoperatively identifying the location of the disk herniation relative to the nerve root (central, axillary, foraminal, etc).[47]

Crossed Straight Leg Raise Sign, Crossed Lasègue Sign

The crossed SLR sign, or well-leg raise sign, utilizes the fact that the SLR not only stretches the ipsilateral nerve root but also causes lateral pull on the dural sac, which subsequently causes contralateral nerve root stretch.[51,52] With this examination, a SLR is performed on the contralateral side, but symptoms are produced in the symptomatic leg. Sensitivity has been shown to be low, ranging from 4% to 42% but with specificity higher at 85% to 100%.[46,47] The crossed Lasègue sign has been associated with accurate preoperative classification of contained versus uncontained disk herniation.[53]

Femoral Nerve Stretch Test

The reverse SLR, or femoral nerve stretch test, can be used to evaluate lesions involving the more proximal L2-L4 nerve roots that innervate the femoral nerve.[54] Because the more proximal nerve roots have less gliding excursion, the supine SLR is not effective in localizing them. However, the femoral nerve can be more specifically tested by placing the patient prone, passively flexing the knee, and then extending the hip. This maneuver places tension on the femoral nerve and should recreate anterior thigh pain coming from L2-L4 nerve root irritation. Sensitivity for detecting proximal lumbar nerve root compression is 50%, with 100% specificity.[44] Because this maneuver reduces tension on the sciatic nerve, pain radiating down the leg should be reduced. Hence, complaints of exacerbation of distal pain with this test may indicate a nonorganic etiology of pain.[50] Similar to the crossed SLR sign, a crossed femoral nerve stretch test may aid in the diagnosis of proximal lumbar disk herniation.[55]

STRAINS AND SPRAINS

Strains and sprains account for one of the most common causes of low-back pain in the elite athlete. Keene et al examined 333 college-level athletes and found muscle strain to be the largest pain generator with 59% acute and 41% chronic injuries.[19] Likewise, Micheli and Wood showed that lumbar muscular strain accounted for 27% of low-back pain in adolescent athletes and 6% in adult athletes.[18] By definition, a muscle strain is a tear in the muscle fibers at either the muscle belly or musculotendinous junction. Conversely, a sprain is a stretch in 1 or more of the spinal ligaments without disrupting the continuity of the ligament. Inflammation typically peaks at 24 to 48 hours after injury. This may be accompanied by muscle spasms or pain localized to a trigger point. Recurrent strains are defined by having brief asymptomatic periods between exacerbations. Likewise, chronic strains describe long-standing muscular pain due to strains. Despite their commonplace, these diagnoses are often ones of exclusion. Athletes will typically present with acute lumbar pain that is localized and often associated with muscle spasm. Pain is exacerbated with particular motion in the absence of any neurologic deficits. When examining these patients, it is key to palpate the axial skeleton and paraspinal musculature to define the source of pain. Forward- and side-bending test can also help to localize the source of spasm. Plain radiographs are useful to rule out other etiologies such as spondylolisthesis or spondylolysis. In the instances of sprains or strains, plain imaging will be negative. Tenets of treatment for strains and sprains consist of a brief period of rest, activity modification, nonsteroidal anti-inflammatory drugs (NSAIDs), and targeted physical therapy with focus on trunk strengthening.[56]

MANAGER'S TIPS

- The lumbar spine is a common source of pain in the elite athlete
- A focus physical examination will help to guide the clinician as to the source of pain
- Spondylolysis typically presents as axial back pain, made worse with hyperextension of the lumbar spine
- Herniated nucleus pulposus most commonly presents as radicular pain, which can be exacerbated with provocative maneuvers
- Lumbar strains and sprains are most severe 24 to 48 hours after the traumatic event and will commonly present as paraspinal or axial back pain in the setting of negative plain films

REFERENCES

1. Soprano J, Fuchs S. Common overuse injuries in the pediatric and adolescent athlete. *Clin Pediatr Emerg Med.* 2007;8:7-14.

2. Roos KG, Marshall SW, Kerr ZY, et al. Epidemiology of overuse injuries in collegiate and high school athletics in the United States. *Am J Sports Med.* 2015;43:1790-1797.

3. DiFiori JP, Benjamin HJ, Brenner J, et al. Overuse injuries and burnout in youth sports: a position statement from the American Medical Society for Sports Medicine. *Clin J Sport Med.* 2014;24:3-20.

4. Brenner JS, American Academy of Pediatrics Council on Sports, Medicine, and Fitness. Overuse injuries, overtraining, and burnout in child and adolescent athletes. *Pediatrics.* 2007;119:1242-1245.

5. Pengel KB. Common overuse injuries in the young athlete. *Pediatr Ann.* 2014;43:e297-e308.

6. Logan K. Overuse and underutilization in youth sports: time to seek equipoise. *J Pediatr.* 2015;166:517-519.

7. Lysens RJ, Ostyn MS, Vanden Auweele Y, et al. The accident-prone and overuse-prone profiles of the young athlete. *Am J Sports Med.* 1989;17:612-619.

8. Fredrickson BE, Baker D, McHolick W, et al. The natural history of spondylolysis and spondylolisthesis. *J Bone Joint Surg Am.* 1984;66:699-707.

9. Bono CM. Low-back pain in athletes. *J Bone Joint Surg.* 2004;86:382-396.

10. Lawrence JP, Greene HS, Grauer JN. Back pain in athletes. *J Am Acad Orthop Surg.* 2006;14:726-735.

11. Riley LH, An HS. Chapter 4: History and physical exam of the spine. In: *Principles and Techniques of Spine Surgery.* Williams and Wilkins; 1998.

12. Sherping SC, Frymoyer JW, Wiesel SW. Chapter 4: History and physical exam. In: *The Adult and Pediatric Spine.* 3rd ed. Philadelphia: Lippincott Williams & Wilkins; 2004.

13. Yamashita T, Kanaya K, Sekine M, Takebayashi T, Kawaguchi S, Katahira G. A quantitative analysis of sensory function in lumbar radiculopathy using current perception threshold testing. *Spine.* 2002;27(14):1567-1570.

14. Suri P, Hunter DJ, Katz JN, Li L, Rainville J. Bias in the physical examination of patients with lumbar radiculopathy. *BMC Musculoskelet Disord.* 2010;11:275.

15. Bradley WG, Daroff RB, Fenichel GM, eds. *Neurology in Clinical Practice: Principles of Diagnosis and Management.* 5th ed. Boston: Butterworth Heinemann; 2007.

16. Vroomen PC, de Krom MC, Knottnerus JA. Consistency of history taking and physical examination in patients with suspected lumbar nerve root involvement. *Spine.* 2000;25(1):91-96 [discussion 97].

17. Videman T, Sarna S, Battie MC, et al. The long-term effects of physical loading and exercise lifestyles on back-related symptoms, disability, and spinal pathology among men. *Spine.* 1995;20(6):699-709.

18. Micheli LJ, Wood R. Back pain in young athletes. Significant differences from adults in causes and patterns. *Arch Pediatr Adolesc Med.* 1995;149(1):15-18.

19. Keene JS, Albert MJ, Springer SL, Drummond DS, Clancy WG Jr. Back injuries in college athletes. *J Spinal Disord.* 1989;2(3):190-195.

20. McCleary MD, Congeni JA. Current concepts in the diagnosis and treatment of spondylolysis in young athletes. *Curr Sports Med Rep.* 2007;6(1):62-66.

21. ElRassi G, Takemitsu M, Woratanarat P, et al. Lumbar spondylolysis in pediatric and adolescent soccer players. *Am J Sports Med.* 2005;33(11):1688-1693.

22. Sys J, Michielsen J, Bracke P, et al: Nonoperative treatment of active spondylolysis in elite athletes with normal X-ray findings: literature review and results of conservative treatment. *Eur Spine J.* 2001;10(6):498-504.

23. Yamaguchi KT Jr, Skaggs DL, Acevedo DC, et al. Spondylolysis is frequently missed by MRI in adolescents with back pain. *J Child Orthop.* 2012;6(3):237-240.

24. Morita T, Ikata T, Katoh S, et al. Lumbar spondylolysis in children and adolescents. *J Bone Joint Surg Br.* 1995;77(4):620-625.

25. Miller SF, Congeni J, Swanson K. Long-term functional and anatomical follow-up of early detected spondylolysis in young athletes. *Am J Sports Med.* 2004;32(4):928-933.

26. Standaert CJ, Herring SA. Expert opinion and controversies in sports and musculoskeletal medicine: the diagnosis and treatment of spondylolysis in adolescent athletes. *Arch Phys Med Rehabil.* 2007;88(4):537-540.

27. Kurd MF, Patel D, Norton R, et al. Nonoperative treatment of symptomatic spondylolysis. *J Spinal Disord Tech.* 2007;20(8):560-564.

28. d'Hemecourt PA, Zurakowski D, Kriemler S, et al. Spondylolysis: returning the athlete to sports participation with brace treatment. *Orthopedics.* 2002;25(6):653-657.

29. Transfeldt EE, Mehbod AA. Evidence-based medicine analysis of isthmic spondylolisthesis treatment including reduction versus fusion in situ for high-grade slips. *Spine.* 2007;32(suppl 19):S126-S129.

30. Sward L, Hellstrom M, Jacobsson M, et al. Disc degeneration and associated abnormalities of the spine in elite gymnasts: a magnetic resonance imaging study. *Spine.* 1991;16:437-443.

31. Ong A, Anderson J, Roche J. A pilot study of the prevalence of lumbar disc degeneration in elite athletes with lower back pain at the Sydney 2000 Olympic Games. *Br J Sports Med.* 2003;37:263-266.

32. Capel A, Medina FS, Medina D, et al. Magnetic resonance study of lumbar disks in female dancers. *Am J Sports Med.* 2009;37:1208-1213.

33. Bartolozzi C, Caramella D, Zampa V, Dal Pozzo G, Tinacci E, Balducci F. The incidence of disk changes in volleyball players: the magnetic resonance findings. *Radiol Med.* 1991;82:757-760.

34. Cholewicki J, McGill SM, Norman RW. Lumbar spine loads during the lifting of extremely heavy weights. *Med Sci Sports Exerc.* 1991;23:1179-1186.

35. Cappozzo A, Felici F, Figura F, Gazzani F. Lumbar spine loading during half-squat exercises. *Med Sci Sports Exerc.* 1985;17:613-620.

36. Papagelopoulos PJ, Shaughnessy WJ, Ebersold MJ, Bianco AJ Jr, Quast LM. Long-term outcome of lumbar discectomy in children and adolescents sixteen years of age or younger. *J Bone Joint Surg Am.* 1998;80:689-698.

37. Alyas F, Turner M, Connell D. MRI findings in the lumbar spines of asymptomatic, adolescent, elite tennis players. *Br J Sports Med.* 2007;41:836-841.

38. Xin SQ, Zhang QZ, Fan DH. Significance of the straight-leg-raising test in the diagnosis and clinical evaluation of lower lumbar intervertebral-disc protrusion. *J Bone Joint Surg Am.* 1987;69:517-522.

39. Herkowitz H, Garfin S, Eismont F, Bell G, Balderston R. *Rothman-simeone, the Spine.* 6th ed. Philadelphia: Saunders Elsevier; 2011.

40. Charnley J. Orthopaedic signs in the diagnosis of disc protrusion. With special reference to the straight-leg-raising test. *Lancet.* 1951;1(6648):186-192.

41. Andersson GB, Deyo RA. History and physical examination in patients with herniated lumbar discs. *Spine.* 1996;21(24 suppl):10S-18S.

42. Hakelius A. Prognosis in sciatica. A clinical follow-up of surgical and non-surgical treatment. *Acta Orthop Scan. Suppl.* 1970;129:1-76.

43. Kosteljanetz M, Bang F, Schmidt-Olsen S. The clinical significance of straight-leg raising (Lasegue's sign) in the diagnosis of prolapsed lumbar disc. Interobserver variation and correlation with surgical finding. *Spine.* 1988;13(4):393-395.

44. Suri P, Rainville J, Katz JN, et al. The accuracy of the physical examination for the diagnosis of midlumbar and low lumbar nerve root impingement. *Spine.* 2011;36(1):63-73.

45. Cecin HA. Cecin's Sign ("X" Sign): improving the diagnosis of radicular compression by herniated lumbar disks. *Rev Bras Reumatol.* 2010;50(1):44-55.

46. Sugar O. Charles Lasegue and his 'Considerations on Sciatica'. *JAMA.* 1985;253(12):1767-1768.

47. Supik LF, Broom MJ. Sciatic tension signs and lumbar disc herniation. *Spine.* 1994;19(9):1066-1069.

48. Dimitrijevic DT. Lasegue sign. *Neurology.* 1952;2(5):453-454.

49. Cram RH. A sign of sciatic nerve foot pressure. *J Bone Joint Surg Br Vol.* 1953;35-B(2):192-195.

50. Wong DA, Transfeldt E, Macnab I, McCulloch JA. *Macnab's Backache.* 4th ed. Philadelphia: Lippincott Williams & Wilkins; 2007.

51. Hudgins WR. The crossed straight leg raising test: a diagnostic sign of herniated disc. *J Occup Med.* 1979;21(6):407-408.

52. Woodhall B, Hayes G. The well-leg raising test of Fajersztajn in the diagnosis of ruptured lumbar intervertebral disc. *J Bone Joint Surg.* 1950;32(4):786-792.

53. Nikola V, Olle S. Physical signs in lumbar disc hernia. *Clin Orthop Relat Res.* 1997;333:192-201.

54. Dyck P. The femoral nerve traction test with lumbar disc protrusions. *Surg Neurol.* 1976(3):163-166.

55. Rihn JA, Harris EB. *Musculoskeletal Examination of the Spine- Chapter 2: Physical Examination of the Thoracolumbar Spine.* Thorofare, NJ: Slack Incorporated; 2011.

56. Weinstein SM, Herring SA, Cole AJ. Rehabilitation of the patient with spinal pain. In: Delisa JA, Gans BM, Bockenek WL, eds. *Rehabilitation Medicine: Principles and Practice.* 3rd ed. Philadelphia, PA: Lippincott-Raven; 1998:1423-1451.

SECTION 7
Medical Issues in Baseball Players

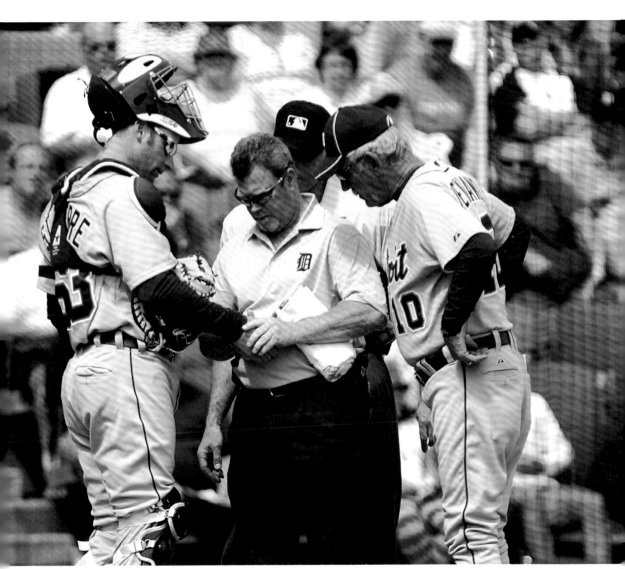

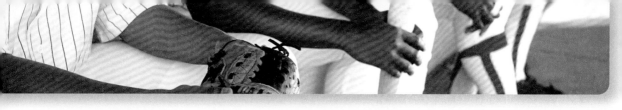

CHAPTER 32

The Preparticipation Evaluation for Baseball Players

John T. Nickless, MD | Kathleen M. Weber, MD

- -

I just want to play baseball.

—*David Ortiz*

INTRODUCTION

The preparticipation evaluation (PPE) is routinely utilized throughout amateur and professional athletics to screen for underlying medical conditions that may place the athlete at risk.[1-7] The primary objective of the PPE is to ensure the safety of athletes by identifying conditions that could potentially be life-threatening or disabling.[1-3,5-16] A thorough history and physical examination performed before participation can expose specific risk factors, allow for prevention of injury, facilitate management of chronic conditions, identify undiagnosed medical conditions, ensure compliance with organizational regulations, and optimize athletic performance.[1,2] Additionally, the PPE allows a rapport and working relationship to be established between the medical staff, coaches, and athletes, while providing an opportunity for the physician to counsel athletes on common health and wellness issues specific to the patient population.[1-3,8] Although the utility of the PPE in predicting or preventing serious injury or death is often debated, most medical organizations support the use of the PPE as an integral tool in maintaining the health and safety of athletes.[16] This is especially true given that the PPE constitutes the sole contact with the health care system for 30% to 88% of student athletes.[5,16]

CLINICAL CONSIDERATIONS

Most states and athletic associations require a thorough PPE to be performed every 1 to 3 years.[3,13,16] Updates with a comprehensive questionnaire and problem focused physical examination should be performed annually to detect and treat any new concerns that may have arisen since the last comprehensive PPE was performed.[16] Ideally, the PPE should be performed at least 5 to 6 weeks before the start of athletic training to allow sufficient time for further evaluation or treatment, if necessary.[3,6,7,13,16] Regulations on who can perform PPEs (physicians, physician assistants, nurse practitioners, etc) vary by state. However, most suggest that the evaluation be performed by a sports medicine–trained physician, who has a firm understanding of the sport, awareness of population specific injuries and conditions, and who will provide ongoing medical care to the athletes as the established team physician.[4,13,16,17] All screening methods, testing, and decisions should be made in the athlete's best interest and should be based on sound scientific evidence and medical criteria that meets or exceeds that established standard of care.[13]

Location

The PPE should be performed in a setting that allows a comprehensive history and physical examination, while also protecting patient privacy.[13] Individual examinations in a physician's office afford the benefit of a quiet, comfortable, and private atmosphere. It also allows more time to build a trusting relationship with the athlete, thoroughly review medical records, and increase the ability to provide general health maintenance counseling.[1,3,13,16] Individual examinations in a physician's clinic are recommended by numerous medical associations including the American Academy of Family Physicians and the American Academy of Pediatrics.[6,16]

Another widely used method involves the use of a coordinated medical team to provide PPEs for a large number of athletes. Mass screenings allow numerous athletes to undergo evaluation in an organized fashion, which allows effective use of time and resources.[6,16] These examinations may be conducted in a gymnasium, athletic training complex, or a community facility that allows for a significant volume of athletes to undergo screening and physical examinations in an efficient manner. However, it should again be emphasized that the chosen facility should allow for separate quiet areas to conduct appropriate medical histories and physical examinations to protect the athlete's privacy.[6,7,16]

When performed in a mass setting, the PPE of athletes should be overseen by a team physician who has a deep understanding of sport-specific conditions and injuries to implement useful and efficient screening methods during the PPE.[17] A primary care physician with a broad medical knowledge will typically direct a team of primary care physicians, subspecialists, and other trained medical staff positioned at various stations to ensure that the PPEs are completed in a resourceful, yet scrupulous, manner.

These large-scale assessments are often station based including designated areas for vital signs, medical examination, orthopedic evaluation, vision screening, and occasionally cardiology-specific examination.[6] Some athletic programs will also incorporate preseason baseline concussion screening as part of the PPE. Physical therapists, nutritionists, and athletic trainers may also be available to provide additional education and counseling on proper nutrition and injury prevention.[6,16] This method allows for a large number of athletes to undergo evaluation, while minimizing cost. It can also expedite additional evaluation as orthopedic physicians, cardiologists, and other subspecialists may be readily accessible for immediate consultation and recommendations, as opposed to outside referral, which may lead to further delays in clearance for athletic participation.[1,16]

It is imperative that the head team physician establishes a chain of command among the medical staff to make certain that any possible medical or musculoskeletal concern is addressed, worked up, and followed up appropriately. Additional effort should also be made by the team physician to communicate any abnormal findings or need for additional workup with the athlete, the athlete's parent or guardian, athletic trainers, the athlete's primary care physician, and appropriate subspecialists.[6]

Medical History

A thorough and systematic approach should be implemented in obtaining a complete medical history for each athlete, as the history alone will identify 68%

to 85% of medical or musculoskeletal issues that may limit initial clearance for unrestricted participation.[6,16,18] A questionnaire may be completed by the athlete and their parents before the PPE to screen for medical or musculoskeletal conditions, which may place the athlete at risk. In addition to a careful review of the screening questionnaire, a detailed medical history should be obtained at the time of the PPE.[1,6,9,19]

The examiner should be meticulous in obtaining a thorough medical history, and ideally, a parent should be present to assist in obtaining a history from any athlete under the age of 18 years. If the athlete is not fluent in the English language, the history should be obtained in the athlete's primary language, with the help of an interpreter, to ensure accuracy and minimize confusion.[16] Fundamental elements of the medical history should include questions in regards to cardiovascular, pulmonary, hematologic, musculoskeletal, neurologic, ear/nose/throat, genitourinary, gastrointestinal, endocrine, dermatologic, ophthalmologic, and dental symptoms.[1,3,13,20,21]

Medical and Surgical History

Athletes should be questioned in regard to their family history and personal medical history, including conditions that they have received treatment for in the past, or those that are currently being monitored or managed by a medical professional. This information allows the medical team to be aware of potential situations that may arise in regard to an athlete's medical condition and also allows the medical staff to assist in the treatment and management of acute and chronic conditions.[5,6] Eliciting a history of heat illness can also be helpful in planning appropriate training regimens and monitoring athletes. Additionally, the athlete should be solicited about any surgical history, as this may reveal a medical disorder, which was not discussed as part of the medical history, or a potential orthopedic condition, which may place the athlete at increased risk for injury.[5]

A review of immunization records should also be included in the comprehensive PPE. This provides an opportunity for the medical team to direct the athlete in regard to vaccine recommendations. Although not typically an area for disqualification from participation, many schools and universities require proof of particular vaccinations for enrollment. Furthermore, athletes who compete internationally may require specific immunizations to gain entry to certain countries and prevent illness from transmittable diseases.[22]

Medications, Supplements, and Allergies

The practitioner should inquire about the use of any prescription medications, which may uncover acute or chronic medical conditions that had been omitted from the patient's medical history. The athlete should also be questioned in regard to the use of over-the-counter medications or other supplements to provide appropriate counseling about medical conditions, avoid potentially harmful medication interactions, and ensure compliance with organizational substance policies.[5-7,22] The medical team should also be aware of any environmental or medication allergies that the athlete has, particularly those that have been associated with angioedema or anaphylaxis, which may prove useful if an emergent situation were to arise.[5,6,16]

Psychosocial History

As the PPE serves as the sole contact with the health care system for many athletes, time should be taken to assess for and provide counseling in regard to high-risk behaviors including sexual activity and the use of recreational drugs, tobacco, and alcohol. Additionally, practitioners should assess the athlete's mental health, living situation, and nutritional status as all these factors can affect the athlete's general well-being and athletic performance.[5,7,16,22]

Family History and Cardiovascular Survey

Particular attention should be paid to the cardiovascular portion of the history and physical examiantion, as cardiovascular conditions are the leading medical cause of sudden death among athletes.[16,23-25] In high school athletes, the frequency of sudden cardiac death (SCD) is estimated to be between 1/100,000 and 1/300,000 per year.[6] In the United States, hypertrophic cardiomyopathy (HCM) is the leading cause of SCD among young athletes.[12,25,26] In athletes <35 years old, HCM accounts for 36% to 44% of SCD among athletes, followed by coronary artery anomalies (17%), myocarditis (6%), arrhythmogenic right ventricular cardiomyopathy (4%), mitral valve prolapse (4%), followed by a variety of other cardiac conditions (Figure 32.1).[10,11] Atherosclerotic coronary artery disease is the leading cause of SCD in athletes >35 years of age.[6]

To screen for potentially life-threatening or disqualifying cardiac conditions, the American Heart Association (AHA) recommends the use of a 14-element preparticipation cardiovascular screening for competitive athletes (Table 32.1).[27] The elements in this comprehensive survey are aimed at eliciting concerning risk factors and symptoms in the individual athlete, inquiring about the possibility of a family history of SCD, and investigating for any physical

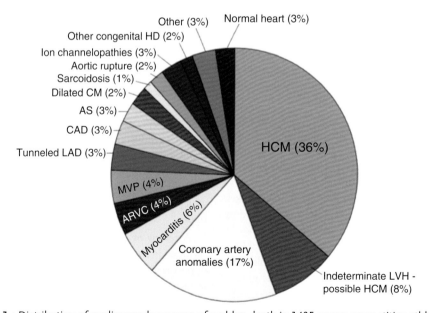

FIGURE 32.1 • Distribution of cardiovascular causes of sudden death in 1435 young competitive athletes. From the Minneapolis Heart Institute Foundation Registry, 1980 to 2005. ARVC, arrhythmogenic right ventricular cardiomyopathy; AS, aortic stenosis; CAD, coronary artery disease; CM, cardiomyopathy; HD, heart disease; LAD, left anterior descending; LVH, left ventricular hypertrophy; MVP, mitral valve prolapse. (Reprinted with permission from Maron BJ, Thompson PD, Ackerman MJ. Recommendations and considerations related to preparticipation screening for cardiovascular abnormalities in competitive athletes: 2007 Update. *Circulation.* 2007;115(12):1643-1655. Copyright ©2007 American Heart Association, Inc.

TABLE 32.1 14-Element American Heart Association (AHA) Recommendations for Preparticipation Cardiovascular Screening in Competitive Athletes

Medical History[a]
Personal History
1. Chest pain/discomfort/tightness/pressure related to exertion 2. Unexplained syncope/near-syncope[b] 3. Excessive and unexplained dyspnea/fatigue or palpitations, associated with exercise 4. Prior recognition of a heart murmur 5. Elevated systemic blood pressure 6. Prior restriction from participation in sports 7. Prior testing for the heart, ordered by a physician
Family History
8. Premature death (sudden and unexpected, or otherwise) before 50 y of age attributable to heart disease in ≥1 relative 9. Disability from heart disease in close relative <50 y of age 10. Hypertrophic or dilated cardiomyopathy, long-QT syndrome, or other ion channelopathies, Marfan syndrome, or clinically significant arrhythmias; specific knowledge of genetic cardiac conditions in family members
Physical Examination
11. Heart murmur[c] 12. Femoral pulses to exclude aortic coarctation 13. Physical stigmata of Marfan syndrome 14. Brachial artery blood pressure (sitting position)[d]

[a]*Parental verification is recommended for high school and middle school athletes.*

[b]*Judged not to be of neurocardiogenic (vasovagal) origin; of particular concern when occurring during or after physical exertion.*

[c]*Refers to heart murmurs judged likely to be organic and unlikely to be innocent; auscultation should be performed with the patient in both the supine and standing positions (or with Valsalva maneuver), specifically to identify murmurs of dynamic left ventricular outflow tract obstruction.*

[d]*Preferably taken in both arms.*

Reprinted with permission from Maron BJ, Friedman RA, Kligfield P, et al. Assessment of the 12-Lead ECG as a screening test for detection of cardiovascular disease in healthy general populations of young people (12 -25 Years of Age). Circulation. 2014;130(15):1303-1334. Copyright © 2014 American Heart Association, Inc.

examination findings that may be worrisome. A positive finding on any component of this cardiovascular screening should prompt further questioning and consideration of advanced testing to investigate for an underlying cardiac condition, which may place the athlete at risk for SCD.

Training Regimen

In addition to obtaining a thorough medical history, the PPE also allows an opportunity for the team physician to assess training routines, as baseball players, particularly pitchers, are at risk for acute traumatic injuries or chronic overuse injuries associated with repetitive microtrauma.[6,28] In the adolescent baseball player, risk factors for injury to the elbow or shoulder include year-round pitching, pitching for multiple teams, high pitch counts, throwing more than 100 innings per year, pitching on consecutive days, pitching while fatigued, throwing breaking pitches, throwing with high velocity, and glenohumeral internal rotation deficit (GIRD).[28-30] These risk factors should be addressed, and the

athletes, parents, and coaches should be educated about appropriate training regimens. Major League Baseball (MLB) and USA Baseball have developed Pitch Smart guidelines, which designate limitations for pitching workloads for youth and adolescent baseball players with the aim of preventing injury (Table 32.2).

PHYSICAL EXAMINATION

Vital Signs

The physical examination should begin with obtaining vital signs, including height, weight, pulse, and blood pressure (BP), and follow a systems-based approach during examination.[3,5-7] Hypertension is one of the most common cardiovascular conditions and has been noted in 6.4% of athletes during PPEs. When elevated BP is noted, further investigation should involve questioning in regard to family history of hypertension and personal use of stimulants such as caffeine, over-the-counter medications, nicotine, and nutritional or performance enhancing supplements.[16]

TABLE 32.2 Pitching Rest Protocol Based on the Athlete's Age, as Recommended by the Major League Baseball Pitch Smart Organization

			Required Days of Rest After Pitching				Daily Max (Pitches in a Game)
Age (Years)	0 d	1 d	2 d	3 d	4 d	5 d	
7-8	1-20	21-35	36-50	N/A	N/A	N/A	50
9-10	1-20	21-35	36-50	51-65	66+	N/A	75
11-12	1-20	21-35	36-50	51-65	66+	N/A	85
13-14	1-20	21-35	36-50	51-65	66+	N/A	95
15-16	1-30	31-45	46-60	61-75	76+	N/A	95
17-18	1-30	31-45	46-60	61-80	81+	N/A	105
19-22	1-30	31-45	46-60	61-80	81-105+	106+	120

Modified from MLB Pitch Smart guidelines (http://m.mlb.com/pitchsmart/pitching-guidelines/).

In athletes noted to have elevated BP, their BP should be rechecked after lying in a quiet, comfortable room for at least 10 to 15 minutes, ensuring the use of an appropriately sized cuff for the individual.[6] If the BP continues to remain elevated, it should again be rechecked a week later. The diagnosis of hypertension often requires 3 or more abnormal BP readings. Based on the criteria published in the *Seventh Report of the Joint National Committee on Prevention, Detection, Evaluation, and Treatment of High Blood Pressure* (JNC 7), adult BP falls into 4 categories: normal (<120/80), prehypertension (120-139/80-90), stage 1 hypertension (140-159/90-99), and stage 2 hypertension (≥160/100).[31] A more recent update of guidelines based on expert opinion was released in 2014, which not only allows for slight leniency in the management of hypertension in individuals over the age of 60 years, but also concludes the that abovementioned classifications and criteria from JNC 7 remain reasonable to continue following.[32]

A consensus on high blood pressure in children and adolescents places children into 1 of 4 blood pressure categories corresponding to age-, gender-, and height-related standards. In athletes under the age of 18 years, the diagnosis of prehypertension is made when the BP falls between 90% and 95% of the standard for age, gender, and height. Stage 1 hypertension is diagnosed when the BP ranges from 95% to 99% plus 5 mm Hg of the norm, and stage 2 hypertension, when the BP is >99% plus 5 mm Hg of the norm.[33]

Children and adolescents who meet the criteria for the diagnosis of hypertension should undergo additional evaluation investigating for a secondary cause of hypertension or end-organ damage. The workup should include blood testing with glucose, creatinine, thyroid function testing, lipid panel, and hematocrit. A urinalysis (UA) and electrocardiogram (ECG)

should also be obtained as part of the hypertensive workup. In children and adolescents with stage 1 or 2 hypertension, a renal ultrasound is also recommended. Additionally, an echocardiogram and a retinal examination are suggested for all individuals with diabetes mellitus or renal disease with blood pressure ranging between the 90th and 94th percentile, as well as for all patients with BP ≥95th percentile.[33] Athletic participation should be withheld in any patient with stage 2 hypertension or evidence of end-organ damage, until their blood pressure can be further evaluated and better controlled.[16]

Eyes

Examination of the eyes should include testing of visual acuity, extraocular eye motions, pupillary reactions to light and accommodation, pupil symmetry, nystagmus, and near-point convergence.[1,5,6,22] Any pupillary asymmetry (anisocoria) or abnormal pupil shape should be documented, which may be helpful in avoiding unnecessary workup if the athlete experiences a head or eye injury.[6,22] Visual acuity should be tested both with and without corrective lenses. An athlete with best-corrected vision worse than 20/40 in one eye is determined to be functionally 1-eyed. In this case, the athlete should be required to wear protective eyewear approved by the American Society for Testing and Materials during sports which place the athlete at risk for eye injury.[6,7,16,21,22]

Ears, Nose, Neck, and Throat

A brief examination of the ears, nose, neck, and throat should evaluate the tympanic membranes, auditory canals, nasal septum, oral mucosa, posterior pharynx, tonsils, dental hygiene, thyroid gland, and lymph nodes of the head and neck.[1,5,6,22] Any abnormality on examination should prompt further investigation and possible workup. Special attention should be paid to the oral cavity on the examination of baseball players, given the high rate of smokeless tobacco use. It is estimated that 33% to 40% of professional baseball players and 45% to 55% of college baseball players use smokeless tobacco. These athletes may show signs of malignant oral lesions, premalignant oral leukoplakia, gingival regression, or dental caries.[34] Any athlete using smokeless tobacco, also known as chewing tobacco or dip, should be educated about the negative health effects, including elevated BP, nicotine dependence, and oral/throat cancer, and offered assistance in cessation of its use.

Cardiovascular

As previously discussed, the cardiovascular portion of the PPE is often the most important aspect because cardiovascular etiologies are the primary medical cause of sudden death in athletes.[6,16,24,25] The medical history is often the most valuable means of exposing concerning symptoms in the individual athlete, or a family history that may be associated with a cardiovascular condition; however, a thorough physical examination should also be performed including the physical examination elements listed in Table 32.1. In addition to obtaining a blood pressure, the examination should include auscultation of the heart in multiple positions, including squatting, standing, and supine. The examiner should note any murmurs that increase in intensity with either Valsalva maneuver or positions that decrease venous return, as these can be related to hypertrophic cardiomyopathy and require further investigation.[5,6,18,22,27] Additionally, any systolic murmur graded as 3/6 or greater or any diastolic murmur warrants further workup.[5] Radial and femoral pulses should be palpated, and any asymmetry should prompt evaluation for a possible coarctation of the aorta.[5,22,27] The patient should also be observed for any stigmata of Marfan syndrome, which places the athlete at increased risk of aortic rupture and SCD. These features may include being disproportionately tall and slender, an arm span that exceeds the patient's height, long slender fingers, increased flexibility, kyphoscoliosis, a high-arched palate, pectus excavatum or carinatum, or dislocation of the lenses of the eyes.[5,6,22,27]

Pulmonary

While auscultation of the athlete's lungs is often unremarkable, it is an important aspect of the physical examination. The practitioner should auscultate both the anterior and posterior lung fields to ensure good air entry throughout all lung fields. The chest wall should also be observed to confirm symmetric movement of the rib cage.[5] Any cough, rhonchi, wheezes, rales, or prolonged expiratory phase should be noted, as these findings may be associated with an acute medical illness such as a viral or bacterial pneumonia or may be related to an underlying medical condition such as asthma or exercise-induced bronchospasm.[6,16,22] In athletes with a history of asthma or exercise-induced bronchospasm, the physician should inquire about how often the athlete experiences symptoms, discuss the need for medications and compliance with medication use, counsel on exposure to allergens or irritants, and ensure that the athlete has access to a rescue albuterol inhaler at all times during athletic participation.[16] In athletes that complain of symptoms such as shortness of breath or wheezing during activity, yet have a normal examination, provocative laboratory testing such as pre- and postexercise spirometry or pulmonary function testing should be considered to further investigate for exercise induced asthma or bronchospasm.[3,6,16]

Gastrointestinal and Genitourinary

The abdominal examination should be performed with the athlete lying in a supine position. The skin should be exposed to ensure satisfactory inspection of the abdomen. Auscultation of all 4 quadrants should be performed before palpation to avoid palpation-induced cessation of bowel sounds.[5,6] The abdomen should then be palpated in all 4 quadrants, noting any areas of tenderness, guarding, masses, or hepatosplenomegaly.[6,16] Enlargement of the spleen may be a sign of mononucleosis and blood work, and imaging should be considered for the workup of splenomegaly, as this can place the athlete at risk for splenic rupture.[6]

A brief genitourinary examination in the presence of a chaperone should be conducted in all male athletes.[6] The examination is performed with the athlete standing and begins with visualization of the genitals, observing for any skin lesions or other abnormalities. The scrotum is then palpated ensuring the presence of 2 testicles. Any palpable masses or abnormalities in the size or shape of the testicles should be noted. The examiner should also perform a digital palpation of the inguinal canals while the athlete coughs or performs a Valsalva maneuver to check for possible hernias. Any abnormalities noted during the examination should undergo further workup accordingly.[5,6,16,22] The examiner may also consider educating the athlete about monthly self-testicular examinations to screen for testicular cancer.[16,22]

A pelvic examination is not part of a standard PPE in female athletes. However, any complaint of symptoms or concerning findings in the medical history or on physical examination, such as amenorrhea, dysfunctional uterine bleeding, pelvic pain, suprapubic tenderness to palpation, gravid uterus, or other various symptoms, should prompt further workup or referral to a subspecialist for consultation.[16,22]

Musculoskeletal

Musculoskeletal conditions are commonly encountered by the health care provider during the PPE and account for the majority of restrictions or delayed clearance for participation in athletic activity.[6,21] A detailed history is 92% sensitive in detecting significant musculoskeletal injuries, while the physical examination is 51% sensitive and 97% specific in detecting injuries.[16,18] Before examination, the practitioner should inquire about any previous injuries or musculoskeletal conditions that have prevented the athlete from participation. Additionally, the medical provider should discuss the mechanism of specific injuries, time to return to play after the injury, any need for previous medical treatment or physical therapy for musculoskeletal conditions, any prior need for advanced imaging, the use of equipment such as braces or splints, and any previous surgeries.[6,16] By inquiring about these aspects, the physician may be able to uncover acute injuries or chronic conditions that require further attention or place the athlete at

risk for further injury. In the asymptomatic athlete, a screening musculoskeletal exam is appropriate and evaluates the athletes overall range of motion, flexibility, and strength relatively quickly (Table 32.3).[8,18] This general examination also allows the practitioner to assess for asymmetry, hyperlaxity, tenderness to palpation, bruising, swelling, or weakness, which may indicate current injury.[18] A focused physical examination should be conducted in regard to any joint or region that has been previously injured or required surgery. Any athlete that demonstrates ligamentous instability, decreased functional capacity, strength less than 90% of the unaffected side, or significant decrease in range of motion should be restricted from athletic participation until further workup and rehabilitation can be completed.[6]

The practitioner should also assess the throwing arm of the athlete as the high-velocity, repetitive motion associated with throwing requires extremes of rotation and places the overhead baseball athlete at risk for injury of the throwing shoulder or elbow, particularly in pitchers.[28,35-38] Pitching-related shoulder pain has been documented to occur in 30% to 74% of baseball pitchers.[39] The examination should include range of motion and strength testing, as shoulder adductor-abductor muscular imbalances and GIRDs have been linked to increased risk of injury in the throwing extremity, particularly ulnar collateral ligament (UCL) injuries.[28,35,40] Any concerns for chronic or acute

TABLE 32.3 The "90-Second" Musculoskeletal Screening Examination for Use During Preparticipation Physical Evaluations

Instruction	Observations
Stand facing examiner	Acromioclavicular joints: general habitus
Look at ceiling, floor, over both shoulders, touch ears to shoulder	Cervical spine motion
Shrug shoulders (resistance)	Trapezius strength
Abduct shoulders to 90° (resistance at 90°)	Deltoid strength
Full external rotation of arms	Shoulder motion
Flex and extend elbows	Elbow motion
Arms at sides, elbows at 90° flexed; pronate and supinate wrists	Elbow and wrist motion
Spread fingers; make fist	Hand and finger motion, strength, and deformities
Tighten (contract) quadriceps; quadriceps	Symmetry and knee effusions, ankle effusion relax
"Duck walk" away and toward examiner	Hip, knee, and ankle motions
Back to examiner	Shoulder symmetry; scoliosis
Knees straight, touch toes	Scoliosis, hip motion, hamstring tightness
Raise up on toes, heels	Calf symmetry, leg strength

injuries of the shoulder or elbow should prompt further workup and rehabilitation if warranted.

Dermatologic

The athlete should be questioned in regard to any history of infectious skin lesions, and the skin should be thoroughly evaluated for any signs of bacterial, parasitic, fungal, or viral skin lesions, as these typically require treatment.[16,22] Infectious lesions pose a health risk to other athletes, as they can be transferred through skin-to-skin contact or the use of shared equipment.[16] The athlete's skin should also be evaluated for any lesions that may be suspicious for malignancy. If present, a skin biopsy should be performed and sent for pathology, or the athlete should be referred to a dermatologist for additional workup.[16,22] Owing to the frequency of direct sunlight exposure in baseball, the athlete should be counseled on the regular use of sunscreen. The American Academy of Dermatology recommends the use of a sunscreen with a broad spectrum of ultraviolet (UV) light protection with a sun protection factor (SPF) of 15 or higher.[41] However, many dermatologists suggest using a sunscreen with an SPF of 30 or higher.[42] The athlete should be educated on the need to apply the sunscreen before sun exposure and perform reapplication at the product's recommended time intervals.

Neurologic and Concussion

Concussions are a very common condition, with an estimation of 1.8 to 3.6 million concussions occurring each year in the United States related to recreational and athletic participation.[13,43] No standardized screening protocol has been adopted by the sports community, and many athletic association do not require baseline concussion testing as part of their PPE. However, many experts and medical associations agree that there is value in obtaining baseline neurocognitive testing during the PPE, which can be extremely beneficial in assessing an athlete with a suspected concussion and progressing them back into participation after injury.[13,43,44]

A history of concussions should be obtained, and medical records of these injuries should be reviewed if available. The athlete should be questioned in regard to the number of previously diagnosed concussions, possible instances of undiagnosed concussions, mechanism of each injury, severity and duration of symptoms with each episode, and use of protective equipment. Additionally, the practitioner should inquire about the athlete's and family history of mood disorders, migraines, learning disabilities, attention deficit hyperactive disorder/attention deficit disorder, recreational drug use, alcohol use, medications, sleep habits, and stressors, as these factors may confound symptoms often associated with concussions or be associated with a prolonged duration of symptoms.[13,43,44]

As previously mentioned, examination should include visual acuity, extraocular eye motions, pupillary reactions to light and accommodation, and documentation of pupil symmetry.[1] While not part of a typical PPE, the authors also suggest documenting the presence of nystagmus and near-point convergence. Additionally, a baseline balance error scoring system (BESS) test should be obtained, which includes a narrow double-leg stance, single-leg stance, and tandem stance. All these measures help in establishing an individual athlete's baseline and can prove useful when assessing for concussions.[43]

It is imperative to obtain baseline concussion assessments and neuropsychological testing on all athletes, and there are numerous resources available from paper assessments with the Sport Concussion Assessment Tool—5th edition (SCAT5) to more advanced computerized testing with programs such as the Immediate Post-Concussion Assessment and Cognitive Testing (ImPACT) and Cogstate.[45,46] These tools, in addition to many other concussion assessment instruments that are on the market, assist the physician in making the diagnosis of concussion and continuing to monitor the progression of concussive symptoms. The concussion assessment tool used by the team physician should be based on the practitioner's comfort with each system, ability to accurately interpret the results of the test and the resources available.[43,44]

DIAGNOSTIC TESTING

Laboratory Testing

Routine screening with laboratory testing remains controversial. However, the general consensus among most major sports medicine societies is that no routine screening is required for the clearance of asymptomatic individuals.[3,6,7,16] Current studies have not supported the use of laboratory tests including complete blood count (CBC), comprehensive metabolic panel (CMP), UA, lipid panel, ferritin level, or sickle cell trait.[16,47] However, many athletic associations, particularly at the professional and collegiate levels, choose to screen their athletes with laboratory tests to investigate for possible underlying medical conditions, which may place the athlete at risk. For instance, the National Collegiate Athletic Association (NCAA) requires all athletes to present documentation of testing for sickle cell trait, although the athletes do have the option to sign a waiver to opt out of this testing.[48]

Electrocardiogram

The use of ECGs as screening tools during PPEs remains controversial. Some studies have found a significant decrease in mortality associated with SCD by screening for cardiac abnormalities using ECGs during PPEs. However, these results were noted in a small Italian population known to have higher rates of arrhythmogenic disorders when compared with the United States.[11,12,26,27] Multiple international societies including the European Society of Cardiology (ESC) and International Olympic Committee (IOC) have recommended the standardized use of screening ECGs among all athletes. Conversely, the AHA has not supported the use of ECGs as a requirement during the PPE and instead endorses the use of medical history and physical examination alone for cardiovascular screening in athletes (Table 32.1). The basis for this decision relates to the relatively low prevalence of cardiovascular abnormalities associated with sudden death (1/100,000-1/300,000 in US high school athletes), the significant amount of resources required to perform ECG screening for large populations of athletes, the exorbitant cost of mandatory ECG screening, and the high false-positive rate of seemingly abnormal ECG findings associated with the athlete's heart.[6,9,11-13,19,26,27,49]

Despite being recommended against by the AHA, numerous athletic organizations and the majority of professional athletic organizations include ECG screening in their standard PPE protocol. With the introduction of specific criteria, such as the Seattle criteria, as well as expanding knowledge in regard to normal physiologic changes associated with athlete's hearts, ECGs may have increased ability to detect potentially fatal cardiac abnormalities among asymptomatic athletes and may grow in the frequency of use in the PPE.[50-52] Any athlete that reports concerning symptoms, significant family history, or has worrisome findings on physical examination should undergo further cardiac workup with consideration of ECG, echocardiogram, stress testing, referral to cardiology, or cardiac magnetic resonance imaging (MRI) when appropriate.

Disqualifying Conditions

In determining clearance, 3.1% to 13.9% of athletes require further workup before being cleared for participation, with only 0.2% to 1.9% of athletes being completely disqualified from athletic participation. This clearance decision for participation in athletics is typically placed into 1 of 4 categories:

• Cleared for participation without restrictions
• Cleared for participation with recommendations for further evaluation
• Clearance for participation withheld, with reconsideration for participation pending further evaluation or treatment
• Not cleared for participation in a particular sport, or not cleared for any athletic participation[6,16]

This decision is often difficult and must be made on an individual basis, taking the athlete's condition, the sport being played, risk for injury or death, availability of protective equipment, and the wishes of the athletes and their parents into consideration. A team approach may be required to determine clearance, including the input from subspecialists and a review of the most current literature. However, the final decision for participation lies in the hands of the head team physician.[6,16,17] Table 32.4 displays a list of commonly encountered medical conditions and recommendations on clearance for each condition.[53]

TRIP TO THE MOUND

Ethical and Legal Issues

While protecting each athlete's health and wellness is the main priority of the PPE, the team physician must also protect the athlete's privacy. All medical forms, medical information, and decisions in regard to the athlete's eligibility for participation should comply with Health Insurance Portability and Accountability Act (HIPPA) and Federal Education Records Protection Act (FERPA) guidelines. Often, the only information that should be relayed to administrators or coaches is whether or not the athlete is eligible for participation. Any further information in regard to the athlete's medical condition should remain confidential, unless appropriate authorization forms have been completed by the athletes or their guardian to share this information freely.[16,17]

The team physician's determination to clear or restrict participation is also another major medicolegal issue associated with the PPE. As previously mentioned, the decision to restrict clearance is multifactorial and often a very complex decision. In the presence of a medical condition, which places the athletes at increased risk for injury or death, the athletes and their parents should be thoroughly educated on the potential risks of athletic participation. Although the athlete may disagree with the decision, a team physician or institution has the right to withhold an athlete from participation as long as the decision was individualized, reasonable, and based on current and evidence-based medical advice.[16]

In cases when parents or athletes disagree with restrictions from participation, exculpatory waivers have been considered by some institutions.

However, these exculpatory waivers are often standard forms that may include confusing medicolegal terminology and typically do not hold up in court. Some have instead suggested having the athletes and their parents write and sign their own letter discussing their knowledge of the medical condition and associated risks of athletic participation, which demonstrates an understanding of the risks ensued by disregarding medical advice.[6,16] If the athlete is restricted from participation in a particular sport, the team physician should also provide the athlete with acceptable alternatives for recreational activity.

TABLE 32.4 Recommendations for Sports Participation Clearance Based on Medical Conditions

Condition	May Participate
Atlantoaxial instability (instability of the joint between cervical vertebrae 1 and 2) Explanation: Athlete (particularly if he or she has Down syndrome or juvenile rheumatoid arthritis with cervical involvement) needs evaluation to assess the risk of spinal cord injury during sports participation, especially when using a trampoline.	Qualified yes
Bleeding disorder Explanation: Athlete needs evaluation.	Qualified yes
Cardiovascular disease	
Carditis (inflammation of the heart) Explanation: Carditis may result in sudden death with exertion.	No
Hypertension (high blood pressure) Explanation: Those with hypertension >5 mm Hg above the 99th percentile for age, gender, and height should avoid heavy weight lifting and power lifting, bodybuilding, and high-static component sports. Those with sustained hypertension (>95th percentile for age, gender, and height) need evaluation. The National High Blood Pressure Education Program Working Group report defined prehypertension and stage 1 and stage 2 hypertension in children and adolescents younger than 18 y.	Qualified yes
Congenital heart disease (structural heart defects present at birth) Explanation: Consultation with a cardiologist is recommended. Those who have mild forms may participate fully in most cases; those who have moderate or severe forms or who have undergone surgery need evaluation. The 36th Bethesda Conference defined mild, moderate, and severe disease for common cardiac lesions.	Qualified yes

Dysrhythmia (irregular heart rhythm)
    Long-QT syndrome
    Malignant ventricular arrhythmias
    Symptomatic Wolff-Parkinson-White syndrome
    Advanced heart block
    Family history of sudden death or sudden cardiac event
    Implantation of a cardioverter-defibrillator
        Explanation: Consultation with a cardiologist is advised. Those with symptoms (chest pain, syncope, near-syncope, dizziness, shortness of breath, or other symptoms of possible dysrhythmia) or evidence of mitral regurgitation on physical examination need evaluation. All others may participate fully.
	Qualified yes

(continued)

TABLE 32.4 Recommendations for Sports Participation Clearance Based on Medical Conditions (continued)

Condition	May Participate
Heart murmur Explanation: If the murmur is innocent (does not indicate heart disease), full participation is permitted. Otherwise, athlete needs evaluation (see structural heart disease, especially hypertrophic cardiomyopathy and mitral valve prolapse).	Qualified yes
Structural/acquired heart disease	
Hypertrophic cardiomyopathy	Qualified no
Coronary artery anomalies	Qualified no
Arrhythmogenic right ventricular cardiomyopathy	Qualified no
Acute rheumatic fever with carditis	Qualified no
Ehlers-Danlos syndrome, vascular form	Qualified no
Marfan syndrome	Qualified yes
Mitral valve prolapse	Qualified yes
Anthracycline use	Qualified yes
Explanation: Consultation with a cardiologist is recommended. The 36th Bethesda Conference provided detailed recommendations. Most of these conditions carry a significant risk of sudden cardiac death associated with intense physical exercise. Hypertrophic cardiomyopathy requires thorough and repeated evaluations, because disease may change manifestations during later adolescence. Marfan syndrome with an aortic aneurysm also can cause sudden death during intense physical exercise. Athlete who has ever received chemotherapy with anthracyclines may be at increased risk of cardiac problems because of the cardiotoxic effects of the medications, and resistance training in this population should be approached with caution; strength training that avoids isometric contractions may be permitted. Athlete needs evaluation.	

Vasculitis/vascular disease
    Kawasaki disease (coronary artery vasculitis)
Pulmonary hypertension
    Explanation: Consultation with a cardiologist is recommended. Athlete needs individual evaluation to assess risk on the basis of disease activity, pathologic changes, and medical regimen.
	Qualified yes

Cerebral palsy Explanation: Athlete needs evaluation to assess functional capacity to perform sports-specific activity.	Qualified yes
Diabetes mellitus Explanation: All sports can be played with proper attention and appropriate adjustments to diet (particularly carbohydrate intake), blood glucose concentrations, hydration, and insulin therapy. Blood glucose concentrations should be monitored before exercise, every 30 min during continuous exercise, 15 min after completion of exercise, and at bedtime.	Yes
Diarrhea, infectious Explanation: Unless symptoms are mild and athlete is fully hydrated, no participation is permitted, because diarrhea may increase risk of dehydration and heat illness (see fever).	Qualified no

TABLE 32.4 Recommendations for Sports Participation Clearance Based on Medical Conditions   (continued)

Condition	May Participate
Eating disorders Explanation: Athlete with an eating disorder needs medical and psychiatric assessment before participation.	Qualified yes
Eyes	
Functionally 1-eyed athlete Loss of an eye Detached retina or family history of retinal detachment at young age High myopia Connective tissue disorder, such as Marfan or Stickler syndrome Previous intraocular eye surgery or serious eye injury Explanation: A functionally 1-eyed athlete is defined as having best-corrected visual acuity worse than 20/40 in the poorer-seeing eye. Such an athlete would suffer significant disability if the better eye were seriously injured, as would an athlete with loss of an eye. Specifically, boxing and full-contact martial arts are not recommended for functionally 1-eyed athletes, because eye protection is impractical and/or not permitted. Some athletes who previously underwent intraocular eye surgery or had a serious eye injury may have increased risk of injury because of weakened eye tissue. Availability of eye guards approved by the American Society for Testing and Materials and other protective equipment may allow participation in most sports, but this must be judged on an individual basis.	Qualified yes
Conjunctivitis, infectious Explanation: Athlete with active infectious conjunctivitis should be excluded from swimming.	Qualified no
Fever Explanation: Elevated core temperature may be indicative of a pathologic medical condition (infection or disease) that is often manifested by increased resting metabolism and heart rate. Accordingly, during athlete's usual exercise regimen, the presence of fever can result in greater heat storage, decreased heat tolerance, increased risk of heat illness, increased cardiopulmonary effort, reduced maximal exercise capacity, and increased risk of hypotension because of altered vascular tone and dehydration. On rare occasions, fever may accompany myocarditis or other conditions that may make usual exercise dangerous.	No

Gastrointestinal
  Malabsorption syndromes (celiac disease or cystic fibrosis)
    Explanation: Athlete needs individual assessment for general malnutrition or specific deficits resulting in coagulation or other defects; with appropriate treatment, these deficits can be treated adequately to permit normal activities.
  Short-bowel syndrome or other disorders requiring specialized nutritional support, including parenteral or enteral nutrition
    Explanation: Athlete needs individual assessment for collision, contact, or limited-contact sports. Presence of central or peripheral, indwelling, venous catheter may require special considerations for activities and emergency preparedness for unexpected trauma to the device(s).
	Qualified yes

Heat illness, history of Explanation: Because of the likelihood of recurrence, athlete needs individual assessment to determine the presence of predisposing conditions and behaviors and to develop a prevention strategy that includes sufficient acclimatization (to the environment and to exercise intensity and duration), conditioning, hydration, and salt intake, as well as other effective measures to improve heat tolerance and to reduce heat injury risk (such as protective equipment and uniform configurations).	Qualified yes

(continued)

TABLE 32.4 Recommendations for Sports Participation Clearance Based on Medical Conditions   (continued)

Condition	May Participate
Hepatitis, infectious (primarily hepatitis C) Explanation: All athletes should receive hepatitis B vaccination before participation. Because of the apparent minimal risk to others, all sports may be played as athlete's state of health allows. For all athletes, skin lesions should be covered properly, and athletic personnel should use universal precautions when handling wood or body fluids with visible blood.	Yes
HIV infection Explanation: Because of the apparent minimal risk to others, all sports may be played as athlete's state of health allows (especially if viral load is undetectable or very low). For all athletes, skin lesions should be covered properly, and athletic personnel should use universal precautions when handling blood or body fluids with visible blood. However, certain sports (such as wrestling and boxing) may create a situation that favors viral transmission (likely bleeding plus skin breaks). If viral load is detectable, then athletes should be advised to avoid such high-contact sports.	Yes
Kidney, absence of one Explanation: Athlete needs individual assessment for contact, collision, and limited-contact sports. Protective equipment may reduce risk of injury to the remaining kidney sufficiently to allow participation in most sports, providing such equipment remains in place during activity.	Qualified yes
Liver, enlarged Explanation: If the liver is acutely enlarged, then participation should be avoided because of risk of rupture. If the liver is chronically enlarged, then individual assessment is needed before collision, contact, or limited-contact sports are played. Patients with chronic liver disease may have changes in liver function that affect stamina, mental status, coagulation, or nutritional status.	Qualified yes
Malignant neoplasm Explanation: Athlete needs individual assessment.	Qualified yes
Musculoskeletal disorders Explanation: Athlete needs individual assessment.	Qualified yes
Neurologic disorders	
History of serious head or spine trauma or abnormality, including craniotomy, epidural bleeding, subdural hematoma, intracerebral hemorrhage, second-impact syndrome, vascular malformation, and neck fracture Explanation: Athlete needs individual assessment for collision, contact, or limited-contact sports.	Qualified yes
History of simple concussion (mild traumatic brain injury), multiple simple concussions, and/or complex conclusion Explanation: Athlete needs individual assessment. Research supports a conservative approach to concussion management, including no athletic participation while symptomatic or when deficits in judgment or cognition are detected, followed by graduated return to full activity.	Qualified yes
Myopathies Explanation: Athlete needs individual assessment.	Qualified yes
Recurrent headaches Explanation: Athlete needs individual assessment.	Yes

TABLE 32.4 Recommendations for Sports Participation Clearance Based on Medical Conditions   (continued)

Condition	May Participate
Recurrent plexopathy (burner or stinger) and cervical cord neuropraxia with persistent defects Explanation: Athlete needs individual assessment for collision, contact, or limited-contact sports. Regaining normal strength is important benchmark for return to play.	Qualified yes
Seizure disorder, well controlled Explanation: Risk of seizure during participation is minimal.	Yes
Seizure disorder, poorly controlled Explanation: Athlete needs individual assessment for collision, contact, or limited-contact sports. The following noncontact sports should be avoided: archery, riflery, swimming, weightlifting, power lifting, strength training, and sports involving heights. In these sports, occurrence of a seizure during activity may pose a risk to self or others.	Qualified yes
Obesity Explanation: Because of the increased risk of heat illness and cardiovascular strain, obese athlete particularly needs careful acclimatization (to the environment and to exercise intensity and duration), sufficient hydration, and potential activity and recovery modifications during competition and training.	Yes
Organ transplant recipient (and those taking immunosuppressive medications) Explanation: Athlete needs individual assessment for contact, collision, and limited-contact sports. In addition to potential risk of infections, some medications (eg, prednisone) may increase tendency for bruising.	Qualified yes
Ovary, absence of one Explanation: Risk of severe injury to remaining ovary is minimal.	Yes
Pregnancy/postpartum Explanation: Athlete needs individual assessment. As pregnancy progresses, modifications to usual exercise routines will become necessary. Activities with high risk of falling or abdominal trauma should be avoided. Scuba diving and activities posing risk of altitude sickness should also be avoided during pregnancy. After the birth, physiological and morphologic changes of pregnancy take 4-6 wk to return to baseline.	Qualified yes
Respiratory conditions	
Pulmonary compromise, including cystic fibrosis Explanation: Athlete needs individual assessment, but, generally, all sports may be played if oxygenation remains satisfactory during graded exercise test. Athletes with cystic fibrosis need acclimatization and good hydration to reduce risk of heat illness.	Qualified yes
Asthma Explanation: With proper medication and education, only athletes with severe asthma need to modify their participation. For those using inhalers, recommend having a written action plan and using a peak flowmeter daily. Athletes with asthma may encounter risks when scuba diving.	Yes
Acute upper respiratory infection Explanation: Upper respiratory obstruction may affect pulmonary function. Athletes need individual assessment for all except mild disease (see fever).	Qualified yes

(continued)

TABLE 32.4 Recommendations for Sports Participation Clearance Based on Medical Conditions   (continued)

Condition	May Participate

Rheumatologic diseases
  Juvenile rheumatoid arthritis
    Explanation: Athletes with systemic or polyarticular juvenile rheumatoid arthritis and history of cervical spine involvement need radiographs of vertebrae C1 and C2 to assess risk of spinal cord injury. Athletes with systemic or HLA-B27-associated arthritis require cardiovascular assessment for possible cardiac complications during exercise. For those with micrognathia (open bite and exposed teeth), mouth guards are helpful. If uveitis is present, risk of eye damage from trauma is increased; ophthalmologic assessment is recommended. If visually impaired, guidelines for functionally 1-eyed athletes should be followed.
  Juvenile dermatomyositis, idiopathic myositis
  Systemic lupus erythematosus
  Raynaud phenomenon
    Explanation: Athlete with juvenile dermatomyositis or systemic lupus erythematosus with cardiac involvement requires cardiology assessment before participation. Athletes receiving systemic corticosteroid therapy are at higher risk of osteoporotic fractures and avascular necrosis, which should be assessed before clearance; those receiving immunosuppressive medications are at higher risk of serious infection. Sports activities should be avoided when myositis is active. Rhabdomyolysis during intensive exercise may cause renal injury in athletes with idiopathic myositis and other myopathies. Because of photosensitivity with juvenile dermatomyositis and systemic lupus erythematosus, sun protection is necessary during outdoor activities. With Raynaud phenomenon, exposure to the cold presents risk to hands and feet.
	Qualified yes

Sickle cell disease Explanation: Athlete needs individual assessment. In general, if illness status permits, all sports may be played; however, any sport or activity that entails overexertion, overheating, dehydration, or chilling should be avoided. Participation at high altitude, especially when not acclimatized, also poses risk of sickle cell crisis.	Qualified yes
Sickle cell trait Explanation: Athletes with sickle cell trait generally do not have increased risk of sudden death or other medical problems during athlete participation under normal environmental conditions. However, when high exertional activity is performed under extreme conditions of heat and humidity or increased altitude, such catastrophic complications have occurred rarely. Athletes with sickle cell trait, like all athletes, should be progressively acclimatized to the environment and to the intensity and duration of activities and should be sufficiently hydrated to reduce the risk of exertional heat illness and/or rhabdomyolysis. According to National Institutes of Health management guidelines, sickle cell trait is not a contraindication to participation in competitive athletics, and there is no requirement for screening before participation. More research is needed to assess fully potential risks and benefits of screening athletes for sickle cell trait.	Yes
Skin infections, including herpes simplex, molluscum contagiosum, verrucae (warts), staphylococcal and streptococcal infections (furuncles [boils], carbuncles, impetigo, methicillin-resistant *Staphylococcus aureus* [cellulitis and/or abscesses]), scabies, and tinea Explanation: During contagious periods, participation in gymnastics or cheerleading with mats, martial arts, wresting, or other collision, contact, or limited-contact sports is not allowed.	Qualified yes

TABLE 32.4 Recommendations for Sports Participation Clearance Based on Medical Conditions   (continued)

Condition	May Participate
Spleen, enlarged Explanation: If the spleen is acutely enlarged, then participation should be avoided because of risk of rupture. If the spleen is chronically enlarged, then individual assessment is needed before collision, contact, or limited-contact sports are played.	Qualified yes
Testicle, undescended or absence of one Explanation: Certain sports may require a protective cup.	Yes

This table is designed for use by medical and nonmedical personnel. "Needs evaluation" means that a physician with appropriate knowledge and experience should assess the safety of a given sport for an athlete with the listed medical condition. Unless otherwise noted, this need for special consideration is because of variability in the severity of the disease, the risk of injury for the specific sports listed in Table 32.4, or both.

Reproduced with permission from Rice SG. Medical conditions affecting sports participation. Pediatrics. 2008;121(4):841-848. Copyright © 2008 by the AAP.

MANAGER'S TIPS

- Primary goal of the PPE is to identify medical conditions or risk factors, which could lead to injury or death

- PPEs should be conducted by a qualified practitioner in an appropriate clinical setting

- Athletes may be evaluated with an individual examination in a physician's office or mass screening using a station-based method

- Include a comprehensive medical history and thorough physical examination

- Conduct PPEs at least 5 to 6 weeks before the start of training to allow sufficient time for additional evaluation or testing, if required

- Final decisions for athletic participation and restrictions are determined by the team physician

- Decisions should be made on an individual basis, consider the potential harm of participation, and be based on current medical evidence

- Protect patient confidentiality by abiding by HIPPA and FERPA regulations

REFERENCES

1. Hoffmann S, Macri E. The preparticipation physical evaluation. In: Brukner P, Khan K, eds. *Brukner & Khan's Clinical Sports Medicine*. 4th ed. Sydney, Australia: McGraw-Hill Education; 2011:1176-1184.

2. Iqbal Z, Coles P. Screening the elite sportsperson. In: Brukner P, Khan K, eds. *Brukner & Khan's Clinical Sports Medicine*. 4th ed. Sydney, Australia: McGraw-Hill Education; 2011:1185-1202.

3. Mirabelli MH, Devine MJ, Singh J, et al. The preparticipation sports evaluation. *Am Fam Physician*. 2015;92(5):371-376.

4. Casa DJ, Ferrara MS, Adams WM, et al. Developing safety policies for organized sports. In: Casa DJ, Stearns RL, eds. *Preventing Sudden Death in Sports & Physical Activity*. 2nd ed. Burlington: Jones & Bartlett Publishers; 2016:1-16.

5. Conley KM, Bolin DJ, Carek PJ, et al. National Athletic Trainers' Association position statement: preparticipation physical examinations and disqualifying conditions. *J Athl Train*. 2014;49(1):102-120. doi:10.4085/1062-6050-48.6.05.

6. Gayagoy JJ, Foster KW, Tucker JB. Preparticipation examination. In: Birrer RB, O'Connor FG, Kane SF, eds. *Musculoskeletal and Sports Medicine for the Primary Care Practitioner*. 4th ed. Boca Raton: CRC Press; 2016:49-62.

7. Landry GL, Bernhardt DT. Preparticipation physical examination. In: *Essentials of Primary Care Sports Medicine*. Champaign: Human Kinetics; 2003:287-301.

8. Kibler WB, Chandler TJ, Uhl T, et al. A musculoskeletal approach to the preparticipation physical examination. Preventing injury and improving performance. *Am J Sports Med*. 1989;17(4):525-531. doi:10.1177/036354658901700413.

9. Wingfield K, Matheson GO, Meeuwisse WH. Preparticipation evaluation: an evidence-based review. *Clin J Sport Med*. 2004;14(3):109-122.

10. Thompson PD. Preparticipation screening of competitive athletes. *Circulation*. 2009;119(8):1072-1074. doi:10.1161/CIRCULATIONAHA.108.843862.

11. Maron BJ, Thompson PD, Ackerman MJ, et al. Recommendations and considerations related to preparticipation screening for cardiovascular abnormalities in competitive athletes: 2007 update. *Circulation*. 2007;115(12):1643-1655. doi:10.1161/CIRCULATIONAHA.107.181423.

12. Harmon KG, Zigman M, Drezner JA. The effectiveness of screening history, physical exam, and ECG to detect potentially lethal cardiac disorders in athletes: a systematic review/meta-analysis. *J Electrocardiol*. 2015;48(3):329-338. doi:10.1016/j.jelectrocard.2015.02.001.

13. Ljungqvist A, Jenoure P, Engebretsen L, et al. The International Olympic Committee (IOC) Consensus Statement on periodic health evaluation of elite athletes, March 2009. *Br J Sports Med*. 2009;43(9):631-643. doi:10.1136/bjsm.2009.064394.

14. Madsen NL, Drezner JA, Salerno JC. The preparticipation physical evaluation: an analysis of clinical practice. *Clin J Sport Med*. 2014;24(2):142-149. doi:10.1097/JSM.0000000000000008.

15. Carek PJ, Mainous A. The preparticipation physical examination for athletics: a systematic review of current recommendations. *Br Med J (Clin Res Ed)*. 2003;327(7418):E170. doi:10.1136/bmjusa.02120003.

16. American Academy of Family Physicians, American Academy of Pediatrics, American College of Sports Medicine, American Orthopaedic Society for Sports Medicine, American Osteopathic Academy for Sports Medicine, American Medical Society for Sports Medicine. Bernhardt DT, Roberts WO, eds. *Preparticipation Physical Evaluation*. 4th ed. American Academy of Pediatrics; 2010.

17. Herring SA, Ben Kibler W, Putukian M. Team physician consensus statement: 2013 update. *Med Sci Sports Exerc*. 2013;45(8):1618-1622. doi:10.1249/MSS.0b013e31829ba437.

18. Carek PJ, Mainous AG. A thorough yet efficient exam identifies most problems in school athletes. *J Fam Pract*. 2003;52(2):127-134.

19. Maron BJ, Levine BD, Washington RL, et al. Eligibility and disqualification recommendations for competitive athletes with cardiovascular abnormalities: Task Force 2: preparticipation screening for cardiovascular disease in competitive athletes: a scientific statement from the American Heart Association and American College of Cardiology. *Circulation*. 2015;132(22):e267-e272. doi:10.1161/CIR.0000000000000238.

20. Magee DJ. Primary care assessment. In: *Orthopedic Physical Assessment*. 6th ed. St. Louis: Elsevier Health Sciences; 2008:1072-1104.

21. Kurowski K, Chandran S. The preparticipation athletic evaluation. *Am Fam Physician*. 2000;61(9):2683-2690 and 2696-2698.

22. Peterson AR, Bernhardt DT. The preparticipation sports evaluation. *Pediatr Rev*. 2011;32(5):e53-e65. doi:10.1542/pir.32-5-e53.

23. Maron BJ, Doerer JJ, Haas TS, et al. Sudden deaths in young competitive athletes. *Circulation*. 2009;119(8):1085-1092. doi:10.1161/CIRCULATIONAHA.108.804617.

24. Maron BJ. Sudden death in young athletes. *N Engl J Med*. 2003;349(11):1064-1075. doi:10.1056/NEJMra022783.

25. Harmon KG, Asif IM, Maleszewski JJ, et al. Incidence, cause, and comparative frequency of sudden cardiac death in National Collegiate Athletic Association athletes: a decade in review. *Circulation*. 2015;132(1):10-19. doi:10.1161/CIRCULATIONAHA.115.015431.

26. Pelliccia A, Zipes DP, Maron BJ. Bethesda conference #36 and the European Society of Cardiology Consensus Recommendations revisited. *J Am Coll Cardiol*. 2008;52(24):1990-1996. doi:10.1016/j.jacc.2008.08.055.

27. Maron BJ, Friedman RA, Kligfield P, et al. Assessment of the 12-lead ECG as a screening test for detection of cardiovascular disease in healthy general populations of young people (12-25 years of age). *Circulation*. 2014;130(15):1303-1334. doi:10.1161/CIR.0000000000000025.

28. Erickson BJ, Chalmers PN, Bush-Joseph CA, et al. Predicting and preventing injury in major League baseball. *Am J Orthop*. 2016;45(3):152-156.

29. Lyman S, Fleisig GS, Andrews JR, et al. Effect of pitch type, pitch count, and pitching mechanics on risk of elbow and shoulder pain in youth baseball pitchers. *Am J Sports Med*. 2002;30(4):463-468. doi:10.1177/03635465020300040201.

30. Erickson BJ, Chalmers PN, Axe MJ, et al. Exceeding pitch count recommendations in little league baseball increases the chance of requiring Tommy John surgery as a professional baseball pitcher. *Orthop J Sports Med*. 2017;5(3):2325967117695085. doi:10.1177/2325967117695085.

31. Chobanian AV, Bakris GL, Black HR, et al. Seventh report of the Joint National Committee on prevention, detection, evaluation, and treatment of high blood pressure. *Hypertension*. 2003;42(6):1206-1252. doi:10.1161/01.HYP.0000107251.49515.c2.

32. James PA, Oparil S, Carter BL, et al. 2014 Evidence-based guideline for the management of high blood pressure in adults: report from the panel members appointed to the Eighth Joint National Committee (JNC 8). *J Am Med Assoc*. 2014;311(5):507-520. doi:10.1001/jama.2013.284427.

33. National High Blood Pressure Education Program Working Group on High Blood Pressure in Children and Adolescents. The fourth report on the diagnosis, evaluation, and treatment of high blood pressure in children and adolescents. *Pediatrics*. 2004;114(2):555-576. doi:10.1542/peds.114.2.S2.555.

34. Cooper J, Ellison JA, Walsh MM. Spit (smokeless)-tobacco use by baseball players entering the professional ranks. *J Athl Train*. 2003;38(2):126-132.

35. Wilk KE, Andrews JR, Arrigo CA. The abductor and adductor strength characteristics of professional baseball pitchers. *Am J Sports Med*. April 2016. doi:10.1177/036354659502300309.

36. Seroyer ST, Nho SJ, Bach BR, et al. The kinetic chain in overhand pitching: its potential role for performance enhancement and injury prevention. *Sports Health*. 2010;2(2):135-146. doi:10.1177/1941738110362656.

37. Fronek J, Yang JG, Osbahr DC, et al. Shoulder functional performance status of minor league professional baseball pitchers. *J Shoulder Elbow Surg*. 2015;24(1):17-23. doi:10.1016/j.jse.2014.04.019.

38. Bigliani LU, Codd TP, Connor PM, et al. Shoulder motion and laxity in the professional baseball player. *Am J Sports Med*. 2016;25(5):609-613. doi:10.1177/036354659702500504.

39. Chalmers PN, Erickson BJ, Ball B, et al. fastball pitch velocity helps predict ulnar collateral ligament reconstruction in major league baseball pitchers. *Am J Sports Med.* 2016;44(8):2130-2135. doi:10.1177/0363546516634305.

40. Harris JD, Frank JM, Jordan MA, et al. Return to sport following shoulder surgery in the elite pitcher: a systematic review. *Sports Health.* 2013;5(4):367-376. doi:10.1177/1941738113482673.

41. Lim HW, Naylor M, Hönigsmann H, et al. American Academy of Dermatology consensus conference on UVA protection of sunscreens: summary and recommendations. Washington, DC, Feb 4, 2000. *J Am Acad Dermatol.* 2001;44:505-508. doi:10.1067/mjd.2001.112913.

42. Farberg AS, Glazer AM, Rigel AC, et al. Dermatologists' perceptions, recommendations, and use of sunscreen. *JAMA Dermatol.* 2017;153(1):99-101. doi:10.1001/jamadermatol.2016.3698.

43. Harmon KG, Drezner JA, Gammons M, et al. American medical society for sports medicine position statement: concussion in sport. *Br J Sports Med.* 2013;47(1):15-26. doi:10.1136/bjsports-2012-091941.

44. McCrory P. Preparticipation assessment for head injury. *Clin J Sport Med.* 2004;14(3):139-144.

45. McCrory P, Meeuwisse W, Dvorak J, et al. Consensus statement on concussion in sport-the 5th international conference on concussion in sport held in Berlin, October 2016. *Br J Sports Med.* 2017;51(11):838-847. doi:10.1136/bjsports-2017-097699.

46. Echemendia RJ, Meeuwisse W, McCrory P, et al. The sport concussion assessment tool 5th edition (SCAT5). *Br J Sports Med.* April 2017. doi:10.1136/bjsports-2017-097506.

47. Jordan LB, Smith-Whitley K, Treadwell MJ, et al. Screening U.S. college athletes for their sickle cell disease carrier status. *Am J Prev Med.* 2011;41(6):S406-S412. doi:10.1016/j.amepre.2011.09.014.

48. Parsons JT. *NCAA Sports Medicine Handbook.* 25th ed. Indianapolis: National Collegiate Athletic Association; 2014.

49. Drezner J, Corrado D. Is there evidence for recommending electrocardiogram as part of the pre-participation examination? *Clin J Sport Med.* 2011;21(1):18-24. doi:10.1097/JSM.0b013e318205dfb2.

50. Drezner JA, Ackerman MJ, Anderson J, et al. Electrocardiographic interpretation in athletes: the 'Seattle criteria'. *Br J Sports Med.* 2013;47(3):122-124. doi:10.1136/bjsports-2012-092067.

51. Brosnan M, La Gerche A, Kalman J, et al. The Seattle Criteria increase the specificity of preparticipation ECG screening among elite athletes. *Br J Sports Med.* 2014;48(15):1144-1150. doi:10.1136/bjsports-2013-092420.

52. Maron BJ, Pelliccia A. The heart of trained athletes. *Circulation.* 2006;114(15):1633-1644. doi:10.1161/CIRCULATIONAHA.106.613562.

53. Rice SG. Medical conditions affecting sports participation. *Pediatrics.* 2008;121(4):841-848. doi:10.1542/peds.2008-0080.

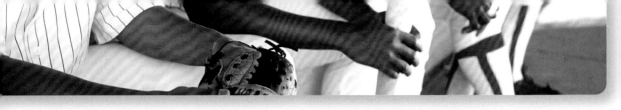

CHAPTER 33

Nutrition for the Elite Baseball Athlete

Heidi Skolnik, MS, CDN, FACSM

A hot dog at the game beats roast beef at the Ritz.

—*Humphrey Bogart*

INTRODUCTION

Baseball is an anaerobic sport that requires precision skill. Fueled by phosphocreatine and glycogen, baseball requires split-second reaction time. As a sport that requires constant shifting of strategy based on who is up to bat or on base, baseball players need to stay alert through 9 innings and be ready for longer games should a tie take place. Often played in hot, humid conditions and at night, the schedule demands days on the road as well as back-to-back games. Air travel or long bus rides bring their own challenges. Resiliency to get through a long season healthy can be supported by specific nutritional patterns and choices. With continuously changing schedules, erratic patterns of food consumption, and disrupted sleep, baseball athletes can find themselves in a negative cyclical pattern of eating. Too often, players eat too little before a game and then overconsume food and alcohol afterward. This habit interferes with needed sleep and adequate recovery and can challenge weight maintenance goals. Players need to stay fueled to perform. Even though long hours are required, baseball is not a high-energy expenditure sport. Players must remain focused and alert, not lethargic from either underfueling or overeating. As power athletes, baseball players are often concerned with putting on muscle and decreasing body fat. The actual energy output varies based on position with catchers and pitchers needing the greatest amount of fuel and to pay close attention to recovery efforts. Because most games are played at night, players are often misaligned with the general population in terms of daily schedule. Many restaurants and take-out places may be closed postgame. This limits players'

options and can be particularly difficult for collegiate and minor league players who have less resources and access to healthful food selections. Additionally, these teams often play in smaller towns that shut down earlier than big cities. Language barriers and cultural food preferences may also need to be taken into account. Of course, supplements are always changing and players are often curious about the ability for these products to enhance their performance.[1]

NUTRIENT TIMING: CONDITIONING, PREGAME, DURING GAME, POSTGAME

Nutrient timing refers to manipulating and planning specific quantity, selection, and timing of intake of food and/or supplements to maximize performance results. Although there is a lot of attention given to how to eat around game time, eating habits during training and conditioning are equally as important to maximize efforts and preparedness in athletes. Conditioning demands are markedly different than game demands.[2]

Fundamentals: Baseline Dietary Needs

Consistency off the field contributes to consistency on the field. Patterns of caloric distribution influence the stability of energy, mood, body composition, hormone levels (including cortisol production and insulin/blood glucose levels), immune function, injury risk, and hydration. Many baseball players underfuel during the day, showing up at practice or a game having eaten a fraction of their daily requirements. This can lead to distracted play and overeating after the game. Overeating late at

TABLE 33.1 Macronutrient Needs

	Carbohydrate	Protein	Fat
Pitchers and catchers	6-8 g/kg	1.2-1.7 g/kg	1.0 g/kg or more
Fielders	4-7 g/kg	1.2-1.7 g/kg	1.0 g/kg or more

night can interfere with sleep as well as morning hunger, continuing a negative cycle of under- and overeating. This is true for both the high school and college athlete (skip breakfast, eat a moderate lunch at noon, play an afternoon game, upload all calories at night) as well as the professional athlete who sleeps in, grabs an egg and cheese breakfast sandwich (300 calories of a needed 3500-calorie/day), and heads to the field.

There is an art and science to these recommendations, as the athlete's entire individual profile must be considered. Health risk factors such as metabolic syndrome, weight, habits, food preferences, and family history should all be taken into account. Table 33.1 depicts general macronutrient recommendations for baseball players based on the position played. These recommendations do not distinguish the quality, quantity, or timing of food selection, merely the amount of each to consume. These details can be very important; for example, consuming protein (20 to 40 g) at regular intervals throughout the day has been shown to stimulate and maximize muscle protein repair and building.[3] Grabbing a buttered bagel for breakfast provides calories but no protein, vitamin C, or calcium. The egg and cheese muffin does provide some protein and calcium but not enough calories. Adding even an orange juice (100 calories and vitamin C, potassium, and other phytonutrients) or cup of fruit helps round out this selection. Add a yogurt too, and the player is now better aligned with caloric and nutrient needs.

Carbohydrate uptake is also best managed when distributed more evenly throughout the day. Many athletes think of bread, pasta, and sweets as carbohydrates instead of also identifying milk, yogurt, fruit, vegetables, beans, potatoes, and all grains as a part of this category. This may seem insignificant, but it is, in fact, extremely important, as it is impossible to know if you are eating too much or too little of a something when you cannot identify it! Baseball players need appropriate amounts of carbohydrate to fuel their power and strength, whereas excessive amounts of starch and fat are unnecessary. Planning meals and snacks that contain fruits, nonstarch vegetables, whole grains/beans, lean protein, and healthy fats, along with proper hydration, is important not just for proper

fueling but also for adequate nourishment. This can prevent unintended weight gain while providing nutrients that will support immune function, muscle integrity, strength, and power.

Dietary fat, once shunned, has now been embraced. Necessary for absorption of all fat-soluble vitamins, helpful with taste and satiety, and an integral part of hormone development, fat is an essential component of a healthy athlete's diet. Nuts, avocado, and oils remain "healthy" fats with the understanding that all fats can fit into a healthy meal plan. Still, limiting saturated fat in abundance is considered beneficial by many health organizations.[4]

It has been shown that an athlete's attitude toward eating well influences his food choices. Knowledge regarding how to eat a well-balanced diet, the convenience and availability of healthful foods, the ability to afford these foods, and the motivation to seek them out were salient facilitating factors related to perceived behavioral control. Intention to eat a healthful diet was a predictor of healthful dietary behavior.[5]

The fundamental and easiest depiction of a baseball player's diet can be seen in the "athlete's plate model" for moderate training as pictured in Figure 33.1.[6] This can mean a turkey sandwich (protein and starch) with a side salad with sliced avocado (vegetable plus fat), a glass of milk (dairy = protein and carbohydrate), and 2 pieces of fruit (carbohydrate); or a stir fry (oil/fat plus vegetables plus protein over rice/starch) and fruit; or wild salmon with a mango salsa, sesame broccoli with red pepper, and roasted potatoes; or minestrone soup and pasta with spinach and chicken in garlic and oil. There can be many variations of "the plate."

Training and Conditioning

To maximize resistance-training efforts, eating carbohydrate and protein before training, either through solid, whole foods (eggs, toast, and fruit; Greek yogurt parfait with fruit and nuts, etc), a protein/carb shake, or other supplement (bars, Ready To Drink beverages), will help increase energy and may help stimulate maximal protein synthesis. Consuming carbohydrate solely or in combination with protein during resistance exercise increases muscle glycogen stores, ameliorates muscle damage, and facilitates greater acute and chronic training adaptations.[7] Size, intensity, volume, frequency of training, and timing of intake will determine the amounts of carbohydrate and protein needed before, during, and after a training bout. Still, regular mealtimes and appropriate calories are the greatest influencers on growth and adaptation. Consuming 20 to 40 g of protein every 3 to 4 hours seems to stimulate muscle protein synthesis along with training.[3]

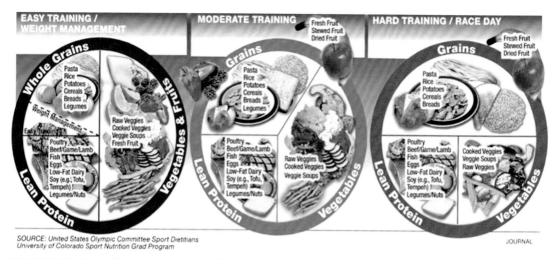

SOURCE: United States Olympic Committee Sport Dietitians
University of Colorado Sport Nutrition Grad Program

JOURNAL

FIGURE 33.1 • The Athlete's Plates are a collaboration between the United States Olympic Committee Sport Dietitians and the University of Colorado (UCCS) Sport Nutrition Graduate Program.

Consuming fruits, vegetables, and whole grains are crucial in providing macronutrients for tissue repair and immune function.[8] Ingestion of amino acids, primarily essential amino acids, immediately to 2 hours after exercise, has been shown to stimulate muscle protein synthesis. These benefits may be increased by adding carbohydrate.[7] Recovery drinks can be as easy as chocolate milk or a protein shake with 1 to 1.5 scoops of a whey protein powder (if vegan and using a pea protein, make sure it has added leucine).

PREGAME

If the athlete has managed time well and is organized, he will have eaten anywhere from one-third to two-thirds of his daily calorie needs by game time. For a 1:00 PM game, breakfast and a snack; 4:00 PM game, breakfast and lunch; 7:00 PM game, breakfast, lunch, and snack should all be eaten before the game begins. Adjusting the schedule based on game time is essential, yet keeping as much consistency as possible is also helpful. Even as nonathletes, we all know what it feels like if all you have eaten all day is a light breakfast and a banana. Consistency in timing meals throughout the day will help energy and concentration throughout the game. It is simple; the player needs to be fueled to perform at his best. sample meal timing based on a 7:00 PM home game.

DURING GAME

It can be beneficial to eat 25 to 30 g of carbohydrate during a game to help keep energy and focus. This can be especially important for catchers and pitchers and during very intense games. If a moderate mixed snack is consumed within an hour of taking the field, mostly likely drinking just water up to the 6th inning will suffice. If athletes do not enter the game well fueled, they may need to experiment with taking in more fuel during the game. This is where the differentiation between fuel and nutrition must be made. Easy-to-digest foods in 15 to 30 g of carbohydrate portions: applesauce squeeze pack, sports drinks, Chex (rice or corn cereal), salted pretzels, GU, gels or sports beans, piece of a bar, etc, all can provide a boost to energy in these situations.

POSTGAME

The intent of a postgame recovery snack is to help replace depleted glycogen stores, stimulate muscle repair, help maintain immune function, modulate hunger, and contribute to rehydration. Depleted glycogen stores may not happen in 1 game, but over the course of several days of training and playing; this may be more crucial for catchers and pitchers. Recovery begins 1 hour after a game or workout but is not completed within this time frame. Rather all food consumed between the end of the game and the beginning of the next game will contribute to overall energy stores and functions. Although all players may not have expended the same energy, or caused the same muscle damage, it is a smart practice to provide a recovery snack or beverage even if only to take the edge off hunger until players can eat a meal.

Weight and effort determines the protein and carbohydrate content of a recovery snack. For players

TABLE 33.2 Sample Meal Timing Based on 7:00 PM Game Time

Meal	Time	Calories	Notes
Breakfast	11:00 am	600+ calories	Eat more, not less, during this meal! Some athletes skip this meal and then "pound food" when they get to the stadium at one or two o'clock.
Lunch	2:00-3:00 pm	700-800 calories	Eat a "traditional dinner" with time to digest before the game. Eating heartier here will provide energy for the game and help appetite management later at night.
Pre-Game snack	5:30 pm	200-400 calories	Moderate snack. Simple with mixed protein and carbohydrate. Trick is not to get bored and overeat while waiting for game to start. This can be a smoothie.
During snack	8:30 pm	100 calories	Sports drink or water with salted snack
Postsnack/ recovery	10:15 pm	300-500 calories	Mix of protein and carbohydrate, takes edge off hunger until dinner. If club provides a full meal, can skip recovery snack here and just eat meal. Or have recovery snack, shower, change and have the meal provided.
Dinner	11:30 pm	600-800 calories	May seem smaller than usual due to distributing calories earlier in the day. Will help athletes calm down and be able to sleep better than if they consume a large amount postgame
Sleep	2:00 am		

weighing between 180 and 205 lbs, approximately 8 to 25 g of protein and 60 to 100 g of carbohydrate are indicated. Catchers and pitchers may go higher on the carbohydrate (0.1-0.25 g/kg protein and 0.7-1.5 g/kg carbohydrate). See Table 33.3 for sample recovery options.

TABLE 33.3 Sample Recovery Options

	Grams Protein	Carbohydrate
Greek yogurt (1 cup)	20	9
Pineapple with cottage cheese (1 cup)	24	32
Chocolate milk (20 oz)	20	65
Whey protein powder	20 g/scoop	1
Cliff bar	10	45
Peanut butter and banana sandwich	12	43
Granola bar[2]	3	29
Applesauce, sweetened (1 cup)	0.5	50
Super pretzel	5	34
Beef jerky	13	4

Pair protein options with carbohydrate options to meet recovery parameter suggestion.

Double check the label of the specific product you choose.

NA, not available.

OFF-SEASON AND IN-SEASON: TIME MANAGEMENT AND SKILL ATTAINMENT

Off-season conditioning may be more intense than during season, and following nutrient timing guidelines may be of even greater benefit. Although performance is not at stake, seeing training adaptation is. The off-season is the ideal time to focus on altering bodyweight and composition. After allowing for adequate rest and recuperation from the season, separating the off-season into goal-specific time periods will allow the athlete to come back ready for spring training.

Off-season is a great time to hone basic nutrition skills such as shopping, planning, and meal preparation. Menu literacy is helpful, enabling athletes on the road to determine which fast food and fast causal restaurant selections are best. Players can check each restaurant's website for nutritional information. However, learning which singular food items might be deemed "most nutritious" does not a meal make; therefore, having a sports nutritionist to refer to on staff is best. Although not specific to athletes:

https://www.healthydiningfinder.com/Home might offer some insights and

http://www.eatthis.com/restaurants has some great comparisons to learn from.

Learning how to stock a pantry with staples and how to utilize the freezer will help athletes have food available when they need it. Today there are many food delivery options and ways to have groceries delivered to the home. This convenience can make a big difference. There are also many apps available that can help: meal planning app, recipe organizers, and even an app to help you figure out how to use ingredients from leftovers!

- cheftap.com = recipe organizer
- pepperplate.com = recipe manager
- foodily.com

Obviously, as income grows, so too does access to more healthful food options. Single players have different challenges than their married or partnered counterparts. Booster clubs might also be a resource. In the minor league, sensitivity, acknowledgment, and help for players from other countries to manage food selection are helpful.

DO NOT SWEAT IT: HYDRATION RULES

Dehydration impairs performance, hastens fatigue, can induce cramping, lessens mental acuity, and can inhibit glycogen processing. When dehydrated, the ability to think and react slows, stamina and recuperation becomes suppressed, power and strength output drops, and the risk of injury increases dramatically![9]

Dehydration is preventable. Because baseball is played under the hot sun and in humid weather, coupled with travel and, for many, frequent alcohol ingestion, baseball players are at risk for dehydration on a daily basis. It is easy to spot-check players' hydration levels using urine specific gravity test, and a medical professional or even athletes themselves can be taught to use dip sticks or a refractometer to monitor their own hydration levels. According to Armstrong et al, checking urine color is as valid as checking osmolarity or urine specific gravity.[10] To gauge hydration status, see Figure 33.2 for a urine color reference chart.

Manager's Tip: Some Reminders for Players

- Drink often throughout the day—players will absorb more liquid when their stomach is partially full than when empty
- An easy way to check hydration, players should be peeing every 3 to 4 hours and pee should be ample. If pee is dense and smells, the player is probably

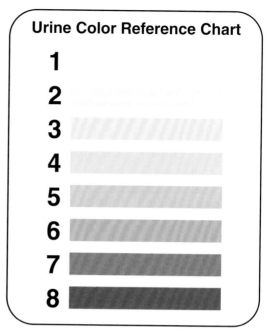

FIGURE 33.2 • **Urine color reference chart.** Adapted from http://www.budgetforhealth.com/wp-content/uploads/2011/12/Pee-chart.jpg.

dehydrated. Although urine can become darker because of supplements or some foods, usually, if pee looks like apple juice and is not of good volume, the player is dehydrated

- Eat all meals as food contributes approximately one-third of daily hydration needs. Skipping meals hurts hydration efforts
- Rehydrate before alcohol is consumed. Alcohol is a diuretic (coffee is not)
- Drink at least 16 oz of fluid with each meal. All fluid, except alcohol, counts. Milk, juice, seltzer, flavored seltzers, sports drinks, iced tea, and coffee all count toward fulfilling fluid needs. Drink 15 to 22 oz 4 hours before play and 8 to 16 oz 2 hours before. This leaves enough time to pee before the game starts.
- Sip water or a sports drink while in the dugout
- Replenish 16 to 24 oz of nonalcoholic fluid for every pound lost during a game (or practice)
- Players should be within 2 lbs of yesterday's playing weight by next day's game
- Sports drinks provide sodium and taste, as well as fluid. Sodium helps with fluid balance and taste helps athletes drink more. Sodium can be consumed other ways (eg, pretzels or salted sunflower seeds) during a game when water only is imbibed

THREE STRIKES: CAFFEINE, ALCOHOL, AND SLEEP

Caffeine

Caffeine is seen as an ergogenic aid, helping athletes be alert and improve RPE (rating of perceived exertion). There is evidence that caffeine have a positive or negative influence with a wide individual variability based on genetics and the gene variant CYP1A2, which controls the enzyme that breaks down caffeine.[11] For some, caffeine has ergogenic effect. Others are nonresponders. And yet, there are those for whom caffeine can actually hurt performance. Additionally, based on schedule, as well as habituation, sleep schedules, and culture, there are those players who rely on coffee and energy drinks to stimulate them and to help them be alert during the day/game and then overindulge in alcohol at night, a depressant, creating a cycle of up and down that interferes with any natural circadian rhythm, sleep, and healing/recovery.

Alcohol

Late nights, open bars, the culture of sports, and age of players often lean toward overconsumption of alcohol at night. The impact on recovery and performance is still being unearthed. What has been established is that consuming 5 or more alcoholic beverages in 1 night can affect brain and body activities for up to 3 days. Two consecutive nights of drinking 5 or more alcoholic beverages can affect brain and body activities for up to 5 days. Attention span is shorter for periods up to 48 hours after drinking.[12] Additionally, alcohol consumption reduces rates of muscle protein synthesis following a bout of concurrent exercise, even when coingested with protein. Alcohol ingestion suppresses the anabolic response in skeletal muscle and may therefore impair recovery and adaptation to training and/or subsequent performance.[13] This is true even for moderate amounts of alcohol consumption, which has been shown to magnify the loss of force associated with strenuous eccentric exercise. This resulting weakness seems to be the result of the damaging effects of alcohol on muscle recovery rather than merely the overall effects of acute alcohol consumption.[14] Of course, alcohol also is a diuretic and compounds the difficulty of staying hydrated or rehydrating.

An additional consequence of even acute alcohol consumption is it can negatively affect sleep, both in quantity and quality, all of which affect recovery, resiliency, and mental clarity for games.

Sleep

Poor sleep can lead to decreases in performance and recovery for athletes. Sleep deprivation may impair muscle glycogen repletion, impair muscle damage repair, cause alterations in cognitive function, and lead to an increase in mental fatigue.[15] Additionally, lack of sleep can interfere with appetite regulating hormones and contribute to overconsumption of calories in subsequent days. Behaviors related to evening games (eg, napping, caffeine consumption, alcohol consumption), as well the need to "come down" from being jazzed up for a game, can all negatively affect sleep. Overeating late at night often pushes bed time further back. Baseball also has an inconsistent schedule with interspersed day and night games. Travel and travel fatigue may also contribute to sleep debt.

Sleep disorders and symptoms are common in athletes and may be go unrecognized. It is important to educate athletes on adequate duration, quality, and timing of sleep. It is important to screen and treat sleep disorders such as sleep apnea and insomnia that are seen in some athletes.[16] Although sleep disturbance may not seem to be a nutritional issue, what, when, and how much you eat and drink can, in fact, affect sleep and lack of sleep can affect appetite regulating hormones and therefore food selection.

TRENDS AND FADS

Ketogenic Diet

As of now, the literature on ketogenic diets does not support its use for anaerobic performance. Some of the studies that support its use were conducted on ultraendurance athletes who run at submaximal intensity. Additionally, the shift in metabolic fuel utilization, as seen in these studies, does not necessarily equate to improved performance. During off-season, there may be a place for use in weight loss or to help regulate metabolic syndrome (and in the broader medical community for different medical reasons, ie, epilepsy or seizure disorders), but it is NOT recommended for performance improvement especially in high-intensity, power sports.[17-20]

Nutritional Supplements

New products hit the market every day. Major League Baseball (MLB) provides a list of banned substances for its players. NCAA (National Collegiate Athletic Association) has a list as well. Still, it is a challenge for doctors, athletic trainers, and even nutritionists to keep up with all the claims made by every manufacturer.

There are a few resources that can lend some insight into the legitimacy of claims or purity of the product.

> https://www.aegislabs.com
> https://www.consumerlab.com
> http://www.naturaldatabase.com
> https://www.drugfreesport.com
> http://www.nsfsport.com

- NSF Certified on label assures the product does not have any banned substances in the supplements; it does not ensure efficacy. NSF includes screening for more than 270 substances banned by most major athletic organizations, including stimulants, narcotics, steroids, diuretics, beta-2 agonists, masking agents, and other substances

Probiotics

The understanding of the gut microbiome is expanding. The gut is home to trillions of microorganisms that have fundamental roles in many aspects of human biology, including metabolism, endocrine, neuronal, and immune function.[21]

The bacteria in the gut plays an important role in which nutrients are extracted from foods during digestion, so 2 players eating the same food may extract a different proportion of nutrients based on their microbiota. Additionally, preliminary data are showing that the microbiota acts like an endocrine organ (eg, secreting serotonin, dopamine, or other neurotransmitters) and there may a gut-brain axis. Training may have a direct influence on affecting the composition of the gut microbiota and vice versa.[21]

Being the first line of defense, after skin, in screening out viruses and dangerous bacteria, a healthy gut plays an important role in the immune system. In a sport where athletes share a locker room, an upper respiratory infection can easily spread from one player to another; reducing this risk is wise. With athletes on the road and eating food that may be unfamiliar, probiotics may help to reduce risk of occurrence, severity, or length of gastrointestinal distress.[22] Consuming adequate fiber and fermented foods (yogurt is one) helps keep the gut rich in bacteria that supports these functions. Because many athletes diets may lack foods that support a healthy microbiome, taking a probiotic may be helpful. As more is studied and learned, it may be discovered that a simple probiotic supplement is not nearly enough; however, at this point, it would be recommended over nothing, especially for players with poor diets. Still, as Pyne points out "Practical issues to consider include medical and dietary screening of athletes, sourcing of recommended probiotics and formulations, dose-response requirements for different probiotic strains, storage, handling and transport of supplements and timing of supplementation in relation to travel and competition."[22]

Tart Cherry Juice

Best used during season/competition when recovery is preferred over adaptation, cherry juice has been found to lessen pain, improve sleep, accelerate return to strength/decrease the decrease in strength experienced after heavy loading, and decrease blood markers of inflammation.[23,24] There is some evidence that exogenous antioxidant consumption can thwart muscle adaption desired during conditioning workouts. Antioxidants interrupt or squelch the signaling pathways needed for optimal adaption and strength attainment.[25] It is hypothesized that the naturally occurring melatonin in tart cherry juice helps athletes sleep better.[26,27] There are several products on the market including tart cherry juice and a powdered supplement.

Vitamin D

In a 2017 systematic review, looking at the effects of vitamin D supplementation, there did not seem to be a performance-enhancing aspect.[28] However, perhaps the more correct way to look at this is whether a deficiency leads to decreased performance and increased risk of injury. It is difficult to eat enough vitamin D through food alone; the skin converts vitamin D from sun. Obviously, baseball athletes spend plenty of time in the sun during season, although mostly covered up. In one study where 103 NCAA collegiate athletes in Southern States were studied, 23% were insufficient and 9%, predominately non-Caucasian, were deficient. Those with lower vitamin D status as measured by serum 25-OH D had lower scores on assessment of muscular strength and anaerobic power.[29] A general recommendation of 600 to 800 IU a day of vitamin D3 with higher dose indicated based on laboratory values seems warranted. Vitamin D deficiency is often defined as <20 ng/mL (50 nmol/L), and insufficiency defined as 20 to 32 ng/mL (50-80 nmol/L), and optimal levels are >40 ng/mL (100 nmol/L).

SUMMARY

A long season with back-to-back games and travel can make staying well fueled, well nourished, and well hydrated a challenge. Baseball athletes can help themselves perform at their peak by paying attention to some very basic sports nutrition strategies. Attention to nutrient timing and caloric distribution is an important part of optimal performance for the elite baseball player. The power, strength, skill, and concentration required to be elite will be better expressed when the athlete pays attention to the quality, quantity and timing of food intake, is selective when it comes to supplements, and is able to monitor hydration status.

REFERENCES

1. Dines JS, Altchek DW, Andrews J, ElAttrach NS, Wilk KE, Yocum LA. *Sports Medicine of Baseball*. 1st ed. Philadelphia: Lippincott Williams & Wilkins; 2012.

2. Skolnik H, Chernus A. *Nutrient Timing for Peak Performance*. 1st ed. Human Kinetics; 2010.

3. Jäger R, Kerksick CM, Campbell BI, et al. International society of sports nutrition position stand: protein and exercise. *J Int Soc Sports Nutr [Internet]*. 2017;14:20.

4. Saturated Fats [Internet]. American Heart Association. Cited December 7, 2017. Available at http://www.heart.org/HEARTORG/HealthyLiving/FatsAndOils/Fats101/Saturated-Fats_UCM_301110_Article.jsp#.

5. Backman DR, Haddad EH, Lee JW, Johnston PK, Hodgkin GE. Psychosocial predictors of healthful dietary behavior in adolescents. *J Nutr Educ Behav [Internet]*. 2002;34:184-193.

6. Athlete Factsheets and Resources [Internet]. Team USA, United States Olympic Committee. 2017. Cited December 7, 2017. Available at https://www.teamusa.org/About-the-USOC/Athlete-Development/Sport-Performance/Nutrition/Athlete-Factsheets-and-Resources.

7. Kerksick CM, Arent S, Schoenfeld BJ, et al. International society of sports nutrition position stand: nutrient timing. *J Int Soc Sports Nutr [Internet]*. 2017;14:33. Cited September 13, 2017.

8. Izaki T, Omori M. Eating behaviors of high school baseball players in Japan. *J Int Soc Sports Nutr*. 2010;7(suppl 1): P18.

9. Nutritional Guidelines [Internet]. Playball, USA Baseball. Cited September 2, 2017.

10. Armstrong LE, Herrera Soto JA, Hacker FT, et al. *J sport Nutr [Internet]*. 1998;8:345-355. Cited September 6, 2017.

11. Guest NS, Jamnik J, Womack C, El-Sohemy A. Genetic variation related to caffeine metabolism or response during exercise. *J Int Soc Sports Nutr [Internet]*. 2015;12:P53.

12. Gulhane TF. Effect of alcohol on athletic performance. *Int J Appl Res [Internet]*. 2015;1:131-133. Cited September 4, 2017].

13. Parr EB, Camera DM, Areta JL, et al. Alcohol ingestion impairs maximal post-exercise rates of myofibrillar protein synthesis following a single bout of concurrent training. Alway SE, ed. *PLoS One [Internet]*. 2014;9:e88384. Cited September 10, 2017.

14. Barnes MJ, Mündel T, Stannard SR. Post-exercise alcohol ingestion exacerbates eccentric-exercise induced losses in performance. *Eur J Appl Physiol [Internet]*. 2010;108:1009-1014. Cited Sep 10, 2017.

15. Nédélec M, Halson S, Abaidia AE, Ahmaidi S, Dupont G. Stress, sleep and recovery in elite soccer: a critical review of the literature. *Sports Med*. 2015:1387-1400.

16. Malhotra RK. Sleep, recovery, and performance in sports. *Neurol Clin [Internet]*. 2017;35:547-557. Cited September 10, 2017.

17. Burke LM, Ross ML, Garvican-Lewis LA, et al. Low carbohydrate, high fat diet impairs exercise economy and negates the performance benefit from intensified training in elite race walkers. *J Physiol [Internet]*. 2017;595:2785-2807.

18. McSwiney FT, Wardrop B, Hyde PN, Lafountain RA, Volek JS, Doyle L. Keto-adaptation enhances exercise performance and body composition responses to training in endurance athletes. *Metabolism [Internet]*. 2018;81:25-34.

19. O'Malley T, Myette-Cote E, Durrer C, Little JP. Nutritional ketone salts increase fat oxidation but impair high-intensity exercise performance in healthy adult males. *Appl Physiol Nutr Metab [Internet]*. 2017;42:1031-1035.

20. Leckey JJ, Ross ML, Quod M, Hawley JA, Burke LM. Ketone diester ingestion impairs time-trial performance in professional cyclists. *Front Physiol*. 2017;8.

21. Clark A, Mach N. Exercise-induced stress behavior, gut-microbiota-brain axis and diet: a systematic review for athletes. *J Int Soc Sports Nutr [Internet]*. 2016;13:43.

22. Pyne DB, West NP, Cox AJ, Cripps AW. Probiotics supplementation for athletes – clinical and physiological effects. *Eur J Sport Sci*. 2015;15(1):63-72.

23. Vitale KC, Hueglin S, Broad E. Tart cherry juice in athletes: a literature review and commentary. *Curr Sports Med Rep*. 2017:230-239.

24. Levers K, Dalton R, Galvan E, et al. Effects of powdered Montmorency tart cherry supplementation on an acute bout of intense lower body strength exercise in resistance trained males. *J Int Soc Sports Nutr [Internet]*. 2015;12:41.

25. Merry TL, Ristow M. Do antioxidant supplements interfere with skeletal muscle adaptation to exercise training? *J Physiol [Internet]*. 2016;594:5135-5147.

26. Losso JN, Finley JW, Karki N, et al. Pilot study of the tart cherry juice for the treatment of insomnia and investigation of mechanisms. *Am J Ther [Internet]*. 2017;8:1.

27. Howatson G, Bell PG, Tallent J, Middleton B, McHugh MP, Ellis J. Effect of tart cherry juice (Prunus cerasus) on melatonin levels and enhanced sleep quality. *Eur J Nutr*. 2012;51:909-916.

28. Farrokhyar F, Sivakumar G, Savage K, et al. Effects of vitamin D supplementation on serum 25-hydroxyvitamin D concentrations and physical performance in athletes: a systematic review and meta-analysis of randomized controlled trials. *Sports Med*. 2017:2323-2339.

29. Hildebrand RA, Miller B, Warren A, Hildebrand D, Smith BJ. Compromised vitamin D status negatively affects muscular strength and power of collegiate athletes. *Int J Sport Nutr Exerc Metab*. 2016;26:558-564.

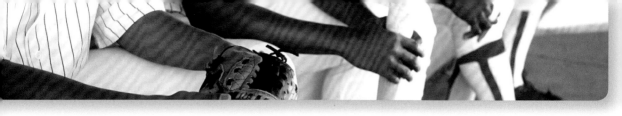

CHAPTER 34

Performance-Enhancing Drug Use in Baseball

Gary Green, MD

The ballplayer who loses his head, who can't keep his cool, is worse than no ballplayer at all.

—Lou Gehrig

INTRODUCTION

All sports are unique in that each requires distinctive sets of skills and talents. However, no sport is immune from the temptation to use performance-enhancing drugs (PEDs). Indeed, the recent McLaren reports[1,2] on the state-sponsored doping program in Russia revealed that athletes from 20 sports were involved with PED use, including curling and table tennis (see Table 34.1). Even non-Olympic regional sports, such as Kabaddi, have seen anabolic steroid scandals in their tournaments. As chairman of the NCAA drug testing committee, the author has observed positive drug tests in diverse sports such as a Division I male, football player to a Division III female, cross-country runner. It appears that regardless of the sport or level of play, there is an inherent desire in athletes to try to improve performance in any way possible, legal or not. To have a complete understanding of PED use in athletes, it is imperative to be familiar with the effects of particular drugs and the unique demands of a particular sport. This allows some ability to predict the patterns of drug use for a sport. This chapter will explore the common PEDs in sport with an emphasis on those drugs that have particular appeal in the sport of baseball.

Before delving into specific substances, it is important to have an understanding of sports pharmacology. Sports pharmacology is a construct that groups drugs according to their reason for use. Whereas traditional pharmacology categorizes drugs according to their chemical structures, sports pharmacology is based on an understanding of why athletes use drugs and hopefully methods of deterrence. The 3 categories of use are ergogenic (performance-enhancing), recreational, and therapeutic drugs. For those who work with athletes, the reasons behind this distinction are clear. As an example, consider a drug class such as amphetamines. They can be used as an ergogenic aid, recreationally (eg, methamphetamine) or as a therapeutic drug (eg, dextroamphetamine/amphetamine salts). In the case of an athlete, all 3 uses should be addressed very differently.

There are several methods that antidoping programs use to categorize banned substances. Table 34.2 (the World Anti-Doping Agency, WADA) and Table 34.3 (Major League Baseball, MLB) are examples of how these may be organized. Regardless of categorization, a hallmark of all antidoping programs is that change is constant and antidoping programs need to continually evolve in order to keep pace with the changes in a particular sport. Professional baseball offers an excellent example. Although the pitcher's mound is 60 feet, 6 inches from home plate and the bases 90 feet apart just as they were 100 years ago, the sport has evolved in many ways. MLB originally comprised 2, separate 8-team leagues in which the farthest trip was from Boston to St. Louis and the season comprised 154 games. Train travel necessitated rest days, and there was the opportunity to adjust to travel. In the present schedule with 162 games played in 187 calendar days, teams travel from New York to Seattle in 5 hours crossing 4 time zones and can play a few hours later.

TABLE 34.1 Number of Disappearing Positive Test Results by Sport Russian Athletes[5]

From Richard H. McLaren Independent Investigation of Sochi Olympic Allegations, Part I. https://www.wada-ama.org/sites/default/files/resources/files/20160718_ip_report_newfinal.pdf. Reprinted with permission from World Anti-Doping Agency.

TABLE 34.2 WADA Prohibited List at All Times

S0: Nonapproved substances
S1: Anabolic agents
S2: Peptide hormones, growth factors, related substances, and mimetics
S3: Beta-2 agonists
S4: Hormones and metabolic modulators
S5: Diuretics and masking agents

From WADA Prohibited List. https://www.wada-ama.org/en/content/what-is-prohibited/prohibited-at-all-times/non-approved-substances. Reprinted with permission from World Anti-Doping Agency.

TABLE 34.3 Major League Baseball Prohibited Substances

Drugs of abuse
Performance-enhancing drugs
Stimulants
DHEA
Diuretics and masking agents

Data from Major League Baseball Joint Drug Prevention and Treatment Program. http://www.mlb.com/pa/pdf/jda.pdf.

DEFINITION

In discussing PED use, all antidoping programs begin with a prohibited list of drugs that are banned in a particular sport. WADA developed an international standard and most sports organizations use this as a basis for their programs. Many sports organizations, especially professional North American sports, are not signatories to the WADA Code, yet share many of the same principles, testing protocols, and laboratories. Once a prohibited list is drafted and approved, an antidoping program defines what constitutes a doping offense. The traditional definition of doping is the presence of a prohibited substance or its metabolites or markers in an athlete's bodily specimen. This would be the classic case of an athlete having an adverse analytical finding in a bodily fluid, ie, "failing a drug test."

However, the definition of a doping offense has expanded to include many scenarios that do not involve an adverse analytical finding, ie, positive drug test. It is worth emphasizing that one of the newest and more effective tools in the efforts to curtail PED use is the use of the "nonanalytical" positive test, or evidence of PED use without a positive drug test.

A single drug test only reveals what was in the body at that particular moment and is limited in terms of details concerning route of administration, time course, number of times used, and dosage. In the case of a "nonanalytical" positive test, evidence may demonstrate the schedule of drug use, dosages, routes, and patterns that were much more revealing than a single doping test. The expansion of investigative capabilities has increased the deterrence effect of antidoping programs and probably represents the biggest recent advance to the field. The aforementioned McLaren report is an example of this type of work.[1,2] Indeed, following the release of the Mitchell Report on PED use in MLB, the Office of the Commissioner of Baseball established a Department of Investigations and has conducted multiple major PED investigations since it was established.

WHY CARE ABOUT THE USE OF PERFORMANCE-ENHANCING DRUGS IN ATHLETES?

Amateur and professional sports organizations annually spend millions of dollars and devote countless resources to antidoping programs. PEDs can threaten the integrity of a sport and thus any use or risks associated with their use are not acceptable. There are numerous examples of what happens when there are either no PED regulations in sport or they are not enforced. A laissez faire policy with a lack of regulation quickly leads to a loss of what is valued about sport.[5]

SPECIFIC PEDs IN BASEBALL

WADA and MLB list hundreds of substances on their banned lists. These lists are amended annually so that it is imperative for players and medical professionals to be aware of any changes. Every organization has its own specific banned list, eg, the National Collegiate Athletic Association (NCAA) differs from many other organizations, with its own method of determining which substances are banned. Although it is beyond the scope of this chapter to discuss every banned substance category, it is worthwhile to highlight a few of the more commonly used PEDs in baseball.

ANABOLIC-ANDROGENIC STEROIDS

Anabolic-androgenic steroids (AASs) are drugs that are testosterone or testosterone-like synthetic drugs that result in both anabolic and androgenic effects.

These drugs have both anabolic (increased protein synthesis or muscle building) and androgenic (male secondary sex characteristics) effects to varying degrees, but all of the drugs in this class have the ability for both. These drugs act by transport to the cell nucleus by cytoplasmic proteins and result in the production of messenger RNA for protein synthesis. Studies have documented that supraphysiologic doses of AAS in conjunction with strength training and a high-protein diet can increase muscle mass and result in true muscle hypertrophy and strength gains.[6] AASs may also have anticatabolic effects and increase aggressiveness that leads to improved workouts.

Although AASs have been shown to have anabolic effects by increasing muscle, there are also significant adverse effects of these drugs mainly from their androgenic properties. Androgen receptors are located throughout the body and thus AASs affect almost all bodily systems to some degree. Although there are some adverse reactions that can affect all users, many of the side effects depend to some degree on the amount of naturally produced androgens, ie, whether the user is an adult male, adult female, or developing adolescent. Table 34.4 summarizes some of the common adverse effects that have been reported from the use and misuse of AASs.[7]

Drug testing for AASs is mainly conducted by gas chromatography/mass spectrometry (GC/MS) on collected urine samples. This method is efficient at detecting exogenous anabolic steroids, and advances in the sensitivity of this procedure have allowed for the detection of long-acting metabolites of parent compounds. For some drugs, such as nandrolone decanoate, metabolites can be detected for up to a year or more after the last use, thus providing an effective deterrent. However, the improved detection of exogenous AASs led athletes to using designer AASs and testosterone in order to avoid a positive test. Designer AASs represent an ongoing challenge to antidoping programs and the need for continued research in this area. The use of testosterone creates a different issue, as all athletes naturally produce testosterone. Initially, this was addressed by the testosterone:epitestosterone ratio (T/E) in which an elevated ratio (above 4:1) was considered evidence of exogenous testosterone use. However, there are significant limitations to that ratio, and this led to the development of isotope ratio mass spectrometry (IRMS) or carbon isotope ratio testing. IRMS is able to detect subtle variations between endogenous and exogenous testosterone that can determine if an athlete has used exogenous testosterone. Table 34.5 contains a list of the AASs that have been detected as part of the MLB Joint Drug Testing Program since 2007.

TABLE 34.4 Selected Adverse Effects of Anabolic-Androgenic Steroids

General
Decreased high-density lipoprotein (HDL)
Increased low-density lipoprotein (LDL)
Thrombosis
Myocardial infarction
Compartment syndrome
Tendon ruptures
Peliosis hepatis
Hepatocellular dysfunction
Acne
Psychological dependence
Adult Males
Impotence
Oligo-azoo-spermia
Decreased testicular size
Gynecomastia
Prostate dysfunction and carcinoma
Adult Females
Reduced level LH/FSH
Menstrual irregularities
Hirsutism
Clitoromegaly
Deepening of the voice
Male pattern alopecia
Youths
Premature epiphyseal closure
Depression and suicide
Premature puberty

TABLE 34.5 Summary of Positive Testing in MLB Joint Drug Program 2007-2017

Anabolic-Androgenic Steroids	38
Stanozolol	8
Testosterone	6
Boldenone	6
Dehydrochlormethyltestosterone	6
Nandrolone	4
Androstenedione	2
Methenolone	1
Methandienone	1
Clostebol	1
Drostanolone	1
DHEA	1
Oxandrolone	1
Stimulants	85
Adderall	68
Clobenzorex	8
Amphetamine	5
Methylhexanamine	3
Oxilofrine	1
Nonanalytic positive	16
Miscellaneous	9
Clenbuterol	2
Ipamorelin	2
GHRP-2	1
SARMs	1
Modafinil	1
Tamoxifen	1
Clomiphene	1

Data from Publicly Released Annual Reports from the MLB Independent Program Administrator 2007-2017.

SYSTEMIC ANDROGEN RECEPTOR MODIFIERS

In the never-ending search for drugs that can build muscle, have limited androgenic effects, and avoid drug testing, athletes have turned to systemic androgen receptor modifiers (SARMs). These are nonsteroidal compounds that affect the androgen receptors in muscle, bone, and prostate, much like an AAS. Although research has been conducted on these compounds for legitimate medical uses, to date the United States Food and Drug Administration has not approved these for human use. Despite that, they are readily sold on the Internet for "research purposes" and have been found in multiple dietary supplements. Adverse effects have been reported for these substances that include testosterone suppression, adverse effects on cholesterol, and androgenic effects. All SARMs are banned by most drug testing programs with some of the more popular ones being andarine and ostarine. SARMs are readily detectable by antidoping drug testing.

HUMAN GROWTH HORMONE

The combination of more sophisticated testing for AASs, the development of recombinant human growth hormone (rhGH), and the lack of an available test for rhGH led athletes to using this compound. Natural growth hormone (GH) is produced by the anterior pituitary and made up of several different isoforms. The rhGH is similar to natural GH, but typically contains only the 22 kilodalton (22 kDa) isomer of GH. Although much is known about the effects of GH in patients with acromegaly and the therapeutic use of rhGH in GH-deficient patients, there is little information on normal adults abusing rhGH in supraphysiologic doses. GH does appear to increase lean body mass, although combining it with AASs seems to multiply its effects. There is also a paucity of information on the adverse effects in a normal population abusing the drug in high doses for short periods. The reported risks of rhGH include glucose intolerance, tumors, and the development of acromegaly, arthralgias, myalgias, pseudotumor, and carpal tunnel syndrome. It is also significant that rhGH occupies a particular position in the United States Pharmacopeia in that it is the only drug that cannot be given for an off-label use. The only approved uses in adults are HIV wasting syndrome, hGH deficiency, and short-bowel syndrome.

Developing a drug test for rhGH proved challenging to scientists owing to its similarities to natural GH, the pulsatile nature of GH release, its short half-life, and extremely minute quantities in the urine. The first widely available test for rhGH utilized a blood test that compared the ratio of the 22 kDa isomer of rhGH with all other isomers. Although this isomer test was developed for use at the 2004 and 2008 Olympics, the first positive test was not confirmed until 2010 in an English Rugby player. This test was significant in that it ushered in the use of blood testing in an antidoping setting that had previously exclusively relied on urine testing. The isomer test was of limited use because the window of detection is approximately 48 hours after use. The biomarker test was developed in order to extend the detection of rhGH for up to 2 weeks. This blood test relied on the fact that administration of rhGH increases the production of insulin-like growth factor-1 (IGF-1) from the liver and (procollagen type III) P-III-NP from bone. By comparing rhGH users with controls, an algorithm was developed that can effectively discriminate users from nonusers. Two Russian paralympic weight lifters tested positive with the biomarker test during the 2012 Paralympics and later admitted using rhGH.

OTHER GROWTH FACTORS

As has now become evident, the antidoping world is a cat-and-mouse game whereby the users try to stay one step ahead of the testers. With the advent of testing for rhGH, athletes turned to GH-releasing peptides and secretagogues to obtain the effect of GH. These are synthetic peptides containing a small fraction of GH that are potentially releasers of GH. As with the previously mentioned SARMs, these are not approved for human use, yet are readily available online and have been found in dietary supplements. Some of the common ones are alexamorelin, GHRP-2, GHRP-6, ipamorelin, and ghrelin. These are all detectable through drug testing, and several athletes from a variety of sports have been sanctioned for their use. Although there are limited data on their adverse effects, there are reports of reactivation of cancers and GH-related effects.

STIMULANTS AND SYMPATHOMIMETIC AMINES

Stimulants have been associated with sports since the 1800s with their obvious appeal of increased energy. Baseball has not been immune to that, and the demands of the travel schedule have certainly fueled their use. Stimulants are a broad class of sympathomimetic amines that have both central and peripheral effects. Their use is complicated by the fact that they can be used for ergogenic, recreational, or therapeutic reasons. These drugs generally have varying amounts of (1) alpha effects on smooth muscle contraction and vasoconstriction, (2) beta 1 effects with tachycardia, and (3) beta 2 effects with bronchodilation. The best-known stimulant is amphetamine, but others include ephedrine, synephrine, heptaminol, methylhexanamine, methylphenidate, and clobenzorex. Table 34.5 lists stimulants that have been detected as part of the MLB Joint Drug Testing Program since 2007. Many of these can be found in dietary supplements and are frequently not listed on the label of ingredients. These compounds typically have relatively short half-lives, making detection difficult, but they are banned by most sporting organizations. In addition to the above effects, stimulants can be particularly dangerous in athletes owing to the risk of heat illness and tachyarrhythmias. Athletes who require these drugs to treat an underlying medical condition, such as attention deficit hyperactivity disorder (ADHD), need to be fully evaluated in order to determine if a true indication exists. Athletes who are shown to require these drugs should be carefully monitored for adverse effects and to determine if they have an ongoing need for the medication.

DIETARY SUPPLEMENTS

It is estimated that Americans annually spend about $30 billion on dietary supplements, with a considerable percentage of that devoted to "sports" supplements. The passage of the Dietary Supplement Health Education Act (DSHEA) in 1994 led to a marked explosion in the types of products that are considered dietary supplements and a corresponding lack of oversight as to their quality. Multiple studies have revealed frequent contamination of dietary supplements, inaccurate labeling, and supplements containing pharmaceuticals.[7] As a result, it is difficult for consumers and athletes alike to have confidence in the contents of their supplements. Recognizing that some supplements can assist athletes with the demands of their sport, athletes are faced with a difficult dilemma, as athletes have been suspended owing to an unlabeled substance in their supplement causing a positive drug test. It is further complicated by the "strict liability" code of many drug testing programs that an athlete is responsible for what is in his body, regardless of how it entered (with few rare exceptions). Several programs have been developed to assist athletes. The United States Anti-Doping Agency (USADA) provides "Supplement 411" to inform athletes about high-risk dietary supplements and provide education in this area.[8] MLB relies on the NSF Certified for Sport program, which certifies that dietary supplements do not contain any substances on the prohibited list. As of 2018, they have certified more than 700 products that are available for MLB players to safely use without risking a positive drug test.[9] Although these programs and similar ones have been helpful in reducing the risks (not only for positive drug tests, but potentially serious health consequences), dietary supplements continue to be an area of significant concern for consumers and athletes.

THERAPEUTIC USE EXEMPTION

As demonstrated in the case of amphetamines, several banned drugs have legitimate medical indications. It is a challenge for antidoping programs to develop a protocol to determine whether an athlete has a reasonable need for the drug. In general, the athlete needs to have a diagnosed medical condition and a demonstrable need for the medication, has tried nonbanned alternatives, would suffer significant adverse effects if the drug were to be withheld, and would not enhance performance above a normal level. Many programs also specify that the application to use the banned substance cannot be a direct result of use of prohibited drugs. In many cases the diagnosis and treatment is relatively straightforward. For example, insulin is on the WADA banned list

and it is relatively simple to confirm that a diabetic athlete requires insulin. However, conditions such as ADHD are more complicated owing to the difficulty in diagnosis and treatment options. All antidoping programs need a therapeutic use exemption (TUE) process in order to allow those with medical conditions to take medications that allow them to compete on an even level and exclude those who wish to gain an unfair advantage.

MLB DRUG TESTING PROGRAMS

MLB oversees a comprehensive program comprising 5 separate drug programs that include Major League and Minor League players, international and domestic prospect players, as well as programs that cover Umpires and all League and Club nonplaying personnel. These programs were either established or improved by the 2007 Mitchell Report that investigated the use of PED in baseball players during the 1990s and 2000s. In the decade since the publication of that report, MLB has conducted over 65,000 blood and urine tests in the Major League Program alone (publicly available). MLB was the first professional league to institute blood testing for hGH and has also established a Department of Investigations, increased the penalties for use, conducted year-round testing, expanded the banned substance list to mirror the WADA code, and contributed millions of dollars to antidoping research. MLB is a founding member of the Partnership for Clean Competition, which has become the world's leading funders of antidoping research.

Although the Major League Program gets the majority of media attention, the Minor League Program is an important facet of the overall antidoping program. The Major League Program is called the "Joint Drug Program" because it is the result of collective bargaining between MLB and the MLB Players Association. All players under this program are part of the MLB Players Association, and collective bargaining is required before any changes are made to the drug testing policy and procedures. As part of the agreement, a yearly annual report is released to the public. Under this program, the number of annual tests has increased from 3486 in 2007 to 10,237 in 2017 (publicly available). Minor Leaguers are not union members and thus their program is not subject to collective bargaining. Just as MLB Clubs use their Minor League affiliates to groom their players to graduate to the Major

Leagues, the Minor League drug testing program prepares players to conform to the Major League drug testing regulations.

As the recent Russian Olympic doping scandal demonstrates, being a signatory to the WADA Code does not necessarily prevent an organized doping scandal. The effectiveness of any program depends on the quality of the program and the commitment of the organization and all stakeholders toward maintaining clean sport.

THE ROLE OF NONATHLETE PROFESSIONALS IN DOPING CONTROL

Physicians

Physicians play a unique role in the use of PEDs in athletes. On one hand, physicians are entrusted with an athlete's health and safety and are cognizant that many PEDs have harmful adverse effects. However, athletes also consult with physicians in order to improve their performance, whether it is career-saving surgery, eg, ulnar collateral reconstruction (Tommy John Surgery), or medications to treat an underlying medical condition. This can sometimes lead physicians to cross the line with respect to PEDs. There is evidence that athletes have sought out physicians' advice on performance enhancement since the ancient Greek Olympics, and this trend continues in modern times. It is incumbent to remember that none of the recent doping scandals, German Democratic Republic, the Tour de France drug use, the recent Russian revelations, and many more, could have occurred without the active participation of physicians. While the athlete with a positive drug test makes headlines, it is important to remember that certified athletic trainers, physicians, sports scientists, coaches, and a host of other professionals influence an athlete's decision whether or not to take PEDs.

Of course, physicians also play a key role in the antidoping movement. Physicians are integral to testing programs, the development of the prohibited list, TUEs, and counseling athletes on the adverse effects and ethics of PED use. It is clear that the ethics of medicine, "First do no harm" precludes advising and prescribing banned PEDs to athletes. Physicians who work with athletes need to be intimately familiar with the prohibited list in that specific sport before prescribing any medications, recommending OTC medications or dietary supplements.

SUMMARY

The responsibility for maintaining integrity in sport falls to a number of entities. Antidoping programs are an important part of that and require a great deal of expense and vigilance if the ethics of sport are to be maintained. There are numerous examples, eg, the former East Germany, Tour de France, of the consequences of inaction in this area. It is important to remember in the face of these scandals that the majority of athletes compete cleanly and wish to continue to do so. These are the real losers when PED use is allowed unchecked. Doping has the potential to reduce the ethic and value that is placed on sport in society. As potential doping agents evolve into the realm of genetic manipulation, it will be incumbent among those who care about the integrity of sport to speak up and push for clean sports.

ACKNOWLEDGMENTS

I would like to thank MLB for their dedication to antidoping efforts. I would specifically cite former Commissioner Bud Selig, current Commissioner Rob Manfred, deputy Commissioner Dan Halem, and MLB vice-president Jon Coyles for their unwavering support in this area. I would also like to thank my wife Debbie for her commitment, love, and support of my career, and my parents who gave me the opportunity to achieve my dreams. The opinions expressed in this chapter are those of the author and do not represent the position of MLB.

REFERENCES

1. Richard H. *McLaren Independent Investigation of Sochi Olympic Allegations, Part I.* https://www.wada-ama.org/sites/default/files/resources/files/20160718_ip_report_newfinal.pdf.

2. Richard H. *McLaren Independent Investigation of Sochi Olympic Allegations, Part II.* https://www.wada-ama.org/sites/default/files/resources/files/mclaren_report_part_ii_2.pdf.

3. *WADA Prohibited List.* https://www.wada-ama.org/en/content/what-is-prohibited/prohibited-at-all-times/non-approved-substances.

4. *Major League Baseball Joint Drug Prevention and Treatment Program.* http://www.mlb.com/pa/pdf/jda.pdf.

5. Murray T. *Good Sport: Why Our Games Matter-and How Doping Undermines Them.* New York: Oxford University Press; 2017.

6. Bhasin S, Storer TW, Berman N, et al. The effects of supraphysiologic doses of testosterone on muscle size and strength in normal men. *N Engl J Med*. 1996;335:1-7.

7. Green GA, Patel A, Puffer JC. Drugs and doping in athletes. In: Madden C, et al, eds. *Netter's Sports Medicine*. 2nd ed. Philadelphia: Elsevier; 2017 [chapter 26].

8. *US Anti-Doping Supplement 411 Program*. https://www.usada.org/substances/supplement-411/.

9. *NSF International Certified for Sport Program*. http://www.nsfsport.com/.

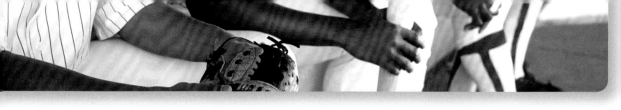

CHAPTER **35**

Mental Conditioning for Baseball Players

Gregory Chertok, MEd, CMPC

Baseball is ninety percent mental and the other half is physical.

—*Yogi Berra*

INTRODUCTION

Athletes in every sport will swear theirs is inherently the most mentally challenging. It makes sense that we tend to think of the mental demands within our own sport as the greatest—after all, we are intimately familiar with its intricacies and idiosyncrasies. However, baseball is arguably one of the more mentally taxing sports for several reasons.

For one, there are large amounts of "downtime"—time between pitches, time between innings, and time spent away from physical action owing to injury or rehabilitation efforts—to manage. A ballplayer typically begins to question, doubt, worry, fear, anticipate, catastrophize, and judge during moments of solitude and inactivity. There is no time to engage in this type of thinking when we are distracted by turning a double play or stealing third. Unfortunately, a baseball game contains more moments of downtime than intense action; a position player can spend mere minutes with the ball in his glove or off his bat in a game that lasts 3 hours—that is only roughly 10% of the game.

Secondly, most competitive athletes are excellence seeking by nature, which makes accepting anything other than perfection a challenge. Within baseball, imperfection is guaranteed: we lionize those who are able to fail only 70% of the time.

To manage the downtime and to deal with the failure-laden nature of the game are the mental challenges inherent in baseball. These as well as staying present with every pitch, staying in control in key moments, and adjusting to constantly shifting on-field situations are the focus of this chapter. Although medical professionals should not be tasked as the sole dispensers of mental game information, they can play a key role in helping athletes overcome injury and maintain confidence throughout a season.

In my consulting with baseball players, those who typically make the most noticeable improvements in their mental game have the greatest **self-awareness**. That is, they understand the internal environment—particular moods, emotions, thoughts, bodily sensations, and goals—needed to thrive on the field and are willing to ask themselves, "Am I really thinking in a way that will give me the best chance of success?"[1] For example, a self-aware batter might be most comfortable on pitches low and inside and will stay disciplined to keep his attention on swinging at balls only in that zone early in the count rather than awkwardly lunging at a ball off the plate because of nerves or anxiety. A self-aware pitcher knows he must be relaxed before pitches, even though the intensity of the situation might tempt him to rush his motion, tense his body, or overthrow. An injured player with great self-awareness will rationally heed the advice of medical experts and follow the course of rehab despite his feelings of jittery impatience away from his starting role. Consider the following as questions you can pose to help cultivate honest self-awareness in your players. Those with limited awareness might not yet be able to accurately answer some of them, although encouraging them to reflect on past games as well as simple journaling targeting these questions will begin to help.

- *Do your breathing patterns change based on the situation? Are you breathing similarly in the box on a 1-0 count in the first inning as you would on a 3-2 count with 2 outs in the last inning of a 1-run game?*

- *After making an error or striking out, what happens to your body as a result? Do your fists clench, shoulders raise, or jaw tighten? Do you pace in the dugout, droop your posture, or tense your muscles?*

- *While injured or out of action, what is your self-talk like as a baseball player? Hopeful and optimistic? Gloomy and apathetic? What messages are you giving yourself about who you are as an athlete and a person?*

- *In the field between pitches, where are you choosing to put your focus? On distractions—such as fans, personal statistics, or the dinner menu after tonight's game—or something else that might help your mind and body better prepare for the next pitch?*

- *How do you spend your between-pitch time on the mound? Does what you do help you feel ready and in control for every pitch?*

- *How do you prepare for the game beforehand? Talk to teammates casually, listen to music (if so, what genres?), or sit alone with your thoughts? And does this help get you into your ideal performance state?*

- *Does your preparation change based on outside factors such as weather or the timing of the game? It might have to; research from several years ago reveals that a Major League Baseball pitcher's natural sleep preference might affect how he performs in day and night games. For instance, in early games that started before 7 pm, the earned run average (ERA) of pitchers who were morning types (3.06) was lower than the average ERA of pitchers who were evening types (3.49).[2] Do you account for this while getting ready for your outing that day/night?*

Or what about asking this simple question for facilitating self-awareness: *what's your number?* That is, how emotionally aroused you have to be—your internal energy level—to play your best. It might help for him to visualize a thermometer inside his body that represents the numbers, ranging from 1 (lowest energy, at the bottom of the thermometer) to 10 (highest energy or the red boiling point at the very top) (Figure 35.1). Everyone is different; all athletes require varying states of arousal to feel and perform optimally.[3] I have worked with ballplayers who claim that to play their best, their number must be a 9: thinking fast, their bodies quivering with energy and power, almost frenzied with excitement. These players tend to be vocal leaders and highly demonstrative after a good (or bad) play. Other ballplayers assert they must be at a much lower number, say, a 2, to play their best: typically very calm and controlled; their thinking is more measured, breathing patterns are perhaps slower, and they generally look relaxed on the field. Those who must be at a lower number maintain their intensity and competitiveness; they just know that to

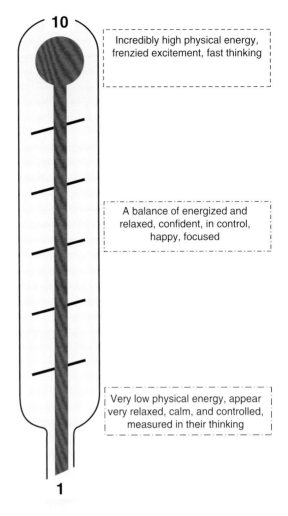

FIGURE 35.1 • The internal thermometer representing your "number," or your ideal emotional arousal level.

give themselves the best chance of playing well, they have got to get themselves under control and achieve a relaxed state of being.

Most of us have to be somewhere around the middle, enjoying a balance of energy and control. Have your players consider where they might need to be and if their number changes depending on the task (ie, a 3 during pregame taping and stretching, 6 while hitting, 8 while on the bases, 4 on the bench, and 9 in the weight room).

Having the awareness of where one's mental state is in comparison with where it should be is a critical first step; we are never open to changing our number if we are unaware that change is needed. Ultimately, every ballplayer at the highest level must then be able to effectively monitor and manage his own thoughts, feelings, and behaviors to return to that ideal state, an ability termed **self-regulation**.[4] Being able to successfully regulate how one thinks, feels, and acts begins with simple **focusing**.

We claim to know what focus means; it is a word we commonly use to make attributions about our players' poor performance ("What are you doing out there!? Come on, focus!"; "He got taken out in the 4th because he just wasn't focused on the mound today"). When someone is instructed to "focus," the suggestion is that their focus is presently off—that they aren't focused—as though referring to a light switch (focus on–focus off). However, this is an unhelpful and inaccurate model of our attention. As living, breathing humans, our focus is more like a flashlight: it is always "on"—we are always focused on *something*—it is just a question of where we choose to shine the light of our attention. When your math teacher scolds you for staring absentmindedly out the classroom window and claims you "aren't focused," you can accurately retort, "Oh, no, Mrs Johnson, I'm very focused. You see those ducklings in the pond out there? I'm just not focused on you." (One cannot guarantee, however, that Mrs Johnson appreciates the validity of your comment.)

This is a powerful shift for many ballplayers, on realizing that they have the ability to control where they place their attention and that being "unfocused" is simply a matter of intentionally shining the flashlight back onto something more productive. Focus does not "just happen": the responsibility is on the player himself to redirect his focus, as that is one of the only things he can truly control on the field and in the training room.

Our focus can only be directed in 1 of 2 ways: either internally (eg, on thoughts, feelings, one's breathing) or externally (eg, on the ball, the catcher's glove, signs from a coach).[5] In reading this chapter, your attention naturally shifts from the text on the page (external) to reflecting on how it relates to your own interaction with players (internal), to perhaps noticing the time on the clock overhead (external), and back again to the text (external). Our flashlight is fluid, in that it is constantly shifting and redirecting. The game's mentally disciplined players understand where the light should be shining at particular times and are able to redirect it there.

For instance, as a hitter, while in the dugout, he may direct his focus *externally* on picking up the pitcher's tendencies and patterns during the delivery. Then, in the on-deck circle his flashlight might alternate between *external*, on timing the pitcher and developing rhythm, and *internal*, on mentally rehearsing how he would like to approach the at-bat and putting a great swing on a particular pitch or perhaps on taking a few deep breaths to relax. Once in the box, the flashlight is *external*, on the pitcher's motion or spin of the ball, and is rarely shining on something internal, such as the

mechanics of the swing or excessive thinking. A related study showed that batting performance of elite players is best when their focus is on the effect of the swing or on the ball leaving the bat (external) and directed away from the actual swing itself (internal).[6] Highly skilled hitters have thousands of hours of practice and countless reps in the box–the neural connections in the brain associated with hitting strengthen and thicken in response to such practice, allowing messages to be sent from the brain to the body quickly and efficiently. There is little benefit trying to control something in which we are so well practiced, so players must develop trust in their abilities and stay externally focused on the pitcher's cues and ball path.

When navigating through a dark room in your house equipped with a flashlight, unrelated noises or distractions might prompt you to shine the flashlight away from your path and onto the origin of the sound. It is only natural to do so; once you realize the noise is innocuous you would calmly shine the light back onto your path. Similarly, it is never a problem when the flashlight of our players shines onto baseball's unrelated distractions or the "uncontrollables": things that they do not have the power to change (think bad calls, field conditions, fans, poor weather, past injuries, or future playing time). It is part of the normal human condition to stray from the path, at least temporarily, when other stimuli are demanding our attention. It is only problematic if we do not quickly identify the errant direction of our flashlight (ie, poor self-awareness) nor shine it back onto what is really important in this present moment (ie, poor self-regulation). The farther a player strays off course, the more arduous the journey back will be: when a player chooses to spend several innings lamenting his deteriorating batting average after starting the game 0-for-2, it becomes even more difficult to effectively prepare for his third at-bat with sound body and mind. A player who is still heard grumbling about his current state of health 1 month after his shoulder injury may have difficulty adhering to his rehab protocol and therefore may prolong his recovery time.

Strengthening the control of our flashlight helps us think about mistakes—and injuries—differently and therefore improve our reactions to them. It is amateurish to strike out on a changeup and interpret that as indication you are "just not a good off-speed hitter," give up a home run and begin questioning your stuff on the mound that day, or experience a short-term overuse injury and conclude that your career will not ever return to where it was: all are examples of poor control over how we choose to interpret events on the field. In a game rife with mistakes and injuries—assuming we cannot eliminate all of them—our task is to improve our relationship to them. This is logical advice for anyone who must bear some inconvenience: an early morning commuter who sits in unavoidable traffic or an apartment dweller who lives below an oft-practicing rock drummer cannot get rid of the annoyances but must change how they relate to them.

Each mistake, if viewed the right way, has something to teach us as ballplayers. Shakespeare might as well have been describing the athlete's interior life when he said, "Nothing is either good or bad, but thinking makes it so." No event is factually good or bad, but how we choose to think about it makes that event appear either way. Your living is determined not so much by what happens to you as by the way your mind looks at what happens. Realizing that we control how we interpret the events in our lives, which ultimately shapes how we react to them, is empowering. Strikeouts no longer must diminish our worth as a hitter but can be seen as opportunities for learning and growth. Getting picked off first base does not have to be interpreted in strictly negative terms; it may reveal your need to further develop lateral agility or quicken your reaction time, which, eventually, becomes a rather enlightening and performance-enhancing mistake. Injuries provide opportunities for greater reflection, a change in perspective, and the development of other nonphysical baseball skills. What a competitive advantage it is to be able to shift to a learning mindset, to think of mistakes as teachers, and calmly bring our full selves back to the here and now with our new-found knowledge.

While our flashlight can attend to internal or external cues, it can also shine on different moments in time. Although it is enticing for a player to berate himself for a bad at-bat last inning (past) or envision how sparkling his ERA will become after pitching a shutout tomorrow (future), success is most possible when he is present with what he is doing. Consider ways in which you can help your players bring themselves back to what is right in front of them—back to where their feet are.

- *Choose a "focal point"* or a fixed reference point somewhere in the stadium—a banner, sign, foul pole—to look at during points of the game when you have lost control of your emotions or your body, as a reminder to redirect the flashlight back onto getting ready for this pitch
- *Produce a sensation in your body.* Shawn Green, as chronicled in his book "The Way of Baseball," would step out of the box when he caught himself listening to his negative voice and hit the sides of his cleats firmly with his bat. The action was not intended to

be punishment for a reckless swing; "I was hitting my shoes to make my feet tingle, to feel my feet, to move my awareness into my feet, and out of my mind".[7] The tingling sensation was being felt "now," which brought him back to focusing on this moment: on preparing for the pitch to come. Clapping your hands, tugging on a wristband, or tapping your temples—or something more meaningful to you—can satisfy this too

- *Breathe deeply.* We average between 16 and 18 breath cycles per minute. As anxiety swells within us moments before a critical pitch or anger rages in response to an error on the field, our breath cycles increase exponentially and become shallow from the upper chest, often without us realizing it, preventing a healthy flow of oxygen into the bloodstream and the brain. Slow, deep breaths help us think clearly, make better decisions, and shine the flashlight on the present moment—breathing can only happen right now

- *Use your self-talk effectively.* Our own voice acts as a guide—it influences our mood, confidence levels, ability to learn, and throwing accuracy, among others. Hordes of research reveal that self-talk is consistently positively related to performance improvements.[8] Being aware of what you are thinking about—even talking out loud to yourself—helps us recognize if our thoughts are off-path, which allows us to bring our attention back to the present

Many of us tend to listen to the unhelpful content of our self-talk—the doubting words, the angry self-criticisms, the sarcastic questioning—especially if our performance is poor. Imagine for a moment walking down the dark, empty streets of a large city late at night, when you encounter a small alley off the main road. As you peer down, you see an eerie-looking cloaked man staring at you who says, "Hey, you. Come over here; I've got something to show you." Surely none of us would even entertain the idea of voluntarily walking toward him; we have been instructed, rightly, from a young age not to follow people who are potentially dangerous, so we would pretend to ignore his words or perhaps walk away from him with more hurried footsteps. However, when it comes to a player's own menacing words—"Don't screw up," "You're a bum," "You'll never be able to start on this team, you're just not good enough"—he listens. He may follow this negative voice down the alley, blindly and obediently, and soon enough begin to believe what it is telling him.

Surely this does not mean we can eliminate all negativity from our thoughts. However, as with our flashlight, we have got control over which thoughts we decide to listen to. Thoughts are like waves: you cannot choose when they come, but you can choose which ones to surf. Assist your players in identifying the kind of self-talk that will produce smooth, focused performance and understanding their ability to choose not to follow the kind of talk that will produce tense, analytical, fearful performance. Typically, here is what effective self-talk looks like:

- *Calm, measured tone, as you would speak to a young-ster with limited experience*
- *Simple and direct words. The words can be **motivational**, intended to ramp up energy levels and arousal, or **instructional**, to remind us how to execute the task without excessive analysis. "Let's go!" and "Hit it to me, I want the ball" are examples of motivational talk in baseball. "Attack the ball," "Smooth and easy swing," and "Stay low" are examples of instructional talk*
- *Positive. Not meant in the optimistic sense, but as far as how you phrase commands to yourself. "See ball, hit ball" is better than "Don't strike out," and "Hit my spot low and in" is better than "Don't put this curve out over the plate"*
- *Present focused*

Self-talk is likely to stay productive and focus is likely to stay present if we are performing some task that is well practiced. The inner voice of a power hitter is calmer and reassured when swinging away than squaring around to bunt; he has swung away far more times than he has attempted to bunt. To be able to remark "I feel like I've been here before" is key, then, to effective self-talk and positive mood.

However, practice should not be limited to the body. Miraculously, the same neural pathways in the brain are activated when you physically execute a skill as when you mentally rehearse that same skill. In other words, go out onto the baseball field and swing a bat 10 times. Then, step off the field, close your eyes, and simply imagine swinging 10 times. Your brain does a poor job of distinguishing between these 2 activities and will respond almost identically to both the physical and mental rehearsal of the swing. It will consider both modalities of practice nearly equally beneficial.

Most players will consider imagery in rigidly positive terms: picturing hoisting up the trophy, hitting a home run, or otherwise doing something triumphant. However, the goal of imagery is to feel ready for anything and everything and to be able to enter any situation on the field and say, "I feel like I've been here before." After all, we never want to arrive anywhere on our own professional field where we have not already been for a few seconds in our mind. Encourage your players to think of some of the commonly occurring moments that would serve them well to mentally

practice before having to physically face it again. Task them to imagine their perfect reaction to the imperfect situation. Here is a list of a few.

- *Playing through injury or fatigue/not feeling at your best*

Most of us are not often feeling physically flawless going into game day. It is guaranteed that we will be scratched, scraped, sore, strained, or sprained in some part of our body, which diverts our attention away from the task of performance and onto dealing with the discomfort. If you are experiencing injury, do not hope it away. Assume it will be present, and take time to mentally rehearse how you would want to cope with it.

- *Dealing with a bad call by the umpire*

Umpires—who are human (and fallible)—will inevitably make poor calls. It seems prudent to prepare for this. The typical reaction to a bad call is resentment and rushed, sloppy play. Imagine a healthier reaction, one that exudes calmness and control, and rehearse it routinely so that the response is programed in your brain and retrievable when needed.

- *Faulty equipment*

Glove strings break, wooden bats splinter, shoelaces untie, and batting gloves rip. Train yourself to visualize and plan for both good and bad outcomes.

- *External distractions*

Crowd noise, coaches watching your every move, and trash-talking opponents. Many athletes claim to invest energy in avoiding or distracting themselves from it, "not focusing on it," as if it does not exist. Such distractions are not going anywhere, but what should change is how we respond to them. And 1 way to confront the distractions is through imagery, by mentally rehearsing what it looks and feels like to steady our breathing and give a gentle reminder to keep our attention grounded on the task at hand.

Some players find it easier to control their actions rather than their thinking patterns. In other words, it is simpler for some to focus on improving on-field behaviors over improving the content of our self-talk (behavior is easier to "see" than thought). There is plenty of research demonstrating how changing our physical state can influence our attitudes and thoughts, just as research suggests changing our thinking can influence behaviors; the relationship is reciprocal. There is a landmark psychology study from nearly 3 decades ago that comes to mind: in the study, 1 group of participants was told to hold a pencil between their teeth while performing a task that involved rating the degree of humor in cartoons. Holding the pencil in the mouth this way forced the individuals to smile, without being consciously aware they were doing so. Another group of participants was instructed to hold the pencil between their lips without it touching their teeth, forcing the muscles to contract downward and form a frown. The participants who were led to smile judged the cartoons as funnier than participants who were led to frown. It was argued that the simple act of subconsciously adopting certain facial postures affected their mood, which in turn affected their perception of the video.[9]

How a ballplayer carries himself, then, matters. His posture in the on-deck circle, for instance, can affect whether he enters the batter's box with confidence or fear; his posture on the mound can help him feel either dominant or subordinate to the hitter; how he leads off first base can make him more or less eager to take the extra base on a hit into the outfield. I had worked once with a player who, after recording an out at the plate the inning before, would lazily jog to his position, throw the ball during preinning warm-ups with unnecessary velocity, and sulk his body between pitches once the inning began. These actions, naturally, were performed out of anger in response to his previous at-bat. However, as the player would later admit, those behaviors would serve to "feed" the negativity. With each lazy step and each anger-infused throw, the negativity would build, and it would become even more difficult to rid himself of that feeling as he prepared for his next at-bat, which required relaxed concentration. Only once he changed his behaviors—running confidently onto the field, keeping his body posture dominant and expansive, throwing warm-ups from his position more casually—was he able to change his attitude.

MANAGER'S TIPS

- Facilitate awareness in your players by challenging them with questions. Most players have not considered how their bodies feel under stress, or what thoughts they should choose to focus on, or what their psychophysiologic reaction is after a strikeout (let alone what it should be). Start a conversation and pose simple questions to see how self-aware they really are

- "What's your number?" is a convenient and straightforward way to help your players check in with themselves. We each have an optimal internal energy level that helps us hit, field, train, or recover our best

- Your players will feel greater control over their "number" when they understand its relationship with their flashlight, that is, that their number can move up or down depending on where we choose to shine the light of our attention. Have them think about past performances they were proud of and encourage them to consider where their focus actually was. Have them deliberately shift their focus during a lifting session in the weight room or rehab in the training room—from something internal (such as their breathing or the movement of their legs during the squat) to something external (such as the image of their quivering muscle in the mirror or the movement of the weight itself moving up and down). See if changing their focus actually changes the experience for them

- We gain control over our flashlight by using a variety of skills including behavioral cues (ie, deep breathing to relax and stay present or producing a bodily sensation to bring awareness out of our thinking mind and into the body) as well as cognitive cues (choosing a focal point as a mental reminder of where you want to put your attention or using the kind of self-talk that will guide your focus onto the right things)

- Help your players realize the way they are talking to themselves actually influences performance (both on the field and through injury recovery). For most, that means assuming a calm and measured tone, simple words, positive language, and a focus on the present moment

- Assist your players in using mental imagery, so they feel ready for success—and feel ready for the inevitable barriers and bits of adversity that they will have to deal with, such as playing through physical discomfort, reacting well to bad calls, and staying focused on their task amid outside distractions

- Teach your players the importance of physically carrying themselves the right way; it not only promotes power and confidence to others but also influences our own emotional state

REFERENCES

1. Zinsser N, Bunker LK, Williams JM. Cognitive techniques for improving performance and building confidence. In: Williams JM, ed. *Applied Sport Psychology: Personal Growth to Peak Performance*. 5th ed. McGraw-Hill College; 2006:353.

2. American Academy of Sleep Medicine. *Sleep Preference can Predict Performance of Major League Baseball Pitchers*. ScienceDaily; June 11, 2010. Retrieved May 31, 2017 at www.sciencedaily.com/releases/2010/06/100609083223.htm.

3. Hanin YL. Emotions and athletic performance: individual zones of optimal functioning. In: *European Yearbook of Sport Psychology*. Vol 1. 1997:29-72.

4. Weinberg R, Gould D. Introduction to psychological skills training. In: *Foundations of Sport and Exercise Psychology*. 6th ed. Human Kinetics; 2015:257.

5. Weinberg R, Gould D. Introduction to psychological skills training. In: *Foundations of Sport and Exercise Psychology*. 6th ed. Human Kinetics; 2015:379.

6. Castaneda B, Gray R. Effects of focus of attention on baseball batting performance in players of differing skill levels. *J Sport Exerc Psychol.* 2007;29:60-77.

7. Green S. *The Way of Baseball: Finding Stillness at 95 MPH*. New York: Simon & Schuster; 2011.

8. Hatzigeorgiadis A, Zourbanos N, Galanis E, Theodorakis Y. Self-talk and sports performance: a meta-analysis. *Perspect Psychol Sci.* 2011;6:348-356.

9. Strack F, Martin LL, Stepper S. Inhibiting and facilitating conditions of the human smile: a nonobtrusive test of the facial feedback hypothesis. *J Pers Soc Psychol.* 1988;54(5):768-777.

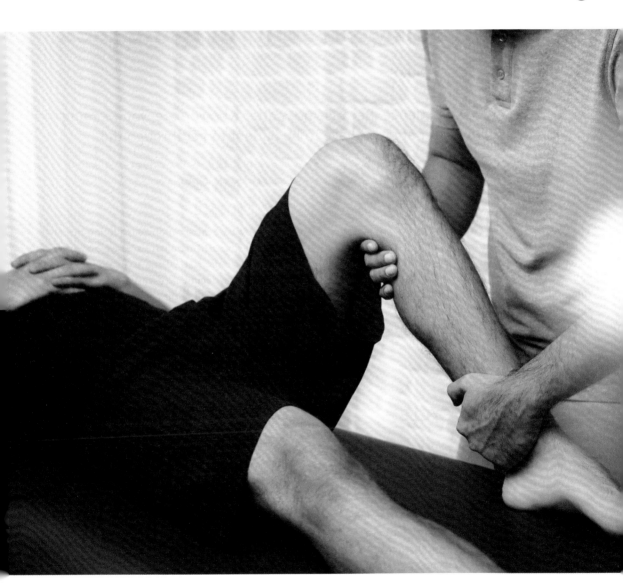

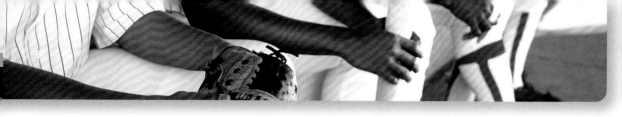

CHAPTER 36

Rehabilitation of the Overhead Throwing Athlete: General Principles

Bernard Li, DPT, OCS, SCS, LAT

Work hard. And have patience. Because no matter who you are, you're going to get hurt in your career and you have to be patient to get through the injuries.

—*Randy Johnson*

INTRODUCTION

Rehabilitation follows a structured, multistage approach with emphasis on breaking the inflammation cycle, restoring muscle length tension relationships, improving soft tissue adaptability, enhancing proprioception and optimization of neuromuscular control, and systematically returning the athlete to competitive throwing.[8,9,10]

CONTROLLING INFLAMMATORY CYCLE

Activity Modification

Modalities: ice, contrast, heat, ultrasound, phonophoresis, electrical stimulation, iontophoresis, transcutaneous electrical stimulation, laser therapy, cryotherapy, electrotherapeutics, vasopneumatic compression, manual therapy, therapeutic soft tissue techniques, postural training, body mechanics/ergonomics, neuromuscular reeducation, therapeutic exercise prescription, and athlete education.

Monitor the inflammatory cycle and patient physiologic response over time to break potential for chronic inflammation.

RANGE OF MOTION

Improving soft tissue flexibility, scapulothoracic mobility, spinal movement, posture, and hip mobility.

Most throwers exhibit an obvious motion disparity whereby external rotation is excessive and internal rotation is limited at 90° of abduction. Several investigators have documented that pitchers exhibit greater external rotation of the shoulder than position players.[1,3,6]

We have noted from literature that pitchers exhibit an average of 129.9°·10° of external rotation and 62.6°·9° of internal rotation when passively assessed at 90° of abduction. In pitchers, the external rotation is approximately 7° greater in the throwing shoulder when compared with the nonthrowing shoulder, while internal rotation is 7° greater in the nonthrowing shoulder.[5]

If external rotation of the throwing arm is less than 5° greater than the nonthrowing arm, that is a red flag.

Scapulohumeral rhythm looking for appropriate timing and coordination of the shoulder muscles.

Scapula Dyskinesia

Scapulohumeral Ratio

Target muscles: The muscle groups targeted in this conditioning program include the following (Table 36.1):

- Deltoids (front, back, and over the shoulder)
- Trapezius muscles (upper, middle, lower)
- Rhomboid muscles (upper back)
- Teres muscles (supporting the shoulder joint)
- Supraspinatus (supporting the shoulder joint)
- Infraspinatus (supporting the shoulder joint)
- Subscapularis (front of shoulder)

TABLE 36.1 Muscles that Position the Pectoral Girdle

Position in the Thorax	Movement	Target	Target Motion Direction	Prime Mover	Origin	Insertion
Anterior thorax	Stabilizes clavicle during movement by depressing it	Clavicle	Depression	Subclavius	First rib	Inferior surface of clavicle
Anterior thorax	Rotates shoulder anteriorly (throwing motion); assists with inhalation	Scapula; ribs	Scapula: depresses; ribs: elevates	Pectoralis minor	Anterior surfaces of certain ribs (2-4 or 3-5)	Coracoid process of scapula
Anterior thorax	Moves arm from side of body to front of body; assists with inhalation	Scapula; ribs	Scapula: protracts; ribs: elevates	Serratus anterior	Muscle slips from certain ribs (1-8 or 1-9)	Anterior surface of vertebral border of scapula
Posterior thorax	Elevates shoulders (shrugging); pulls shoulder blades together; tilts head backward	Scapula; cervical spine	Scapula: rotates inferiorly, retracts, elevates, and depresses; spine: extends	Trapezius	Skull; vertebral column	Acromion and spine of scapula; clavicle
Posterior thorax	Stabilizes scapula during pectoral girdle movement	Scapula	Retracts; rotates inferiorly	Rhomboid major	Thoracic vertebrae (T2-T5)	Medial border of scapula
Posterior thorax	Stabilizes scapula during pectoral girdle movement	Scapula	Retracts; rotates inferiorly	Rhomboid minor	Cervical and thoracic vertebrae (C7 and T1)	Medial border of scapula

- Biceps (front of upper arm)
- Triceps (back of upper arm)
  - Pectoralis
  - Latissimus
  - Serratus anterior

LAXITY

Most throwers exhibit significant laxity of the glenohumeral joint, which permits excessive range of motion. The hypermobility of the thrower's shoulder has been referred to as "thrower's laxity."[5,9] "Acquired laxity" (J. R. Andrews, 1996), while others have documented that the overhead thrower exhibits congenital laxity.[5,9]

Bigliani et al[8] examined laxity in 72 professional baseball pitchers and 76 position players. The investigators noted a high degree of inferior glenohumeral joint laxity, with 61% of pitchers and 47% of position players exhibiting a positive sulcus sign in the throwing shoulder. Additionally, in the players who also exhibited a positive sulcus sign in the dominant shoulder, 89% of the pitchers and 100% of the position players exhibited a positive sulcus sign in the nondominant shoulder. Thus, it would appear that some baseball players exhibit inherent or congenital laxity, with superimposed acquired laxity, as a result of adaptive changes from throwing.[9]

The overhead thrower frequently experiences shoulder pain because of anterior capsular laxity and increased demands placed on the dynamic stabilizers.[9]

MUSCLE STRENGTH

Investigators demonstrated that the external rotation strength of the pitcher's throwing shoulder is significantly weaker than the nonthrowing shoulder, by 6%. Conversely, internal rotation strength of the throwing shoulder was significantly stronger, by 3%, compared with the nonthrowing shoulder. In addition, adduction strength of the throwing shoulder is also significantly stronger than in the nonthrowing shoulder, by approximately 9% to 10%. We believe that an important isokinetic value is the unilateral muscle ratio, which describes the antagonist/agonist muscle strength ratio. A proper balance between agonist and antagonist muscle groups is thought to provide dynamic stabilization to the shoulder joint.[2,4,5,9]

To provide proper muscle balance, the external rotator muscles should be at least 65% the strength of the internal rotator muscles.[94] Optimally, the external-to-internal rotator muscles strength ratio should be 66% to 75%.[4,5,7,8,9]

Proper scapular movement and stability are imperative for asymptomatic shoulder function.[8,9] The scapular muscles work in a synchronized fashion and act as force couples about the scapula, providing both movement and stabilization.[8,9]

PROPRIOCEPTION

The thrower relies on enhanced proprioception to influence the neuromuscular system to dynamically stabilize the glenohumeral joint in the presence of significant capsular laxity and excessive range of motion.[9]

Each stage represents a progression from the prior phase: the exercises become more aggressive and demanding, and the stresses applied to the shoulder joint gradually increase.[9]

Clinical examination of the shoulder complex:

1. Posture eval (resting position of the scapula)
2. Spine eval (rounded shoulders, forward head)
3. Scapulothoracic mobility (protraction, anterior tilt)
4. Range of motion (ER/IR [internal rotation], muscle length)
5. MMT
6. Special tests: laxity, proprioception
7. Movement analysis
   a. Immediate motion (IR, adduction)
   b. Intermediate
   c. Advanced strengthening
   d. Biomechanical analysis
   e. Return to activity, throwing mechanics, throwing program

REHABILITATION OF THE OVERHEAD THROWER— PHASES AND GOALS[9]

Phase 1—Acute Phase Goals
- Break the pain and inflammation cycle
- Regain optimal motion
- Prevent excessive muscular atrophy—restore strength

- Reestablish dynamic stability (muscular balance)
- Control functional stress/strain
- Restore muscle balance

Exercises and Modalities
- Cryotherapy, ultrasound, electrical stimulation
- Flexibility and stretching for posterior shoulder muscles and capsule (improve internal rotation and horizontal adduction)
- Rotator cuff strengthening (especially external rotator muscles)
- Scapular muscles strengthening (especially retractor, protractor, depressor muscles)
- Dynamic stabilization exercises (rhythmic stabilization)
- Closed kinetic chain exercises
- Proprioception training
- Activity modification
- Abstain from throwing

Phase 2—Intermediate Phase Goals

(Progress the strengthening program, continue to improve flexibility, and facilitate neuromuscular control. Emphasis on the restoration of muscle balance.)
- Progress strengthening and mobility program
- Therapeutic exercise
- Restore muscular balance (external/internal rotation)
- Enhance dynamic stability
- Control flexibility and stretches

Exercises and Modalities
- Continue stretching and flexibility (especially internal rotation and horizontal adduction)
- Progress isotonic strengthening
- Complete shoulder program
- Thrower's Ten program
- Scapulothoracic mobility program
- Rhythmic stabilization drills
- Initiate hip and core mobility and strengthening program
- Initiate leg program

Phase 3—Advanced Strengthening Phase Goals
- Aggressive strengthening
- Progress neuromuscular control

- Improve strength, power, and endurance
- Perform functional exercises
- Plyometric training
- Initiate light throwing activities (dry drills)

The interval throwing program is initiated once the athlete can fulfill these specific criteria: (1) satisfactory clinical examination, (2) nonpainful range of motion, (3) satisfactory isokinetic test results, and (4) appropriate rehabilitation progress.

Exercises and Modalities

- Flexibility and stretching
- Rhythmic stabilization drills
- Thrower's Ten program
- Dynamic rotator cuff program
- Initiate plyometric program
- Initiate endurance drills
- Initiate throwing program (phases?)

Phase 4—Return to Activity Phase Goals

- Progress to throwing program
- Return to competitive throwing
- Continue strengthening and flexibility drills

Exercises

- Stretching and flexibility drills
- Thrower's Ten program[11]
- Plyometric program
- Progress interval throwing program to competitive throwing

PRINCIPLES OF REHABILITATION IN THE THROWER[9]

1. Never overstress healing tissue
2. Prevent negative effects of immobilization
3. Emphasize external rotation muscular strength
4. Establish muscular balance
5. Emphasize scapular muscle strength
6. Improve posterior shoulder flexibility (internal rotation range of motion)
7. Enhance proprioception and neuromuscular control
8. Establish biomechanically efficient throwing
9. Gradually return to throwing activities
10. Use established criteria to progress

Differential Diagnosis

- Posterosuperior glenoid impingement
- Overuse syndrome tendinitis
- Posterior rotator cuff musculature tendinitis
- SLAP lesions
- Subacromial impingement
- Bennett lesion
- Primary instability
- Acute traumatic instability
- Thoracic outlet
- Cervical radiculopathy
- Fracture
- Improper mechanics

REFERENCES

1. Bigliani LU, Codd TP, Connor PM, et al. Shoulder motion and laxity in the professional baseball player. *Am J Sports Med*. 1997;25:609-613.
2. Brown LP, Niehues SL, Harrah A, et al. Upper extremity range of motion and isokinetic strength of the internal and external shoulder rotators in major league baseball players. *Am J Sports Med*. 1988;16:577-585.
3. Johnson L. Patterns of shoulder flexibility among college baseball players. *J Athl Train*. 1992;27:44-49.
4. Wilk KE, Andrews JR, Arrigo CA, et al. The strength characteristics of internal and external rotator muscles in professional baseball pitchers. *Am J Sports Med*. 1993;21:61-66.
5. Wilk KE, Arrigo C. Current concepts in the rehabilitation of the athletic shoulder. *J Orthop Sports Phys Ther*. 1993;18:365-378.
6. Wilk KE, Arrigo CA. An integrated approach to upper extremity exercises. *Orthop Phys Ther Clin North Am*. 1992;1:337-360.
7. Wilk KE, Arrigo CA, Andrews JR. Current concepts: the stabilizing structures of the glenohumeral joint. *J Orthop Sports Phys Ther*. 1997;25:364-379.
8. Wilk KE, Arrigo CA, Andrews JR. *Functional Training for the Overhead Athlete*. LaCrosse, WI: Sports Phys Therapy Home Study Course; 1995.
9. Wilk KE, Meister K, Andrews JR. Current concepts in the rehabilitation of the overhead throwing athlete. *Am J Sports Med*. 2002;30(1).
10. Wilk KE, Suarez K, Reed J. Scapular muscular strength values in professional baseball players [abstract]. *Phys Ther*. 1999;79(5 suppl):S81-S82.
11. Wilk KE. Advanced throwers' ten program. In: *Physical Rehabilitation of the Injured Athlete*. 2012:e16-e20. **Modified from Wilk KE. Preventive and rehabilitative exercises for the shoulder and elbow. 2011. Available at www.kevinwilk.com. Accessed November 22, 2011.

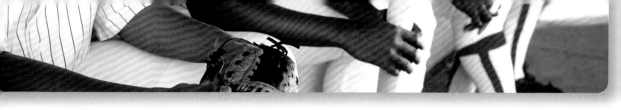

CHAPTER 37

Rehabilitation Strategies for the Shoulder and Scapula

Michael Schuk, PT, DPT, ATC | Steve Donohue, ATC | Timothy Lentych, MS, ATC/L | David Colvin, PT, DPT, MS, ATC

INTRODUCTION

The complex shoulder anatomy combined with the intricate and repetitive and forceful nature of throwing places baseball players at an increased risk of shoulder injuries compared with other athletes. Ciccotti et al recently conducted a study by means of the MLB Health and Injury Tracking System (HITS) and displayed that from the 2011 to 2014 baseball seasons, shoulder injuries were the most prevalently injured body in all professional baseball players (Major and Minor Leagues).[1] Similarly, Conte et al reported that 28% of all injuries sustained to professional baseball pitchers involve the shoulder.[2,3]

During overhead throwing, rotator cuff (RTC) muscle activity resists the high shoulder distractive forces (80%-120% bodyweight) during the arm cocking and deceleration phases.[4] These forces are rapid and acute. The acceleration phase of the baseball pitch is the fastest recorded human movement and occurs at an excess of 7250°/s.[2,5-7] Pitching at competitive levels requires tremendous shoulder and scapular stability within a healthy range of flexibility. The glenohumeral joint capsule must be loose enough to allow the extreme motions required for successful completion of sporting activities and, at the same time, exhibit the ability to dynamically stabilize the humeral head via RTC force couples.[8,9] Wilk et al have termed this challenge as the "thrower's paradox" and suggests that inability to successfully balance this "paradox" is the primary reason for injury.[9,10]

It is important for the overhead athlete to maintain supple soft tissue to facilitate necessary motion of the throwing shoulder. It is equally important to keep a functional balance of muscular strength and stability throughout a full range of motion and while muscular endurance, synergistic muscular activation, and neuromuscular control and coordination also play an integral role in keeping the shoulder healthy.

The clinician with a sound background of the biomechanics involved with the throwing motion will have an advantage in understanding the underlying causative factors related to specific injuries and similarly will have an advantage in guiding both the rehabilitation and injury prevention. This chapter outlines a series of rehabilitation strategies for the shoulder and scapula in the overhead athlete.

REHABILITATION PROGRAM

It is widely acknowledged that there are numerous structural (musculoskeletal and osseous) adaptations that may occur at an early age due to the high-volume, repetitive nature, and extreme positions the overhead thrower assumes. Shoulder positioning is also influenced by daily tasks that may impede posture, thereby affecting both resting and functional positions alike.[8] Regardless of a surgical versus conservative approach, a rehabilitation program is comprehensive and individualized to the needs of the player. Core, trunk, and the lower extremities are included in all shoulder rehabilitation programs.

A thorough examination should at minimum include a detailed history to best appreciate the nature of the injury, the mechanism of injury, and the demands of the athlete's specific positional requirements along with a detailed and comprehensive physical assessment that measures both passive and active range of motion, strength, and function. A connective tissue assessment through manual therapy will also assist in providing valuable information regarding the athletes' available motion, and the clinician will likely find tension in different planes of movement that can be addressed during the treatment. The initial findings should be compared with baseline or preinjury measurements to be used as a guideline for objectively quantifying progress along with presenting the clinician with a list of functional impairments to address during the rehabilitation. A rehab program should contain a few key elements, which are unwavering: prevent further injury; promote healing of damaged and distorted tissue; restore normal range of motion, mobility, strength, and stability; and regain neuromuscular control before returning to play.

The program should be progressive in nature, following the natural healing process and allowing the athlete to adapt to higher loads and volume gradually while being cautious not to advance too rapidly. Before returning to play, the athlete should receive approval from the physician along with the physical therapist and/or certified athletic trainer. The end goal of a rehab program is to assist the athlete in returning to sport at a physical well-being level equal to or greater than prior capabilities. As clinicians, it is also important to educate athletes during the rehabilitation process, so they are more aware of their bodies and how to better care for themselves during the course of their careers and in the event they are without clinician supervision.

Phase 1: Acute Phase

Following injury, the athlete typically experiences frustration from physical injury itself (pain, inflammation, and functional limitations) along with abruptly being removed from sport participation. If a mental skills coach or sports psychologist is available, integrating him or her into the rehab process at this time will benefit the athlete.

Successful athletes are highly adaptable throughout their careers, and their bodies are even more so capable of adapting when they are injured. Almost immediately after an injury, skilled athletes will find other ways to achieve similar levels of function by compensating with healthier joints and limbs and using other compensation strategies. As health care professionals, we expect compensatory mechanisms will likely lead to bad habits and therefore create further chaos on the body and lead to further injury. While function is our primary goal as rehabilitation experts, understanding pain generators and utilizing modalities and techniques to minimize pain should be of high regard in this initial phase of rehabilitation. Along with this, preventing further damage, limiting atrophy, improving range of motion and flexibility, and maintaining core and cardiovascular status are important in this beginning phase.

Preventing further damage is of primary concern and can be accomplished with activity modification or avoidance. For the throwing athlete, that may mean refraining from throwing for a predetermined period. Depending on the injury, the athlete's injury history, level of competition, and the doctors' orders, that time will vary. For instance, RTC inflammation can mean no throwing for 2 to 4 weeks (depending on severity), while ulnar collateral ligament reconstruction (UCLR) will push the athlete closer to the 5-month mark before initiating a return to throwing program. Similarly, the athlete with a clean injury history to the said extremity should normally not take as long as the athlete with a long list of injuries and/or surgeries to that same body part.

There are many therapeutic modalities to assist with pain and inflammation, most notably cryotherapy, topical analgesics, laser, iontophoresis, kinesiology taping, anti-inflammatory medications, and occasionally even injections. Soft tissue mobilization and lymphatic flow techniques after injury can be beneficial to assist with decreasing local edema and inflammation. Conservative manual techniques in this phase can decrease pain and muscular guarding for the patient while allowing the clinician to get a sense of and improve on the soft tissue (connective tissue) pliability and extensibility surrounding the injured area from the onset of injury. In addition to the abovementioned modalities, light stretching, low-grade joint mobilizations, and active-assisted range of motion exercises have been shown to assist in reducing the athlete's pain.[2,12]

With activity modification or avoidance, the player will quickly lose mobility in the impacted joints, most notably the glenohumeral, sternoclavicular, acromioclavicular, and scapulothoracic joints for the overhead athlete. This could have a compounding effect as loss of mobility in one joint will subsequently require compensation in another joint. In the overhead athlete, most commonly we see a loss of internal rotation and horizontal adduction.[2] The loss of internal rotation is referred to as glenohumeral internal rotation deficit (GIRD) and is more specifically a loss of greater than or equal to 17° of the throwing shoulder compared with the opposite shoulder. Occasionally, a loss of external rotation may be present as well and a loss of greater than 5° ER of the throwing shoulder compared with the nonthrowing shoulder is referred to as external rotation deficit. Along with activity modification, muscle inflexibility due to significant and repetitive eccentric muscle forces during arm deceleration can cause

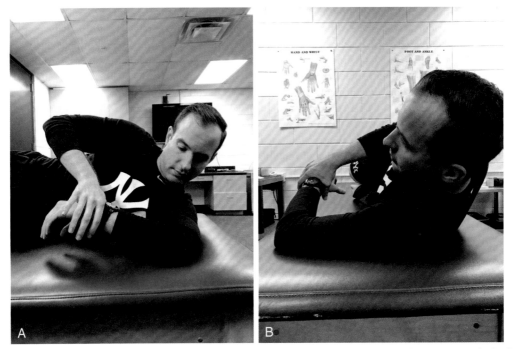

FIGURE 37.1 • A, Self sleeper stretch for internal rotation. B, Modified sleeper position demonstrates the body rotated posteriorly to position the arm in the scapular plane.

the overhead thrower to exhibit a significant loss of motion (especially internal rotation), particularly closely after pitching.[10] Determining the cause of the lack of motion and which structures are involved will help guide the treatment. If diagnostic imaging is available, it may be helpful in further understanding the loss of internal rotation, especially if there are osseous adaptations that have occurred. If the posterior shoulder musculature has tightened, soft tissue mobilization followed by stretching the soft tissue structures in the posterior shoulder will likely improve the flexibility. The 2 most common stretches we use in this situation are the sleeper stretch (Figure 37.1) and horizontal adduction stretch (Figure 37.2). If the posterior joint capsule has been determined to be hypomobile, a specific joint mobilization (posterolateral) will be beneficial (Figure 37.3).[2] Shoulder flexion motion is also frequently restricted in the throwing athlete and should be assessed and treated if needed. Figure 37.4 demonstrates a shoulder flexion stretching technique.

During the examination, the clinician should assess the patient's resting posture along with shoulder, clavicular, and scapular mobility and stability. It is very common to see rounded shoulders and a forward head posture in this population. This posture is associated with muscle weakness of the scapular

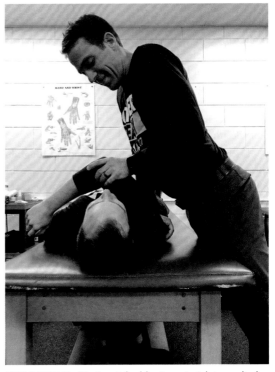

FIGURE 37.2 • Horizontal adduction stretch is applied by the clinician while simultaneously providing a slight internal rotation force while stabilizing the lateral scapular border.

retractors owing to prolonged elongation and altered length tension relationships between synergistic muscle groups that elevate, posteriorly tilt, abduct, and protract the scapula during active arm elevation.[9]

Performing pectoralis minor stretching (Figure 37.5) and myofascial release techniques along with strengthening the scapular retractors, protractors, and depressors will be of major benefit to our injured athletes.

In this first phase, it is also imperative to prevent further muscular atrophy with a return to muscular strengthening via isometrics and low-level strengthening and stabilization exercises. For many athletes, this is a much needed and often overlooked phase of rehab, as they may not have had a good foundational strengthening program to begin with and therefore will benefit greatly with education on proper shoulder and scapular positioning with no to minimal resistance necessary. To provide proper muscle balance, the external rotator muscles should be at least 65% the strength of the internal rotator muscles.[11] Instructing the athlete to perform small but important movements, such as a scapular retraction, may take time and repetition but should be the foundation to any strengthening program. An example of an isometric exercise that can be used for both the external and internal rotators is the "walkout" exercise with tubing resistance (Figure 37.6). This can be progressed by band resistance and be done with or without the utilization of blood flow restriction (BFR). Once the patterns have been mastered and the patient is pain free, progressive load can be added. Refer to chapter 43 for further discussion on BFR.

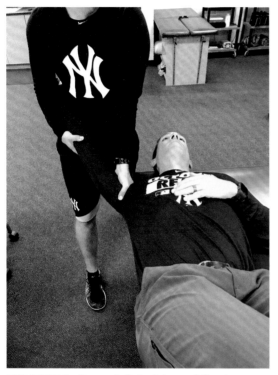

FIGURE 37.3 • Posteroinferior joint mobilization.

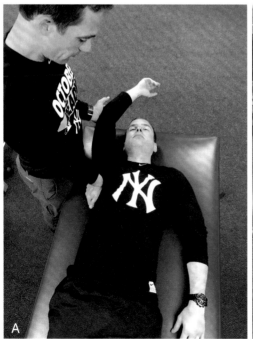
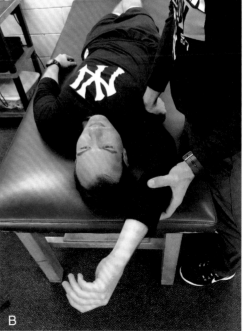

FIGURE 37.4 • A, Shoulder flexion motion assessment. B, A shoulder flexion stretch while stabilizing the scapula.

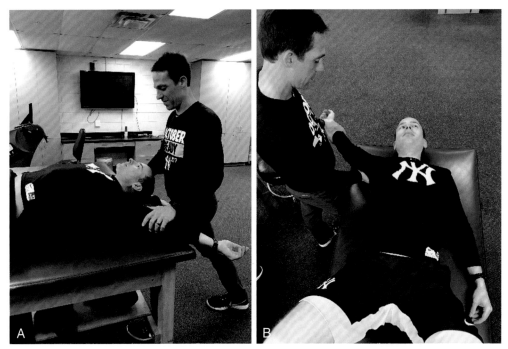

FIGURE 37.5 • A, Clinician-assisted pec stretch using a foam roller. B, Isometric contraction into clinicians hand along the distal forearm.

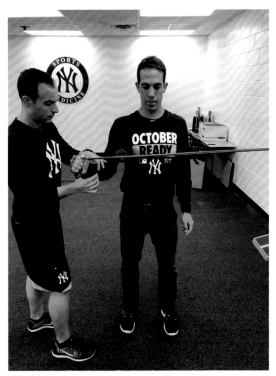

FIGURE 37.6 • Clinician-provided rhythmic stabilization drills while patient performs "walkout" exercise with tubing.

Occasionally, neuromuscular drills will begin toward the end of this phase or at the beginning of phase 2. These include proprioceptive neuromuscular facilitation (PNF) drills, upper extremity rhythmic stabilization drills, and slow reversal hold exercises. Begin with light resistance and in linear planes in this phase before advancing to higher resistance and multiplanar positions in phases 2 and 3, which more closely mimic the arms positions during the throwing motion. Performing these in different planes allows the athlete to reestablish proprioception and joint stabilization by facilitating agonist/antagonist muscular coactivation.[2] Mostly, before initiating PNF drills, we will have the athlete's begin with active motion through desired patterns with no resistance. Once the player is comfortable and demonstrates proper pattern recognition, resistance can be applied.

Phase 2: Intermediate Phase

In this phase, emphasis is placed on normalizing mobility and flexibility and increasing strength and neuromuscular control of the shoulder and scapula. Strengthening of the shoulder prime movers (accelerators) and stabilizers (decelerators) is emphasized with a general weakness typically present in the external rotators of the overhead thrower.

Performing isotonic exercises both eccentrically and concentrically is of high importance, as these muscles work to generate force in the acceleration phase of throwing along with working to slow force down in the deceleration phase (eccentrically). Both muscle groups are important to the throwing athlete; however, the decelerators are subjected to larger deleterious stresses and are more frequently injured in overhead sporting activities.[8] The "Thrower's Ten" program was specifically designed to address weakness in the muscle groups listed earlier.[2,13,13] Begin these exercises on a stable surface and with a solid base of support before progressing to more challenging positions, such as on a physio ball with a decreased base of support. This is a good time to progress this program (along with other exercises) with lighter weights and higher reps to ensure proper form and in preparation for advanced exercises in later phases.

A highly functional shoulder also requires great neuromuscular control. Rhythmic stabilization, PNF, and other drills with oscillatory movements are excellent exercises to incorporate during this phase. These drills promote endurance training and dynamic stabilization of the RTC.[9] Combining isotonic exercises with rhythmic stabilization drills is an advancement of coordination and strength that can be accomplished toward the end of this phase and into the next. An example of an exercise that combines isotonics with neuromuscular control is tubing PNF patterns with concurrent rhythmic stabilizations throughout various ranges of motion following ROM guidelines (Figure 37.7). To further challenge the athlete's core and engage the lower extremity, perform this same exercise in a closed kinetic chain position such as a side plank. Rhythmic stabilization drills can be performed every rep or every few reps. Muscle groups of importance to strengthen via neuromuscular exercise are the scapular retractors, protractors, and depressors. These muscles also tend to be weaker in the overhead throwing athlete and when strong and balanced allow the arm to be functionally mobile through a normalization of force couples and proprioceptive and kinesthetic awareness.[9] As mentioned earlier, this is also the time to advance core and lower extremity strengthening and balancing exercises into the athletes' program. Typically, during this phase, the athlete can also progress away from stationary cardiovascular activities such as stationary biking and initiate or transition to land-based jogging or, if appropriate, machine-based antigravity running. If they have not already, now is a good time to begin a regimented lower extremity–based lifting program as well.

Phase 3: Strengthening Phase

Improving muscular strength, power, and endurance is the main goal of this phase along with progressing functional activities and initiating sport-specific activity. For the overhead athlete, a throwing program is oftentimes the first initiated sport-specific program. In preparation for throwing, upper extremity plyometric exercises should be initiated at least a few weeks prior. Advance prior neuromuscular and proprioceptive exercises with dynamic stabilization drills including rhythmic stabilization at end ranges and manual resistance exercises with perturbations and other core challenged exercises.

Progressing specific exercises and challenging the core simultaneously can be accomplished by advancing from double-leg support to single leg and/or performing exercises on an uneven surface such as a foam mat or BOSU Ball. Advancing to a physio ball from prone on a standard treatment table will also increase the demands of the core musculature and prove to be more challenging to the athlete during this phase of rehab. Adding in sustained holds and alternating arm movements will improve the muscular endurance of the throwing shoulder and scapula (Figure 37.8). These are also great drills to assist the athlete suffering from muscular fatigue, as more motor units will be recruited with sustained holds, which will help to improve the strength.

Initiating plyometric drills will begin with a solid base of support and 2-hand throws and advance to single-leg (decreased base of support) or mimic a thrower's stride position with single-arm tosses. Exercises will also advance from linear planes to multidirectional planes that closely mimic the thrower's pitching mechanics. Plyometric drills improve joint proprioception and dynamic stability while also gradually increasing the stresses on the shoulder through the transfer of energy from the legs and trunk to the upper extremity.[10] Once the Thrower's Ten exercises are mastered, the athlete should be progressed to the Advanced Thrower's Ten program. The additional exercises as described by Wilk et al are prone bilateral full can, horizontal abduction, and prone 90/90 with external rotation.[2,13] These exercises can be performed with free weights including dumbbells or ankle/wrist cuff weights and manual resistance or tubing alike. The clinician should be cautiously progressive in nature but not until the athlete has mastered the prior level of resistance or endurance with proper form.

Performing higher repetitions (25-50) with lighter weight will allow the athlete to improve muscular endurance. However, the athlete's level of play, age, and

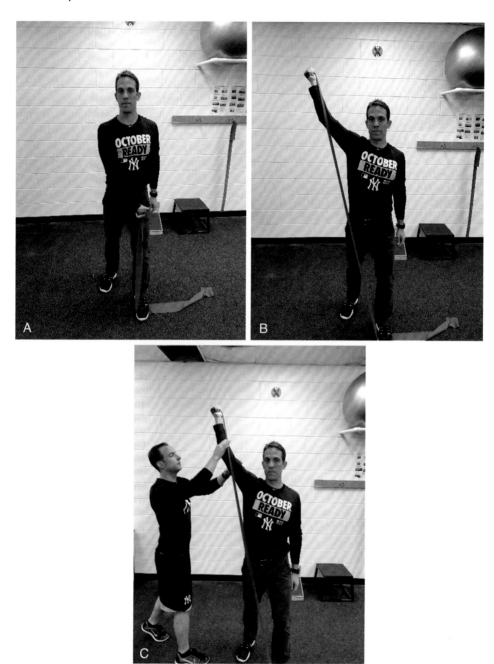

FIGURE 37.7 • Functional D2 pattern (A) flexion and (B) extension using tubing and (C) rhythmic stabilization drills at end range.

stage of muscular strength and endurance building will dictate the range of repetitions used.

Phase 4: Advanced Strengthening and Function/Return to Throwing Phase

Before initiating any sport-specific programs, it is vital for the athlete to receive clearance from the treating physician and rehab clinician. The physician will perform his or her own examination but also will rely heavily on the rehabilitation expert, as we spend the most time with the athlete throughout the rehab process. For return to throwing clearance and at a minimum, the athlete should be pain free; demonstrate full range of motion, strength, and stability; and exhibit excellent neuromuscular control, which should be demonstrated through a comprehensive physical assessment that incorporates a functional testing

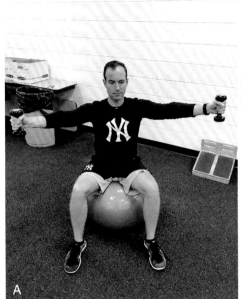
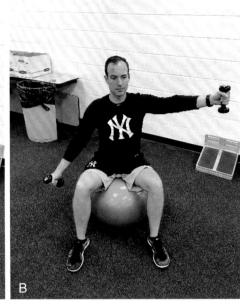

FIGURE 37.8 • Sustained holds (A) and alternating arm movements (B) on an unstable surface to engage core and improve muscular endurance.

protocol. Examples of functional testing exercises for the upper extremity may include activities such as wall ball endurance with perturbation (timed), wall dribbles (12-3 o'clock positions) for high reps, 90/90 wall ball toss, and a plyometric progression including 90/90 throws for accuracy. This program should also include a scapular assessment and an abdominal endurance/lower extremity strength assessment. The throwing program is further discussed and presented in chapter 39. As discussed earlier, it is vital for the athlete to continue with a structured exercise program throughout the remainder of and beyond the rehabilitation program.

Phase 5: Return to Play

Once the athlete has successfully completed the return to play programs, including throwing, hitting, and running (as necessary based on positional requirements), advanced progression into team activities should come next. For the pitcher, after fulfilling bullpen requirements, live batting practice (BP) and a simulated game will be the next progression before competing in a live game. Depending on the level of play before injury, the pitcher should also partake in rehab games at lower levels to build up arm strength and endurance preceding a return to the prior highest level of play. For the position player, a progression would include cage hitting (dry swings, tee, and toss), cage BP, field BP progressing to full BP and, perhaps next, a simulated game before competing at a lower-level game. Once the

player successfully completes lower-level rehab games and is both completely physically and mentally prepared for more activity, he should be declared ready for return to the prior level of competition after a final medical clearance from the physician.

REFERENCES

1. Ciccotti MG, Pollack KM, Ciccotti MC. Elbow injuries in professional baseball. *Am J Sports Med.* 2017;45:2319-2328.
2. Wilk KE, Macrina LC. Nonoperative and postoperative rehabilitation for injuries of the throwing shoulder. *Sports Med Arthrosc Rev.* 2014;22(2):137-150.
3. Conte S, Requa RK, Garrick JG. Disability days in major league baseball. *Am J Sports Med.* 2001;29:431-436.
4. Escamilla RF, Andrews JR. Shoulder muscle recruitment patterns and related biomechanics during upper extremity sports. *Sports Med.* 2009;39(7):569-590.
5. Wilk KE, Macrina LC, Yenchak AJ. Chapter 40: Shoulder rehabilitation for the overhead athlete. In: *Sports Medicine of Baseball.* 2012:429-447.
6. Fleisig GS, Andrews JR, Dillman CJ, et al. Kinetics of baseball pitching with implications about injury mechanisms. *Am J Sports Med.* 1995;23:233-239.
7. Fleisig GS, Barrentine SW, Escamilla RF, et al. Biomechanics of overhand throwing with implications for injuries. *Sports Med.* 1996;21:421-437.
8. Wilk KE, Arrigo C. Current concepts in the rehabilitation of the athletic shoulder. *J Orthop Sports Phys Ther.* 1993;18:366.

9. Wilk KE, Arrigo CA, Hooks TR, et al. Rehabilitation of the overhead throwing athlete: there is more to it than just external/internal rotation strengthening. *PM R.* 2016;8:S78-S90.

10. Wilk KE, Meister K, Andrews J. Current concepts in the rehabilitation of the overhead throwing athlete. *Am J Sports Med.* 2002;30:136-151.

11. Wilk KE, Arrigo CA, Andrews JR. Current concepts: the stabilizing structures of the glenohumeral joint. *J Orthop Sports Phys Ther.* 1997;25:364-379.

12. Noyes FR, Mangine RE, Barber S. Early knee motion after open and arthroscopic anterior cruciate ligament reconstruction. *Am J Sports Med.* 1987;15:149-160.

13. Wilk KE, Yenchak AJ, Arrigo CA, et al. The advanced throwers ten exercise program: a new exercise series or enhanced dynamic shoulder control in the overhead throwing athlete. *Phys Sports Med.* 2011;39:90-97.

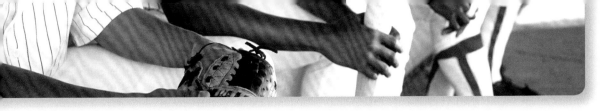

CHAPTER 38

Rehabilitation Strategies for the Elbow

Kevin E. Wilk, PT, DPT, FAPTA | Christopher A. Arrigo, MS, PT, ATC | Leonard C. Macrina, MSPT, SCS, CSCS | E. Lyle Cain, Jr, MD | Jeffrey R. Dugas, MD | James R. Andrews, MD

You're going to feel good. But no matter how much you rehab you do, you can't speed up the healing process. I would rather see a guy come back in 14 months and pitch seven, eight or nine more years then come back in 10 months and get hurt again. You cannot mess with mother nature and father time. Nature will heal it if you give it time.

—*Tommy John*

INTRODUCTION

Injuries to the elbow in the overhead athlete, particularly the baseball pitcher, occur commonly and continue to increase in frequency.[20] Pitchers sustain most baseball-related injuries, accounting for 61% of all injuries in Major League Baseball, with 72% of these injuries affecting the throwing shoulder and elbow.[21] Elbow injuries account for between 22% and 26% of all Major League Baseball pitching injuries.[21,74] Conte et al[21] reported that 25% of all major league pitchers, and 14% of all minor league pitchers on active rosters have undergone ulnar collateral ligament (UCL) surgery.

These elbow injury rates occur in part because the joint is subjected to severe and repetitive valgus stress during throwing that is responsible for unique and sport-specific injury patterns.[36,38] These injuries are caused by chronic stress overload or repetitive microtraumatic stress imparted across the joint during the overhead pitching motion as the elbow extends at over 2300°/s, resulting in a medial sheer force of 300 N and compressive force of 900 N.[8,38,98] In addition, the valgus stress applied to the elbow during the acceleration phase of throwing is 64 Nm,[38,98] which exceeds the ultimate tensile strength of the UCL.[29] Thus, the medial aspect of the elbow undergoes tremendous tension (distraction) forces, and the lateral aspect is forcefully compressed during throwing.

The overhead athlete is susceptible to a specific set of elbow injuries induced by the various forces placed on the elbow during throwing.[33,98] Valgus stress created during the acceleration phase of throwing places tension across the medial aspect of the elbow and is responsible for injuries to the flexor-pronator complex and UCL.[38] Compression forces are also applied to the lateral aspect of the elbow during the throwing motion, which may result in osteochondritis dissecans (OCD). The posterior compartment is subject to tensile, compressive, and torsional forces during both the acceleration and deceleration phases of throwing. This may result in valgus extension overload (VEO) and lead to osteophyte formation, stress fractures of the olecranon, or physeal injury.[7,108]

This chapter will provide an overview of the rehabilitation principles and guidelines used to manage the overhead athlete's elbow, as well as detail specific nonoperative and postoperative treatment guidelines for the injuries most commonly seen at the thrower's elbow.

GENERAL REHABILITATION GUIDELINES

Rehabilitation after any elbow injury or surgery needs to follow a sequential and progressive multiphased approach to be successful. The goal of elbow rehabilitation is to return the athletes to their previous functional level as quickly and safely as possible. An outline of the multiphased, criteria-based rehabilitation process detailed below is presented for both elbow injury (Table 38.1) and after surgery (Table 38.2).

Phase I—Immediate Motion Phase

The first phase of elbow rehabilitation is the immediate motion or acute phase. The goals of this phase are to minimize the effects of immobilization, reestablish nonpainful range of motion (ROM), decrease pain and inflammation, and retard muscular atrophy.

Early ROM activities are performed to nourish the articular cartilage and assist in the synthesis, alignment, and organization of collagen tissue.[23,28,45,70,72,84,85,99] ROM activities are performed for all planes of elbow and wrist motions to prevent the formation of scar tissue and adhesions. Active-assisted and passive ROM exercises are performed for the humeroulnar joint to restore elbow flexion/extension as well as for the humeroradial and radioulnar joints to restore forearm supination/pronation. Reestablishing full elbow extension or,

more frequently in the throwing athlete, preinjury motion is the primary goal of early ROM activities to minimize the occurrence of elbow flexion contractures.[1,43,68] In surgical cases, the preoperative elbow motion must be carefully assessed and recorded. Postoperatively, if the athlete was not seen before injury or surgery, the clinician should ask whether full elbow extension has been present in the past 2 to 3 years. Postoperative ROM is often related to preoperative motion, especially in the case of UCL reconstructions. Wright et al[110] reported on 33 professional baseball players before the competitive season noting an average loss of throwing elbow extension of 7° and flexion of 5.5° when compared with the nonthrowing side. The loss of elbow extension can be a deleterious side effect for the overhead athlete. The elbow is predisposed to flexion contractures due to the intimate congruency of the joint articulations, the tightness of the joint capsule, and the tendency of the anterior capsule to develop adhesions after injury.[99] The brachialis muscle also attaches to the capsule and crosses the elbow joint before becoming a tendinous structure further contributing to the propensity for joint contracture.

TABLE 38.1 Nonoperative Rehabilitation Program for Elbow Injuries

I. Acute Phase (Week 1)
Goals:
• Improve motion
• Diminish pain and inflammation
• Retard muscle atrophy
Exercises:
1. Stretching for wrist and elbow joint, stretches for shoulder joint
2. Strengthening exercises isometrics for wrist elbow, and shoulder musculature
3. Pain and inflammation control cryotherapy, HVGS, ultrasound, and whirlpool

II. Subacute Phase (Weeks 2-4)
Goals:
• Normalize motion
• Improve muscular strength, power, and endurance
Week 2
1. Initiate isotonic strengthening for wrist and elbow muscles
2. Initiate exercise tubing exercises for shoulder
3. Continue use of cryotherapy, etc
Week 3
1. Initiate rhythmic stabilization drills for elbow and shoulder joint
2. Progress isotonic strengthening for entire upper extremity
3. Initiate isokinetic strengthening exercises for elbow flexion/extension
Week 4
1. Initiate Throwers' Ten program
2. Emphasize eccentric biceps work, concentric triceps, and wrist flexor work
3. Program endurance training
4. Initiate light plyometric drills
5. Initiate swinging drills

TABLE 38.1 Nonoperative Rehabilitation Program for Elbow Injuries   (continued)

III. Advanced Phase (Weeks 4-6)

Goals:
  Preparation of athlete for return to functional activities
Criteria to progress to advanced phase:
  1. Full nonpainful ROM
  2. No pain or tenderness
  3. Satisfactory isokinetic test
  4. Satisfactory clinical exam
Weeks 4-5
  1. Continue strengthening exercises, endurance drills, and flexibility exercises daily
  2. Thrower's Ten program
  3. Progress plyometric drills
  4. Emphasize maintenance program based on pathology
  5. Progress swinging drills (ie, hitting)
Weeks 6-8
  Initiate interval sport program once determined by physician
    Phase I program

IV. Return to Activity Phase (Weeks 6-9)
Weeks 6 through 9—when you return to play depends on your condition and progress, your physician will determine when it is safe. 1. Continue strengthening program Thrower's Ten program 2. Continue flexibility program 3. Progress functional drills to unrestricted play

TABLE 38.2 Postoperative Rehabilitative Protocol for Elbow Arthroscopy

I. Initial Phase (Week 1)

Goal:
  • Full wrizst and elbow ROM
  • Decrease swelling
  • Decrease pain
  • Retardation or muscle atrophy
A. Day of surgery
  Begin gently moving elbow in bulky dressing
B. Post-op Days 1 and 2
  1. Remove bulky dressing and replace with elastic bandages
  2. Immediate post-op hand, wrist, and elbow exercises
    a. Putty/grip strengthening
    b. Wrist flexor stretching
    c. Wrist extensor stretching
    d. Wrist curls
    e. Reverse wrist curls
    f. Neutral wrist curls
    g. Pronation/supination
    h. AIAAROM elbow extension/flexion
C. Post-op days 3 through 7
  1. PROM elbow extension/flexion (motion to tolerance)
  2. Begin PRE exercises with 1 lb weight
    a. Wrist curls
    b. Reverse wrist curls
    c. Neutral wrist curls
    d. Pronation/supination
    e. Broomstick rollup

(continued)

TABLE 38.2 Postoperative Rehabilitative Protocol for Elbow Arthroscopy   (continued)

II. Intermediate Phase (Week 2-4)

Goal:
 • Improve muscular strength and endurance
 • Normalize joint arthrokinematics
 A. Week 2 range of motion exercises (overpressure into extension)
  1. Addition of biceps cud and triceps extension
  2. Continue to progress PRE weight and repetitions as tolerable
 B. Week 3
  1. Initiate biceps and biceps eccentric exercise program
  2. Initiate rotator cuff exercises program
   a. External rotators
   b. Internal rotators
   c. Deltoid
   d. Supraspinatus
   e. Scapulothoracic strengthening

III. Advanced Phase (Week 4-8)

Goals:
  Preparation of athlete for return to functional activities
 Criteria to progress to advanced phase:
  1. Full nonpainful ROM
  2. No pain or tenderness
  3. Isokinetic test that fulfills criteria to throw
  4. Satisfactory clinical examination
 A. Weeks 4 through 6
  1. Continue maintenance program, emphasizing muscular strength, endurance, and flexibility
  2. Initiate interval throwing program phase

Injury to the elbow may cause excessive scar tissue formation of the brachialis muscle as well as functional splinting of the elbow limiting full extension.[99]

In addition to ROM exercises, joint mobilizations of the humeroulnar joint is performed as tolerated to aid in minimizing the occurrence of flexion contractures. Posterior glides with oscillations are performed at the end range of available motion to assist in regaining full elbow extension. Grade I and II mobilizations are initially used, progressing to more aggressive grade III and IV mobilization techniques in end range during later stages of rehabilitation when acute symptoms have subsided. Joint mobilization should also include the restoration of radiocapitellar and radioulnar joint accessory motion.

If the athlete continues to have difficulty achieving full extension using ROM and mobilization techniques, a low-load, long-duration (LLLD) stretch may be incorporated to produce a deformation (creep) of the collagen tissue, resulting in tissue elongation.[52,88,96,97] We have found this technique to be extremely beneficial for restoring full elbow extension. The athlete lies supine with a towel roll or foam pad placed under the distal brachium to act as a cushion and fulcrum. Light resistance exercise tubing is

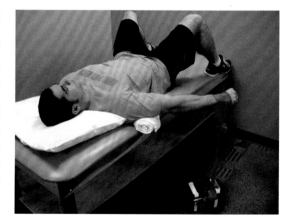

FIGURE 38.1 ● A low-load, long duration stretch into elbow extension is performed using light resistance. The shoulder is internally rotated while the forearm is pronated to best isolate and maximize the stretch on the elbow joint.

applied to the athlete's wrist and secured to the table or a dumbbell on the ground (Figure 38.1). The athlete is instructed to relax as much as possible for 10 to 15 minutes per treatment. The amount of resistance applied should be of a low enough magnitude to enable the athlete to perform the stretch for the

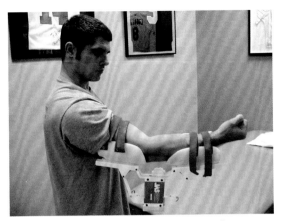

FIGURE 38.2 • Commercial device used by the patient at home to work on knee extension range of motion.

entire duration without pain, muscle spasm, or reflexive guarding. The technique should impart a tolerable low load combined with a comfortable long-duration stretch. Athletes are instructed to perform the LLLD stretch several times per day for a total of at least 60 minutes. Generally, we instruct athletes to perform a 15-minute LLLD stretch, 4 times per day. This type of stretching is often referred to as the TERT program (total end range time).[60] LLLD stretching combined with joint mobilization, passive ROM and stretching is extremely effective in treating athletes with a stiff elbow. However, in some instances it may be beneficial to include the use of an additional splint or brace to create an additional LLLD stretch. The brace is worn at night for several hours while sleeping (Figure 38.2).

The aggressiveness of stretching and mobilization techniques is dictated by the healing constraints of the involved tissues, the specific pathology/surgery, the amount of available motion, and end feel. It is imperative to never overstress healing tissue. When the athlete presents with a decrease in motion and a hard end feel without pain, aggressive stretching and mobilization technique may be used. Conversely, a patient exhibiting pain before resistance or an empty end feel should be progressed slowly with gentle mobilization and stretching. In addition, it is beneficial to be aggressive with glenohumeral rehabilitation to improve ROM through internal rotation (IR) and external rotation (ER) stretching.

Another goal of this phase is to decrease the pain and inflammation. In addition to the performance of grade I and II joint mobilization techniques to neuromodulate pain by stimulating type I and type II articular joint receptors,[58,111] cryotherapy and high-voltage electrical stimulation are incorporated to further assist in reducing pain and inflammation. Once the acute inflammatory response has subsided, moist heat, warm whirlpool, and ultrasound are used at the onset of treatment to prepare the tissue for stretching and improve the extensibility of the capsule and musculotendinous structures. Additionally, joint mobilization techniques are advanced to grade III and IV mobilizations.

The early phases of rehabilitation also focus on voluntary activation of muscle and retarding muscular atrophy. Subpainful and submaximal isometrics are performed initially for the elbow flexors and extensors, as well as the wrist flexor, extensor, pronator, and supinator muscle groups. Shoulder isometrics are also performed during this phase with caution regarding the use of IR and ER exercises if painful. Alternating rhythmic stabilization drills for shoulder flexion/extension/horizontal abduction/adduction, shoulder IR/ER, and elbow flexion/extension/supination/pronation are performed to begin reestablishing proprioception and neuromuscular control of the upper extremity. Furthermore, the athlete's shoulder joint ROM should be addressed during this phase of the rehabilitation process and a stretching program included to improve IR and horizontal adduction, which are typically limited in the throwing athlete.

Phase II—Intermediate Phase

The intermediate phase is initiated when the athlete exhibits full ROM, minimal pain and tenderness, and a good (4/5) manual muscle test of the elbow flexor and extensor musculature. The emphasis of this phase includes enhancing elbow and upper extremity mobility, improving muscular strength and endurance, and reestablishing neuromuscular control of the elbow complex.

Stretching, mobilization, and flexibility activities are continued to maintain full elbow and wrist ROM. Mobilization techniques are progressed to more aggressive grade III and IV techniques as needed to apply a stretch to capsular tissue at end range. Flexibility exercises are advanced during this phase to focus on wrist flexion, extension, pronation, and supination. Elbow extension and forearm pronation flexibility is emphasized in throwing athletes to reduce joint stress and improve movement efficiency. Shoulder flexibility must also be maintained, and often improved, in overhead athletes during elbow rehabilitation with emphasis placed on ER and IR at 90° of abduction, flexion, and horizontal adduction. Shoulder ER at 90° of abduction is emphasized because any loss of throwing specific ER may result in increased strain on the medial elbow structures during the overhead throwing motion; however, the greater passive ER is beyond throwing normal, the more stress there is on the UCL and the greater the risk of UCL injury.[38,39,74,102]

The available passive ER in the throwing shoulder should be 125° to 130°.[100-104] IR flexibility must also be diligently addressed with a goal of 50° to 55° in the thrower.[100-104] Horizontal adduction flexibility in the throwing shoulder should be between 40° and 45°.[100-104] The normalization of shoulder joint ROM in the throwing athlete should also consider the total range of motion (TROM) of combined shoulder ER and IR with a throwing shoulder goal of 180° to 185°.[100-104]

Strengthening exercises are advanced from isometrics to isotonic contractions, beginning with concentric movements and progressing to include eccentric contractions as the athlete tolerates. Emphasis is placed on elbow flexion and extension, wrist flexion and extension, and forearm pronation and supination. The glenohumeral and scapulothoracic muscles are also placed on a progressive resistance program during the later stages of this phase with a focus on strengthening shoulder ER and the periscapular muscles. This program includes ER and IR with exercise tubing at 0° of abduction and isotonic resistive active ROM exercises against gravity. Initially these exercises include standing scaption in ER (full can),[77-79] standing abduction, side-lying ER, and prone rowing. As strength returns, the program is advanced to include a full range of upper extremity strengthening exercises with emphasis on the posterior rotator cuff muscles and scapular strengthening, focused on the lower trapezius. The upper extremity strengthening program we use is called the Thrower's Ten program[105] (Table 38.3). It has been designed based on electromyographic studies to illicit the greatest activity of the muscles most needed to provide dynamic upper limb stability.[78,79]

TABLE 38.3 Thrower's Ten Exercise Program

Diagonal pattern D2 extension
Diagonal pattern D2 flexion
External rotation at 0° abduction
Internal rotation at 0° abduction
Shoulder abduction to 90°
Scapular abduction, external rotation ("full cans")
Side-lying external rotation
Prone horizontal abduction
Prone horizontal abduction (full external rotation, 100° abduction)
Prone rowing
Prone rowing into external rotation
Press-ups
Push-ups
Elbow flexion
Elbow extension
Wrist extension
Wrist supination
Wrist pronation

Neuromuscular control exercises are initiated in this phase to enhance the muscles ability to control the elbow joint during athletic activities. These exercises include proprioceptive neuromuscular facilitation exercises with rhythmic stabilization and manual resistance elbow/wrist flexion drills (Figure 38.3).

Phase III—Advanced Strengthening Phase

The third phase involves a progression of activities to prepare the athlete for sport participation. The goals of this phase are to progressively increase strength, power, endurance, and neuromuscular control to prepare for a gradual return to sport. Specific criteria that must be met before entering this phase include full nonpainful ROM, no pain or tenderness on clinical examination, and strength that is 70% of the contralateral extremity.

Activities during this phase include aggressive strengthening exercises, emphasizing higher resistance, functional movements, eccentric contractions, plyometric activities, and longer bouts of exercise. Elbow flexion exercises are progressed to emphasize eccentric control. The biceps muscle is an important stabilizer during the follow-through phase of overhead

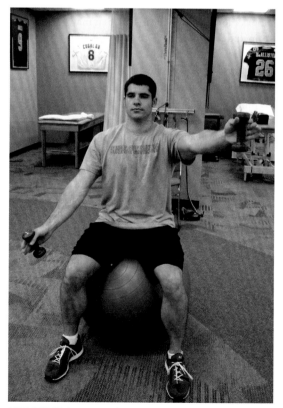

FIGURE 38.3 • Manual concentric and eccentric resistance exercises for the elbow flexors and wrist flexor-pronators.

throwing to eccentrically control the deceleration of the elbow, preventing pathologic abutting of the olecranon within the fossa.[10,38] Elbow flexion can be performed with elastic tubing to emphasis both slow and fast speed concentric and eccentric contractions. Manual resistance is also incorporated for concentric and eccentric strengthening of the elbow flexors. Strengthening exercises with weight machines are also incorporated during this phase beginning with bench press, seated rowing, and front latissimus dorsi pulldowns. The triceps must also be a focus of aggressive strengthening in this phase. Empirically we often note weak triceps musculature in athletes that develop pain when returned to throwing prematurely. Elbow extension is primarily exercised with a concentric contraction because the triceps functions this way during the acceleration phase of throwing.

The overhead athlete is placed on the Advanced Thrower's Ten program in this phase[107] (Table 38.4). This program incorporates throwing motion–specific exercises and movement patterns, performed in a discrete series, utilizing principles of coactivation, high-level neuromuscular control, dynamic stabilization, muscular facilitation, endurance, and coordination that serve to restore muscle balance and symmetry in the throwing athlete.[107] Examples include the full can raise with sustained holds while seated on a stability ball (Figure 38.4) or prone horizontal abduction on a stability ball while performing sustained holds (Figure 38.5).

TABLE 38.4 Advanced Thrower's Ten Exercise Program

1A	Seated stability ball external rotation at 0° abduction
1B	Seated stability ball internal rotation at 0° abduction
2	Seated stability ball full can
3	Seated stability ball lateral raise to 90°
4	Side-lying external rotation
5	Prone T's on stability ball
6	Prone Y's on stability ball
7	Prone row into external rotation on stability ball
8	Shoulder extensions on stability ball
9	Lower trapezius isolation on stability ball
10	Seated high row into external rotation on stability ball
11	Seated biceps/triceps on stability ball
12	Wrist flexion/extension and supination/pronation

Exercises 1 through 11 are performed with sustained holds.

Neuromuscular control exercises are progressed to include side-lying ER with manual resistance. Concentric and eccentric ER is performed against the clinician's resistance with the addition of rhythmic stabilization cocontractions at the end range of ER. This manual resistance exercise may be progressed to standing ER with exercise tubing at 0° and finally at 90° (Figure 38.6).

Plyometric drills are an extremely beneficial form of functional exercise for training the elbow in the overhead athlete and are incorporated at this point in the rehabilitation program.[89,106] Plyometric exercises are performed using a weighted medicine ball during the later stages of this phase to train the shoulder and elbow to develop and withstand the high levels of stress throwing imparts on the arm. Plyometric exercises are initially performed with 2 hands using a chest pass, side-to-side throw, and overhead soccer throw. These are progressed to include 1-handed

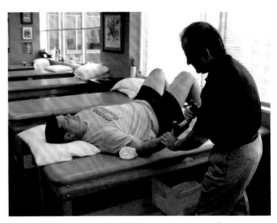

FIGURE 38.4 • Advanced Thrower's Ten: Full can raises with sustained holds while seated on a stability ball.

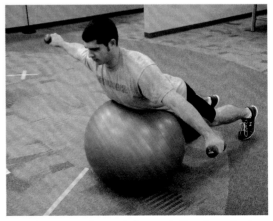

FIGURE 38.5 • Advanced Thrower's Ten: Prone horizontal abduction on a stability ball while performing sustained holds.

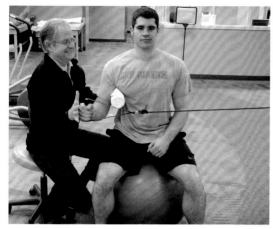

FIGURE 38.6 • External rotation at 90° abduction with exercise tubing, manual resistance, and rhythmic stabilizations, while the athlete is seated on a stability ball.

activities such as 90°/90° throws with rhythmic stabilization at end range (Figure 38.7), external and IR throws at 0° of abduction into a trampoline, and wall dribbles to improve the musculature endurance of the entire throwing arm. Specific plyometric drills for the forearm musculature include wrist flexion flips (Figure 38.8) and extension grips. These last 2 plyometric drills are a vital component to include in an elbow rehabilitation program because they emphasize dynamic strength and functional endurance of the forearm and hand musculature.

Phase IV—Return to Activity Phase

The final phase of elbow rehabilitation, the return to activity phase, allows the athlete to progressively return to full competition using an interval return to throwing program. Other interval programs are used for various other sports including tennis and golf.[80]

Before an athlete can be advanced to the return to activity phase of rehabilitation, they must exhibit full ROM, no pain or tenderness, a satisfactory isokinetic test, and a satisfactory clinical examination. Isokinetic testing at 180° and 300°/s is commonly utilized to determine the readiness of the athlete to begin an interval sport program.[80] Our data indicate that a bilateral comparison of elbow flexion at 180°/s should be 10% to 20% stronger and elbow extensors 5% to 15% stronger in the throwing arm when compared with the nonthrowing arm. We have established a set of return to throwing criteria that must be met before the initiation of an interval throwing program (ITP) (Table 38.5).

Once these criteria have been met, we initiate a formal interval sport program as described by Reinold et al.[80] The first step in the return to throwing process is

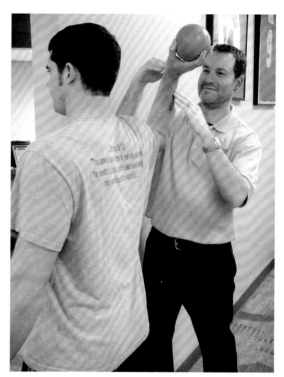

FIGURE 38.7 • Plyometric wall throws with a 2-pound ball while the rehabilitation specialist performs a rhythmic stabilization at end range.

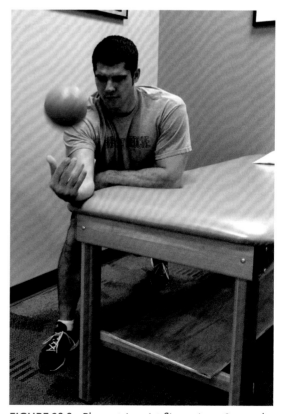

FIGURE 38.8 • Plyometric wrist flips using a 2-pound medicine ball to strengthen the wrist flexors.

the implementation of a long-toss ITP that is player and position dependent, beginning at 45 feet and gradually progressing to 120 or 180 feet. Throwing should be performed without pain or significant increase in symptoms. During the long-toss program, as intensity and distance progress, the stresses significantly increase on the athlete's medial elbow and anterior shoulder joint.[37] We believe it is important for the overhead athlete to perform stretching and an abbreviated strengthening program before and after performing their ITP. Typically, our overhead throwers warm-up, stretch, and perform 1 set of their exercise program before throwing, followed by 2 additional sets of exercises after completing their program. This provides an adequate warm-up while also ensuring maintenance of necessary ROM and flexibility of both the elbow and shoulder joints. The following day, the throwers will exercise their scapular muscles, external rotators, and perform a core stabilization program.[80]

TRIP TO THE MOUND

Phase I Long-Toss Interval Throwing Program

The ITP is designed to gradually return motion, strength, and confidence in the throwing arm after injury or surgery by slowly progressing through graduated throwing distances. The ITP is initiated upon clearance by the athlete's physician to resume throwing and performed under the supervision of the rehabilitation team (physician, physical therapist, and athletic trainer).

The program is set up to minimize the chance of reinjury and emphasize prethrowing warm-up and stretching. In development of the ITP, the following factors are considered most important.

1. The act of throwing the baseball involves the transfer of energy from the feet through the legs, pelvis, trunk, and shoulder through the elbow and hand. Therefore, any return to throwing after injury must include attention to the entire body

2. The chance for reinjury is lessened by a graduate progression of interval throwing

3. Proper warm-up is essential

4. Most injuries occur as the result of fatigue

5. Proper throwing mechanics lessen the incidence of reinjury

6. Baseline requirements for throwing include pain-free ROM, adequate muscle power, adequate muscle resistance to fatigue

Because there is an individual variability in all throwing athletes, there is no set timetable for completion of the program. Most athletes, by nature, are highly competitive individuals and wish to return to competition at the earliest possible moment. While this is a necessary quality of all athletes, the proper channeling of the athlete's energies into a rigidly controlled throwing program is essential to lessen the chance of reinjury during the rehabilitation period. The athlete may have the tendency to want to increase the intensity of the throwing program. This will increase the incidence of reinjury and may greatly retard the rehabilitation process. It is recommended to follow the program rigidly, as this will be the safest route to return to competition.

During the recovery process, the athlete will probably experience soreness and a dull, diffuse, aching sensation in the muscles and tendons. If the athlete experiences sharp pain, particularly in the joint, stop all throwing activity until this pain ceases. If continued pain persists, the physician should be contacted.

Weight training: The athlete should supplement the ITP with a high-repetition, low-weight, exercise program. Strengthening should address a good balance between anterior and posterior musculature so that the shoulder will not be predisposed to injury. Special emphasis must be given to posterior rotator cuff musculature for any strengthening program. Weight training will not increase throwing velocity but will increase the resistance of the arm to fatigue and injury. Weight training should be done the same day as you throw; however, it should be after your throwing is completed, using the day in between for flexibility exercises and a recovery period. A weight training pattern or routine should be stressed at this point as a "maintenance program." This pattern can and should accompany the athlete into and throughout the season as a deterrent to further injury. It must be stressed that weight training is of no benefit unless accompanied by a sound flexibility program.

Individual variability: The ITP is designed so that each level is achieved without pain or complications before the next level is started. This sets up a progression that a goal is achieved before advancement instead of advancing to a specific time frame. Because of this design, the ITP may be used for different levels of skills and abilities from those in high school to professional levels. The reasons for being in the ITP will vary from person to person. Example: One athlete may wish to use alternate days throwing with or without using weights in-between; another athlete may have to throw every third or fourth day due to pain or swelling. "Listen to your body—it will tell you when to slow down." Again, completion of the steps of the ITP will vary from person to person. There is no set timetable in terms of days to completion.

Warm-up: Jogging increases blood flow to the muscles and joints, thus increasing their flexibility and decreasing the chance of reinjury. Because the amount of warm-up will vary from person to person, the athlete should jog until developing a light sweat, then progress to the stretching phase.

Stretching: Because throwing involves all muscles in the body, all muscle groups should be stretched before throwing. This should be done in a systematic fashion beginning with the legs and including the trunk, back, neck, and arms. Continue with capsular stretches and L-bar ROM exercises.

Throwing mechanics: A critical aspect of the ITP is maintenance of proper throwing mechanics throughout the advancement. The use of the crowhop method simulates the throwing act, allowing emphasis of the proper body mechanics. This throwing method should be adopted from the start of the ITP. Throwing flat-footed encourages improper body mechanics, placing increase stress on the throwing arm and therefore predisposing the arm to reinjury. The pitching coach and sports biomechanist (if available) may be valuable allies to the rehabilitation team with their knowledge of throwing mechanics.

Components of the crowhop method are first a hop, then a skip, followed by the throw. The velocity of the throw is determined by the distance, whereas the ball should have only enough momentum to travel each designed distance. Again, emphasis should be placed upon proper throwing mechanics when the athlete begins phase II: "throwing off the mound" or from the athlete's respective position, to decrease the chance of reinjury.

Throwing: Using the crowhop method, the athlete should begin warm-up throws at a comfortable distance (approximately 30-45 feet) and then progress to the distance indicated for that phase (Table 38.1). The program consists of throwing at each step 2 to 3 times without pain or symptoms before progressing to the next step. The object of each phase is for the athlete to be able to throw the ball without pain the specified distance (45, 60, 90, 120, 150, 180 feet), 75 times at each distance. After the athlete can throw at the prescribed distance without pain, they will be ready for throwing from flat ground 60 feet, 6 inches in the normal pitching mechanics or return to their respective position (step 14). At this point, full strength and confidence should be restored in the athlete's arm. It is important to stress the crowhop method and proper mechanics with each throw. Just as the advancement to this point has been gradual and progressive, the return to unrestricted throwing must follow the same principles. A pitcher should first throw only fast balls at 50%, progressing to 75% and 100%. At this time, the athlete may start more stressful pitches such as breaking balls. The position player should simulate a game situation, again progressing at 50% to 75% to 100%. Once again, if an athlete has increased pain, particularly at the joint, the throwing program should be backed off and readvanced as tolerated, under the direction of the rehabilitation team.

Batting: Depending on the type of injury that the athlete has, the time of return to batting should be determined by the physician. It should be noted that stress placed on the arm and shoulder in the batting motion is very different from the throwing motion. Return to unrestricted use of the bat should also follow the same progression guidelines as seen in the training program. Begin with dry swings progressing to hitting off the tee, then soft toss, and finally live pitching.

Summary: In using the ITP in conjunction with a structured rehabilitation program, the athlete should be able to return to full competition status, minimizing any chance of reinjury. The program and its progression should be modified to meet the specific needs of each individual athlete. A comprehensive program consisting of a maintenance strength and flexibility program, appropriate warm-up and cool-down procedures, proper pitching mechanics, and progressive throwing and batting will assist the baseball player in returning safely to competition.

45′ Phase	60′ Phase	90′ Phase	120′ Phase

Step 1:
  A. Warm-up throwing
  B. 45′ (25 throws)
  C. Rest 5-10 min
  D. Warm-up throwing
  E. 45′ (25 throws)
Step 2:
  A. Warm-up throwing
  B. 45′ (25 throws)
  C. Rest 5-10 min
  D. Warm-up throwing
  E. 45′ (25 throws)
  F. Rest 5-10 min
  G. Warm-up throwing
  H. 45′ (25 throws)
	Step 3:
	  A. Warm-up throwing
	  B. 60′ (25 throws)
	  C. Rest 5-10 min
	  D. Warm-up throwing
	  E. 60′ (25 throws)
	Step 4:
	  A. Warm-up throwing
	  B. 60′ (25 throws)
	  C. Rest 5-10 min
	  D. Warm-up throwing
	  E. 60′ (25 throws)
	  F. Rest 5-10 min
	  G. Warm-up throwing
	  H. 60′ (25 throws)
		Step 5:
		  A. Warm-up throwing
		  B. 90′ (25 throws)
		  C. Rest 5-10 min
		  D. Warm-up throwing
		  E. 90′ (25 throws)
		Step 6:
		  A. Warm-up throwing
		  B. 90′ (25 throws)
		  C. Rest 5-10 min
		  D. Warm-up throwing
		  E. 90′ (25 throws)
		  F. Rest 5-10 min
		  G. Warm-up throwing
		  H. 90′ (25 throws)
			Step 7:
			  A. Warm-up throwing
			  B. 120′ (25 throws)
			  C. Rest 5-10 min
			  D. Warm-up throwing
			  E. 120′ (25 throws)
			Step 8:
			  A. Warm-up throwing
			  B. 120′ (25 throws)
			  C. Rest 5-10 min
			  D. Warm-up throwing
			  E. 120′ (25 throws)
			  F. Rest 5-10 min
			  G. Warm-up throwing
			  H. 120′ (25 throws)

150′ Phase	**180′ Phase**		**Throwing program should be performed every other day, unless otherwise specified by your physician or rehabilitation specialist.** Perform each step ___ times before progressing to the next step.

Step 9:
  A. Warm-up throwing
  B. 150′ (25 throws)
  C. Rest 5-10 min
  D. Warm-up throwing
  E. 150′ (25 throws)
Step 10:
  A. Warm-up throwing
  B. 150′ (25 throws)
  C. Rest 5-10 min
  D. Warm-up throwing
  E. 150′ (25 throws)
  F. Rest 5-10 min
  G. Warm-up throwing
  H. 150′ (25 throws)
	Step 11:
	  A. Warm-up throwing
	  B. 180′ (25 throws)
	  C. Rest 5-10 min
	  D. Warm-up throwing
	  E. 180′ (25 throws)
	Step 12:
	  A. Warm-up throwing
	  B. 180′ (25 throws)
	  C. Rest 5-10 min
	  D. Warm-up throwing
	  E. 180′ (25 throws)
	  F. Rest 5-10 min
	  G. Warm-up throwing
	  H. 180′ (25 throws)
	Step 13:
	  A. Warm-up throwing
	  B. 180′ (25 throws)
	  C. Rest 5-10 min
	  D. Warm-up throwing
	  E. 180′ (25 throws)
	Step 14: Begin throwing off the mound or return to respective position.		

Flat Ground Throwing	Flat Throwing
A. Warm-up throwing	A. Warm-up throwing
B. Throw 60 feet (10-15 throws)	B. Throw 60 feet (10-15 throws)
C. Throw 90 feet (10 throws)	C. Throw 90 feet (10 throws)
D. Throw 120 feet (10 throws)	D. Throw 120 feet (10 throws)
E. Throw 60 feet (flat ground) using pitching mechanics (20-30 throws)	E. Throw 60 feet (flat ground) using pitching mechanics (20-30 throws)
	F. Throw 60-90 feet (10-15 throws)
	G. Throw 60 feet (flat ground) using pitching mechanics (20 throws)

TABLE 38.5 Return to Throwing

Criteria to Initiate Phase I Throwing (Long Toss)

- Full nonpainful ROM
  - Shoulder total ROM within 50 of nonthrowing shoulder
  - Shoulder horizontal adduction 400> on throwing shoulder
  - GIRD of <150
  - Elbow and wrist PROM within normal limits
- Satisfactory shoulder, elbow, and wrist strength based on manual muscle test, handheld dynamometer, or isokinetic testing
  - ER/IR ratio: 72%-76%
  - ER/ABD ratio: 68%-73%
  - Throwing shoulder IR 115%> compared with nonthrowing shoulder
  - Throwing shoulder ER 95%> compared with nonthrowing shoulder
  - Throwing arm elbow flexion/extension 100%-115% compared with nonthrowing arm
  - Throwing arm wrist flexion/extension and forearm pronation/supination 100%-115% compared with nonthrowing arm
- Satisfactory clinical examination
  - Physician clearance
- Successfully completed appropriate rehabilitation program
  - Completed all steps of rehabilitation
- Satisfactory functional test scores
  - Prone ball drop test (throwing side 110%>)
  - One-arm ball throws against the wall using 1 kg (2-pound) Plyoball for 30 s without pain
  - Single-leg step down for 30 s (20 cm [8 inches] step)
- Satisfactory score on the KJOC throwers' assessment

After completion of a long-toss program, pitchers will progress to phase II of the throwing program, throwing off a mound.[80] In phase II the number of throws, intensity, and type of pitch are purposefully progressed to gradually increase the stress placed on the elbow and shoulder joints. Pitcher's begins at 50% intensity and gradually progress to 75%, 90%, and 100% over a 4- to 6-week period. Breaking balls are initiated once the pitcher can throw 40 to 50 pitches at 80% intensity without symptoms. Successful completion of the throwing program from the mound prepares the athlete to return to unrestricted throwing.

TRIP TO THE MOUND

Phase II Off The Mound Interval Throwing Program

After the completion of phase I of the ITP and the athlete can throw to the prescribed distance without pain, the athlete will be ready for throwing off the mound or return to his respective position. At this point, full strength and confidence should be restored in the athlete's arm. Just as the advancement to this point has been gradual and progressive, the return to unrestricted throwing must follow the same principles. A pitcher should first throw only fast ball at 50%, progressing to 75% and 100%. At this time, the athlete may start more stressful pitches such as breaking balls. The position player should simulate a game situation, again progressing at 50% to 75% to 100%. Once again, if an athlete has increased pain, particularly at the joint, the throwing program should be backed off and readvanced as tolerated, under the direction of the rehabilitation team.

Summary: In using the ITP in conjunction with a structured rehabilitation program, the athlete should be able to return to full competition status, minimizing any chance of reinjury. The program and its progression should be modified to meet the specific needs of each individual athlete. A comprehensive program consisting of a maintenance strength and flexibility program, appropriate warm-up and cool-down procedures, proper pitching mechanics, and progressive throwing and batting will assist the baseball player in returning safely to competition.

Stage 1: Fastballs Only

Step 1: Interval throwing (use interval throwing to 120′ phase as warm-up)

15 Throws off mound 50%

Step 2: Interval throwing

30 throws off mound 50%

Step 3: Interval throwing

45 throws off mound 50%

Step 4: Interval throwing

60 throws off mound 50%

Step 5: Interval throwing (use speed gun to aid in effort control)

70 throws off mound 50%

Step 6: 45 throws off mound 50%

30 throws off mound 75%

Step 7: 30 throws off mound 50%

45 throws off mound 75%

Step 8: 65 throws off mound 75%

10 throws off mound 50%

All throwing off the mound should be done in the presence of your pitching coach to stress proper throwing mechanics.

Stage 2: Fastballs Only

Step 9: 60 throws off mound 75%

15 throws in batting practice

Step 10: 50 to 60 throws off mound 75%

30 throws in batting practice

Step 11: 45 to 50 throws off mound 75%

45 throws in batting practice

Stage 3

Step 12: 30 throws off mound 75% warm-up

15 throws off mound 50% breaking balls

45 to 60 throws in batting practice (fastball only)

Step 13: 30 throws off mound 75%

30 breaking balls 75%

30 throws in batting practice

Step 14: 30 throws off mound 75%

60 to 90 throws in batting practice (gradually increase breaking balls)

Step 15: Simulated game: Progressing by 15 throws per workout (pitch count)

SPECIFIC NONOPERATIVE REHABILITATION GUIDELINES

Ulnar Collateral Ligament Injury

The initial treatment of UCL injury is generally nonoperative[81] and consists of rest from the overhead sport, anti-inflammatory medications, and rehabilitation. Rettig et al[81] report that about half of these individuals can be treated successfully without surgery and are able to return to the same level of athletic activity. The use of platelet-rich plasma (PRP) with nonoperative management has also been proposed as a viable option.[73] When PRP is incorporated in the treatment approach, there is an initial rest period of 2 weeks when only physical agents and gentle passive ROM exercises are allowed. This is followed by the initiation of more comprehensive physical therapy management with a gradual progression of activity estimated to last around 10 to 15 weeks in total duration.[73] Podesta et al[73] reported an 88% rate of return to play without symptoms following the use of PRP in combination with supervised physical therapy.

Our nonoperative rehabilitation program is outlined in Table 38.6. ROM is initially permitted in a nonpainful arc, usually from 10° to 100°, to allow for a decrease in inflammation and the appropriate alignment of collagen tissue as the UCL heals. A hinged ROM brace is used to restrict motion and prevent valgus loading during the acute phase of rehabilitation. Additionally, it may be beneficial to rest the UCL immediately following an initial painful episode of throwing to prevent additional harmful stresses on the ligament. Isometric exercises are performed for the shoulder, elbow, and wrist to prevent muscular atrophy. Ice and anti-inflammatory medications are prescribed to control pain and inflammation.

ROM of both flexion and extension is gradually increased by 5° to 10° per week during the second phase of treatment with full ROM achieved by 3 to 4 weeks after injury. Pain-free elbow flexion/extension

TABLE 38.6 Conservative Treatment After Ulnar Collateral Sprains of the Elbow

I. Immediate Motion Phase (Weeks 0 Through 2)

Goals:
• Increase range of motion
• Promote healing of ulnar collateral ligament
• Retard muscular atrophy
• Decrease pain and inflammation
ROM:
  1. Brace (optional) nonpainful ROM (20°-90°)
  2. AAROM, PROM elbow and wrist (nonpainful range)
Exercises:
  1. Isometrics—wrist and elbow musculature
  2. Shoulder strengthening (no external rotation strengthening)
Ice and compression

II. Intermediate Phase (Weeks 3 Through 6)

Goals:
• Increase range of motion
• Improve strength/endurance
• Decrease pain and inflammation
• Promote stability
ROM:
  Gradually increase motion 00-135 inches (increase 100 per week)
Exercises:
  Initiate isotonic exercises: wrist curls, wrist extensions pronation/supination, biceps/triceps dumbbells: external rotation, deltoid, supraspinatus, rhomboids, internal rotation
Ice and compression

III. Advanced Phase (Weeks 6 and 7 Through 12 and 14)

Criteria to progress:
  1. Full range of motion
  2. No pain or tenderness
  3. No increase in laxity
  4. Strength 4/5 of elbow flexor/extensor
Goals:
• Increase strength, power, and endurance
• Improve neuromuscular control
• Initiate high-speed exercise drills
Exercises:
  Initiate exercises: tubing, shoulder program, Thrower's Ten program, biceps/triceps program, supination/pronation, wrist extension/flexion, plyometrics throwing drills

IV. Return to Activity Phase (Weeks 12 Through 14)

Criteria to progress to return to throwing:
  1. Full nonpainful ROM
  2. No increase in laxity
  3. Isokinetic test fulfills criteria
  4. Satisfactory clinical examination
Exercises:
  1. Initiate interval throwing
  2. Continue Thrower's Ten program
  3. Continue plyometrics

motion is encouraged to assist in collagen formation and alignment. Valgus loading at the elbow should be controlled for the first 4 to 6 weeks to control stress on the UCL. Rhythmic stabilization exercises are initiated to develop dynamic stabilization and neuromuscular control of the upper extremity. As dynamic stability is advanced, isotonic exercises are incorporated for the entire upper extremity.

The advanced strengthening phase is usually initiated at 6 to 7 weeks postinjury. During this phase, the athlete is progressed to the Thrower's Ten isotonic strengthening program and plyometric exercises are slowly incorporated. An ITP is initiated once the athlete regains full motion, exhibits adequate strength, and has dynamic stability of the elbow. The athlete can return to competition following the asymptomatic completion of the appropriate interval sport program. If symptoms reoccur during the ITP, it is usually at longer distances, greater intensities, or with throwing off the mound. If symptoms persist and unrestricted throwing is not attained, the athlete should be reassessed, and surgical intervention should be considered.

Medial Epicondylitis and Flexor-Pronator Tendinitis

Medial epicondylitis occurs due to changes within the flexor-pronator musculotendinous unit. The underlying pathology is a microscopic or macroscopic tear within the flexor carpi radialis or pronator teres near the origin on the medial epicondyle. Ulnar neuropathy has been reported in 25% to 60% of athletes with medial epicondylitis.[40,65,93] Overhead throwers who exhibit flexor-pronator tendinitis may have an associated UCL injury. Tendinitis can develop as a secondary pathology in the throwing athlete because of the underlying increased laxity within the UCL. Therefore, before initiating a rehabilitation program for medial epicondylitis, it is important that the UCL be accurately examined for the presence of any instability, lesion, or pathology. It is also beneficial to determine the number of episodes and chronicity of medial epicondylar complaints. Athletes with long histories of medial epicondylitis may exhibit chronic degeneration in the form of tendinosis or tendinopathy, not true tendonitis. Conversely, patients with first-time episodes probably exhibit paratendonitis or tendinitis. The treatment is significantly different for these 2 classifications of pathology. Nirschl et al[66] reported 4 stages of epicondylitis beginning with an early inflammatory reaction followed by angiofibroblastic degeneration, leading to structural failure and ultimately fibrosis or calcification. The appropriate treatment of tendinopathy must focus on a careful examination to determine the exact pathology present and address the correct stage of the involved tissue. Often an athlete is diagnosed with "tendonitis" only later to discover that the tendon had already undergone a degenerative process and evolved to tendonosis.[53,65,67] The differential diagnosis of tendonosis is made through MRI, ultrasound examination, or tissue biopsy.

The nonoperative approach used in the treatment of epicondylitis (ie, tendinitis and/or paratendonitis) focuses on diminishing pain and inflammation combined with the gradual improvement of muscular strength (Table 38.7). The primary goals of rehabilitation are to control the applied loads and create an environment that stimulates a healing response. The initial treatment consists of warm whirlpool, iontophoresis, stretching, and light strengthening exercises. Therapeutic modalities are often utilized by rehabilitation specialists to decrease inflammation and promote healing. There is very limited evidence to support the use of these modalities in isolation. Common modalities may include cold laser therapy, class IV deep tissue laser, iontophoresis, ultrasound, electrical stimulation, nitric oxide, and extracorporeal shockwave therapy.

TABLE 38.7 Epicondylitis Rehabilitation Protocol

Phase I Acute Phase
Goals: • Decrease inflammation   • Promote tissue healing   • Retard muscular atrophy   Cryotherapy   Whirlpool   Stretching to increase flexibility wrist extension/flexion elbow extension/flexion forearm supination/pronation   Isometrics wrist extension/flexion elbow extension/flexion forearm supination/pronation   HVGS   Phonophoresis   Friction massage   Iontophoresis (with anti-inflammatory, ie, dexamethasone)   Avoid painful movements (ie, gripping, etc)

(continued)

TABLE 38.7 Epicondylitis Rehabilitation Protocol   (continued)

Phase II Subacute Phase
Goals: • Improve flexibility   • Increase muscular strength/endurance   • Increase functional activities/return to function   Exercises: 1. Emphasize concentric/eccentric strengthening   2. Concentration on involved muscle group   3. Wrist extension/flexion   4. Forearm pronation/supination   5. Elbow flexion/extension   6. Initiate shoulder strengthening (if deficiencies are noted)   7. Continue flexibility exercises   8. May use counterforce brace   9. Continue use of cryotherapy after exercise/function   10. Gradual return to stressful activities   11. Gradually reinitiate once painful movements
Phase III Chronic Phase
Goals: • Improve muscular strength and endurance   • Maintain/enhance flexibility   • Gradual return to sport/high-level activities   Exercises: 1. Continue strengthening exercises (emphasize eccentric/concentric)   2. Continue to emphasize deficiencies in shoulder and elbow strength   3. Continue flexibility exercises   4. Gradually decrease use of counterforce brace   5. Use of cryotherapy as needed   6. Gradual return to sport activity   7. Equipment modification (grip size, string tension, playing surface)   8. Emphasize maintenance program

However, when used in combination with exercise, manual soft tissue interventions, and other modalities, studies have shown improved tissue quality and outcomes.[2,16,17,33-35,44,46,47,51,54,64,69,71,75,76,91,93-95]

The authors have utilized the disposable iontophoresis patch (Hybresis DJO Global, Vista, CA) successfully in the treatment of tendinitis in the throwing athlete. The patch is worn for 2 hours with dexamethasone applied. We have observed excellent results clinically, particularly when point tenderness can be narrowed to one specific location. The depth of penetration of dexamethasone when used in iontophoresis has been reported to range from 12 to 18 mm.[5,42] Gangarosa et al[41] reported a 1 to 3 cm depth of penetration of lidocaine during iontophoresis. High-voltage electrical stimulation and cryotherapy are used following treatment to decrease pain and postexercise inflammation. The athlete should also be cautioned against excessive gripping activities and to minimize repetitive stress during the treatment process.

Conversely, the treatment for tendonosis focuses on increasing blood flow and circulation to the involved area to promote tendon healing, collagen synthesis, and alignment. Modalities to promote a heating affect and improve blood flow such as class IV deep tissue laser,[16,33,54,91] moist heat, extracorporeal shockwave therapy,[9,51,93] instrumented assisted soft tissue mobilization, transverse friction massage, and dry needling[48,92] are utilized to promote tendon regeneration. Tendon loading by eccentric exercise and strength training has been shown to improve results in this patient population by increasing collagen synthesis[55] and realigning fiber orientation.[3,19,90] The use of pain stimulation or noxious stimulation is gaining popularity as a treatment before strength training to aide in the management of degenerative tissue. The primary goal of this modality is to produce pain at the site of the degenerative tissue encouraging the body to respond by releasing endorphins, which will block any pain response felt by the involved tissue. Once the pain has been reduced, the athlete will perform specific exercises designed to progressive load the tendon through eccentric contractions to produce collagen synthesis and collagen alignment. The authors of this chapter have found the use of pain stimulation to be extremely successful in the treatment of patellar and Achilles tendinopathies. Use of this treatment may be limited for the elbow because of the surrounding contractile tissues of the flexors and extensors that would become activated when the electrical stimulation intensity is increased.

Once the athlete's symptoms have subsided, an aggressive stretching and strengthening program with emphasis on high-load, low-repetition eccentric contractions is initiated. Wrist flexion and extension activities should be performed initially with the elbow flexed between 30° and 45°, progressing to full elbow extension as symptoms allow. The athlete is advanced to plyometric exercises and then into an ITP, as the criteria to advance to the return to activity phase are exhibited. Because poor mechanics are often a cause of this condition, an analysis of sport mechanics and proper supervision as the athlete progresses through the ITP are critical. If nonoperative treatment fails, then a surgical debridement of the necrotic tissue may be warranted.

PRP is a promising intervention for the treatment of chronic tendinopathy in which a small sample of the athlete's own blood is separated out and the platelet-rich layer is injected into the sight of injury. The goal of PRP treatments is to stimulate a regenerative response that has otherwise been difficult to elicit thus far. The proposed mechanism delivers humoral mediators and growth factors locally into the involved tissue to induce a healing response. PRP has the advantage of being minimally invasive, produces only a local tissue response, and avoids an inflammatory reaction. Some disadvantages may include the cost of treatment, lack of supporting evidence, and staffing time to withdraw the blood, spin it down, and reinject it into the site of pathology.

Early research on the clinical application of PRP to promote healing and adaptive responses is promising.[24,26,27,50,56,57,61,62,86,87] Mishra et al[61] showed significant benefits to PRP in patients with chronic lateral epicondylitis. Basic science and controlled studies have yet to truly surmise the efficacy of PRP as a treatment for elbow flexor-pronator tendinopathy.

Ulnar Neuropathy

There are numerous theories regarding the cause of ulnar neuropathy of the elbow in throwing athletes. Ulnar nerve changes can result from tensile forces, compressive forces, or nerve instability. Any one or combination of these mechanisms may be responsible for ulnar nerve symptoms.

A leading mechanism for tensile force on the ulnar nerve is valgus stress. This may be coupled with an ER-supination stress overload mechanism. The traction forces are further magnified when underlying valgus instability from UCL injury is present. Ulnar neuropathy is often a secondary pathology of UCL insufficiency. Compression of the ulnar nerve is often due to hypertrophy of the surrounding soft tissues or the presence of scar tissue. The nerve may also be trapped between the 2 heads of the flexor carpi ulnaris. Repetitive flexion and extension of the elbow with an unstable nerve can irritate or inflame the nerve. The nerve may sublux in and out of the groove or rest on the medial epicondyle rendering it vulnerable to direct trauma.

There are 3 stages of ulnar neuropathy.[4] The first stage includes an acute onset of radicular symptoms. The second stage is manifested by a recurrence of symptoms, as the athlete attempts to return to competition. The third stage is associated with persistent motor weakness and sensory changes. Once the athlete presents in the third stage of injury, conservative management may not be effective.

The nonoperative treatment of ulnar neuropathy focuses on diminishing ulnar nerve irritation, enhancing dynamic medial elbow joint stability, and gradually returning the athlete to competition. Nonsteroidal anti-inflammatory drugs are often prescribed, and rehabilitation includes iontophoresis disposable patch and cryotherapy. After the diagnosis of ulnar neuropathy, throwing athletes are instructed to discontinue throwing activities for at least 4 weeks, depending on the severity and chronicity of their symptoms. The use of a night splint with the elbow flexed to 45° may be beneficial to rest and calm down the irritated nerve. The athlete progresses through the immediate motion and intermediate phases of rehabilitation over the course of 4 to 6 weeks with emphasis placed on eccentric resistance exercises and dynamic stabilization drills. Plyometric exercises are utilized to facilitate further dynamic stabilization of the medial elbow. The athlete begins an ITP when full pain-free ROM and satisfactory muscle performance is exhibited without neurologic symptoms. The athlete may gradually return to play if neurologic symptoms do not recur, as they are progressed through the interval throwing process.[80]

Valgus Extension Overload

VEO occurs in repetitive sport activities, such as throwing, and is produced during the acceleration or deceleration phases as the olecranon wedges up against the medial olecranon fossa during elbow extension.[108]

This mechanism may result in osteophyte formation on the posteromedial olecranon and potentially loose bodies within the elbow joint. Repetitive extension stress from the triceps may further contribute to this injury. There is often a certain degree of underlying valgus laxity of the elbow in these athletes, further facilitating osteophyte formation through compression of the radiocapitellar joint and the posteromedial elbow.[6,13] Overhead athletes typically present with pain at the posteromedial aspect of the elbow that is exacerbated with forced elbow extension and valgus stress.

A conservative treatment approach is often attempted before considering surgical intervention. Initial treatment involves relieving the posterior elbow of pain and inflammation. The authors recommend the use of ice, class IV deep tissue laser, and iontophoresis to control inflammation. As symptoms subside and ROM normalizes, dynamic stabilization and strengthening exercises are initiated and progressively advanced. Emphasis is placed on improving eccentric strength of the elbow flexors to control the rapid extension that occurs at the elbow during athletics. Manual resistance exercises of concentric and eccentric elbow and wrist flexion are incorporated along with resisted elbow flexion with exercise tubing. The athlete's throwing mechanics should be carefully assessed to determine if mechanical faults are causing the VEO symptoms or if an underlying UCL instability exists.

Osteochondritis Dissecans

OCD of the elbow may develop owing to the valgus strain placed on the elbow joint during throwing, which produces not only medial tension but also a lateral compressive force.[12] This is observed as the capitellum of the humerus compresses against the radial head. Athletes often complain of lateral elbow pain upon palpation and valgus stress. Morrey[63] described a 3-stage classification characterizing the pathologic progression of OCD lesions. Stage 1 describes patients without evidence of subchondral displacement or fracture, whereas stage 2 lesions show evidence of subchondral detachment or articular cartilage fracture. Stage 3 lesions involve detached osteochondral fragments, resulting in intra-articular loose bodies. Nonsurgical treatment is attempted for stage 1 patients only and consists of relative rest and immobilization until elbow symptoms have resolved.

Nonoperative treatment includes 3 to 6 weeks of immobilization at 90° of elbow flexion. The splint or brace should be removed 3 to 4 times a day for ROM activities of the shoulder, elbow, and wrist. As symptoms resolve a strengthening program is initiated with isometric exercises. Isotonic exercises are included

after approximately 1 week of pain-free isometric exercise. Aggressive high-speed, eccentric, and plyometric exercises are progressively included to prepare the athlete for the start of an ITP.

If nonoperative treatment fails or evidence of loose bodies exist, surgical intervention including arthroscopic abrading and drilling of the lesion with fixation or removal of the loose body is indicated.[14,82,109] Long-term follow-up studies regarding the outcome of patients undergoing surgery to drill or reattach the lesions have not produced favorable results, suggesting that prevention and early detection of symptoms may be the best form of treatment.[14]

Little League Elbow

"Little League elbow" is a collective term used to describe a spectrum of medial epicondylar apophyseal injuries that ranges from microtrauma of the physis to fracture and displacement of the medial epicondyle through the apophysis. Pain of the medial elbow is common is adolescent throwers. The medial epicondyle physis is subject to repetitive tensile and valgus forces during both the cocking and acceleration phases of throwing. These forces may result in microtraumatic injury to the physis with potential fragmentation, hypertrophy, separation of the epiphysis, or avulsion of the medial epicondyle. Treatment varies based on the extent of injury.

In the absence of an avulsion, a rehabilitation program like the nonoperative treatment of UCL sprains is utilized. Emphasis is placed initially on the reduction of pain and inflammation along with the restoration of motion and strength. Strengthening exercises are performed in a gradual fashion, beginning with isometrics and progressing to light isotonic strengthening exercises. In young throwing athletes, we emphasize core, legs, and shoulder strengthening along with elbow and forearm exercises. Often these individuals exhibit poor core, hip, and scapular muscle control along with weak shoulder musculature. In addition, stretching exercises are performed to normalize shoulder ROM, especially into IR and horizontal adduction. No heavy lifting is permitted for 12 to 14 weeks. An ITP is initiated and advanced as tolerated once symptoms subside.

In the presence of a nondisplaced or minimally displaced avulsion, a brief period of immobilization for approximately 7 days is encouraged, followed by a gradual progression of ROM, flexibility, and strength exercises. An ITP is usually allowed at weeks 6 to 8. If the avulsion is displaced, an open reduction, internal fixation procedure may be required to appropriately address the lesion.

SPECIFIC POSTOPERATIVE REHABILITATION GUIDELINES

Ulnar Collateral Ligament Reconstruction

Surgical reconstruction of the UCL attempts to restore the stabilizing functions of the anterior bundle of the UCL.[9] Several types of surgical procedures to reconstruct the UCL exist, including the Jobe procedure,[49] the docking procedure,[31,83] and the DANE procedure.[11,13,30] At our center, the procedure that is used is a modified Jobe procedure in which a palmaris longus or gracilis graft is taken and passed in a figure 8 pattern through drill holes in the sublime tubercle of the ulna and the medial epicondyle.[45] A subcutaneous ulnar nerve transposition is also performed at the time of reconstruction.

The rehabilitation program we currently use after UCL reconstruction is based on the figure 8 surgical procedure with an ulnar nerve transposition (Table 38.8). Immediately after surgery, the athlete is placed in a posterior splint with the elbow immobilized at 90° of flexion. This splint is utilized for the first 7 days postoperatively to allow early healing of the UCL graft and fascial slings involved in the nerve transposition. The athlete can perform wrist ROM, gripping, and submaximal isometrics for the wrist and elbow during this time frame. After a week, the posterior splint is discontinued, and a hinged elbow ROM brace is initiated to protect the healing tissues from detrimental valgus stress (Figure 38.9). The brace is discontinued at the beginning of postoperative week 5.

Passive ROM activities are initiated immediately to decrease pain and slowly apply appropriate stress the healing tissues. Initially, the focus of rehabilitation is in obtaining full passive elbow extension while gradually progressing flexion. Elbow extension is encouraged early on to at least 15°, but if full extension is comfortably available and pain free, it is allowed. Bernas et al[15] demonstrated that there was 3% or less strain in both bands of the reconstructed ligament and approximately 1% strain for the anterior band of the UCL in full extension. The authors determined that in the immediate postoperative period, full elbow extension is safe and does not place excessive stress on the healing graft. Conversely, elbow flexion to 100° is allowed and should be brought along at about 10° per week until full ROM is achieved by 4 to 6 weeks after surgery.

Isometric exercises are progressed to include light resistive isotonic exercises at week 4 and to the full Thrower's Ten program by week 6 after surgery.

Focus is again placed on developing dynamic stabilization of the medial elbow. Owing to the anatomical orientation of the flexor carpi ulnaris and flexor digitorum superficialis overlaying the UCL, isotonic and stabilization activities for these muscles may assist the UCL in stabilizing valgus stress at the medial elbow.[25] We incorporate concentric and eccentric strengthening of these muscles beginning 4 to 5 weeks after surgery.

Aggressive exercises involving eccentric and plyometric contractions are included in the advanced phase, usually weeks 12 through 16. The Advanced Thrower's Ten program is initiated at week 12 after surgery. Two-hand plyometric drills are initiated at week 12, and one-hand drills, at week 14. An ITP is not permitted until at least 16 weeks postoperatively when the athlete can exhibit all the previously outlined criteria to begin throwing. In most cases, throwing from a mound is progressed within 4 to 6 weeks after the initiation of an ITP, and a return to competitive throwing begins at approximately 9 months after surgery.

Cain et al[18] reported on the outcome of UCL reconstruction of the elbow in 743 athletes during a 2-year minimum follow-up. The authors went on to report that UCL reconstruction with subcutaneous ulnar nerve transposition was found to be effective in correcting valgus elbow instability in the overhead athlete and allowed most athletes (83%) to return to previous or higher level of competition in less than 1 year. Major complications were noted in only 4% of the subjects.

The rehabilitation program after UCL reconstruction utilizing the docking procedure is slightly different. Dodson et al[31] advocated an elbow brace with ROM from 30° to 60° for the first 3 weeks then 15° to 90° at week 4 postoperatively. The athlete should obtain full ROM by 6 weeks after the surgery. Isotonic strengthening exercises are also initiated at week 6 to improve glenohumeral and scapulothoracic strength. Plyometric activities may be performed at approximately 10 weeks after the surgery to further stress the healing tissues in preparation for the ITP. The athlete may also incorporate heavier strengthening exercise utilizing machine weights at this time. A positional layer may begin a hitting program at 12 weeks postoperatively, which includes first hitting off a tee, progressing to soft-toss throws and finally formal batting practice. The ITP is permitted at 4 months postoperatively and formal pitching is typically accomplished at 9 months after the surgery.

TABLE 38.8 Postoperative Rehabilitation Protocol After Ulnar Collateral Ligament Reconstruction Using Autogenous Palmaris Longus Graft (Accelerated ROM)

I. Immediate Postoperative Phase (Weeks 0-3)

Goals:
- Protect healing tissue
- Decrease pain/inflammation
- Retard muscular atrophy
- Protect graft site, allow healing

A. Postoperative week 1
  1. Brace: Posterior splint at 90° elbow flexion
  2. Range of motion: Wrist AROM extension/flexion immediately postoperative
  3. Elbow postoperative compression dressing (5-7 d)
  4. Wrist (graft site) compression dressing 7-10 d as needed
  5. Exercises:
      a. Gripping exercises
      b. Wrist ROM
      c. Shoulder isometrics (no shoulder ER)
      d. Biceps isometrics
  6. Cryotherapy: To elbow joint and to graft site at wrist

B. Postoperative week 2
  1. Brace:
      a. Elbow ROM 15°-105° or tolerance
      b. Motion to tolerance
  2. Exercises:
      a. Continue all exercises listed earlier
      b. Elbow range of motion in brace (30°-105°)
      c. Initiate elbow extension isometrics
      d. Continue wrist ROM exercises
      e. Initiate light scar mobilization over distal incision (graft)
  3. Cryotherapy: Continue ice to elbow and graft site

C. Postoperative week 3
  1. Brace:
      a. Elbow ROM 5°/10° to 115°/120°
      b. Motion to tolerance
  2. Exercises:
      a. Continue all exercises listed earlier
      b. Elbow ROM in brace
      c. Initiate active ROM wrist and elbow (no resistance)
      d. Initiate light wrist flexion stretching
      e. Initiate active ROM shoulder:
          i. Full can
          ii. Lateral raises
          iii. ER/IR tubing
          iv. Elbow flexion/extension
      f. Initiate light scapular strengthening exercises
      g. May incorporate bicycle for lower extremity strength and endurance

II. Intermediate Phase (Weeks 4-7)

Goals:
- Gradual increase to full ROM
- Promote healing of repaired tissue
- Regain and improve muscular strength
- Restore full function of graft site

TABLE 38.8 Postoperative Rehabilitation Protocol After Ulnar Collateral Ligament Reconstruction Using Autogenous Palmaris Longus Graft (Accelerated ROM) *(continued)*

A. Week 4
    1. Brace:
        a. Elbow ROM 0°-135°
        b. Motion to tolerance
    2. Exercises:
        a. Begin light resistance exercises for arm (1 lb)
            i. Wrist curls, extensions, pronation, supination
            ii. Elbow extension/flexion
        b. Progress shoulder program emphasize rotator cuff and scapular strengthening
        c. Initiate shoulder strengthening with light dumbbells
B. Week 5
    1. ROM: Elbow ROM 0°-135°
    2. Discontinue brace
    3. Maintain full ROM
    4. Continue all exercises: Progress all shoulder and UE exercises (progress weight 1 lb)
C. Week 6
    1. AROM: 0°-145° without brace or full ROM
    2. Exercises:
        a. Initiate Thrower's Ten program
        b. Progress elbow strengthening exercises
        c. Initiate shoulder external rotation strengthening
        d. Progress shoulder program
D. Week 7
    1. Progress Thrower's Ten program (progress weights)
    2. Initiate PNF diagonal patterns (light)

III. Advanced Strengthening Phase (Weeks 8-14)

Goals:
- Increase strength, power, endurance
- Maintain full elbow ROM
- Gradually initiate sporting activities

A. Week 8
    1. Exercises:
        a. Initiate eccentric elbow flexion/extension
        b. Continue isotonic program: forearm and wrist
        c. Continue shoulder program—Thrower's Ten program
        d. Manual resistance diagonal patterns
        e. Initiate plyometric exercise program (2-hand plyos close to body only)
            i. Chest pass
            ii. Side throw close to body
        f. Continue stretching calf and hamstrings
B. Week 10
    1. Exercises:
        a. Continue all exercises listed earlier
        b. Program plyometrics to 2 hand drills away from body
            i. Side-to-side throws
            ii. Soccer throws
            iii. Side throws
C. Weeks 12-14
    1. Continue all exercises
    2. Initiate isotonic machines strengthening exercises (if desired)
        a. Bench press (seated)
        b. Lat pull down
    3. Initiate golf, swimming
    4. Initiate interval hitting program

(continued)

TABLE 38.8 Postoperative Rehabilitation Protocol After Ulnar Collateral Ligament Reconstruction Using Autogenous Palmaris Longus Graft (Accelerated ROM)   (continued)

IV. Return to Activity Phase (Weeks 14-32)

Goals:
  • Continue to increase strength, power, and endurance of upper extremity musculature
  • Gradual return to sport activities
A. Week 14
   1. Exercises:
     a. Continue strengthening program
     b. Emphasis on elbow and wrist strengthening and flexibility exercises
     c. Maintain full elbow ROM
     d. Initiate 1-hand plyometric throwing (stationary throws)
     e. Initiate 1-hand wall dribble
     f. Initiate 1-hand baseball throws into wall
B. Week 16
   1. Exercises:
     a. Initiate interval throwing program (phase I) (long-toss program)
     b. Continue Thrower's Ten program and plyos
     c. Continue to stretch before and after throwing
C. Weeks 22-24
   1. Exercises:
     a. Progress to phase II throwing (once successfully completed phase I)
D. Weeks 30-32
   1. Exercises:
     a. Gradually progress to competitive throwing/sports

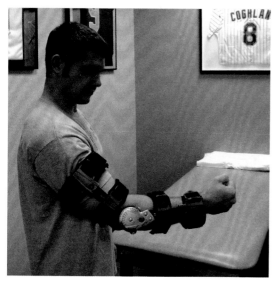

FIGURE 38.9 • Hinged elbow brace utilized postoperatively to protect the graft from deleterious valgus stresses.

Ulnar Collateral Ligament Repair With Internal Brace

Recent advances in surgical technology coupled with a desire to reduce the return to play time after UCL reconstruction have spurred a renewed interest in repair techniques for the UCL. A surgical procedure referred to as the UCL repair with internal brace (Internal Brace; Arthrex Inc.) was developed in part based on the work of Conway et al[22] and is reserved for specific types of UCL injury: partial or complete tears at the origin or insertion of the UCL with good ligament tissue and low-grade midsubstance partial UCL tears.[32] Reconstruction remains the most appropriate surgical option for athletes with chronic, attritional damage to the UCL and associated elbow joint instability.[13,18,22,32] Therefore, injured athletes with good joint stability and high-quality native ligament tissue are the ideal candidates for UCL repair with internal brace.

The surgical technique for UCL repair with internal brace was described in 2016 and includes augmentation of the native ligament repair with a spanning tape dipped in collagen (Internal Brace) that is anchored on each end of the native UCL.[32] Dugas et al[32] reported on the biomechanical analysis comparing gap formation upon valgus stress and maximal torque to failure of the augmented UCL repair and the typical modified Jobe UCL reconstruction technique. This study demonstrated a significantly greater resistance to gapping with valgus stress with the UCL repair (mean ± SD: 0.35 ± 0 16 mm) compared with UCL reconstruction (0.53 ± 0.23 mm). The results of this study suggest that the augmented UCL repair technique replicates failure strength of the traditional UCL reconstruction and provides greater elbow stability at low cyclic loads. When extrapolated to patients undergoing elbow surgery at an early age, this may represent a viable treatment option for long-term elbow stability.

Rehabilitation after UCL repair with internal brace follows a similar course to that described for reconstruction of the UCL, with a few significant differences, most notably the amount of time required to return to play after UCL repair with internal brace is approximately 5 months (7 months less) than after UCL reconstruction surgery (Table 38.9). The initial postoperative course is slightly different with the athlete placed in a ROM brace locked in 90° immediately after surgery. The ROM progression is slightly faster than that seen after UCL reconstruction with full ROM generally obtained about 1 week sooner after UCL repair with internal brace. In conjunction with quicker ROM progression, light concentric shoulder and elbow strengthening exercises are initiated 10 days to 2 weeks after surgery and the Thrower's Ten program started at week 3. Generally, the athlete reaches the intermediate phase of rehabilitation 4 weeks after surgery and is in this phase until approximately week 8. The Advanced Thrower's Ten program is initiated between weeks 4 and 6, with 2-handed plyometric drills beginning 6 weeks after surgery and 1-handed drills 2 months postoperatively. The advanced strengthening phase spans 9 to 14 weeks with a focus on high-speed,

eccentric and plyometric resistive exercises. Resistive weight machine exercises are typically begun 10 weeks after surgery. An ITP is permitted at week 10 while an ITP for the overhead athlete is allowed at week 12 if the athlete is ready.[101,103,107] Athletes generally require 6 to 8 weeks to progress through the first phase of the ITP and begin throwing off the mound between 16 and 20 weeks after surgery. Return to competitive participation ranges from 20 to 28 weeks after surgery for UCL repair with internal brace.

At our center, 212 UCL repairs with internal brace have been performed thus far by one of the authors (JRD). Of these, 1-year follow-up data are available for 47 patients showing a 98% return to preinjury level. Seventy-five percent of the patients were baseball players exhibiting an average Kerlan-Jobe Orthopaedic Clinic Overhead Athlete Shoulder and Elbow score of 93.5%.

Ulnar Nerve Transposition

At our center, an ulnar nerve transposition is performed in a subcutaneous fashion using fascial slings. Caution is taken to not overstress the soft tissue structures involved with relocating the nerve while healing occurs.[99] The rehabilitation after an ulnar nerve transposition is outlined in Table 38.10. A posterior splint at 90° of elbow flexion is used for the first week postoperatively to prevent excessive extension ROM and tension on the healing fascial slings and ulnar nerve. The splint is discharged at

TABLE 38.9 Postoperative Rehabilitation After Ulnar Collateral Ligament Repair With Internal Brace

Phase I: Immediate Postoperative Phase (Week 1)

Goals:
    Protect healing tissue; reduce pain and inflammation; retard muscle atrophy; full wrist range of motion (ROM)
Day of surgery
    1. Elbow ROM brace locked at 90° for 7 d
    2. Passive ROM (PROM) wrist and hand
Post-op days 1 and 2: Add
    1. Shoulder PROM: all directions
    2. Pendulum exercises
    3. Wrist flexor stretching
    4. Wrist extensor stretching
    5. Putty/griping exercises
Post-op days 3 through 7:
    1. Continue previous exercises
        a. External rotation (ER) and internal rotation (IR) PROM exercises
        b. Shoulder flexion to tolerance
    2. Add the following exercises:
        a. Shoulder isometrics: ER, IR, abduction, flexion, and extension
        b. Scapular strengthening (seated neuromuscular control drills with manual resistance)

(continued)

TABLE 38.9 Postoperative Rehabilitation After Ulnar Collateral Ligament Repair With Internal Brace   (continued)

II Acute Phase (Weeks 2-4)
Goals:
• Gradually restore elbow joint ROM
• Improve muscular strength and endurance
• Normalize joint arthrokinematics
Beginning week 2 (day 8):
1. Progress elbow ROM brace to 30°-110°
2. Begin elbow PROM and AAROM 30°-110°
3. Initiate AROM elbow
4. Initiate AROM shoulder joint
5. Scapular strengthening exercises
6. Progress to light isotonic strengthening at day 10
Beginning week 3:
1. Progress elbow ROM to 10°-125°
2. Initiate Thrower's Ten exercise program

III Intermediate Phase (Weeks 4-8)
Goals:
• Restore full elbow ROM
• Progress upper extremity strength
• Continue with functional progression
Beginning week 4:
1. Progress elbow ROM to 0°-145°
2. Progress to Advanced Thrower's Ten Program
3. Progress elbow and wrist strengthening exercises
4. Wrist flexion and elbow flexion movements against manual resistance
Beginning week 6:
1. Initiate 2-hand plyometrics
2. Discontinue brace at week 6
3. Prone planks
Beginning week 8:
1. Progress to 1-hand plyometrics
2. Continue with Advanced Thrower's Ten program
3. Side planks with ER strengthening

IV Advanced Phase (Weeks 9-14)
Criteria to progress to advanced phase:
1. Full nonpainful ROM
2. No pain or tenderness
3. Isokinetic test that fulfills criteria to throw
4. Satisfactory clinical exam
5. Completion of rehab phases without difficulty
Goals:
• Advanced strengthening exercises
• Initiate interval throwing program
• Gradual return to throwing
Beginning week 9:
1. Continue all strengthening exercises
2. Advanced Thrower's Ten program
3. Plyometrics program (1- and 2-hand program)
Beginning week 10:
1. Seated chest press machine
2. Initiate interval hitting program at week 10
3. Seated rowing
4. Biceps/triceps strengthening

TABLE 38.9 Postoperative Rehabilitation After Ulnar Collateral Ligament Repair With Internal Brace   (continued)

Beginning weeks 11-16:
  1. Initiate interval throwing program phase I—long toss (week 12)
  2. Continue all exercises as in weeks 9-10
Beginning weeks 16-20:
  1. Initiate interval throwing phase II (off the mound) when phase I is complete and athlete is ready
  2. Continue Advanced Thrower's Ten program
  3. Continue plyometrics
  4. Continue ROM and stretching programs

V Return to Play Phase (Weeks 20+):

Goals:
  • Gradual return to competitive throwing
  • Continue all exercises and stretches
Week 20+:
  1. Initiate gradual return to competitive throwing
  2. Perform dynamic warm-ups and stretches
  3. Continue Thrower's Ten program
  4. Return to competition when athlete is ready (physician decision)
Note: Each athlete may progress through ITP at different rates/pace
       Should complete 0-90 feet within 3 wk of starting it and complete 120 feet within 8 wk, then begin mound program

TABLE 38.10 Postoperative Rehabilitation Following Ulnar Nerve Transposition

Phase I. Immediate Postoperative Phase (Weeks 0-1)

Goals:
  • Allow soft tissue healing of relocated nerve
  • Decrease pain and inflammation
  • Retard muscular atrophy
A. Week 1
  1. Posterior splint at 900 elbow flexion with wrist free for motion (sling for comfort)
  2. Compression dressing
  3. Exercises such as gripping exercises, wrist ROM, and shoulder isometrics
B. Week 2
  1. Remove posterior splint for exercise and bathing
  2. Progress elbow ROM (PROM 150-1200)
  3. Initiate elbow and wrist isometrics
  4. Continue shoulder isometrics

Phase II. Intermediate Phase (Weeks 3-7)

Goals:
  • Restore full pain-free range of motion
  • Improve strength, power, and endurance of upper extremity musculature
  • Gradually increase functional demands
A. Week 3
  1. Discontinue posterior splint
  2. Progress elbow ROM, emphasize full extension
  3. Initiate flexibility exercise for wrist extension/flexion, forearm supination/pronation, and elbow extension/flexion
  4. Initiate strengthening exercises for wrist extension/flexion, forearm supination/pronation, elbow extensors/flexors, and a shoulder program
B. Week 6
  1. Continue all exercises listed earlier
  2. Initiate light sport activities

(continued)

TABLE 38.10 Postoperative Rehabilitation Following Ulnar Nerve Transposition   (continued)

Phase III. Advanced Strengthening Phase (Weeks 8-12)

Goals:
  • Increase strength, power, endurance
  • Gradually initiate sporting activities
A. Week 8
  1. Initiate eccentric exercise program
  2. Initiate plyometric exercise drills
  3. Continue shoulder and elbow strengthening and flexibility exercises
  4. Initiate interval throwing program

Phase IV. Return to Activity Phase (Weeks 12-16)

Goals:
  • Gradually return to sporting activities
A. Week 12
  1. Return to competitive throwing
  2. Continue Thrower's Ten exercise program

the beginning of week 2 and light ROM activities are initiated. Full ROM is usually restored by 3 to 4 weeks after surgery. Gentle isotonic strengthening is begun during week 3 to 4 and progressed to the full Thrower's Ten program by 4 to 6 weeks after surgery. Aggressive strengthening including eccentric, Advanced Thrower's Ten, and plyometric training is incorporated at week 8 and an ITP at week 8 to 9, if all the criteria to begin throwing is met. A return to competition usually occurs between weeks 12 and 16 postoperatively.

Posterior Olecranon Osteophyte Excision

Surgical excision of posterior olecranon osteophytes is performed arthroscopically using an osteotome or motorized burr. Approximately 5 to 10 mm of the olecranon tip is removed concomitantly, and a motorized burr is used to contour the coronoid, olecranon tip and fossa to prevent further impingement with extreme flexion and extension.[59] Caution is exercised not to remove too much bone and destabilize the elbow, resulting in increased loads on the UCL during forceful throwing.[8]

The rehabilitation program after arthroscopic posterior olecranon osteophyte excision is slightly more conservative in restoring full elbow extension secondary to postsurgical pain. ROM is progressed by athlete tolerance, but by 10 days postsurgery, the athlete should exhibit at least 15° to 105°/110° of ROM, and 5° to 10° to 115° by day 14. Full ROM (0°-145°) is typically restored by 20 to 25 days postsurgery. The rate of ROM progression is most often limited by osseous pain and synovial joint inflammation, usually located at the top of the olecranon.

The strengthening program used after olecranon osteophyte excision follows a similar course to the previously discussed progression. Isometrics are performed for the first 10 to 14 days and isotonic strengthening from week 2 to 6. Initially, especially during the first 2 weeks, forceful triceps contractions may produce posterior elbow pain. If this is present, it should be avoided or at a minimum the force produced by the triceps muscle reduced to pain-free levels. The full Thrower's Ten program is initiated by week 6. An ITP is included by weeks 10 to 12. The rehabilitation focus is like the nonoperative treatment of VEO. Emphasis is placed on eccentric control of the elbow flexors and dynamic stabilization of the medial elbow.

Andrews and Timmerman[11] reported on the outcome of elbow surgery in 72 professional baseball players. Of these athletes, 65% exhibited a posterior olecranon osteophyte and 25% of the athletes who underwent an isolated olecranon excision later required an UCL reconstruction.[11] This may suggest that subtle medial instability may accelerate osteophyte formation.

MANAGER'S TIPS

- The elbow joint is a common site of injury in athletes, especially the overhead athlete
- In the overhead throwing athlete, injuries are usually a result of the repetitive microtraumatic stress imparted during the act of throwing. Rehabilitation of the elbow, whether postinjury or postsurgery, must follow a progressive and sequential order to ensure that healing tissues are not overstressed, and the athlete is returned to sport participation as efficiently as possible

- The rehabilitation program should limit immobilization and achieve full ROM early, especially elbow extension and progressively restore strength, power, and neuromuscular control while gradually incorporating sport-specific activities essential to successfully return the athletes to their previous level of competition as quickly and safely as possible
- The rehabilitation of the elbow must include interventions for the entire kinetic chain (scapula, shoulder, hand, core/hips and legs) to facilitate the athletes' ability to return to high-level participation in throwing

REFERENCES

1. Akeson WH, Amiel D, Woo SL. Immobility effects on synovial joints the pathomechanics of joint contracture. *Biorheology*. 1980;17(1-2):95-110.

2. Alfredson H. Chronic midportion Achilles tendinopathy: an update on research and treatment. *Clin Sports Med*. 2003;22(4):727-741.

3. Alfredson H, Pietila T, Jonsson P, Lorentzon R. Heavy-load eccentric calf muscle training for the treatment of chronic Achilles tendinosis. *Am J Sports Med*. 1998;26(3):360-366.

4. Alley RM, Pappas AM. Acute and performance related injuries of the elbow. In: Pappas AM, ed. *Upper Extremity Injuries in the Athlete*. New York: Churchill Livingstone; 1995:339-364.

5. Anderson CR, Morris RL, Boeh SD, Panus PC, Sembrowich WL. Effects of iontophoresis current magnitude and duration on dexamethasone deposition and localized drug retention. *Phys Ther*. 2003;83(2):161-170.

6. Anderson K. Elbow arthritis and removal of loose bodies and spurs and techniques for restoration of motion. In: Altchek DW, Andrews JR, eds. *The Athlete's Elbow*. Philadelphia: Lippincott, Williams & Wilkins; 2001:219-230.

7. Andrews JR, Craven WM. Lesions of the posterior compartment of the elbow. *Clin Sports Med*. 1991;10(3):637-652.

8. Andrews JR, Heggland EJ, Fleisig GS, Zheng N. Relationship of ulnar collateral ligament strain to amount of medial olecranon osteotomy. *Am J Sports Med*. 2001;29(6):716-721.

9. Andrews JR, Jelsma RD, Joyse ME, Timmerman LA. Open surgical procedures for injuries of the elbow in throwers. *Op Tech Sports Med*. 1996;4(2):109-113.

10. Andrews JR, Jobe FW. Valgus extension overload in the pitching elbow. In: Andrews JR, Zarins B, Carson WB, eds. *Injuries to the Throwing Arm*. Philadelphia: Saunders; 1985:250-257.

11. Andrews JR, Timmerman LA. Outcome of elbow surgery in professional baseball players. *Am J Sports Med*. 1995;23(4):407-413.

12. Andrews JR, Whiteside JA. Common elbow problems in the athlete. *J Orthop Sports Phys Ther*. 1993;17(6):289-295.

13. Azar FM, Andrews JR, Wilk KE, Groh D. Operative treatment of ulnar collateral ligament injuries of the elbow in athletes. *Am J Sports Med*. 2000;28(1):16-23.

14. Bauer M, Jonsson K, Josefsson PO, Linden B. Osteochondritis dissecans of the elbow. A long-term follow-up study. *Clin Orthop Relat Res*. 1992(284):156-160.

15. Bernas GA, Ruberte Thiele RA, Kinnaman KA, Hughes RE, Miller BS, Carpenter JE. Defining safe rehabilitation for ulnar collateral ligament reconstruction of the elbow: a biomechanical study. *Am J Sports Med*. 2009;37(12):2392-2400.

16. Bjordal JM, Lopes-Martins RA, Iversen VV. A randomised, placebo controlled trial of low level laser therapy for activated Achilles tendinitis with microdialysis measurement of peritendinous prostaglandin E2 concentrations. *Br J Sports Med*. 2006;40(1):76-80 [discussion 76-80].

17. Borsa PA, Larkin KA, True JM. Does phototherapy enhance skeletal muscle contractile function and postexercise recovery? A systematic review. *J Athl Train*. 2013;48:57-67.

18. Cain EL Jr, Andrews JR, Dugas JR, et al. Outcome of ulnar collateral ligament reconstruction of the elbow in 1281 athletes: results in 743 athletes with minimum 2-year follow-up. *Am J Sports Med*. 2010;38(12):2426-2434.

19. Clement DB, Taunton JE, Smart GW. Achilles tendinitis and peritendinitis: etiology and treatment. *Am J Sports Med*. 1984;12(3):179-184.

20. Conte SA, Fleisig GS, Dines JS, et al. Prevalence of ulnar collateral ligament surgery in professional baseball players. *Am J Sports Med*. 20: 1-6, 2015.

21. Conte S, Requa RK, Garrick JG. Disability days in major league baseball. *Am J Sports Med*. 29(4):431-436, 2001.

22. Conway JE, Jobe FW, Glousman RE, Pink M. Medial instability of the elbow in throwing athletes: treatment by repair or reconstruction of the ulnar collateral ligament. *J Bone Joint Surg Am*. 1992;74:67-83.

23. Coutts RD, Toth C, Kaita JH. The role of continuous passive motion in the rehabilitation of the total knee patient. In: Hungerford DS, Krackow KA, Kenna RV, eds. *Total Knee Arthroplasty: A Comprehensive Approach*. Baltimore: Williams and Wilkins; 1984:126-132.

24. Creaney L, Hamilton B. Growth factor delivery methods in the management of sports injuries: the state of play. *Br J Sports Med*. 2008;42(5):314-320.

25. Davidson PA, Pink M, Perry J, Jobe FW. Functional anatomy of the flexor pronator muscle group in relation to the medial collateral ligament of the elbow. *Am J Sports Med*. 1995;23(2):245-250.

26. de Mos M, Koevoet W, van Schie HT, et al. In vitro model to study chondrogenic differentiation in tendinopathy. *Am J Sports Med.* 2009;37(6):1214-1222.

27. de Mos M, van der Windt AE, Jahr H, et al. Can platelet-rich plasma enhance tendon repair? A cell culture study. *Am J Sports Med.* 2008;36(6):1171-1178.

28. Dehne E, Torp RP. Treatment of joint injuries by immediate mobilization. Based upon the spinal adaptation concept. *Clin Orthop Relat Res.* 1971;77:218-232.

29. Dillman CJ, Smutz P, Werner S. Valgus extension overload in baseball pitching. *Med Sci Sports Exerc.* 1991;23:S135.

30. Dines JS, ElAttrache NS, Conway JE, Smith W, Ahmad CS. Clinical outcomes of the DANE TJ technique to treat ulnar collateral ligament insufficiency of the elbow. *Am J Sports Med.* 2007;35(12): 2039-2044.

31. Dodson CC, Thomas A, Dines JS, Nho SJ, Williams RJ III, Altchek DW. Medial ulnar collateral ligament reconstruction of the elbow in throwing athletes. *Am J Sports Med.* 2006;34(12):1926-1932.

32. Dugas JR, Walters BL, Beason DP, Fleisig GS, Chronister JE. Biomechanical comparison of ulnar collateral ligament repair with internal bracing versus modified Jobe reconstruction. *Am J Sports Med.* 2016;44(3):735-741.

33. England S, Farrell AJ, Coppock JS, Struthers G, Bacon PA. Low power laser therapy of shoulder tendonitis. *Scand J Rheumatol.* 1989;18(6):427-431.

34. Enwemeka CS. The effects of therapeutic ultrasound on tendon healing. A biomechanical study. *Am J Phys Med Rehabil.* 1989;68(6):283-287.

35. Enwemeka CS. Inflammation, cellularity, and fibrillogenesis in regenerating tendon: implications for tendon rehabilitation. *Phys Ther.* 1989;69(10): 816-825.

36. Fleisig GS, Barrentine SW, Escamilla RF, Andrews JR. Biomechanics of overhand throwing with implications for injuries. *Sports Med.* 1996;21(6):421-437.

37. Fleisig GS, Bolt B, Fortenbaugh D, Wilk KE, Andrews JR. Biomechanical comparison of baseball pitching and long-toss: implications for training and rehabilitation. *J Orthop Sports Phys Ther.* 2011;41(5):296-303.

38. Fleisig GS, Escamilla RF. Biomechanics of the elbow in the throwing athlete. *Op Tech Sports Med.* 1996;4(2):62-68.

39. Ford GM, Genuerio J, Kinkartz J, Githens T, Noonan T. Return-to-play outcomes in professional baseball players after medial ulnar collateral ligament injuries: comparison of operative versus nonoperative treatment based on magnetic resonance imaging findings. *Am J Sports Med.* 2016;44(3):723-728.

40. Gabel GT, Morrey BF. Operative treatment of medial epicondylitis. Influence of concomitant ulnar neuropathy at the elbow. *J Bone Joint Surg Am.* 1995;77(7):1065-1069.

41. Gangarosa LP Sr, Ozawa A, Ohkido M, Shimomura Y, Hill JM. Iontophoresis for enhancing penetration of dermatologic and antiviral drugs. *J Dermatol.* 1995;22(11):865-875.

42. Glass JM, Stephen RL, Jacobson SC. The quantity and distribution of radiolabeled dexamethasone delivered to tissue by iontophoresis. *Int J Dermatol.* 1980;19(9):519-525.

43. Green DP, McCoy H. Turnbuckle orthotic correction of elbow-flexion contractures after acute injuries. *J Bone Joint Surg Am.* 1979;61(7):1092-1095.

44. Gum SL, Reddy GK, Stehno-Bittel L, Enwemeka CS. Combined ultrasound, electrical stimulation, and laser promote collagen synthesis with moderate changes in tendon biomechanics. *Am J Phys Med Rehabil.* 1997;76(4):288-296.

45. Haggmark T, Eriksson E. Cylinder or mobile cast brace after knee ligament surgery. A clinical analysis and morphologic and enzymatic studies of changes in the quadriceps muscle. *Am J Sports Med.* 1979;7(1):48-56.

46. Harvey W, Dyson M, Pond JB, Grahame R. The stimulation of protein synthesis in human fibroblasts by therapeutic ultrasound. *Rheumatol Rehabil.* 1975;14(4):237.

47. Jackson BA, Schwane JA, Starcher BC. Effect of ultrasound therapy on the repair of Achilles tendon injuries in rats. *Med Sci Sports Exerc.* 1991;23(2):171-176.

48. James SL, Ali K, Pocock C, et al. Ultrasound guided dry needling and autologous blood injection for patellar tendinosis. *Br J Sports Med.* 2007;41(8):518-521 [discussion 522].

49. Jobe FW, Stark H, Lombardo SJ. Reconstruction of the ulnar collateral ligament in athletes. *J Bone Joint Surg Am.* 1986;68(8):1158-1163.

50. Kajikawa Y, Morihara T, Sakamoto H, et al. Platelet-rich plasma enhances the initial mobilization of circulation-derived cells for tendon healing. *J Cell Physiol.* 2008;215(3):837-845.

51. Ko JY, Chen HS, Chen LM. Treatment of lateral epicondylitis of the elbow with shock waves. *Clin Orthop Relat Res.* 2001(387):60-67.

52. Kottke FJ, Pauley DL, Ptak RA. The rationale for prolonged stretching for correction of shortening of connective tissue. *Arch Phys Med Rehabil.* 1966;47(6):345-352.

53. Kraushaar BS, Nirschl RP. Tendinosis of the elbow (tennis elbow). Clinical features and findings of histological, immunohistochemical, and electron microscopy studies. *J Bone Joint Surg Am.* 1999;81(2):259-278.

54. Lam LK, Cheing GL. Effects of 904-nm low-level laser therapy in the management of lateral epicondylitis: a randomized controlled trial. *Photomed Laser Surg.* 2007;25(2):65-71.

55. Langberg H, Ellingsgaard H, Madsen T, et al. Eccentric rehabilitation exercise increases peritendinous type I collagen synthesis in humans with Achilles tendinosis. *Scand J Med Sci Sports.* 2007;17(1):61-66.

56. Lyras D, Kazakos K, Verettas D, et al. Immunohistochemical study of angiogenesis after local administration of platelet-rich plasma in a patellar tendon defect. *Int Orthop*. 2010;34(1):143-148.

57. Lyras DN, Kazakos K, Verettas D, et al. The effect of platelet-rich plasma gel in the early phase of patellar tendon healing. *Arch Orthop Trauma Surg*. 2009;129(11):1577-1582.

58. Maitland GD. *Vertebral Manipulation*. 4th ed. London, Boston: Butterworth; 1977.

59. Martin SD, Baumgarten TE. Elbow injuries in the throwing athlete: diagnosis and arthroscopic treatment. *Op Tech Sports Med*. 1996;4(2):100.

60. McClure PW, Blackburn LG, Dusold C. The use of splints in the treatment of joint stiffness: biologic rationale and an algorithm for making clinical decisions. *Phys Ther*. 1994;74(12):1101-1107.

61. Mishra A, Pavelko T. Treatment of chronic elbow tendinosis with buffered platelet-rich plasma. *Am J Sports Med*. 2006;34(11):1774-1778.

62. Mishra A, Woodall J Jr, Vieira A. Treatment of tendon and muscle using platelet-rich plasma. *Clin Sports Med*. 2009;28(1):113-125.

63. Morrey BF. Osteochondritis dessicans. In: DeLee JC, Drez D, eds. *Orthopedic Sports Medicine*. Philadelphia: Saunders; 1994:908-912.

64. Murrell GA, Szabo C, Hannafin JA, et al. Modulation of tendon healing by nitric oxide. *Inflamm Res*. 1997;46(1):19-27.

65. Nirschl RP. Medial tennis elbow: surgical treatment. *Orthop Trans*. 1983;7:298.

66. Nirschl RP. Prevention and treatment of elbow and shoulder injuries in the tennis player. *Clin Sports Med*. 1988;7(2):289-308.

67. Nirschl RP, Ashman ES. Tennis elbow tendinosis (epicondylitis). *Instr Course Lect*. 2004;53:587-598.

68. Nirschl RP, Morrey BF. Rehabilitation. In: Morrey BF, ed. *The Elbow and its Disorders*. Philadelphia: WB Saunders; 1985:147-152.

69. Nowicki KD, Hummer CD III, Heidt RS Jr, Colosimo AJ. Effects of iontophoretic versus injection administration of dexamethasone. *Med Sci Sports Exerc*. 2002;34(8):1294-1301.

70. Noyes FR, Mangine RE, Barber S. Early knee motion after open and arthroscopic anterior cruciate ligament reconstruction. *Am J Sports Med*. 1987;15(2):149-160.

71. Paoloni JA, Appleyard RC, Nelson J, Murrell GA. Topical nitric oxide application in the treatment of chronic extensor tendinosis at the elbow: a randomized, double-blinded, placebo-controlled clinical trial. *Am J Sports Med*. 2003;31(6):915-920.

72. Perkins G. Rest and movement. *J Bone Joint Surg Br*. 1953;35-B(4):521-539.

73. Podesta L, Crow S, Volkmer D, Bert T, Yocum LA, Treatment of partial ulnar collateral ligament tears in the elbow with platelet-rich plasma, *Am J Sports Med*. 2013;41(7):1689-1694.

74. Posner M, Cameron KL, Wolf JM, Belmont PJ Jr, Owens BD. Epidemiology of major league baseball injuries. *Am J Sports Med*. 2011;39(8):1676-1680.

75. Reddy GK, Gum S, Stehno-Bittel L, Enwemeka CS. Biochemistry and biomechanics of healing tendon: part II. effects of combined laser therapy and electrical stimulation. *Med Sci Sports Exerc*. 1998;30(6):794-800.

76. Reddy GK, Stehno-Bittel L, Enwemeka CS. Laser photostimulation of collagen production in healing rabbit Achilles tendons. *Lasers Surg Med*. 1998;22(5):281-287.

77. Reinold MM, Escamilla RF, Wilk KE. Current concepts in the scientific and clinical rationale behind exercises for glenohumeral and scapulothoracic musculature. *J Orthop Sports Phys Ther*. 2009;39(2):105-117.

78. Reinold MM, Macrina LC, Wilk KE, et al. Electromyographic analysis of the supraspinatus and deltoid muscles during 3 common rehabilitation exercises. *J Athl Train*. 2007;42(4):464-469.

79. Reinold MM, Wilk KE, Fleisig GS, et al. Electromyographic analysis of the rotator cuff and deltoid musculature during common shoulder external rotation exercises. *J Orthop Sports Phys Ther*. 2004;34(7):385-394.

80. Reinold MM, Wilk KE, Reed J, Crenshaw K, Andrews JR. Interval sport programs: guidelines for baseball, tennis, and golf. *J Orthop Sports Phys Ther*. 2002;32(6):293-298.

81. Rettig AC, Sherrill C, Snead DS, et al. Nonoperative treatment of ulnar collateral ligament injuries in throwing athletes. *Am J Sports Med*. 2001;29:15-17.

82. Roberts N, Hughes R. Osteochondritis dissecans of the elbow joint; a clinical study. *J Bone Joint Surg Br*. 1950;32-B(3):348-360.

83. Rohrbough JT, Altchek DW, Hyman J, Williams RJ III, Botts JD. Medial collateral ligament reconstruction of the elbow using the docking technique. *Am J Sports Med*. 2002;30(4):541-548.

84. Salter RB, Hamilton HW, Wedge JH, et al. Clinical application of basic research on continuous passive motion for disorders and injuries of synovial joints: a preliminary report of a feasibility study. *J Orthop Res*. 1984;1(3):325-342.

85. Salter RB, Simmonds DF, Malcolm BW, Rumble EJ, MacMichael D, Clements ND. The biological effect of continuous passive motion on the healing of full-thickness defects in articular cartilage. An experimental investigation in the rabbit. *J Bone Joint Surg Am*. 1980;62(8):1232-1251.

86. Sampson S, Gerhardt M, Mandelbaum B. Platelet rich plasma injection grafts for musculoskeletal injuries: a review. *Curr Rev Musculoskelet Med*. 2008;1(3-4):165-174.

87. Sanchez M, Anitua E, Orive G, Mujika I, Andia I. Platelet-rich therapies in the treatment of orthopaedic sport injuries. *Sports Med.* 2009;39(5):345-354.

88. Sapega AA, Quedenfeld TC, Moyer RA, Butler RA. Biophysical factors in range-of-motion exercise. *Phys Sports Med.* 1981;9(12):57-65.

89. Schulte-Edelmann JA, Davies GJ, Kernozek TW, Gerberding ED. The effects of plyometric training of the posterior shoulder and elbow. *J Strength Cond Res.* 2005;19(1):129-134.

90. Shalabi A, Kristoffersen-Wilberg M, Svensson L, Aspelin P, Movin T. Eccentric training of the gastrocnemius-soleus complex in chronic Achilles tendinopathy results in decreased tendon volume and intratendinous signal as evaluated by MRI. *Am J Sports Med.* 2004;32(5):1286-1296.

91. Stergioulas A, Stergioula M, Aarskog R, Lopes-Martins RA, Bjordal JM. Effects of low-level laser therapy and eccentric exercises in the treatment of recreational athletes with chronic achilles tendinopathy. *Am J Sports Med.* 2008;36(5):881-887.

92. Suresh SP, Ali KE, Jones H, Connell DA. Medial epicondylitis: is ultrasound guided autologous blood injection an effective treatment? *Br J Sports Med.* 2006;40(11):935-939 [discussion 939].

93. Wang CJ, Chen HS. Shock wave therapy for patients with lateral epicondylitis of the elbow: a one- to two-year follow-up study. *Am J Sports Med.* 2002;30(3):422-425.

94. Wang CJ, Ko JY, Chen HS. Treatment of calcifying tendinitis of the shoulder with shock wave therapy. *Clin Orthop Relat Res.* 2001;(387):83-89.

95. Wang L, Qin L, Lu HB, et al. Extracorporeal shock wave therapy in treatment of delayed bone-tendon healing. *Am J Sports Med.* 2008;36(2):340-347.

96. Warren CG, Lehmann JF, Koblanski JN. Elongation of rat tail tendon: effect of load and temperature. *Arch Phys Med Rehabil.* 1971;52(10):465-474 [passim].

97. Warren CG, Lehmann JF, Koblanski JN. Heat and stretch procedures: an evaluation using rat tail tendon. *Arch Phys Med Rehabil.* 1976;57(3):122-126.

98. Werner SL, Fleisig GS, Dillman CJ, Andrews JR. Biomechanics of the elbow during baseball pitching. *J Orthop Sports Phys Ther.* 1993;17(6):274-278.

99. Wilk KE, Arrigo C, Andrews JR. Rehabilitation of the elbow in the throwing athlete. *J Orthop Sports Phys Ther.* 1993;17(6):305-317.

100. Wilk KE, Macrina LC, Arrigo CA. Passive range of motion characteristics in the overhead baseball pitcher & their implications for rehabilitation. *Clin Orthop Relat Res.* 2012;470(6):1586-1594.

101. Wilk KE, Macrina LC, Cain EL, Dugas JR, Andrews JR, Rehabilitation of the overhead athlete's elbow. *Sports Health.* 2012; 4(5):404-414.

102. Wilk KE, Macrina LC, Fleisig GS, et al. Deficits in glenohumeral passive range of motion increase risk of elbow injury in professional baseball pitchers: a prospective study. *Am J Sports Med.* 42(9):2075-2081, 2014 [PMID:24944295].

103. Wilk K, Macrina L, Fleisig G, et al. Correlation of glenohumeral internal rotation deficit and total rotational motion to shoulder injuries in professional baseball pitchers. *Am J Sports Med.* 2011;39(2):329-335.

104. Wilk KE, Meister K, Andrews JR. Current concepts in the rehabilitation of the overhead throwing athlete. *Am J Sports Med.* 2002;30(1):136-151.

105. Wilk KE, Obma P, Simpson CD, Cain EL, Dugas JR, Andrews JR. Shoulder injuries in the overhead athlete. *J Orthop Sports Phys Ther.* 2009;39(2):38-54.

106. Wilk KE, Voight ML, Keirns MA, Gambetta V, Andrews JR, Dillman CJ. Stretch-shortening drills for the upper extremities: theory and clinical application. *J Orthop Sports Phys Ther.* 1993;17(5):225-239.

107. Wilk KE, Yenchak AJ, Arrigo CA, Andrews JR. The advanced throwers ten exercise program: a new exercise series for enhanced dynamic shoulder control in the overhead throwing athlete. *Phys Sportsmed.* 2011;39(4):90-97.

108. Wilson FD, Andrews JR, Blackburn TA, McCluskey G. Valgus extension overload in the pitching elbow. *Am J Sports Med.* 1983;11(2):83-88.

109. Woodward AH, Bianco AJ Jr. Osteochondritis dissecans of the elbow. *Clin Orthop Relat Res.* 1975;(110):35-41.

110. Wright RW, Steger-May K, Wasserlauf BL, O'Neal ME, Weinberg BW, Paletta GA. Elbow range of motion in professional baseball pitchers. *Am J Sports Med.* 2006;34(2):190-193.

111. Wyke BD. The neurology of joints. *Ann Roy Coll Surg.* 1966;41:25-29.

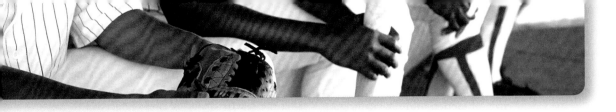

CHAPTER 39

Progressive Throwing Programs—
Science and Rationale

Timothy Lentych, MS, ATC/L | Steve Donohue, ATC | Michael Schuk, PT, DPT, ATC |
David Colvin, PT, DPT, MS, ATC

It's been a grind.

—John Smoltz

INTRODUCTION

A progressive throwing program gradually returns function after injury or a period of rest by slowly progressing through graduated sport-specific activities.[1] In terms of baseball, the progressive throwing program is a gradual progression of throwing in combination with therapeutic exercises and overall conditioning. The programs that are designed are individualized to apply forces to specific healed joints/structures intending to return athletes to their same level of competition as safe and quick as possible. The chance of reinjury is lessened by a graduated progression. Programs should be supervised and with great attention to the details. Ideally a pitching coach or coordinator should be in attendance during the throwing program to ensure appropriate throwing mechanics. For position players, a hitting coach and/or coordinator should be present.

Compliance to the number of throws and weekly schedule is necessary for safe return without reinjury. Timetables can be individualized to account for different player circumstances and established throwing variations in throwing routines. A general time frame in either weeks, months or years can be used as a broad estimate to return. The majority of athletes are highly competitive and uniformly desire to return as early as possible.

Upper extremity injuries that are most prevalent in baseball involve the shoulder and elbow. Most of these injuries are cumulative microtrauma from the repetitive, dynamic overhead throwing motion and create unique predictable injury patterns to baseball. Fortunately, advances in postoperative and nonoperative treatments have allowed players to return to competition after sustaining what previously would have been considered a career-ending injury.[2]

Once the athlete has performed and completed an intensive nonoperative or operative rehabilitation, range of motion, strength, adequate dynamic stabilization, and restoration of confidence should return to baseline or equal bilaterally with the player being asymptomatic. In addition, the athlete must have clearance by the team's physician to proceed to a progressive throwing program. Once cleared, several guidelines may need to be considered while developing a progressive throwing program for that particular athlete:

1. Return to sport activities after injury that include attention to the entire body

2. A gradual progression of applied forces to lessen the chance of reinjury

3. Proper warm-up and maintenance exercises

4. Individualization—starter, reliever, position player, catcher

5. Awareness that most injuries occur due to fatigue

6. Proper biomechanics to minimize the incidence of reinjury[1]

The overhead throwing motion is complex and requires total body strength and coordination from the initiation to follow-through phases. Kinematics is a branch of classical mechanics that describes the motion of points, bodies (objects), and systems of bodies (groups of objects) without considering the mass of each or the forces that caused the motion. Typically, the kinetic chain begins in the lower body and trunk with force and momentum that then transmits the energy distally to the shoulder, elbow, and hand, ending with kinetic energy transfer to the ball.[3]

The kinetic chain of motion in throwing includes stride, pelvis rotation, upper torso rotation, elbow extension, shoulder internal rotation, and wrist flexion. There are 6 phases of the throwing motion. These include windup, early arm cocking, late arm cocking, arm acceleration, arm deceleration, and follow-through. Proper throwing mechanics are essential and should not be unsupervised. There is value to having a pitching coach present along with the rehab expert to emphasize proper mechanics to help limit any flaws and reduce to risk for reinjury. Discussing mechanics with a pitching coach and watching video on the throwing session are an effective tool. Each individual athlete has different mechanics, and proper techniques and training methods will vary from athlete to athlete throughout the throwing program.

INDIVIDUAL VARIABILITY

"Listen to your body." Every athlete can handle certain stresses different ways. Before throwing, an athlete is required to be pain free and cleared by a physician to begin a progressive throwing program. During the throwing program, some athletes may experience soreness or a dull achy feeling in their muscles, and others may not experience any soreness. Each athlete will recover differently. If the soreness is too much, then "listen to your body" or listen to the subjective reporting of the athlete and slow the intensity, volume, and distance of the throwing program or stop the program to rest. This is an example of attempting to set up timetables for each athlete. Timetables have a high risk of changing and should not be compared with other athletes. Each level or phase of the progressive throwing program is to be completed pain free and without complication before starting the next level.[2] Varying skill level of each athlete will be different, which will result in the progression changing from athlete to athlete. The goals are to adhere to the program based on the individual as best as you can to prevent from reinjury and overeagerness of the athlete. Timetables must be flexible, and this can create frustration for athletes.[4]

WARM-UP

An adequate active warm-up is recommended before throwing. The athlete should develop a light sweat by jogging, biking, elliptical, etc. This will create blood flow to the muscles, which will increase flexibility to decrease the risk of reinjury. After perspiring, the athlete will progress to a stretching/flexibility of not only the shoulder or elbow but also the muscles of the whole body. Therefore, all muscle groups should be stretched beginning with the legs and working distally along the kinetic chain.[2] It is recommended to continue capsular stretches and range of motion exercises that began in the early phases of rehab before throwing. One key thing to remember is that the required amount of warm-up will vary from athlete to athlete.

HISTORY

Tom House has stated, "In 60's and 70's, there wasn't a throwing program, the closest thing to it was long toss. The more you threw, the better your arm got." Before 1996, players threw based on instinct and according to how the arm felt. Players often stated that the more and the longer they threw, the better their arm felt.

The throwing program consisted of players on the foul line throwing to their partner who is standing by a "cone" or in line with the "cone," which marks off the distance they are currently receiving the baseball. The program was marked off by cones at distances of 60, 90, and 120 feet, which approximately lasted 10 to 12 minutes. This program capped all players from throwing past 120 feet and did not take in consideration the different backgrounds, routines, body types, and arm strength of each individual player. Each player had their own opinions to the program. Those who did not like the program stated that it reverted players to throw shortened distances even though they trained at throwing a baseball 300 to 330 feet. Individuals who trained at throwing long toss were losing velocity, endurance, feel, recovery, and being undertrained according to Yaeger's article.

Each year went by since 1996 and the throwing program became a part of baseball's culture. The leading experts have researched throwing programs. No matter what type of a throwing program is followed and completed, both the nonoperative and operative programs should start out slowly and build/progress. Slowly build and progress the workloads by increasing the distance, volume, and/or time of the programs. Because there are numerous programs to follow, find a program that best fits the athlete based on history, age, experience (level of play), and position. By following certain guidelines based on the organization or school and individualizing each program, the chance of reinjury is lessened.

THROWING PROGRAMS

Progressive throwing programs are progressive, sport-specific regimens that gradually expose an athlete to the demands they will experience upon a return to sport.[2] Usually a traditional nonoperative or operative rehab will attempt to mimic or reproduce the speed or the joint forces generated by throwing. Strengthening the surrounding musculature postthrowing and individualizing each athlete's program will decrease the risk of reinjury. Regarding a postoperative throwing program, the athlete should advance when that particular phase is completed and no soreness is present. The phases are divided into 2 sections: phase 1 is flat ground throwing (Table 39.1) and phase 2 (Table 39.2) is the mound progression. The first initial phase usually consists throwing at distances of 60, 90, and 120 feet. Depending on the organization, school, or physician, the program will require the athlete to throw 3 times a week on a Monday, Wednesday, and Friday schedule. On those days, throwing should be supplemented with a weight-training program that focuses on the anterior and posterior musculature to help build and maintain strength, avoid injury, and aid in recovery. Special emphasis must be made to the posterior musculature. The postoperative throwing program in Table 39.1 starts off by throwing 60 feet (25 throws) for a total of

2 weeks. Perform each week without pain and progress to the next step, which is 60 feet (50 throws). This step along with the next 3 steps are 4 weeks long to complete without pain before progressing to the next step (refer to Table 39.1); however, the total weeks for flat ground throwing would be 18 weeks.

One key point is to individualize the throwing program. For example, an athlete can be pain free and just finished the fourth week of throwing at 60 to 90 feet (25 throws each for a total of 50) and may not be strong enough to advance to the next step. For that athlete, an adjustment will be made to throw an extra week at 60 to 90 feet (25 throws each for a total of 50) and changes are made to the weight-training program (shoulder exercises). This should be discussed among the athlete, the pitching coordinator/coach, physician, and athletic trainer/physical therapist.

The days in-between throwing are designated for flexibility and soft tissue of the shoulder and elbow complexes in addition to scapular musculature motion/strength to aid in prevention of anterior musculature tightness. The individual and the phase the athlete is at in the throwing program should determine what type of exercise schema that is performed after throwing, for instance, high reps-low weights, low weights-high reps, rotator cuff exercises, stabilization exercises (body blade, wall ball exercises, or rhythmic), timed exercises, plyometric exercises, and scapular exercises. Saturdays are designed as a recovery day as well until the athlete is on the mound progression. Continue to work on soft tissue and flexibility or any individualized program for that particular day. Typically, Sundays are designed for a complete day off.

TABLE 39.1 Flat Ground Throwing Progression

Frequency	Distance	Number of Throws
2 wk	60 feet	25
4 wk	60 feet	50
4 wk	60-90 feet	25 each distance
4 wk	90 feet	50
4 wk	90-120 feet	25 each distance

Throwing progression will be 3 times a week—Mondays, Wednesdays, Fridays.

Flat ground throwing—total 18 wk.

TABLE 39.2 Mound Throwing Progression

Frequency	Distance (Long Toss)	Number of Pitches	Pitch	Mound Size	New Pitch (Additional)
2 wk	120 feet	25	FBs	5 inches (half)	None
2 wk	120 feet	25	FBs	10 inches (full)	CH
2 wk	135 feet	30	FB/CH	10 inches (full)	Spin
2 wk	135 feet	35	ALL	10 inches (full)	None
2 wk	150 feet	45*	ALL	10 inches (full)	None
1 wk	150 feet	1/20**	ALL	10 inches (full)	None
1 wk	150 feet	2/35**	ALL	10 inches (full)	None

Progress to simulated games, then regular season games (starters vs relievers).

FBs, fastballs; CH, changeup; Spin/ALL, sliders, breaking ball, split, etc.

"New pitch" means the athlete will work on throwing the pitch on flat ground 2 wk before throwing it on the mound.

Distance (long toss)—As the number of pitches increases on the mound, the distance on long toss before the mound increases.

Bullpens/side will be twice a week—Tuesdays and Fridays.

*, Bullpens/side of 45—All for starters only; relievers progress to live B.P. **, Live B.P.—1 inning/20 pitches; 2 innings/35 pitches.

Distance (long toss) days will be twice a week—Mondays and Thursdays.

During the flat ground phase, the athlete should develop the use of the crow hop method. Crow hop method simulates the throwing act emphasizing proper body mechanics while using the legs for momentum forward. The goal of using the crow hop method is to use the legs to throw to reduce the stress of the shoulder or elbow and perform proper mechanics. The components of the crow hop are to first hop, then skip, followed by the throw. A pitching coordinator is valuable to ensure the use of proper mechanics during both the postoperative and nonoperative throwing programs.

The second phase is the mound progression. The mound progression lasts between 10 and 12 weeks long depending whether the athlete is a starter or reliever, a setback occurs, or the athlete needs to repeat the session again. Mound progression begins when the athlete is pain free from the flat ground progression. It starts off at an intensity of 50% to 60% effort and throwing fastballs only. Fleisig and colleagues studied healthy pitchers' ability to estimate their throwing efforts, and when targeting 50% effort, the pitchers' generated speeds of 85% with forces and torque approaching 75% of maximum.[2] The use of a radar gun may be valuable during the mound progression even though it can be used during phase 1 as well.

Bullpens or sides will be thrown on Tuesdays and Fridays. Each mound session will be performed for 2 weeks to move to the next step. Again, the athlete has to be pain free and feel strong to move on. The first 2 weeks are thrown from a half mound using fastballs only for 25 pitches. The elevation of a normal game used mound is 10 inches. The use of a half mound for the 2 weeks will be 5 inches in elevation. The idea of using a half mound is to limit the stress and to be a progression for the athlete. After performing 2 pain free weeks, the athlete can progress to the full mound using fastballs only again. Beginning with the full mound phase, the athlete can start throwing a changeup during his flat ground session before the throwing on the mound. As the weeks progress, more pitches are added to the mound sessions; addition of a pitch is performed on the mound and the distance during the flat ground session is increasing. At the end of the mound progression, the athlete will face hitters in live batting practice (B.P.) and then progress to simulated games and finally progress to pitching in regular season games. The progression does not stop when a pitcher is in regular season games. The pitchers will be charted based on innings pitches, number of pitches, intensity during the game/effort level, etc. The athlete will be charted and monitored for that particular season and the seasons to follow.

The nonoperative program tends to be quicker than the postoperative program owing to the athlete having surgery on the shoulder or elbow. However, this program needs to be monitored and individualized to help reduce to risk of further injury that could lead to surgery. Nonoperative throwing programs are based on the type of injury from lower to upper extremity and how many days the athlete has not thrown. For example, if the athlete has not thrown for 14 days (Table 39.3) owing to shoulder tendinitis, then it could take up to 14 days or longer to build strength in the shoulder from throwing. It is a combination of flat ground, progressing to mound work, then facing hitters in live B.P. or a simulated game, and finally a

TABLE 39.3 Return to Pitch Progression (Example: 14 days of No Throwing)

14 days of No Throwing	
Game	Postgame injury complaint
Day 1-14	No throwing—TX's and COND.
Day 15	60' (50)
Day 16	60'-90' (25)
Day 17	No throwing
Day 18	90' (50)
Day 19	90'-120' (25)
Day 20	No throwing
Day 21	90'-120' (25), Spin 10 flat
Day 22	Light toss out to 60'
Day 23	T.P. 120 feet, side 25 FB/CH, Spin 15 flat (R)/(S)
Day 24	No throwing
Day 25	T.P. 135 feet
Day 26	T.P. 135 feet, side 35 ALL (R)/(S)
Day 27	No throwing
Day 28	T.P. 150 feet
Day 29	T.P. 150 feet, B.P. 1/20/side (with hitters) 35 ALL (R) and (S)
	T.P. 150 feet, B.P. 1/20/side (with hitters) 35 ALL (S)
Day 30	No throwing
Day 31	T.P. 150 feet (R)/(S)
Day 32	Game 1/25 (R)
	T.P. 150 feet, B.P. 2/35/simulated game 2/35 ALL (S)
Day 33	T.P. 90 feet (S)
Day 34	T.P. 120 feet, light side 25 ALL
Day 35	T.P. 90 feet (S)
Day 36	Game 3/45 (S)

R, reliever; S, starter; FBs, fastballs; CH, changeup; Spin/ALL, sliders, breaking ball, split, etc; TX's, treatments; COND, conditioning; B.P., batting practice; T.P., throwing program.

rehab assignment to pitch in games before returning to the same level of competition. Common injuries include shoulder tendinitis, shoulder bursitis, shoulder inflammation, elbow flexor inflammation, elbow flexor tendinosis, and post–cortisone injection. The end goal of the nonoperative program is to return an athlete to pitching in games at the same or higher level of competition from when the injury occurred.

CONCLUSION

Progressive throwing programs are an integral part of training, conditioning, and returning an injured baseball player to the game.[2] Remember, if pain exists at a particular step, the athlete is instructed to stop throwing. A brief period of inactivity from throwing will occur until symptoms subside. Then an attempt to progress in the throwing program can begin again. The goal with each throwing program is that upon completion, the athlete will be prepared for the workload during competition. The major feature with many of the throwing programs these days is data driven and has been developed based on research in laboratories, quantifying and studying the effects of volume, duration, intensity, and the biomechanics of flat ground, long toss, mound pitching, and partial effort throwing. Throwing programs are not only designed and structured to return athletes to competition but also to minimize their risk for reinjury and prepare their bodies for the stresses associated with throwing. Medical personnel and field staff (pitching coordinator/coaches) should familiarize themselves with the nonoperative and postoperative programs to make changes or individualize the program to fit the need of the athlete. Once the athlete has met the ultimate goal of returning to competition, the athlete needs to continue to emphasize a maintenance strengthening program, proper warm-up, proper mechanics (watch video), and flexibility to reduce the risk of reinjury.

REFERENCES

1. Reinold MM, Wilk KE, Reed J, et al. Interval sport programs: guidelines for baseball, tennis, and golf. *J Orthop Sports Phy Ther*. 2002:293-299.
2. Chang ES, Bishop ME, Baker D, West RV. Interval throwing and hitting program in baseball: biomechanics and rehabilitation. *Am J Orthop*. 2016:157-162.
3. Axe M, Hurd W, Snyder-Mackler L. Data-based interval throwing programs for baseball players. *Sports Health*. 2009:145-153.
4. Dines J, Altchek D, Andrews J, ElAttrache N, Wilk K, Yocum L. *Sports Medicine of Baseball*. Philadelphia: Lippincott Williams & Wilkins; 2012.

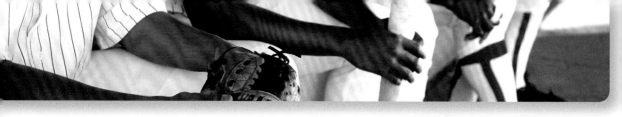

CHAPTER 40

Lower Extremity Rehabilitation and Conditioning

Joseph L. Ciccone, PT, DPT, FAAOMPT, CSCS, OCS, SCS, Cert. DN/SMT, CIMT | AJ Yenchak, PT, DPT, CSCS

I hit big or I miss big. I like to live as big as I can.

—*Babe Ruth*

INTRODUCTION

Baseball-related injuries have traditionally been focused on the upper extremity. The shoulder and elbow have been written and researched extensively, but more recently the lower extremity has gained momentum owing to its influence on the kinetic chain. The trunk is a crucial for generating rotational force, and therefore a massive amount of torque travels through the lower extremity. The lower half of the body is necessary for appropriate positioning of the arm to allow a player to not only generate but also transfer force up through the kinetic chain. Having altered lower extremity mechanics may lead to abnormal movements in the athlete, and pathologic stress on the torso, shoulder, and elbow may originate in the hip.[17] In an 18-season study of Major League Baseball (MLB), it was found that the total cost of players on the disabled list was nearly $700,000,000 and lower extremity injuries accounted for over 30% of all these.[6] Therefore, although upper extremity injuries are the most studied and commented on, there is a need to look at the lower half, as this impacts a large percentage of players and costs a tremendous amount of money. Thigh and knee injuries are in the top 5 most commonly injured areas in professional baseball players, and over 12% of players with knee injuries go on to need surgery.[8,27] Understanding how specific movement patterns affect the lower half of the body allow us to formulate a plan to rehabilitate players and return them to the field.

EXAMINATION

Taking a thorough examination provides a framework to devise a rehabilitation program for each individual athlete. The history is the most important part of the examination and typically the first interaction the clinician has with the athlete. This first interaction may lay the framework for establishing a strong working alliance, which has been shown to predict pain reduction and improvement in physical function.[19] The history will guide a clinician's examination, so they may find the concordant sign most efficiently. It lays the foundation to gain trust and alleviate anxiety with the athlete, which will allow a more open line of communication. Listening and asking appropriate follow-up questions is one of the most important aspects of this interaction, and it allows the athlete to express relevant information without being interrupted, so a clear picture may be formed on factors leading up to the injury. Types of questions a clinician wants to ask are open ended, which provide more information and allow further discussion. Information gathered during the examination should encompass an understanding of an athlete's background of activity levels, mechanism of injury, and what causes the symptoms and try to get a full understanding of condition presentation. This includes pain intensity, how long it lasts, when it occurs, and also what relieves its symptoms, getting a grasp on whether it was traumatic or repetitive and if they have had a similar type of issue before this one. In addition, it is the responsibility of the provider to identity if any red flags come up, which would require a referral to another medical provider.

When providing an examination of the hip and/or lower extremity, we must make sure to address the whole chain, as there are many influencers to other areas. The authors approach when evaluating this area of the body consists of looking at body alignment and gait patterning. Screening the foot, knee, hip, and back are all components that are included and should be evaluated to ensure that all bases are covered and essential information is gathered. All joints of the foot, ankle, knee, and hip are evaluated, especially if there has not been a significant event causing the injury. Obtaining a subjective history with included outcome measures should be done at the start of a visit to obtain foundational information.

The Ottawa ankle and knee rules should be part of the examination procedure, especially if no imaging has been performed and you are the first exposure to the athlete seeing a medical professional. Also included should be ruling out referral pain from more proximal areas such as the lumbar spine, hip, and knee, so a screen to these areas should be performed including repeated motion testing to lumbar spine, facet loading, slump test, and reflex testing. Motion testing should be performed both actively and passively with overpressure being applied to assess end feel. Distinguishing when pain occurs will help differentiate if there is a contractile or noncontractile issue and allow the clinician to get a sense of restrictions in mobility and flexibility. Following this, accessory motion should be performed to joints of the injured area to get a sense of joint play. Once we have a good understanding of joint play, we can assess the soft tissue restrictions by evaluating flexibility of the major musculature for each joint such as gastrocnemius/soleus, hamstring, quadriceps, hip abductors, and hip flexors. Strength testing is then performed for each body area in all planes of motion. It should be noted that strength testing should not only look at muscle strength in a neutral position but should look at an athlete's ability to generate force in shortened and lengthened positions, which is commonly overlooked.

TRIP TO THE MOUND
Range of Motion Testing

With the nature of baseball movements, the lower half is taken through large ranges of motion and therefore should be evaluated in an array of positions that mimic sport-specific movement patterns. Position players have to be able to get into a deep squat to field ground balls, extensive rotational patterns with hitting, and other nontraditional movement patterns such as when sliding or reaching to get a ground ball.

After movement testing is performed, special testing may then be implemented to further the understanding of a patient's diagnosis, but typically a clinician will already have a pretty clear picture of what the issue is based on previous findings during the examination. They are typically more confirmatory in nature. In addition, many special tests that may be utilized do not have sufficient evidence with sensitivity or specificity to give a clear and accurate diagnosis based solely on these maneuvers.

Palpation should be performed to all major muscle groups, ligaments, and bone through the lower half, especially in the area of pain to try and elicit concordant signs. For performance testing: balance, strength, control, and symmetry are inspected with a clinician's preference. Typical tests the authors' use in clinic are squatting, single-leg squatting, anterior step-downs, lunging, hop testing, Y balance test, and single-leg balance. Utilizing an array of these tests will provide information into how the athlete utilizes their system to accomplish specific tasks. We will have them go through movement patterns in sport that they have pain with (if tolerable) to get a deeper understanding of limitations, compensations, and mechanism of injury, which will help the clinician in coming up with a treatment plan strategy. Of course, it is paramount to test the uninvolved side with motion, strength, and performance testing to see what their baseline is. During the examination, it is not only discovering what tissue is affected but also determining the cause. Each individual athlete is a puzzle that we attempt to solve. Factors may have been in place that set this athlete up for injury are investigated and oftentimes may lead up or down the chain from where pain is occurring.

KINETIC CHAIN

Hip range of motion is a critical component when looking at the ability to generate torque and translate force through the body when throwing a ball, swinging a bat, and running. Players with hip, groin, and hamstring injury have been shown to present with hip rotation arc deficit when compared with uninjured group in professional baseball players. These arcs of motion comparing injured with noninjured players were 70° versus 77° on the right and 73° versus 78° on the left.[20] Ellenbecker et al[9] looked at hip rotation range of motion in baseball pitchers and found that there was an expectation of symmetry from left to right. However, they did find that 17% of players had a 10° or greater bilateral difference between limbs in hip internal rotation and 42% of players showed a 10° or greater difference with external rotation. They concluded that with professional baseball players, there was a large variability in the differences between trail and lead legs. This is an evolving topic where much attention and research is being spent, and we will be getting more information on ranges of motion correlating with injury. Just as the shoulder exhibits glenohumeral internal rotation deficit (GIRD) due to the asymmetrical loading patterns, the hip may also develop these types of adaptions.

TRIP TO THE MOUND
Kinetic Chain Influence in Sport

Limitations in the hip may influence a player's ability to rotate their pelvis over the leg. Identifying this is critical and may contribute to injury prevention and rehabilitation. A limitation in hip range of motion may limit an athlete from keeping a firm front leg to pivot over and develop force. You may see a hitter's front foot constantly open up or lose a firm base. One reason for this may simply be a lack of front leg internal rotation. A compensation for this can present as the foot and hip opening up or losing his footing during critical moments during his swing.

In respect to throwing, a pitcher/position player's trail leg must internally rotate to initially develop force, which can then translate up the chain and out into the arm and ball. The lead leg initially will be to externally rotate to set proper foot positioning to accept force and help create a firm front side to stabilize through. As a player begins to accept weight into the front side, the front hip must now accept force, weight, and rotation movements as pelvis rotates over the lead leg. The lead leg must have the ability to internally rotate to accept the force and maintain positioning up the chain. If there is a limitation in the hip with external rotation or internal rotation (IR) through any of the throwing phases, it may place excessive force on articular and soft tissue structures causing the load to become greater than the capacity. When this occurs, breakdown or deviations in movement patterns are unavoidable.

The body is fantastic at making accommodations and compensating for inappropriate movement and loading patterns. However, owing to the high forces, speeds, and repetitions involved in baseball, this can have significant effect on the athlete. It is up to the clinician to identify which structures are hypomobile,

tight, unstable, weak, or not firing in a coordinated movement and then address. It should not be forgotten that a player's arm health may be affected by the lower extremity. It has been seen that a deficit of lead leg hip IR has been seen in players with a history of shoulder injury, as a decrease in IR of the hip affects deceleration and therefore may put greater demands on the arm to slow down.[30]

There are many variables when dealing with lower extremity issues, but once a thorough examination is performed, that information can be used to appropriately direct the treatment approach. Take into account that the body works in harmony to give athletes the ability to generate such exceptional speeds and forces. Although having a specific diagnosis is important, integrating surrounding structures is also a viewpoint that should be implemented in the rehabilitation and performance settings.

Understanding that the hip, knee, and ankle all offer a role in all athletic movements in baseball guides a clinician when developing a treatment plan.

We will address each major body part of the lower extremity into the hip knee and ankle and give treatment approaches, which we use for each specific joint and how we integrate the whole chain as well.

Hip

Mobility

Improving an athlete's pain-free motion in this area significantly influences joint above and below. There can be various pathologies that exist, which limit mobility, and it is important to try and positively influence the hip to allow improved quality of movement. Joint mobilization of the hip joint capsule is a preferred technique to address restrictions. The mobilizations typically performed are inferior, posterior, and lateral.

TRIP TO THE MOUND
End Feel and Motion

There may be radiographic findings that will limit range of motion in an athlete. In these circumstances, one must make sure to not be overly aggressive. Performing a test, treat, and retest to monitor positive changes are suggested. End feel provides important information, and attempts to push or force motions through bony block or hard end feel should be avoided.

It should be noted that the athlete should reenforce passive mobilization actively. Capsular mobility, connective and soft issue areas are addressed initially to improve passive motion and then muscle reeducation is implemented to reinforce this actively and allow the system to hold onto the newly gained range of motion. Passive should be transitioned to active loading to condition the tissue and solidify the motion gained. This loading also conditions the area to accommodate for high stresses at end ranges of motion, which in baseball can be repetitive and cumulative. This will aid an athlete's ability to keep tissue capacity higher than repetitive load. In addition, giving an athlete the ability to allow for variability in motion within a given task will provide further resiliency to injury and maximize performance and freedom of movement.

Mobilizations have been shown to improve hip flexion and IR of the hip,[37] which are the movements that athletes typically have pain and deficit with. Typically with hip mobilization, we start with distraction with oscillations and then progress to inferior, posterior, and lateral distractions (Figures 40.1-40.4). The femur

is progressed from neutral position into restriction. Force of mobilization, directions, and duration should be adjusted to patient's tolerance and therapist preference. Once in desired positions, proprioceptive neuromuscular facilitation techniques are implemented to try and gain more range of motion. Isometric holds of 10 to 20 seconds are typically prescribed and then the new range is taken up. This is done for 3 rounds and then the athlete is asked to actively move his limb into the restriction. This allows him to train his neuromuscular system to actively achieve these ranges as well as strengthen in these end range positions. Multiple rounds and positions may be utilized, and therapists are encouraged to be creative to each individual athlete to achieve desired mobility.

Knee

The knee is a joint that performs flexion, extension, and rotation. The hip should provide sufficient rotation to allow the leg to rotate, but the knee should have the ability to rotate as well and not be overlooked. This is especially important after surgery, as clinicians should be restoring

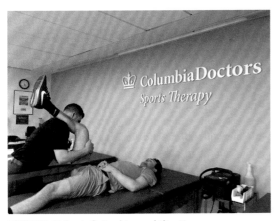

FIGURE 40.1 • Inferior hip mobilization.

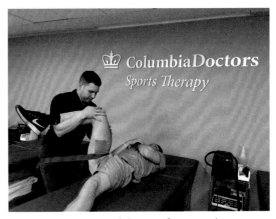

FIGURE 40.3 • Hip mobilization for internal rotation.

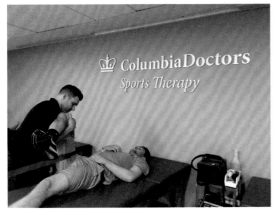

FIGURE 40.2 • Hip mobilization for external rotation.

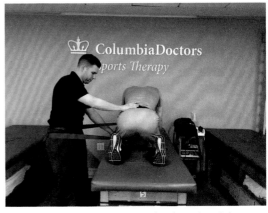

FIGURE 40.4 • Active assistive hip lateral mobilization.

normal rotation. When looking at range of motion, it has been shown that the left and right sides show no difference, and knee internal rotation accounted for 40% and external rotation accounted for 60% of total motion.[2] In addition, the flexion and extension should also be equal on both sides, so the uninvolved can be used as a baseline. When dealing with extension, it should be noted that if a knee hyperextends, then the uninvolved side should hyperextend to similar degrees. In regards to knee mobility, the patella is addressed first followed by the tibiofemoral joint. For patella mobilization, a neutral position is utilized initially in prone or side lying positions and the patella can be mobilized in medial (Figure 40.5A and B), lateral, superior and inferior directions. To improve patella mobility for knee flexion we can bias this motion by placing the knee into a flexed position and then mobilizing the patella inferiorly by hooking the top one's fingertips and then utilizing the other hand to provide force through the fingertips in an inferior direction in line with the tibia (Figure 40.6A-C). When focusing on mobilizing the tibiofemoral joint into flexion we will bring the knee into a flexed position and then oscillate perpendicular to the tibia (Figure 40.7). Switching between the patella mobilization and tibiofemoral is recommended and the knee will then be taken into higher angles and repeated. For extension, the knee is mobilized by placing one hand on distal femur and the other proximally under the calf to oscillate the tibia in a posterior to anterior direction (Figure 40.8A). Another alternative is to place a towel under the heel and proximal tibia and oscillate the distal femur anterior to posterior direction (Figure 40.8B) to facilitate a mobilization for extension. Two towels are utilized to provide extension and anterior glide of the tibia relative to the femur as close to the joint line as possible. Oscillations of variable speed are incorporated to address pain and prolonged end range holds utilized to work on stiffness.

Ankle

When dealing with ankle motion, we have used an inclinometer over the tibial tuberosity in a closed chain position as we ask the athlete to perform a weight bearing lunge for ankle dorsiflexion. This has been shown to be very reliable compared with inclinometer and tape measure technique.[18] Typically a goniometer is used for plantar felxion (PF), inversion, and eversion in an open-chain position, utilizing the fifth metatarsal as a reference for plantarflexion and the second metatarsal for inversion/eversion. The ankle can get stiff very quickly after injury, and it is recommended to start working on motion quickly as long as it is safe for the patient and he is cleared for therapy.

Ankle DF is typically the most restricted movement seen in the ankle, and there is an array of mobilizations that can be performed (Figures 40.9 and 40.10). PF is also critical in restoring for proper push off and drive (Figure 40.11). Having a variety of techniques at your disposal is very helpful, as this can be a challenging joint. In a systematic review it was found that manual therapy consisting of mobilization/manipulation was effective for decreasing pain and improving dorsiflexion range of motion in the acute phase.[21] In addition, for mobility, self-mobilization techniques are utilized as well for an home exercise program to patient tolerance.

Rehabilitation Principles

When treating athletes, we should not assume that they are strong. There are many cases where athletes will come into clinic and have significant deficits in specific musculature but are able to compensate owing to their athletic abilities. Unfortunately, this may place them in a situation that can lead to further injury. In the lower extremity the ankle influences the knee, the

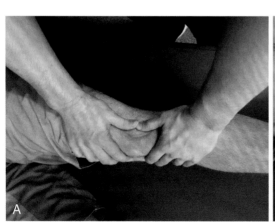
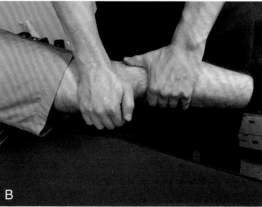

FIGURE 40.5 • A, Prone medial patella mobilization. B, Side-lying medial patella mobilization.

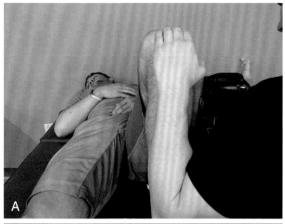

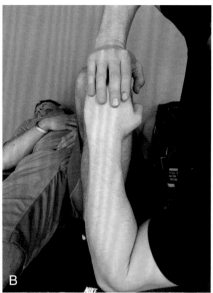

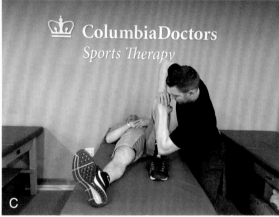

FIGURE 40.6 • A-C, Inferior patella mobilization.

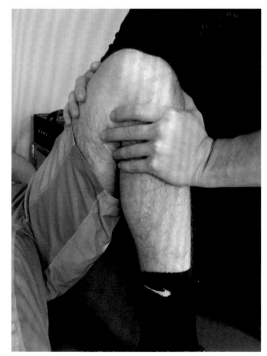

FIGURE 40.7 • Posterior tibiofemoral joint mobilization.

knee influences the hip, and the same in the opposite direction. It is certainly crucial to assess as well as address the area of pain and injury. However, joints above and below should not be neglected, as they have been shown to affect or influence other parts of the lower extremity as previously stated. Looking at the lower extremity as a unit is critical in determining a treatment approach and developing a plan of care for the athlete. The hip significantly influences the knee, and this should be part of the assessment and treatment program. In addition, the ankle can affect the tibia as well as femur and is another area of concern. When it comes time to treating athletes of all ages, we need to understand that there are many ingredients that are needed to maximize outcomes. Soft tissue influences the joints and vice versa. Having a thorough understanding of the movements required for the specific athlete will give the ability to see the demands placed on the lower extremity so that a thorough treatment approach is designed.

It is important to bias specific muscles in isolation, yet it is imperative to have the whole chain work in harmony to allow free-flowing movement to maximize

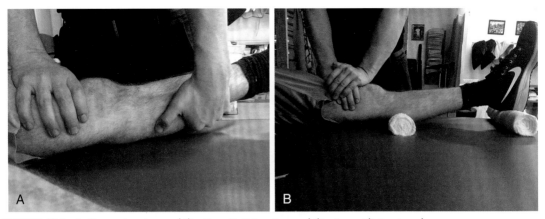

FIGURE 40.8 • A, Knee extension mobilization. B, Extension mobilization utilizing towels.

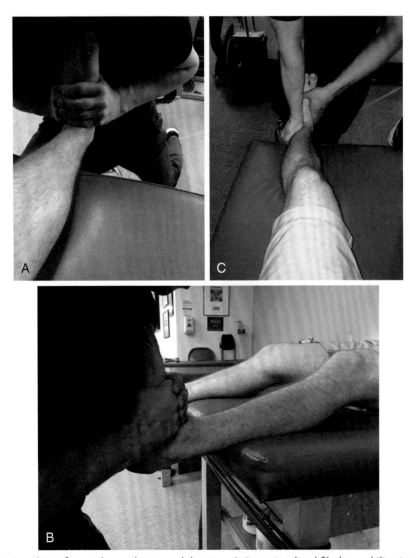

FIGURE 40.9 • A and B, Inferior talocrural joint mobilization. C, Posterior distal fibular mobilization for DF.

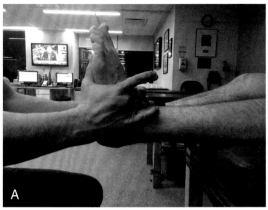 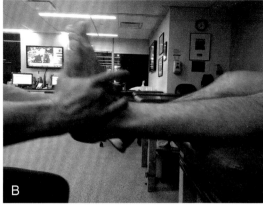

FIGURE 40.10 • A, Talocrural (TC) joint manipulation setup. B, TC joint manipulation thrust inferiorly.

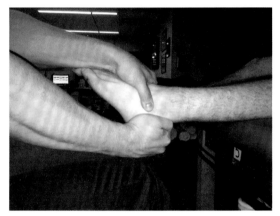

FIGURE 40.11 • Talocrural joint mobilization for plantarflexion.

performance. Before power can be worked on, we must first look at creating strength. Once strength is sufficient, then power can be developed and addressed. And in reality, athletic performance in baseball comes down to generating as much force and speed as possible. When dealing with power, the load should be as high as possible but not be too heavy that it is performed slowly.

Every patient has a unique morphology with accompanied physical attributes. A rehabilitation program should be based on specific findings and clear goals, which are then implemented specifically for that particular patient. We will outline exercises typically used in clinic for specific muscles and then advanced exercises to incorporate the whole chain into athletic movements for baseball specifically.

When dealing with soft tissue injuries, it is important to factor in one's history, as previous injury has shown to be a risk factor for future injury.[10] Three phases are respected with soft tissue injury, which

consists of acute, subacute, and chronic timeliness. All exercises should be progressed to an athlete's tolerance and modified to his response. Understanding tissue healing timelines and exercise progression/regressions will guide the clinician in making appropriate decisions for guiding one's rehabilitation program. After soft tissue injury, athletes may have residual symptoms of weakness, changed neuromuscular control, and soft tissue extensibility, which is why appropriate rehabilitation progression is paramount. Addressing primary area of injury as well as potential factors that could influence the area will always be incorporated into the program.

The acute phase is typically the first 3 days after an injury, and the goal in this point is trying to control pain and swelling while minimizing the loss of motion and strength. Gentle range of motion exercises are incorporated, and if tolerable, gentle isometrics can be integrated. Utilizing compression, electrical stimulation, elevation, and rest to decrease swelling and pain are implemented in the plan of care, so a smooth transition can be made into the subacute phase.

Typically after 3 days through 4 weeks' time, we are in the subacute phase and we are still looking to modulate pain, but now transitioning to increase range of motion and strength/stability. Integrating joint mobilizations to help with pain and range of motion are utilized, and isometric strengthening is progressed to incorporate concentric movements that are light in weight with more reps. Avoiding end range lengthening into painful positions should be avoided until adequate strength is achieved. Incorporating exercises that address surrounding areas that incorporate injured region is preferred before isolating directly. Manual techniques such as soft tissue mobilization may be incorporated but not aggressive to help limit exaggerated scar tissue formation. In addition, gentle cardiovascular activities may be introduced to bring in fresh blood flow, and start to lightly condition the muscles, and maintain fitness levels.

The chronic phase is roughly 4 weeks after soft tissue injury and where the athlete is progressed with exercise training. Concentric loads may be advanced, and starting eccentric-type contractions are added as well. Speed is gradually increased to begin to mimic more sport-related movements in a pain-free manner. Agility drills, plyometric exercises, may be incorporated when an athlete is showing sufficient pain-free strength and movement quality.

TRIP TO THE MOUND

Mobility and Conditioning

An athlete's range of motion and movement should be explored passively as well as actively. Performing isometric contraction at 80% intensity will strengthen the tissue in that position and allow more control of an athlete's body and start to protect against unplanned or repetitive force. The goal is to condition an area so it is strong, stable, fatigue resistant, mobile, and powerful. Simply put, we are making sure that the capacity of the joint, musculature, and supporting structures are greater than loads that will be applied to the system in the athletic event. This is the beauty of rehabilitation. There is freedom to be creative with how this is achieved by applying principles and techniques to the treatment plan.

Returning to sport is a multifactorial decision based on numerous factors, which are objective and subjective. In regard to strength, an athlete must display concentric and eccentric strength within 90% of uninvolved side, sufficient muscle endurance for particular activity he will be returning to with stability in multiple positions of sport, range of motion within 90% of uninvolved side, and showing no fear of returning to activities, which can be addressed using Cincinnati Knee Rating System and Tampa Scale for Kinesiophobia.

Returning to sport is the goal with athletes we treat and can be critical for one's profession. Not only is it important to return to sport, but we should also be implementing a program that will keep the athlete healthy by addressing deficiencies found on examination and having discussions about in-season and off-season programs to minimize chances of reinjury.

Strength and Conditioning

There is an enormous library of exercises that can be implemented for the lower extremity. An athlete's presentation will give lead a clinician to where they should start in regard to addressing joints, muscles, ligaments, and neuromuscular rehabilitation. Here we will go through specific body parts and comment on exercises utilized in clinic. It is recommended that when prescribing exercises that form be performed correctly without compensatory patterns. Once an athlete correctly shows proper movement and control, the difficulty can be elevated.

It should also be noted that exercises are influenced by trunk position, movement direction, and base of support, which affects EMG activity.[28] Modifying positioning of limbs also influence specific musculature to increase or decrease demand on a specific muscle, for example, performing a bridge with large hip abduction angles increases maximal voluntary isometric contraction (MVIC) of gluteus maximus and decreased MVIC of the erector spinae.[16]

Having a strong grasp of strength training principles is mandatory for a therapist, trainer, etc, and can drastically affect exercise prescription. In a meta-analysis for dose response and strength development, it was found that in untrained populations, 60% of 1 repetitions maximum (RM) performed 3 times a week was optimal, and trained individuals utilizing 80% RM performed 2 times a week evoked the greatest strength increases.[29] It can be appropriate to increase volume, and it was shown that untrained individuals are more sensitive to an increase in volume compared with trained. This is a point to consider when developing a treatment plan with a baseball player, as they may need less volume initially based on how long they have been out of competition or not. Also considerations need to be made with a lower extremity injury as to not overexercise them as the baseball season is long and breakdown should be avoided. Training musculature only twice a week is sufficient to get a response in many circumstances.

TRIP TO THE MOUND

Frequency and Variety in Training

When looking specifically at athletes, it was found that 85% of 1 RM 2 days a week was optimal for training. Within a conditioned athletic population, it was seen adding a third day to the routine showed no additional benefit.[26] It should be noted that it is necessary to have variety in training programs in regard to intensity, volume, and frequency to correspond to desired strength requirements.[29]

TRIP TO THE MOUND

Sleep and Injury

Addressing sleep is a variable that gets forgotten. Athletes who got less than 8 hours of sleep a night were 1.7 times more likely to have had an injury compared with athletes who slept for equal to or greater than 8 hours.[23]

Understanding the foundational movements required for specific athletes and their corresponding position gives a clinician information to prescribe the best types of movement, load, speed, volume, and intensity to correspond with demands placed on the players' system. Incorporating a variety of variables, which factor in an athlete's condition, deficits, time lines, and physiological response, is necessary for coming up with an effective approach. There is no cookie-cutter approach taken with an athlete, as the program must be malleable and change depending on response to treatment. In this line of thinking, we must factor in that force production, and tissue protection is not the same throughout ranges of motion. For example, having a symmetrical strong pain-free hamstring contraction against resistance in a prone position with the knee bent at 45° does not mean we can expect similar strength while a pitcher is completing the follow-through phase of throwing. In this instance, there is more length placed on the hamstring and will affect force production. Muscles are angular, speed, and length dependent and should be treated as such by incorporating multiple inputs at a variety of lengths and tensions. We should be trying to expand the muscular strength not only in midrange but also in shortened and lengthened positions to make an athlete's body resilient. Try firing one's hamstring with the hip extended and the knee flexed, and it is most likely the muscle will cramp due to the fact that it is not accustomed to working at that position. Training and adapting the body to multiple positions and end ranges of motion should be a part of the rehab process. Replicating shortened and lengthened ranges of motion creates a more integral neuromuscular connection to be stable in an array of athletic positions.

Treatment of Specific Diagnosis

Exercise prescription needs to be based on the phase of recovery that an athlete is in. Light isometrics may be performed in the acute phase, but performing in a pain-free level is implemented. Once sufficient healing has occurred and we are out of the subacute phase, we may start increasing strength to the injured area with low-level exercises that progress into higher level and then sport-specific movements.

Femoroacetabular Impingement

Femoroacetabular impingement (FAI) presents itself in 2 difference ways. There is cam-type impingement, which is an abnormal femoral head-neck junction that has an increased radius and will cause an impact into the acetabulum. The second one is pincer type, which is acetabular over coverage of the femoral head, which creates an abnormal contact on the acetabular rim. However, it is very common to see a combination of cam and pincer deformity clinically. FAI and labral tears accounted for over 80% of all intra-articular injuries in MLB from 2011 to 2014.[5]

Although intra-articular injuries have gained a lot of press, over 95% of hip injuries are extra-articular, consisting mainly of adductor and iliopsoas strains.[5] It is crucial during the examination to rule out pathologies to then try and focus in on the actual cause. Considering how a baseball player must move in regard to his hip, he needs to be able to accept weight and pivot over the rear leg or front leg. Acutely we will want to work toward accepting weight into the involved side and addressing muscles such as the psoas, adductors, hamstring tensor fascia lata, external rotators, and gluteal musculature. Isometrics of the abdominals and gluteals can be performed, as well as activities such as wall/side planking, gluteal squeezes, and modified planking. As the athlete displays a normalized gait pattern and shows good control with single-leg stance, we may advance to more

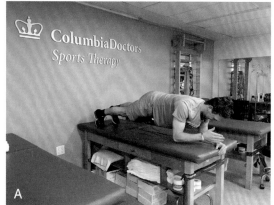

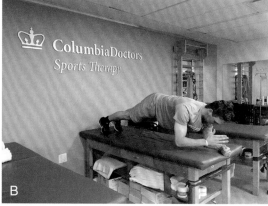

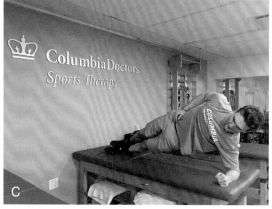

FIGURE 40.12 • A, Standard plank. B, Frontal plank with one arm lift. C, Side plank.

advanced strengthening. Being able to squat without hip shifting or excessive trunk tilt and performing different arrays of step exercises should be addressed, which will put demand on gluteals and external rotators. Strengthening is performed starting from bilateral to unilateral incorporating and progressing core with planks exercises (Figure 40.12A-C). As stated previously, hip motion should be addressed with neuromuscular reeducation and manual therapy techniques, as well as flexibility to needed areas based on the examination. Once an athlete shows excellent single-limb support and control with step exercises without aberrant movement, we can progress to the third phase.

In the third phase, we will advance strength to 5/5 and work on attaining sufficient ROM to perform athletic movement patterns. Advancing strengthening out of sagittal and frontal plane is initiated to transverse exercises such as transverse reaches (Figure 40.13A and B), rotations, and chops (Figure 40.14A-C), which will mimic pivoting over the leg during hitting. Light running progressions are also made during this phase. Depending on an athlete's position, we will introduce exercises such as dynamic movements over the involved extremity such as in following figures (Figure 40.15A and B). Once the athlete is showing 5/5 muscle strength, excellent core control, and dynamic movements, we can start progressing them back to sport with return to throwing and hitting programs.

Adductor Strains

The adductor group consists of adductor magnus, adductor brevis, adductor longus, pectineus, obturator externus, and gracilis. These muscles adduct the thigh as well as help stabilize the pelvis and work eccentrically to stabilize the thigh. Weakness in the hip adduction has been associated with muscle strain as well if the ratio between adduction and abduction is decreased with adduction being only 70% of abduction on commonly injured sides.[35] Therefore it is of high importance to restore strength to this area of the body with isometrics, concentrics, and eccentrics. Performing a strengthening program incorporating adductor/abductor exercises, abdominal sit-ups, back extension strengthening, balance training, and functional movements was much more effective than stretching, massage, and modalities.[14] Overall, strengthening may be progressed from open-chain activities to closed chain,

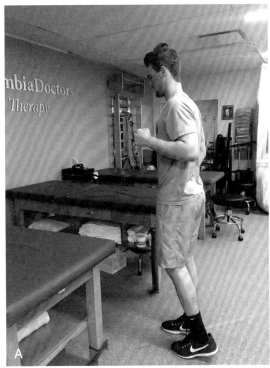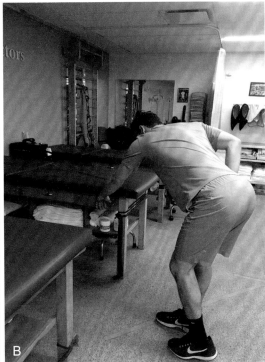

FIGURE 40.13 • Transverse reaches. A, Starting position. B, Finishing position.

consisting of eccentric movements such as sumo squats (Figure 40.16), hip adduction planks (Figure 40.17) balance board, squats, lunges in multiple planes, using a sliding board (Figure 40.18A and B), and increasing load, speed, and volume.[36]

Hamstring Strain

The hamstring is a very common injury seen in a variety of sports and can cause significant time loss to an athlete. It has been documented that recovery of an acute hamstring injury can take anywhere from 9 to 104 weeks.[4] Typically the mechanism is running at max speed or involved extreme stretching. Base running is the primary method of hamstring strain at the major and minor league levels with the majority of injuries running to first base.[1] In addition to an extensive time for recovery, one-third of hamstring injuries will recur, with the greatest risk during the first 2 weeks following return to sport.[13] Time to return to sport can be correlated with location of injury as the more cranial the injury, the longer time it will typically take to return to sport.[3] Many athletes will typically see a change in force-length relationship after injury, as the remodeling and repair of the hamstring achieves a peak force at shorter lengths, which is why a focus should be on eccentric exercises.[31] Restoring symmetrical range of motion and flexibility as well as neuromuscular control of the lumbopelvic region is

addressed. Strengthening of the hamstring and surrounding musculature is the main focus of this type of injury. Slowly biasing lengthening positions into the rehabilitation program for the hamstring should be integrated. In a recent systematic review, it was found that adding lengthening exercises showed a positive effect in rehabilitating this type of injury. Also, progressive agility and trunk stabilization may reduce reinjury rates.[25] Types of exercises that can be started early are bridging exercises, which then progress to walkout bridges to bias the hamstring muscle (Figure 40.19). Starting with exercises that use the hamstring as a secondary or tertiary muscle are utilized and then progressed to more primary demand. Planks may be incorporated early on for trunk stability to hit all surrounding musculature, and once patients begin to show good concentric and isometric control, eccentrics can be integrated, such as the Nordic hamstring curl, Romanian Deadlift (RDL), single-leg RDL, and windmill touches (Figure 40.20). Following these exercises, more baseball-related movements are performed to mimic certain positions or activities, which the athlete will have to return to. Strengthening in end ranges where injury can occur also utilizes performing isometrics in shortened and lengthened positions. Focus should not be on directly stretching the hamstring into extreme lengths, especially early on, as this can cause excessive damage to healing tissue.

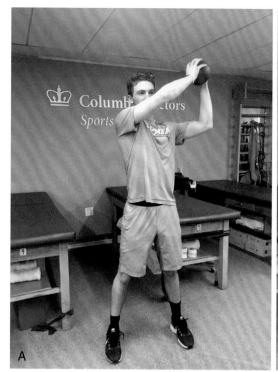
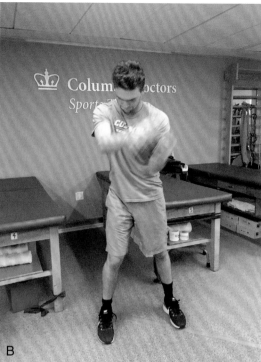
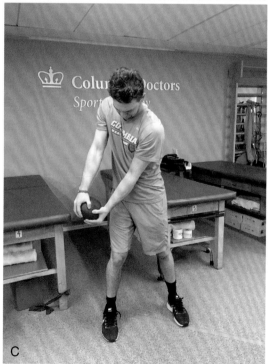

FIGURE 40.14 • Diagonal ball chops. A, Starting position. B, Midposition. C, Finishing position.

Patellofemoral Pain

Patellofemoral pain is pain in the retropatellar or peripatellar area that is caused during loading of the patellofemoral joint. Of all injuries seen in sports medicine, 25% to 30% are attributed to this issue.[12] This can be a very frustrating injury that an athlete deals with and can consist of pain with sitting, squatting, running, jumping, and stair negotiation. This can present when in prolonged positions such as deep squatting in catchers. Dealing with this type of issue

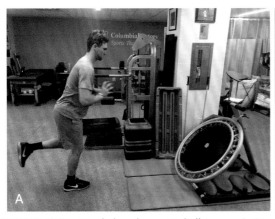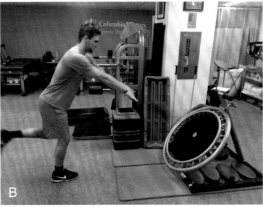

FIGURE 40.15 • Single-leg plyometric ball tosses. A, Starting position. B, Ending position.

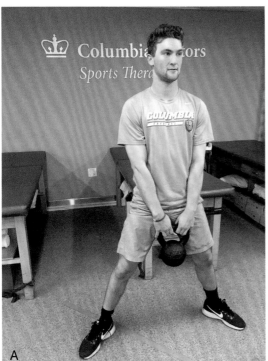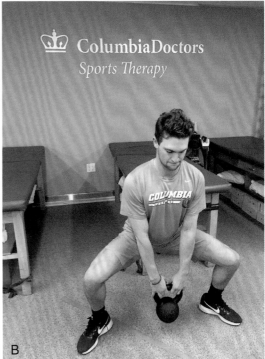

FIGURE 40.16 • Sumo squat. A, Starting position. B, Finishing position.

requires a thorough investigation of the whole chain, as the foot may influence the hip as well as the back or hip. It has been shown that greater lateral patella displacement angles occurred owing to medial femoral rotation as opposed to lateral patella rotation.[32] Addressing factors that may cause excessive femoral and tibial internal rotation must be addressed in the rehab process. Strengthening musculature that fights hip adduction and internal rotation is primary objectives, which is a reason why hip strengthening is a major component. Looking at the ankle for decreased dorsiflexion (DF) whether from talocrural hypomobility or gastrocnemius/soleus restriction is addressed as well as knee range of motion, as lacking full extension may place excessive force on the patellofemoral joint. Unfortunately, in a systematic review, the best exercise to perform for patellofemoral pain was not identified, although pain and function in patients receiving exercise therapy were considerably higher for treating this condition.[11] Depending on how reactive a patient's knee is will dictate the type of exercise that can be performed initially. It is the author's preference to incorporate closed-chain activities for hip and leg strengthening, but open-chain exercises will be performed if closed-chain activities are too painful or not performed with appropriate control. In this type of injury, the examination will really dictate what will be addressed. This is why understanding biomechanics of this joint is critical. In a study comparing open chain versus closed chain forces, it was found that in open-chain activities, less force occurred from 50° to 90° in open chain but from 0° to 46°; closed chain exercises had less stress than open.[33] Initially the therapist should try and reduce swelling and pain with his or her modality of choice and then progress to improving quad and hip strengthening exercises. Macadam et al put together a good systematic review on exercises, which provided the highest EMG activity in gluteal musculature to control dynamic hip abduction and external rotation.[22] What showed to be the highest

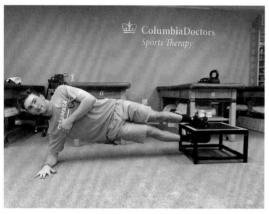

FIGURE 40.17 • Hip adduction planks with step.

level of EMG were closed chain exercises such as the crossover step-up (Figure 40.21) and side bridge with hip abduction. Standing exercises did provide the highest demands of musculature, as weight bearing activities impose greater demands on hip musculature due to the need to stabilize the pelvis and minimize knee valgus. Flexibility is a component that should not be overlooked, and improving hip flexor, quad, hamstring, hip abductors, tensor of fascia lata, gastrocnemius, and soleus is implemented. One other component is providing lumbar manipulation to help improve hip strength and functional testing. In a study conducted that looked at lumbopelvic manipulation, it was found that the manipulation group versus sham group had improvement in EMG activity of the vastus medialis and gluteals medius as well as improvement in a stepdown test and pain intensity[24] (Figure 40.22A and B).

Ankle Sprain

Lateral ankle sprains are typically seen in baseball from awkwardly stepping on a base while running, sliding, or landing awkwardly. It was found that in high school/college athletes, lateral ankle sprains in baseball and softball occurred in almost 80% of the athletes.[34] When looking at sliding specifically, it was found that a feet-first slide may put an athlete at higher risk of ankle injury from the landing phase when the ankle is forced into a plantarflexed position on impact and are subject to high forces.[7] A major change that impacted injuries was the use of breakaway bases, and it was found to decrease injuries by 96%.[15] However, in Major League Baseball, these are not utilized and the risk remains. Ankle injuries are classified by grades I, II, and III. The higher the grade involved typically, the longer the period for recovery. Pain, swelling, motion restriction, and instability are the key factors when

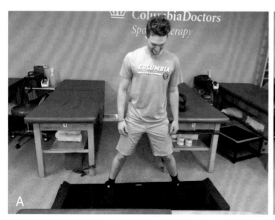
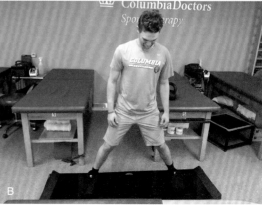

FIGURE 40.18 • A, Hip adduction sliding board starting position. B, Sliding board adductor eccentric/concentric.

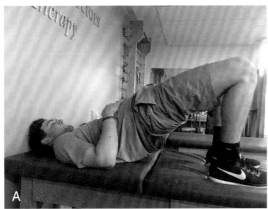 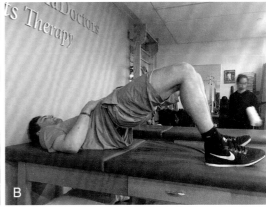

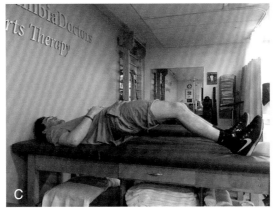

FIGURE 40.19 • A, Bridge least hamstring bias. B, Bridge moderate hamstring bias. C, Bridge most hamstring bias.

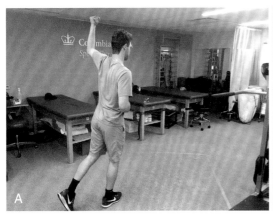 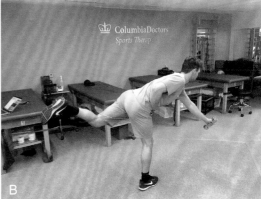

FIGURE 40.20 • Windmill touch. A, Starting position. B, Ending position.

dealing with these types of injuries. Protection occurs initially depending on severity it may range from a cast to no support but limited activities. Initially pain and swelling should be controlled as much as possible with modalities, and motion should be initiated in a pain-free range to minimize motion loss. Early weight bearing and motion are the author's preference as long as the patient tolerates this well to minimize loss of motion, proprioception, balance, and strength. Ankle mobilizations described earlier in this chapter are performed to help restore normal motions. Weight shifting and resistive band exercises

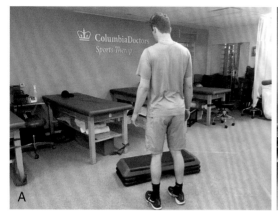
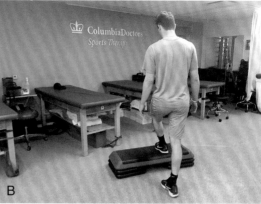
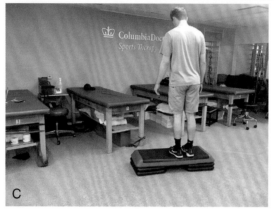

FIGURE 40.21 • Crossover step-ups. A, Starting position. B, Midposition. C, Finishing position.

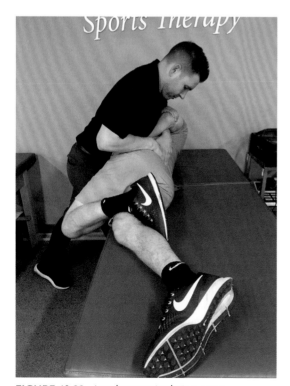

FIGURE 40.22 • Lumbar manipulation setup.

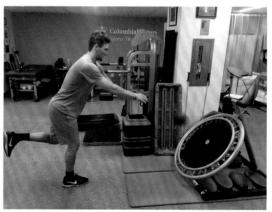

FIGURE 40.23 • Single-leg balance ball tosses.

are begun once the patient can tolerate mild resistance in all ankle directions. Balance exercises are progressed from weight shifting to single-leg balance and then progressed to performing activities while standing on one leg whether ball tossing off a trampoline (Figure 40.23) to performing balance on various surfaces with dynamic movements. Again, it must be addressed to strengthen the ankle and perform balance training in multiple foot ranges of motion to maximize awareness and strengthen to allow full strong mobility. Once the athlete can tolerate lunging, hopping, and showing acceptable pain and strength, a running program may be implemented, as well as more functional positions such as hitting maneuvers and throwing positions (Figures 40.24 and 40.25A and B). Return to sport can be implemented once the athlete is showing nearly symmetrical strength, motion, and pain at a minimum in addition to performing impact and sporting activities up to performance standards.

MANAGER'S TIPS

- Lower extremity injuries are commonplace in the baseball setting, and addressing the whole kinetic chain is critical in establishing a successful rehabilitation program
- Performing a thorough history, physical examination, and functional assessment is crucial in developing a framework to devise a comprehensive program to prescribe appropriate modalities, exercises, and return to sport training

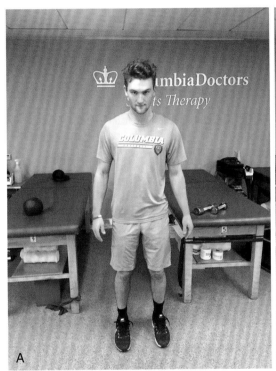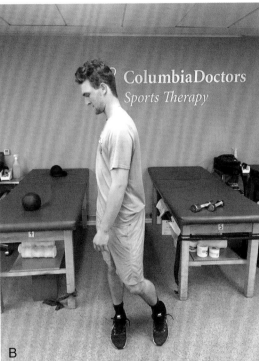

FIGURE 40.24 • Rotating over ankle. A, Starting position. B, Finishing position.

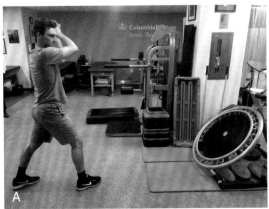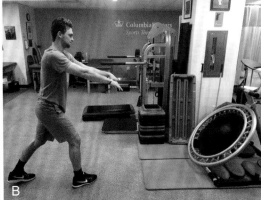

FIGURE 40.25 • Plyometric throws. A, Starting position. B, Finishing position.

- When rehabilitating a baseball athlete, understanding the types of movement patters that his or her position demand will help structure how to lead up to those activities. Remember to provide variability with movement patterns and strengthen in shortened and lengthened positions to minimize risk of injury and provide resiliency to unanticipated movements when they return to play

- Addressing and incorporating surrounding regions above and below the site of an injury pain are important components to examine and integrate within a program. The lower extremity consists of many joints that influence each other and will impact how an athlete progresses and maintains his health through a comprehensive rehabilitation program

REFERENCES

1. Ahmad CS, Dick RW, Snell E, et al. Major and minor league baseball hamstring injuries: epidemiologic findings from the major league baseball injury surveillance system. *Am J Sports Med.* 2014;42(6):1464-1470. doi:10.1177/0363546514529083.

2. Almquist PO, Ekdahl C, Isberg PE, Friden T. Knee rotation in healthy individuals related to age and gender. *J Orthop Res.* 2013;31(1):23-28. doi:10.1002/jor.22184

3. Askling CM, Tengvar M, Saartok T, Thorstensson A. Acute first-time hamstring strains during high-speed running: a longitudinal study including clinical and magnetic resonance imaging findings. *Am J Sports Med.* 2007;35(2):197-206. doi:10.1177/0363546506294679

4. Askling CM, Tengvar M, Saartok T, Thorstensson A. Proximal hamstring strains of stretching type in different sports: injury situations, clinical and magnetic resonance imaging characteristics, and return to sport. *Am J Sports Med.* 2008;36(9):1799-1804. doi:10.1177/0363546508315892.

5. Coleman SH, Mayer SW, Tyson JJ, Pollack KM, Curriero FC. The epidemiology of hip and groin injuries in professional baseball players. *Am J Orthop (Belle Mead NJ).* 2016;45(3):168-175.

6. Conte S, Camp CL, Dines JS. Injury trends in major league baseball over 18 seasons: 1998-2015. *Am J Orthop (Belle Mead NJ).* 2016;45(3):116-123.

7. Corzatt RD, Groppel JL, Pfautsch E, Boscardin J. The biomechanics of head-first versus feet-first sliding. *Am J Sports Med.* 1984;12(3):229-232. doi:10.1177/036354658401200312.

8. Dahm DL, Curriero FC, Camp CL, et al. Epidemiology and impact of knee injuries in major and minor league baseball players. *Am J Orthop (Belle Mead NJ).* 2016;45(3):E54-E62.

9. Ellenbecker TS, Ellenbecker GA, Roetert EP, Silva RT, Keuter G, Sperling F. Descriptive profile of hip rotation range of motion in elite tennis players and professional baseball pitchers. *Am J Sports Med.* 2007;35(8):1371-1376. doi:10.1177/0363546507300260.

10. Engebretsen AH, Myklebust G, Holme I, Engebretsen L, Bahr R. Intrinsic risk factors for hamstring injuries among male soccer players: a prospective cohort study. *Am J Sports Med.* 2010;38(6):1147-1153. doi:10.1177/0363546509358381.

11. Frye JL, Ramey LN, Hart JM. The effects of exercise on decreasing pain and increasing function in patients with patellofemoral pain syndrome: a systematic review. *Sports Health.* 2012;4(3):205-210. doi:10.1177/1941738112441915.

12. Halabchi F, Abolhasani M, Mirshahi M, Alizadeh Z. Patellofemoral pain in athletes: clinical perspectives. *Open Access J Sports Med.* 2017;8:189-203. doi:10.2147/OAJSM.S127359.

13. Heiderscheit BC, Sherry MA, Silder A, Chumanov ES, Thelen DG. Hamstring strain injuries: recommendations for diagnosis, rehabilitation, and injury prevention. *J Orthop Sports Phys Ther.* 2010;40(2):67-81. doi:10.2519/jospt.2010.3047.

14. Hölmich P, Uhrskou P, Ulnits L, et al. Effectiveness of active physical training as treatment for long-standing adductor-related groin pain in athletes: randomised trial. *Lancet.* 1999;353(9151):439-443. doi:10.1016/s0140-6736(98)03340-6.

15. Janda DH, Bir C, Kedroske B. A comparison of standard vs. breakaway bases: an analysis of a preventative intervention for softball and baseball foot and ankle injuries. *Foot Ankle Int.* 2001;22(10):810-816. doi:10.1177/107110070102201006.

16. Kang SY, Choung SD, Jeon HS. Modifying the hip abduction angle during bridging exercise can facilitate gluteus maximus activity. *Man Ther.* 2016;22:211-215. doi:10.1016/j.math.2015.12.010.

17. Klingenstein GG, Martin R, Kivlan B, Kelly BT. Hip injuries in the overhead athlete. *Clin Orthop Relat Res.* 2012;470(6):1579-1585. doi:10.1007/s11999-012-2245-3.

18. Konor MM, Morton S, Eckerson JM, Grindstaff TL. Reliability of three measures of ankle dorsiflexion range of motion. *Int J Sports Phys Ther.* 2012;7(3):279-287.

19. Lakke SE, Meerman S. Does working alliance have an influence on pain and physical functioning in patients with chronic musculoskeletal pain; a systematic review. *J Compassionate Health Care.* 2016;3(1). doi:10.1186/s40639-016-0018-7.

20. Li X, Ma R, Zhou H, et al. Evaluation of hip internal and external rotation range of motion as an injury risk factor for hip, abdominal and groin injuries in professional baseball players. *Orthop Rev.* 2015;7(4):6142. doi:10.4081/or.2015.6142.

21. Loudon JK, Reiman MP, Sylvain J. The efficacy of manual joint mobilisation/manipulation in treatment of lateral ankle sprains: a systematic review. *Br J Sports Med.* 2014;48(5):365-370. doi:10.1136/bjsports-2013-092763.

22. Macadam P, Cronin J, Contreras B. An examination of the gluteal muscle activity associated with dynamic hip abduction and hip external rotation exercise: a systematic review. *Int J Sports Phys Ther.* 2015;10(5):573-591.

23. Milewski MD, Skaggs DL, Bishop GA, et al. Chronic lack of sleep is associated with increased sports injuries in adolescent athletes. *J Pediatr Orthop.* 2014;34(2):129-133. doi:10.1097/BPO.0000000000000151.

24. Motealleh A, Gheysari E, Shokri E, Sobhani S. The immediate effect of lumbopelvic manipulation on EMG of vasti and gluteus medius in athletes with patellofemoral pain syndrome: a randomized controlled trial. *Man Ther.* 2016;22:16-21. doi:10.1016/j.math.2016.02.002.

25. Pas HI, Reurink G, Tol JL, Weir A, Winters M, Moen MH. Efficacy of rehabilitation (lengthening) exercises, platelet-rich plasma injections, and other conservative interventions in acute hamstring injuries: an updated systematic review and meta-analysis. *Br J Sports Med.* 2015;49(18):1197-1205. doi:10.1136/bjsports-2015-094879.

26. Peterson MD, Rhea MR, Alvar BA. Maximizing strength development in athletes: a meta-analysis to determine the dose-response relationship. *J Strength Cond Res.* 2004;18(2):377-382. doi:10.1519/R-12842.1.

27. Pollack KM, D'Angelo J, Green G, et al. Developing and implementing major league baseball's health and injury tracking system. *Am J Epidemiol.* 2016;183(5):490-496. doi:10.1093/aje/kwv348.

28. Reiman M, Bolgla LA, Loudon JK. A literature review of studies evaluating gluteus maximus and gluteus medius activation during rehabilitation exercises. *Physiother Theory Pract.* 2012;28(4):257-268. doi:10.3109/09593985.2011.604981.

29. Rhea MR, Alvar BA, Burkett LN, Ball SD. A meta-analysis to determine the dose response for strength development. *Med Sci Sports Exerc.* 2003;35(3):456-464. doi:10.1249/01.MSS.0000053727.63505.D4.

30. Scher S, Anderson K, Weber N, Bajorek J, Rand K, Bey MJ. Associations among hip and shoulder range of motion and shoulder injury in professional baseball players. *J Athl Train.* 2010;45(2):191-197. doi:10.4085/1062-6050-45.2.191.

31. Sherry MA, Johnston TS, Heiderscheit BC. Rehabilitation of acute hamstring strain injuries. *Clin Sports Med.* 2015;34(2):263-284. doi:10.1016/j.csm.2014.12.009.

32. Souza RB, Draper C, Fredericson M, Powers CM. Femur rotation and patellofemoral joint kinematics: a weight-bearing magnetic resonance imaging analysis. *J Orthop Sports Phys Ther.* 2010;40(5):277-285. doi:10.2519/jospt.2010.3215.

33. Steinkamp LA, Dillingham MF, Markel MD, Hill JA, Kaufman KR. Biomechanical considerations in patellofemoral joint rehabilitation. *Am J Sports Med.* 1993;21(3):438-444. doi:10.1177/036354659302100319.

34. Tanen L, Docherty CL, Van Der Pol B, Simon J, Schrader J. Prevalence of chronic ankle instability in high school and division I athletes. *Foot Ankle Spec.* 2014;7(1):37-44. doi:10.1177/1938640013509670.

35. Tyler TF, Nicholas SJ, Campbell RJ, McHugh MP. The association of hip strength and flexibility with the incidence of adductor muscle strains in professional ice hockey players. *Am J Sports Med.* 2001;29(2):124-128. doi:10.1177/03635465010290020301.

36. Tyler TF, Silvers HJ, Gerhardt MB, Nicholas SJ. Groin injuries in sports medicine. *Sports Health.* 2010;2(3):231-236. doi:10.1177/1941738110366820.

37. Walsh R, Kinsella S. The effects of caudal mobilisation with movement (MWM) and caudal self-mobilisation with movement (SMWM) in relation to restricted internal rotation in the hip: a randomised control pilot study. *Man Ther.* 2016;22:9-15. doi:10.1016/j.math.2016.01.007.

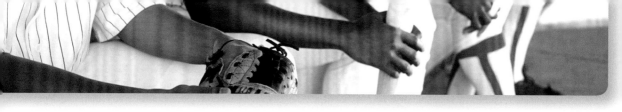

CHAPTER 41

Core Stabilization and Training

Rafael F. Escamilla, PhD, PT, CSCS, FACSM | Kevin E. Wilk, PT, DPT, FAPTA

You can sum up the game of baseball in one word: 'You never know.'
—Joaquin Andujar

INTRODUCTION

The core is an important component to all aspects of the baseball player. The core is critical in throwing a baseball and in hitting a baseball. The core and the effects of the lower extremity provide a kinetic chain effect in transferring energy from the legs up the core and trunk to the shoulder complex. In addition, in hitting, the powerful twisting movement of the hips and legs transfers the kinetic energy up in the core, trunk, and to the shoulders and arms. The importance of the core cannot be overemphasized. To this point, we have seen an increase in abdominal strains and low-back sprains/strains in recent years.

This chapter will examine the scientific literature regarding muscle recruitment patterns of lumbopelvic-hip musculature (commonly referred to as the "core") and loading of the lumbar spine during "core" exercises commonly employed during core-strengthening programs. The chapter will examine the importance of the "core," assess which core muscles are most important for core stability, report the benefits and risks of traditional and nontraditional core stabilization exercises, examine lumbar spinal loading and injury risk during exercises commonly employed to enhance core stability, and examine biomechanical differences between abdominal hollowing and bracing exercises, trunk flexion and extension exercises, and crunch and bent knee sit-up exercises.

WHY IS THE CORE IMPORTANT?

In functional and athletic events the core provides proximal stability for distal mobility.[1] Trunk musculature help stabilize the core by compressing and stiffening the spine, which is important because the osteoligamentous lumbar spine buckles under compressive loads of only 90 N (approximately 20 lbs).[2] Moreover, core muscles act as guy wires around the human spine to prevent spinal buckling.[2] In addition, as core muscles contract, intra-abdominal pressure increases,[3] which further increases spinal stiffness and enhances core stability.[4]

WHAT MUSCLES COMPRISE THE CORE AND WHICH CONTRIBUTE THE MOST TO CORE STABILITY?

There is considerable debate regarding which core muscles are the most important in optimizing core stability (spinal stabilization). Some have suggested that the transversus abdominis and multifidi muscles are key muscles in enhancing spinal stability,[5,6] but others have questioned the importance of these muscles as major stabilizers of the spine.[2,7] Therefore, the effectiveness of the transversus abdominis and multifidi on lumbar stability is not clear. Isolated contractions from the transversus abdominis have not been demonstrated during functional higher demand activities that require all abdominal muscles to become active.[8]

It has previously been reported that in healthy individuals without lumbar pathology, the transversus abdominis contracts before upper extremity motion regardless of the direction of the motion.[9] However, this has been challenged by Morris and colleagues[7] who reported that transversus abdominis activation is directional specific and that symmetrical, bilateral preactivation of the transversus abdominis does not normally occur in healthy individuals without lumbar pathology during rapid unilateral arm movements. This is important because it is postulated that bilaterally preactivation of the transversus abdominis provides lumbar spine stability in anticipation of perturbations of posture.[9] In contrast, transversus abdominis activation is significantly delayed in patients with low-back pain with all movements, indicating a motor control deficit that may result in inefficient muscular stabilization of the spine.[9] However, select low-intensity exercises, such as abdominal hollowing (drawing-in), have been shown to preferentially activate the transversus abdominis in patients with chronic low-back pain during exercises.[10] Moreover, there is evidence that the deep abdominal muscles (transversus abdominis and internal oblique) can be preferentially trained in those with chronic low-back pain by using exercises that target these muscles, such as abdominal hollowing.[11]

To optimize core stabilization, it appears that numerous muscles, including smaller deeper core muscles (eg, transversospinalis, transversus abdominis, internal oblique, quadratus lumborum) and larger superficial core muscles (eg, erector spinae, external oblique, rectus abdominis), must be activated in sequence with appropriate timing and tension.[2] Cholewicki and VanVliet[12] reported that no single core muscle can be identified as most important for lumbar spine stability, that the relative contribution of each core muscle to lumbar spine stability depended on trunk loading direction (spinal instability was greatest during trunk flexion) and magnitude, and that no one muscle contributed more than 30% to overall spine stability. Therefore, lumbar stabilization exercises may be most effective when they involve the entire spinal musculature and its motor control under various spine loading conditions.[12]

BENEFITS AND RISKS OF CORE STABILIZATION EXERCISES

Core strengthening of the lumbopelvic region may decrease injury risk to the thoracolumbar spine by enhancing spinal stability[13] and has been shown to both decrease lower extremity injury risk and enhance performance,[14] although there is not a strong relationship between core stability and performance and results are inconclusive.[15,16] While appropriate spinal loading enhances spinal stability, excessive spinal loading may increase the injury risk to the lumbar spine.[13] Therefore, spinal loading needs to be adequate to maximize core stability but not excessive, which may be injurious to the lumbar spine. For example, lifting extremely heavy weights during the deadlift exercise has resulted in estimated lumbar compressive forces between 18,000 and 36,000 N.[17,18] These extremely high lumbar compressive forces, which result from both the heavy external load being lifted and the high muscle forces that are generated during heavy lifting, may be injurious to the lumbar spine.[17,18]

Unfortunately, there is only a dearth of information in the literature regarding the effectiveness of lumbar stabilization exercises on lumbar pathology, and more research is needed to address this deficit.[19] Although lumbar stabilization exercise programs have been shown to be effective in treating individuals with chronic low-back pain,[20] these programs have not conclusively demonstrated that lumbar stabilization programs are more effective in treating individuals with chronic low-back pain compared with a less specific, more generalized exercise program.[19]

BIOMECHANICAL DIFFERENCES BETWEEN ABDOMINAL HOLLOWING (DRAWING-IN MANEUVER) AND ABDOMINAL BRACING TECHNIQUES

Abdominal hollowing is often performed supine with the hips flexed 45° and the knees flexed 90° (hook lying position), and after taking a deep breath, individuals are instructed to exhale while pulling their navel up and in toward the spine.[21] In abdominal bracing, individuals are instructed to globally activate all abdominal and low-back muscles by tensing all core musculature, without drawing in or pushing out the abdominal cavity.[8,22]

Abdominal hollowing is effective in preferential recruitment of the deeper abdominal (transversus abdominis and internal oblique muscles) and lumbar (multifidi) muscles.[23,24] Hides and colleagues[24] demonstrated that the transversus abdominis and internal oblique contract bilaterally to form a musculofascial "corset" that appears to tighten during abdominal hollowing, enhancing lumbar spine stability and decreasing injury risk to the lumbar spine. Transversus abdominis and internal oblique activity are believed to enhance lumbar stability by increasing intra-abdominal pressure[3] and tensioning the thoracolumbar fascia, and the multifidi provides additional spinal stability by directly controlling lumbar intersegmental movement.[6,25] Moreover, contraction of the transversus abdominis has been shown to significantly decrease the laxity of the sacroiliac joint to a greater extent in abdominal hallowing compared with abdominal bracing.[25] These data provide some evidence that abdominal hollowing may enhance spinal stability and be beneficial for individuals with select lumbar pathologies.

Using biomechanical models, abdominal hollowing has been compared with abdominal bracing with respect to spinal stability and muscle activity.[8,25,21] Grenier and McGill[8] reported that abdominal hollowing was not as effective as abdominal bracing for increasing lumbar spine stability, reporting that abdominal bracing improved lumbar spine stability by 32% with only a 15% increase in lumbar spine compression (higher benefit of lumbar stability with lower risk of lumbar injury). Moreover, these authors demonstrated that the transversus abdominis alone had very little effect on lumbar spine stability. However, when the effects of internal oblique and intra-abdominal pressure are combined with the effects of transversus abdominis, core stability was improved as more core muscles were activated, which is what occurs during abdominal bracing.

Vera-Garcia and colleagues[22] investigated how effective abdominal hollowing and bracing techniques were in controlling spinal mobility and stability against rapid perturbations. They reported that abdominal bracing performed better than abdominal hollowing for spinal stabilization during rapid perturbations. During rapid perturbations, abdominal bracing actively stabilized the spine and reduced lumbar spine displacement, while abdominal hollowing was not effective in spinal stabilization. From these data, it can be inferred that abdominal bracing is more effective than abdominal hollowing during functional activities such as lifting, jumping, pushing, and pressing activities in sport or daily living. However, core muscle cocontraction during abdominal bracing significantly increases lumbar compressive loads compared with abdominal hollowing, which may be problematic in those with lumbar pain and pathology. External oblique and rectus abdominis activity was significantly greater in abdominal bracing compared with abdominal hollowing. Moreover, abdominal hollowing demonstrated a higher spinal compressive loading (cost) to spine stability (benefit) ratio, which implies that abdominal hallowing resulted in higher spinal compressive loads (increased injury risk) with less spinal stability. During abdominal hollowing, individuals were not able to activate the deep abdominal muscles in isolation but always included significant activity from both the external oblique and internal oblique.[22]

Stanton and Kawchuk[26] investigated the effect of abdominal stabilization contractions during abdominal hollowing and bracing on posteroanterior spinal stiffness. Compared with abdominal hollowing, posteroanterior spinal stiffness was significantly greater in abdominal bracing. More work is needed to assess the long-term effects of abdominal hollowing and abdominal bracing on posteroanterior spinal stiffness in individuals with lumbar pain and pathologies.

Abdominal hollowing or bracing techniques have been performed immediately before core-strengthening exercises.[23,27,21] Barnett and Gilleard[23] reported that compared with the curl-up (Crunch) without abdominal hollowing or bracing, the curl-up with abdominal hollowing or bracing resulted in the deep abdominal muscles (transversus abdominis and internal oblique) being recruited earlier than the superficial abdominal muscles (rectus abdominis and external oblique).

Using ultrasound imaging, Teyhen and colleagues[21] examined deep abdominal recruitment patterns during numerous abdominal exercises (crunch, sit back, leg lowering, side plank) and low-back exercises (quadruped opposite arm and leg lift) performed immediately after employing abdominal hollowing. These authors reported that the highest recruitment of the transversus abdominis and internal oblique occurred during the side plank. McGill and colleagues[2,28] reported high activity from several important core muscles (quadratus lumborum, internal oblique, external oblique) during the side plank (resulting in enhanced spinal stability) with moderate spinal compressive loading. Teyhen and colleagues[21] reported high recruitment of the transversus abdominis and internal oblique and low compressive spinal loading during the crunch performed after abdominal hallowing, which is similar to what Axler and McGill reported.[13] Performing the quadruped opposite arm and leg lift after abdominal hallowing preferentially recruited the transversus abdominis with minimal recruitment of the internal oblique, which provides evidence for its use in early phases of motor control exercise programs that emphasize the firing of the transversus abdominis without concomitant high recruitment from other abdominal muscles.[21] From these data, it can be concluded that performing abdominal hallowing before performing abdominal exercises is beneficial to improving core muscle recruitment and spinal stability.

Oh and colleagues[27] investigated the effects of performing abdominal hollowing during prone hip extension exercises on hip and back muscle activity and anterior pelvic tilt. Compared with hip extension without abdominal hollowing, hip extension with abdominal hollowing resulted in significantly less erector spinae activity (17%±12% vs 49%±14% maximum voluntary isometric contraction, MVIC) and significantly greater gluteus maximus (52%±15% vs 24%±8% MVIC) and medial hamstring (58%±20% vs 47%±14% MVIC) activities. Moreover, anterior pelvic tilt was significantly greater without abdominal hollowing (10°±2°) compared with abdominal hollowing

$(3°\pm1°)$. It can be concluded from these data that performing abdominal hollowing with hip extension may be an effective strategy when the goal is to minimize anterior pelvic tilt, lumbar motion, and erector spinae activity and to maximize hip extensor activity.

TRADITIONAL VERSUS NONTRADITIONAL EXERCISES FOR CORE STABILITY

Examples of traditional and nontraditional exercises employed to enhance core stability are shown in Figures 41.1-41.16, and core muscle activity from these exercises are shown in Tables 41.1-41.4. Although these exercises are primarily used to strengthen abdominal musculature, they also recruit additional core muscles such as the latissimus dorsi and lumbar paraspinals.

The abdominal musculature help stabilize the trunk and unload the lumbar spine[13] and are commonly activated by concentric muscle action during trunk flexion such as during the Bent Knee Sit-up or Crunch (Figures 41.5 and 41.6). During the Crunch, the hips remain at a constant angle and the pelvis does not rotate, while during the Bent Knee Sit-up, the hips flex and the pelvis rotates anteriorly. Although the Bent Knee Sit-up has been shown to be effective in activating rectus abdominis and internal and external oblique musculature, the Crunch has been recommended in place of the Bent Knee Sit-up.[29-31] Although the abdominal musculature is activated similarly between the Crunch and Bent Knee Sit-up, unlike during the Crunch there is relatively high hip flexor activity that occurs during the Bent Knee Sit-up, which may increase lumbar spine stress.[13,29-31]

Examples of other traditional abdominal exercises include the Prone Plank on Toes and Side Plank on Toes, and several studies have reported core muscle activity using electromyography (EMG) during these and similar exercises.[29-31] Escamilla et al[30] examined core muscle activity among the Crunch, Bent Knee Sit-up, Prone Plank on Toes, and Side Plank on Toes (Table 41.4). Several significant differences were found: (1) upper rectus abdominis activity was greater in the Crunch compared with the Prone Plank on Toes and Side Plank on Toes, and greater in the Bent Knee Sit-up compared with the Side Plank on Toes; (2) lower rectus abdominis was less in the Side Plank on Toes compared with the remaining 3 exercises; (3) external oblique activity was greater in the Side Plank on Toes compared with the remaining 3 exercises; (4) latissimus dorsi activity was greater in the Prone Plank on Toes compared with the Crunch and Bent Knee Sit-up; (5) lumbar paraspinal activity was greater in the Side Plank on Toes compared with the remaining

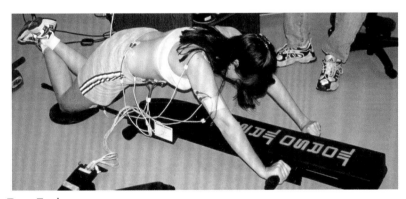

FIGURE 41.1 • Torso Track.

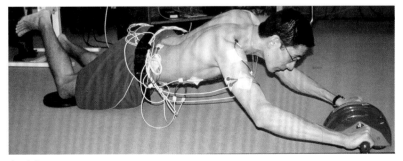

FIGURE 41.2 • Ab Slide.

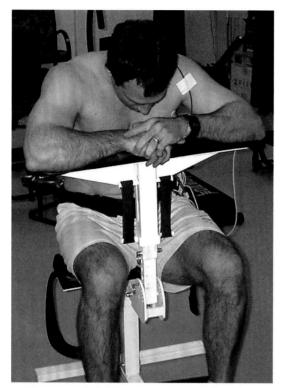

FIGURE 41.3 ▪ Super Abdominal Machine (SAM).

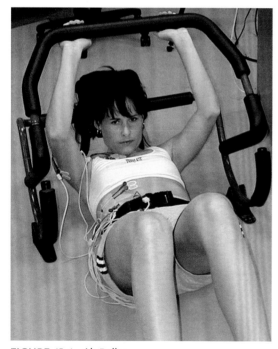

FIGURE 41.4 ▪ Ab Roller.

3 exercises; and (6) rectus femoris activity was greater in the Bent Knee Sit-up compared with the Side Plank on Toes and Crunch, and greater in the Prone Plank on Toes compared with the Crunch.

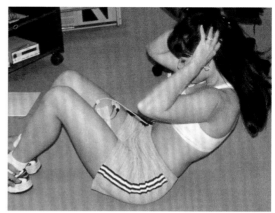

FIGURE 41.5 ▪ Bent Knee Sit-up.

During the Prone Plank on Toes and Side Plank on Toes, Ekstrom et al[32] reported similar rectus abdominis and external oblique activity compared with Table 41.4 and also reported moderate to high longissimus thoracis, lumbar multifidi, gluteus medius, and gluteus maximus activity during the Side Plank on Toes. In addition, internal oblique and quadratus lumborum have demonstrated moderate to high activity during the Side Plank on Toes.[32] Hence, the Side Plank on Toes is a very effective exercise in recruiting core muscles that are important for core stability. However, lumbar compressive force is relatively high in the Side Plank on Toes,[33] which may be problematic for individuals with lumbar pathologies. The Prone Plank on Toes and Crunch produce similar amounts of rectus abdominis, internal oblique, and external oblique activates, but the Prone Plank on Toes was more effective in recruiting the latissimus dorsi and rectus femoris muscles compared with the Crunch.

Abdominal musculature are activated in a different manner during nontraditional core exercises compared with the traditional Crunch and Bent Knee Sit-up. An example is the Reverse Crunch (performing the traditional Crunch in reverse), which involves flexing the trunk by posteriorly rotating the pelvis (Figures 41.11 and 41.12). Nontraditional core exercises may also involve controlling trunk extension (owing to an external force such as gravity) by isometric or eccentric muscle contractions, such as performing the Swiss Ball Decline Push-up (Figure 41.16) by keeping a neutral pelvis and spine.

The Swiss Ball or commercial devices or machines may also be employed during nontraditional core exercises (Figures 41.1-41.4 and 41.7-41.16). Some devices or machines allow only uniplanar motions, such as trunk flexion, whereas others allow multiplanar motions, such as trunk flexion and rotation or trunk extension and rotation.[29-31,34] Adding rotational

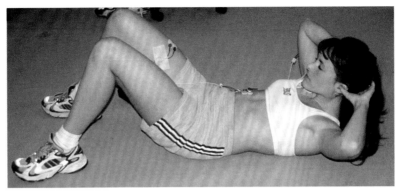

FIGURE 41.6 • Crunch.

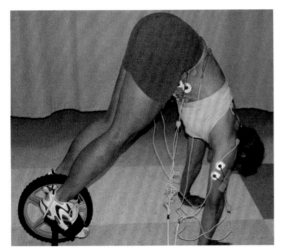

FIGURE 41.7 • Power Wheel Pike.

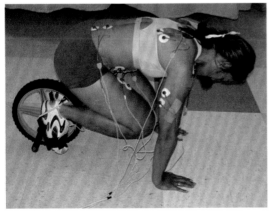

FIGURE 41.8 • Power Wheel Knee-up.

components to trunk flexion can be advantageous in internal or external oblique recruitment. For example, performing the Crunch and Ab Roller with rotation results in simultaneous trunk flexion and rotation. Performing these exercises with left rotation (Crunch Oblique and Ab Roller Oblique) resulted in greater right external oblique activity compared with performing the Crunch and Ab Roller with trunk flexion with no rotation (Crunch Normal and Ab Roller Crunch) (Table 41.1).[31]

EMG data in the scientific literature are limited while performing nontraditional abdominal exercises, with or without abdominal devices.[29-31,35-39] Core muscle activity has been quantified while performing abdominal exercises employing commercial machines or devices, such as the Torso Track, Power Wheel, Hanging Strap, Super Abdominal Machine, Ab Revolutionizer, Ab Slide, Ab Doer, Ab Shaper, Ab Flex, Ab Roller, Ab Rocker, Ab Vice, and Ab Twister.[29-31,34-39] There are several abdominal devices that do not appear to offer any advantage in recruiting abdominal musculature compared with Crunch, Reverse Crunch, and Bent Knee Sit-up, such as the Ab Revolutionizer.[29,31] However, one advantage of the Ab Revolutionizer is that external weight can be added, thereby allowing exercise intensity to be varied. The Reverse Crunch Flat and Ab Revolutionizer Reverse Crunch were performed nearly identical to each, with the only difference is the Reverse Crunch Flat was performed without using an abdominal device. In addition, the Crunch and Ab Roller, which are performed nearly identical to each other, produced similar amounts of abdominal activity (Table 41.1). However, one advantage of the Ab Roller is that the head is supported (Figure 41.4), which may be more comfortable compared with the Crunch, and therefore many individuals may prefer the Ab Roller over the Crunch. Schoffstall et al[34] also reported that performing exercises with abdominal devices that do not appear to offer any advantage in recruiting abdominal musculature compared performing similar exercises without abdominal devices.

Other commercial devices, such as the Ab Twister, Ab Doer, and Ab Rocker, exhibited significantly less abdominal muscle activity compared with the traditional Crunch, Reverse Crunch, and Bent Knee Sit-up, and significantly less abdominal activity compared

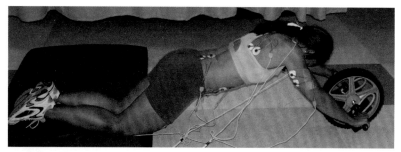

FIGURE 41.9 • Power Wheel Rollout.

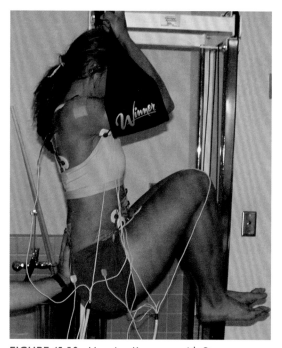

FIGURE 41.10 • Hanging Knee-ups with Straps.

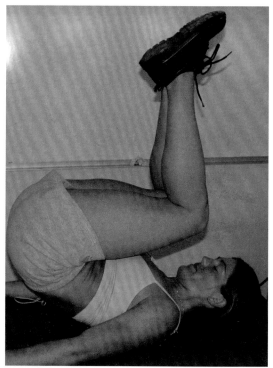

FIGURE 41.11 • Reverse Crunch Flat.

with other commercial abdominal devices, such as the Torso Track, Ab Slide, and Ab Roller.[31] Moreover, the Ab Twister, Ab Doer, and Ab Rocker tend to generate relatively high rectus femoris or lumbar paraspinal activity, which may be contraindicated in individuals with lumbar spine pathologies.[31]

Escamilla et al[29,31] quantified core muscle activity in 27 traditional and nontraditional core exercises with and without various commercial abdominal devices and machines. Of the 27 exercises, 12 are illustrated in Figures 41.1-41.12 with their EMG data shown in Tables 41.1 and 41.2. Among these exercises, upper rectus abdominis activity was highest for the Power Wheel Rollout, Hanging Knee-up with Straps, Reverse Crunch Inclined 30°, Ab Slide, Torso Track, Crunch, and Ab Roller and lowest for the Ab Revolutionizer, Reverse Crunch, Ab Twister, Ab Rocker, and Ab Doer. Lower rectus abdominis activity was highest for the Power Wheel Rollout, Hanging Knee-up with Straps, Ab Slide, and Torso Track and lowest for the Ab Twister, Ab Rocker, and Ab Doer. External oblique activity was highest for the Power Wheel Pike, Power Wheel Knee-up, Hanging Knee-up with Straps, Ab Slide, and Bent Knee Sit-up and lowest for the Crunch, Ab Roller, and Ab Doer. Internal oblique activity was highest for the Power Wheel Rollout, Power Wheel Pike, Power Wheel Knee-up, Hanging Knee-up with Straps, Reverse Crunch Inclined 30°, Ab Slide, Torso Track, Bent Knee Sit-up, and Crunch, and lowest for the Ab Roller, Ab Twister, Ab Rocker, and Ab Doer. These authors concluded that although the traditional Crunch and Bent Knee Sit-up are effective in recruiting abdominal musculature, abdominal recruitment was higher in the Power Wheel Rollout, Power Wheel Pike, Power Wheel Knee-up, Hanging Knee-up with Straps, Reverse Crunch Inclined 30°, Ab Slide, and Torso Track.

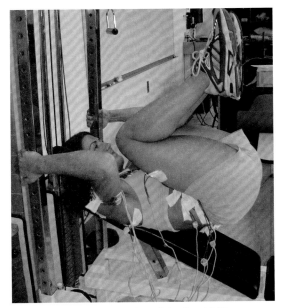

FIGURE 41.12 • Reverse Crunch Inclined 30°.

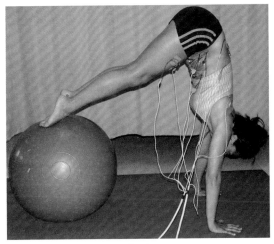

FIGURE 41.13 • Swiss Ball Pike.

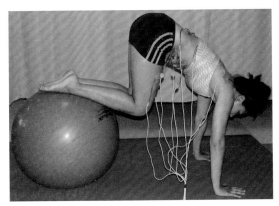

FIGURE 41.14 • Swiss Ball Knee-up.

Many exercises performed with commercial abdominal devices or machines can also be performed using a Swiss Ball, and many studies have quantified core muscle activity during various Swiss Ball exercises.[30,37,40-49] Escamilla et al[30] quantified core muscle activity (Table 41.3) between several Swiss Ball exercises (Figures 41.13-41.16) and the traditional Crunch and Bent Knee Sit-up (Figures 41.5 and 41.6). From Table 41.3, rectus abdominis activity was greatest in the Swiss Ball Rollout, Swiss Ball Pike, and Crunch, while external and internal oblique activities were greatest in the Swiss Ball Rollout, Swiss Ball Pike, and Swiss Ball Knee-up. Latissimus dorsi activity was greatest in the Swiss Ball Pike, Swiss Ball Knee-up, and Swiss Ball Decline Push-up, while rectus femoris activity was greatest in the Swiss Ball Pike, Swiss Ball Knee-up, and Bent Knee Sit-up. Lumbar paraspinal activity was relativity low in all exercises. Although rectus abdominis recruitment is similar among the Crunch, Bent Knee Sit-up, and Swiss Ball exercises, internal and external oblique activities were generally greater in Swiss Ball exercises compared with the Crunch and Bent Knee Sit-up.

Many abdominal exercises traditionally performed on a flat surface can also be performed on a Swiss Ball, such as the Push-up, Bench Press, and Crunch. Several studies have reported an increase in abdominal muscle activity when the Push-up is performed on an unstable surface (eg, Swiss Ball) compared with a stable surface.[44,50-52] Abdominal muscle activity is greater when a Bench Press is performed on a Swiss Ball compared with a flat stable surface.[52,53] Other studies have demonstrated an increase in abdominal muscle activity when performing the Crunch on a Swiss Ball compared with performing the Crunch on a flat surface.[41,48,49] Bridging using an unstable surface (Swiss Ball and BOSU Ball) has also demonstrated greater abdominal activity compared with bridging on a flat surface.[42]

Scott et al[46] reported that compared with a nonlabile surface, using a labile surface, Swiss Ball enhanced lumbar multifidus activity in individuals with chronic low-back pain. However, Paz et al[54] reported that the Swiss Ball may not provide a potential effect on erector spinae activity during Pilates isometric exercises with similar posture when compared with stable surfaces.

In additional to being effective in activating abdominal musculature, the Power Wheel Rollout, Swiss Ball Rollout, Power Wheel Pike, Swiss Ball Pike, Power Wheel Knee-up, Swiss Ball Knee-up, Hanging Knee-up with Straps, and Reverse Crunch Inclined 30°, Reverse Crunch Flat, Ab Slide, Torso Track, Prone Plank on Toes, and Side Plank on Toes are also effective

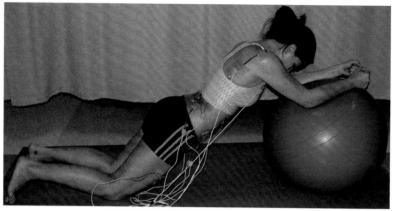

FIGURE 41.15 • Swiss Ball Rollout.

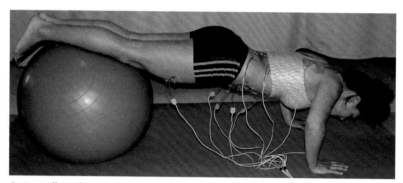

FIGURE 41.16 • Swiss Ball Decline Push-up.

exercises in activating the latissimus dorsi (Tables 41.1-41.4),[29-31] which tenses the thoracolumbar fascia when it contracts and helps stabilize the trunk. Moreover, tension in thoracolumbar fascia from contractions from the internal oblique (and presumably the transversus abdominis) may further enhance lumbar stability, and most of these exercises produce high internal oblique activity (Tables 41.1-41.4). However, all these exercises except for the Power Wheel Rollout, Swiss Ball Rollout, Ab Slide, and Torso Track also exhibited significant rectus femoris activity (and to a lesser extent lumbar paraspinal activity), which may be problematic for some individuals with low-back pathologies owing to the tendency of the hip flexors and lumbar extensors to accentuate lumbar lordosis, lumbar compression, and intradiskal pressure.[3,13] Therefore, the Power Wheel Rollout, Swiss Ball Rollout, Ab Slide, and Torso Track may be the most effective exercise in recruiting abdominal and latissimus dorsi musculature while minimizing rectus femoris and lumbar paraspinal activity. During these "rollout" exercises, the latissimus dorsi contract eccentrically during the initial rollout phase to control the rate of shoulder flexion, and concentrically in the return phase as the shoulders extend. Moreover, although it is logical to assume that the rectus femoris contracts eccentrically during the initial rollout phase (to control the rate of hip extension) and concentrically during the return phase (to cause hip flexion), rectus femoris activity was very low during these 4 exercises. This may partially be explained by the neutral pelvic and spine positions that are maintained while performing these exercises. Workman and colleagues[55] reported that when the pelvis is maintained in neutral or posterior tilted positions compared with an anterior tilted position, there is a tendency for abdominal activity to increase and rectus femoris activity to decrease. Therefore, the latissimus dorsi (and upper extremity muscles in general) may have a greater role in both controlling and causing the rollout and rollback movements during these exercises compared with the hip flexors.

Exercises that recruit the rectus femoris and lumbar paraspinals may be contraindicated for those with weak abdominal muscles or lumbar instability. The forces generated when the hip flexors and lumbar extensors contract act to anteriorly rotate the pelvis and increase the lordotic curve of the lumbar spine, as well as increase L4/L5 compression and intradiskal pressure,[3] and when coupled with weak abdominal musculature, the risk of low-back pathologies increases during these

TABLE 41.1 Machine Device Abdominal Exercises Compared With Traditional Abdominal Crunch and Sit-up Exercises

	Upper Rectus Abdominis	Lower Rectus Abdominis	Internal Oblique	External Oblique	Latissimus Dorsi	Lumbar Paraspinals	Rectus Femoris
Ab Slide	67±26	72±19	53±15	40±16	10±4	3±2	5±3[d]
Torso Track	67±25	72±17	58±14	32±18	10±5	2±2	6±5[d]
Crunch (normal)	51±9	50±8[a,b]	41±9	16±11[a,c]	5±1[d]	2±1	3±2[d]
Crunch (oblique)	50±15	39±14[a,b]	40±11	32±22	8±5	5±3	3±2[d]
Bent Knee Sit-up	38±12[a,b]	44±13[a,b]	49±21	41±16	6±3[d]	4±2	36±16
Super Abdominal Machine (SAM)	42±17[a,b]	50±20[a,b]	36±13[b]	31±21	12±6	4±2	20±15
Ab Roller (crunch)	46±17	42±12[a,b]	38±9[b]	13±8[a,c]	5±2[d]	3±2	1±1[d]
Ab Roller (oblique)	49±12	36±16[a,b]	25±11[a,b,c]	20±9	6±2[d]	3±2	2±2[d]

Average electromyography (EMG) (±SD) for each muscle and exercise expressed as a percentage of maximum isometric voluntary contraction.

Significant difference (P < .001) in EMG activity among abdominal exercises.

Pairwise comparisons (P < .01):

[a]Significantly less EMG activity compared with the Ab Slide (straight and curved).

[b]Significantly less EMG activity compared with the Torso Track.

[c]Significantly less EMG activity compared with the Bent Knee Sit-up.

[d]Significantly less EMG activity compared with the SAM.

Adapted with permission from Escamilla RF, McTaggart MS, Fricklas EJ, et al. An electromyographic analysis of commercial and common abdominal exercises: implications for rehabilitation and training. J Orthop Sports Phys Ther. 2006;36:45-57. doi:10.2519/jospt.2006.36.2.45. ©Journal of Orthopaedic & Sports Physical Therapy®.

conditions.[13] Exercises such as the Bent Knee Sit-up, Power Wheel Pike, Power Wheel Knee-up, Reverse Crunch Inclined 30°, and Reverse Crunch Flat, which have relatively high rectus femoris or lumbar paraspinal activity compared with the Crunch, Ab Roller, Ab Slide, Torso Track, and Power Wheel Rollout, may be contraindicated in individuals with weak abdominal muscles or lumbar instability.[13,29,30] Moreover, during abdominal exercises the EMG magnitude and recruitment pattern of the psoas and iliacus is similar (within 10%) to that of the rectus femoris,[56] which implies that the psoas, iliacus, and rectus femoris may exhibit similar EMG recruitment patterns and magnitudes when performing the aforementioned abdominal exercises. The psoas muscle, by its attachments into the lumbar spine, attempts to hyperextend the spine as it flexes the hip, and this action may be detrimental to some individuals with lumbar instability. The psoas muscle can also generate lumbar compression and anterior shear force at L5-S1,[13,57] which may be problematic for those with lumbar disk pathologies. Although muscle force from the lumbar paraspinals can also increase compression of the lumbar spine, it should be noted that the aforementioned abdominal exercises generated relatively low muscle activity (<10% of a MVIC) from the lumbar paraspinals (Tables 41.1-41.2).[29,31]

BIOMECHANICAL DIFFERENCES BETWEEN ABDOMINAL EXERCISES THAT CAUSE ACTIVE HIP OR TRUNK FLEXION OR CONTROL HIP OR TRUNK EXTENSION

Some core exercises may be appropriate for some individuals but not for others. Some core exercises cause hip and trunk flexion, such as the Bent Knee Sit-up, while other core exercises control hip and trunk extension, such as the Power Wheel Rollout or Swiss Ball Rollout. Core exercises that actively flex the trunk may be problematic for some individuals with lumbar disk pathologies due to increased intradiskal pressure and lumbar spine compression,[3,13] as well as individuals with osteoporosis due to the risk of vertebral compression fractures.[58] In these individuals, it may be more beneficial to maintain a neutral pelvis and spine, such as when performing the Power Wheel or Swiss Ball Rollout, rather than forceful flexion of the lumbar spine, such as when performing the Bent Knee Sit-up. Lumbar stabilization exercises using a Swiss Ball have demonstrated to be an effective interventional therapy for the alleviation of chronic low-back pain and to increase bone mineral density of patients.[59]

TABLE 41.2 Power Wheel and Reverse Crunch Exercises Compared With Traditional Abdominal Crunch and Sit-up Exercises

	Upper Rectus Abdominis	Lower Rectus Abdominis	Internal Oblique	External Oblique	Latissimus Dorsi	Lumbar Paraspinals	Rectus Femoris
Power Wheel Rollout	76±26	81±29	66±25	64±27[b]	15±7[b,c,f]	5±2[b,c,d,e]	6±4[b,c,d,e,h]
Power Wheel Pike	41±11[a,d,e,g]	53±16[a,d]	83±31	96±32	27±16	8±3	26±11[c]
Power Wheel Knee-up	41±18[a,d,e,g]	45±12[a,d]	72±32	80±30	25±12	8±4	43±18
Hanging Knee-up with Straps	69±21	75±16	85±40	79±25	21±12	7±3	15±8[b,c]
Reverse Crunch Inclined 30°	77±27	53±13[a,d]	86±37	50±19[b,c,d]	14±8[b,c,f]	8±4	22±12[c]
Reverse Crunch Flat	41±20[a,d,e,g]	30±13[a,b,c,d,e,g]	52±24[b,c,d,e]	39±16[a,b,c,d]	23±14	6±3[b,c,e]	11±5[b,c,e,h]
Crunch	56±17[a,e]	48±13[a,d]	42±10[b,c,d,e]	27±16[a,b,c,d,e,h]	5±3[a,b,c,d,e,f]	3±1[b,c,d,e,f,h]	3±3[b,c,d,e,h]
Bent Knee Sit-up	39±9[a,d,e,g]	38±11[a,b,d,e]	49±22[b,c,d,e]	50±16[b,c,d]	6±3[a,b,c,d,f]	6±3[b,c,e]	22±12[c]

Average electromyography (EMG) (±SD) for each muscle and exercise expressed as a percentage of maximum isometric voluntary contraction.

Significant difference (P < .001) in EMG activity among abdominal exercises.

Pairwise comparisons (P < .01):

[a]*Significantly less EMG activity compared with the Power Wheel Rollout.*

[b]*Significantly less EMG activity compared with the Power Wheel Pike.*

[c]*Significantly less EMG activity compared with the Power Wheel Knee-up.*

[d]*Significantly less EMG activity compared with the Hanging Knee-up with Straps.*

[e]*Significantly less EMG activity compared with the Reverse Crunch Inclined 30°.*

[f]*Significantly less EMG activity compared with the Reverse Crunch Flat.*

[g]*Significantly less EMG activity compared with the Crunch.*

[h]*Significantly less EMG activity compared with the Bent Knee Sit-up.*

From Escamilla RF, Babb E, DeWitt R, et al. Electromyographic analysis of traditional and nontraditional abdominal exercises: implications for rehabilitation and training. Phys Ther. 2006;86:656-671. Adapted by permission of American Physical Therapy Association.

Some individuals with facet joint syndrome, spondylolisthesis, and vertebral or intervertebral foramen stenosis may not tolerate exercises in which the trunk is maintained in extension but may better tolerate trunk flexion exercises such as the Crunch. In these individuals, trunk flexion–type exercises may decrease facet joint stress and pain and increase vertebral or intervertebral foramina openings, decreasing the risk of spinal cord impingement, nerve root impingement, or facet joint syndrome.

Although "rollout" exercises (eg, Swiss Ball Rollout) and reverse Crunch–type exercises (eg, Hanging Knee-up with Straps) are all effective in activating abdominal musculature, these 2 types of exercises are performed in a different manner.

During rollout exercises, the abdominal musculature contract eccentrically or isometrically to resist the attempt of the force due to gravity to extend the trunk and rotate the pelvis. During the return motion the abdominal musculature contract concentrically or isometrically. If the pelvis and spine are stabilized and maintained in a neutral position throughout the rollout and return movements, then the abdominal musculature primarily contract isometrically. While performing rollout exercises, a relatively neutral pelvis and spine is maintained throughout the movement. In contrast, in reverse Crunch–type exercises, such as the Hanging Knee-up, the abdominal musculature contract concentrically initially as the hips flex, the pelvis rotates

TABLE 41.3 Prone Position Swiss Ball Exercises Compared With Traditional Supine Position Abdominal Crunch and Sit-up Exercises

Exercise	Upper Rectus Abdominis	Lower Rectus Abdominis	Internal Oblique	External Oblique	Latissimus Dorsi	Lumbar Paraspinal	Rectus Femoris
Swiss Ball Rollout	63±30	53±23	46±21	46±18[b]	12±9[b,c]	6±2	8±5[b,c,e]
Swiss Ball Pike	47±18	55±16	56±22	84±37	25±11	8±3	24±6
Swiss Ball Knee-up	32±15[a,d]	35±14	41±16	64±39	22±13	6±3	23±8
Crunch	53±19	39±16	33±13[b]	28±17[b,c]	8±3[b,c,f]	5±2	6±4[b,c,e]
Bent Knee Sit-up	40±13[a]	35±14	31±11[b]	36±14[b,c]	8±3[b,c,f]	6±2	23±12
Swiss Ball Decline push-up	38±20[a]	37±16	33±18[b]	36±24[b,c]	18±12	6±2	10±6[b,c,e]

Average electromyography (EMG) ±SD for each muscle and exercise expressed as a percentage of each muscle's maximum isometric voluntary contraction.

Significant difference (P < .001) in EMG activity among abdominal exercises.

Pairwise comparisons (P < .01):

[a]Significantly less EMG activity compared with the Swiss Ball Rollout.

[b]Significantly less EMG activity compared with the Swiss Ball Pike.

[c]Significantly less EMG activity compared with the Swiss Ball Knee-up.

[d]Significantly less EMG activity compared with the Crunch.

[e]Significantly less EMG activity compared with the Bent Knee Sit-up.

[f]Significantly less EMG activity compared with the Swiss Ball Decline Push-up.

Adapted with permission from Escamilla RF, Lewis C, Bell D, et al. Core muscle activation during Swiss ball and traditional abdominal exercises. J Orthop Sports Phys Ther. 2010;40:265-276. doi:10.2519/jospt.2010.3073. ©Journal of Orthopaedic & Sports Physical Therapy®.

TABLE 41.4 Prone and Side Plank Exercises Compared With Traditional Abdominal Crunch and Sit-up Exercises

Exercise	Upper Rectus Abdominis	Lower Rectus Abdominis	Internal Oblique	External Oblique	Latissimus Dorsi	Lumbar Paraspinal	Rectus Femoris
Prone Plank on Toes	34±15[c]	40±10	29±12	40±21[b]	18±12	5±2[b]	20±7
Side Plank on Toes	26±15[c,d]	21±9[a,c,d]	28±12	62±37	12±10	29±16	14±4[d]
Crunch	53±19	39±16	33±13	28±17[b]	8±3[a]	5±2[b]	6±4[a,d]
Bent Knee Sit-up	40±13	35±14	31±11	36±14[b]	8±3[a]	6±2[b]	23±12

Average electromyography (EMG) ±SD for each muscle and exercise expressed as a percentage of each muscle's maximum isometric voluntary contraction.

Significant difference (P < .001) in EMG activity among abdominal exercises.

Pairwise comparisons (P < .01):

[a]Significantly less EMG activity compared with the Prone Plank on Toes.

[b]Significantly less EMG activity compared with the Side Plank on Toes.

[c]Significantly less EMG activity compared withthe Crunch.

[d]Significantly less EMG activity compared with the Bent Knee Sit-up.

Adapted with permission from Escamilla RF, Lewis C, Bell D, et al. Core muscle activation during Swiss ball and traditional abdominal exercises. J Orthop Sports Phys Ther. 2010;40:265-276 . doi:10.2519/jospt.2010.3073. ©Journal of Orthopaedic & Sports Physical Therapy®.

posteriorly, and the lumbar spine flexes. As the knees are lowered and the hips extend, the reverse movements occur, and the abdominal musculature contracts eccentrically to control the rate of returning to the starting position.

The Hanging Knee-up with Straps, Swiss Ball Pike, Power Wheel Pike, Swiss Ball Knee-up, and Power Wheel Knee-up are all performed similarly by flexing the hips, posteriorly rotating the pelvis, and flattening the lumbar spine, which is basically the reverse action of what occurs during the Bent Knee Sit-up, which involves trunk flexion followed by hip flexion (Bent Knee Sit-up only).[29-31] One limitation to the Hanging Knee-up with Straps is a relatively high L4/L5 disk compression that occurs.[13] However, L4/L5 disk compression has been shown to be slightly higher in the Bent Knee Sit-up compared with the Hanging Knee-up with Straps.[13] Furthermore, EMG from the upper and lower rectus abdominis and internal and external oblique are all significantly greater in the Hanging Knee-up with Straps compared with the Bent Knee Sit-up.[29] Therefore, the Hanging Knee-up with Straps may be preferred over the Bent Knee Sit-up for higher level individuals who want to elicit a higher challenge to the abdominal musculature; however, neither exercise may be appropriate for some individuals with lumbar pathologies due to relatively high L4/L5 compression.

When the lumbar spine is forcefully flexed, which may occur when performing commercial abdominal machine exercises such as the Ab Twister, Ab Rocker, and Ab Doer, the anterior fibers of the intervertebral disk is compressed while the posterior fibers are in tension. In addition, in extreme lumbar flexion, intradiskal pressure may increase several times above the normal intradiskal pressure from a resting supine position.[3] While these stresses on the disk may not be problematic for the normal healthy disk, they may be detrimental to the degenerative disk or pathologic spine.

BIOMECHANICAL DIFFERENCES BETWEEN THE CRUNCH AND BENT KNEE SIT-UP

Not all abdominal exercises involve the same degree of flexion of the lumbar spine. Halpern and Bleck[60] have demonstrated that lumbar spinal flexion was only 3° during the Crunch but approximately 30° during the Bent Knee Sit-up. In addition, the Bent Knee Sit-up has been shown to generate greater lumbar intradiskal pressure[3] and compression[13] compared

with exercises similar to the Crunch, largely due to increased lumbar flexion.[57] This implies the Crunch may be a safer exercise to perform than the Bent Knee Sit-up for some individuals who need minimize lumbar spinal flexion or compressive forces due to lumbar pathology.[13]

Although the Crunch and Bent Knee Sit-up are both effective in recruiting abdominal musculature (Tables 41.1-41.3), there are some differences. Several studies have shown that external oblique activity, and to a lesser extent internal oblique activity, are significantly greater in the Bent Knee Sit-up compared with the Crunch.[13,29-31,57] However, upper rectus abdominis activity has been shown to be greater in the Crunch compared with the Bent Knee Sit-up (Tables 41.1-41.3).[29-31] In addition, rectus femoris and psoas activities have been shown greater in the Bent Knee Sit-up compared with the Crunch.[28,29-31,57] Increased muscle activity from the rectus femoris and psoas may exacerbate low-back pain in some individuals with low-back pathologies.

ABDOMINAL AND OBLIQUE RECRUITMENT BETWEEN THE CRUNCH AND REVERSE CRUNCH

Performing the Reverse Crunch Flat activates the lower abdominals and external oblique to a greater extent than the Crunch.[61] In contrast, Escamilla et al[29,31] and Clark et al[36] reported significantly greater upper and lower rectus abdominis activities in the Crunch compared with the Reverse Crunch Flat, while external and internal oblique activities were not significantly different between these 2 exercises. These discrepancies may be due to methodological differences among studies. For example, in Willett et al,[61] the Reverse Crunch Flat was performed by having subjects raise the lower half of the body off the table as far as possible, while in Escamilla et al[29,31] the subjects were instructed to maximally posteriorly tilt the pelvis and flex the hips. However, during the Reverse Crunch Inclined 30°, which involved a higher degree of difficulty compared with both the Crunch and Reverse Crunch Flat, there was significantly greater upper rectus abdominis, internal oblique, and external oblique activity compared with the Crunch and Reverse Crunch Flat, but there was no significant difference in lower rectus abdominis activity between the Reverse Crunch Inclined 30° and Crunch (Table 41.2).[29] These data show that the increasing difficulty of the Reverse Crunch Inclined 30° results in proportional increases in muscle activity.

MANAGER'S TIPS

- Understanding how different exercises elicit core muscle activity and load the lumbar spine is useful to therapists and other health care or fitness specialists who develop specific core exercises for their patients or clients to facilitate their rehabilitation or training needs

- Core exercises discussed in this chapter activated abdominal muscles and loaded the lumbar spine by a variety of ways, such as actively flexing the trunk, controlling trunk extension, flexing the hips with posterior pelvis rotation, or a combination of flexing the trunk and flexing the hips with spinal and pelvis rotations

- Several nontraditional abdominal exercises generated significantly greater rectus abdominis, internal oblique, and external oblique activity compared with traditional abdominal exercises such as the Crunch and Bent Knee Sit-up. Although both the Crunch and Bent Knee Sit-up demonstrated similar amounts of abdominal activity, the Crunch may be a safer exercise for individuals with low-back pathologies because of relatively high rectus femoris activity and lumbar intradiskal pressure generated during the Bent Knee Sit-up

- Rollout exercises (eg, Power Wheel Rollout, Swiss Ball Rollout, Ab Slide, and Torso Track) were shown to be the most effective exercise in activating rectus abdominis, internal oblique, external oblique, and latissimus dorsi muscles while minimizing lumbar paraspinal and rectus femoris activity

- The Power Wheel Pike, Swiss Ball Pike, Power Wheel Knee-up, Swiss Ball Knee-up, Hanging Knee-up with Straps, and Reverse Crunch Inclined 30° were all shown to be very effective exercises in activating rectus abdominis, internal oblique, external oblique, and latissimus dorsi muscles but at a cost of also producing relatively high rectus femoris or lumbar paraspinal activity (which may be problematic for individuals with lumbar pathologies)

- Many exercises that generated high activity from multiple core muscles, such as abdominal bracing, also produced the greatest core stability as well as relatively high lumbar compressive loads (which may increase injury risk to the lumbar spine)

- Exercises that activated only a few muscles, such as abdominal hallowing, may not be effective in producing the level of core stability needed for many functional activities, such as lifting, running, and jumping. However, these types of exercises may be appropriate early in a core stabilization program, as well as for individuals that cannot tolerate high lumbar compressive loading

- Many individuals, such as athletes training for sport, employ a wide array of sport-specific functional exercises to develop core muscles and enhance core stability. However, there is an absence of research that has been done and reported in the literature involving the effectiveness of performing higher level functional exercises on core stability, and this needs to be the focus of future research

REFERENCES

1. Kibler WB, Press J, Sciascia A. The role of core stability in athletic function. *Sports Med.* 2006;36:189-198.

2. McGill SM. Low back stability: from formal description to issues for performance and rehabilitation. *Exerc Sport Sci Rev.* 2001;29:26-31.

3. Nachemson AL. Disc pressure measurements. *Spine.* 1981;6:93-97.

4. Essendrop M, Andersen TB, Schibye B. Increase in spinal stability obtained at levels of intra-abdominal pressure and back muscle activity realistic to work situations. *Appl Ergon.* 2002;33:471-476.

5. Hodges PW. Is there a role for transversus abdominis in lumbo-pelvic stability? *Man Ther.* 1999;4:74-86.

6. Wilke HJ, Wolf S, Claes LE, Arand M, Wiesend A. Stability increase of the lumbar spine with different muscle groups. A biomechanical in vitro study. *Spine.* 1995;20:192-198.

7. Morris SL, Lay B, Allison GT. Corset hypothesis rebutted—transversus abdominis does not co-contract in unison prior to rapid arm movements. *Clin Biomech.* 2012;27:249-254.

8. Grenier SG, McGill SM. Quantification of lumbar stability by using 2 different abdominal activation strategies. *Arch Phys Med Rehabil.* 2007;88:54-62.

9. Hodges PW, Richardson CA. Inefficient muscular stabilization of the lumbar spine associated with low back pain. A motor control evaluation of transversus abdominis. *Spine.* 1996;21:2640-2650.

10. Teyhen DS, Miltenberger CE, Deiters HM, et al. The use of ultrasound imaging of the abdominal drawing-in maneuver in subjects with low back pain. *J Orthop Sports Phys Ther.* 2005;35:346-355.

11. O'Sullivan PB, Twomey L, Allison GT. Altered abdominal muscle recruitment in patients with chronic back pain following a specific exercise intervention. *J Orthop Sports Phys Ther.* 1998;27:114-124.

12. Cholewicki J, VanVliet JJ IV. Relative contribution of trunk muscles to the stability of the lumbar spine during isometric exertions. *Clin Biomech.* 2002;17:99-105.

13. Axler CT, McGill SM. Low back loads over a variety of abdominal exercises: searching for the safest abdominal challenge. *Med Sci Sports Exerc.* 1997;29:804-811.

14. Willson JD, Dougherty CP, Ireland ML, Davis IM. Core stability and its relationship to lower extremity function and injury. *J Am Acad Orthop Surg*. 2005; 13:316-325.

15. Okada T, Huxel KC, Nesser TW. Relationship between core stability, functional movement, and performance. *J Strength Cond Res*. 2011;25:252-261.

16. Reed CA, Ford KR, Myer GD, Hewett TE. The effects of isolated and integrated 'core stability' training on athletic performance measures: a systematic review. *Sports Med*. 2012;42:697-706.

17. Cholewicki J, McGill SM, Norman RW. Lumbar spine loads during the lifting of extremely heavy weights. *Med Sci Sports Exerc*. 1991;23:1179-1186.

18. Granhed H, Jonson R, Hansson T. The loads on the lumbar spine during extreme weight lifting. *Spine*. 1987;12:146-149.

19. Standaert CJ, Weinstein SM, Rumpeltes J. Evidence-informed management of chronic low back pain with lumbar stabilization exercises. *Spine J*. 2008;8:114-120.

20. Wang XQ, Zheng JJ, Yu ZW, et al. A meta-analysis of core stability exercise versus general exercise for chronic low back pain. *PLoS One*. 2012;7:e52082.

21. Teyhen DS, Rieger JL, Westrick RB, Miller AC, Molloy JM, Childs JD. Changes in deep abdominal muscle thickness during common trunk-strengthening exercises using ultrasound imaging. *J Orthop Sports Phys Ther*. 2008;38:596-605.

22. Vera-Garcia FJ, Elvira JL, Brown SH, McGill SM. Effects of abdominal stabilization maneuvers on the control of spine motion and stability against sudden trunk perturbations. *J Electromyogr Kinesiol*. 2007;17:556-567.

23. Barnett F, Gilleard W. The use of lumbar spinal stabilization techniques during the performance of abdominal strengthening exercise variations. *J Sports Med Phys Fitness*. 2005;45:38-43.

24. Hides J, Wilson S, Stanton W, et al. An MRI investigation into the function of the transversus abdominis muscle during "drawing-in" of the abdominal wall. *Spine*. 2006;31:E175-E178.

25. Richardson CA, Snijders CJ, Hides JA, Damen L, Pas MS, Storm J. The relation between the transversus abdominis muscles, sacroiliac joint mechanics, and low back pain. *Spine*. 2002;27:399-405.

26. Stanton T, Kawchuk G. The effect of abdominal stabilization contractions on posteroanterior spinal stiffness. *Spine*. 2008;33:694-701.

27. Oh JS, Cynn HS, Won JH, Kwon OY, Yi CH. Effects of performing an abdominal drawing-in maneuver during prone hip extension exercises on hip and back extensor muscle activity and amount of anterior pelvic tilt. *J Orthop Sports Phys Ther*. 2007;37:320-324.

28. McGill S, Juker D, Kropf P. Quantitative intramuscular myoelectric activity of quadratus lumborum during a wide variety of tasks. *Clin Biomech*. 1996;11:170-172.

29. Escamilla RF, Babb E, DeWitt R, et al. Electromyographic analysis of traditional and nontraditional abdominal exercises: implications for rehabilitation and training. *Phys Ther*. 2006;86:656-671.

30. Escamilla RF, Lewis C, Bell D, et al. Core muscle activation during Swiss ball and traditional abdominal exercises. *J Orthop Sports Phys Ther*. 2010;40:265-276.

31. Escamilla RF, McTaggart MS, Fricklas EJ, et al. An electromyographic analysis of commercial and common abdominal exercises: implications for rehabilitation and training. *J Orthop Sports Phys Ther*. 2006;36:45-57.

32. Ekstrom RA, Donatelli RA, Carp KC. Electromyographic analysis of core trunk, hip, and thigh muscles during 9 rehabilitation exercises. *J Orthop Sports Phys Ther*. 2007;37:754-762.

33. Kavcic N, Grenier S, McGill SM. Quantifying tissue loads and spine stability while performing commonly prescribed low back stabilization exercises. *Spine*. 2004;29:2319-2329.

34. Schoffstall JE, Titcomb DA, Kilbourne BF. Electromyographic response of the abdominal musculature to varying abdominal exercises. *J Strength Cond Res*. 2010; 24:3422-3426.

35. Avedisian L, Kowalsky DS, Albro RC, Goldner D, Gill RC. Abdominal strengthening using the AbVice machine as measured by surface electromyographic activation levels. *J Strength Cond Res*. 2005;19:709-712.

36. Clark KM, Holt LE, Sinyard J. Electromyographic comparison of the upper and lower rectus abdominis during abdominal exercises. *J Strength Cond Res*. 2003;17:475-483.

37. Hildenbrand K, Noble L. Abdominal muscle activity while performing trunk-flexion exercises using the Ab roller, ABslide, FitBall, and conventionally performed trunk curls. *J Athl Train*. 2004;39:37-43.

38. Sternlicht E, Rugg S. Electromyographic analysis of abdominal muscle activity using portable abdominal exercise devices and a traditional crunch. *J Strength Cond Res*. 2003;17:463-468.

39. Warden SJ, Wajswelner H, Bennell KL. Comparison of Abshaper and conventionally performed abdominal exercises using surface electromyography. *Med Sci Sports Exerc*. 1999;31:1656-1664.

40. Behm DG, Leonard AM, Young WB, Bonsey WA, MacKinnon SN. Trunk muscle electromyographic activity with unstable and unilateral exercises. *J Strength Cond Res*. 2005;19:193-201.

41. Cosio-Lima LM, Reynolds KL, Winter C, Paolone V, Jones MT. Effects of physioball and conventional floor exercises on early phase adaptations in back and abdominal core stability and balance in women. *J Strength Cond Res*. 2003;17:721-725.

42. Czaprowski D, Afeltowicz A, Gebicka A, et al. Abdominal muscle EMG-activity during bridge exercises on stable and unstable surfaces. *Phys Ther Sport*. 2014;15:162-168.

43. Imai A, Kaneoka K, Okubo Y, et al. Trunk muscle activity during lumbar stabilization exercises on both a stable and unstable surface. *J Orthop Sports Phys Ther*. 2010;40:369-375.

44. Marshall PW, Murphy BA. Core stability exercises on and off a Swiss ball. *Arch Phys Med Rehabil*. 2005;86:242-249.

45. Mori A. Electromyographic activity of selected trunk muscles during stabilization exercises using a gym ball. *Electromyogr Clin Neurophysiol*. 2004;44:57-64.

46. Scott IR, Vaughan AR, Hall J. Swiss ball enhances lumbar multifidus activity in chronic low back pain. *Phys Ther Sport*. 2015;16:40-44.

47. Stanton R, Reaburn PR, Humphries B. The effect of short-term Swiss ball training on core stability and running economy. *J Strength Cond Res*. 2004;18:522-528.

48. Sternlicht E, Rugg S, Fujii LL, Tomomitsu KF, Seki MM. Electromyographic comparison of a stability ball crunch with a traditional crunch. *J Strength Cond Res*. 2007;21:506-509.

49. Vera-Garcia FJ, Grenier SG, McGill SM. Abdominal muscle response during curl-ups on both stable and labile surfaces. *Phys Ther*. 2000;80:564-569.

50. Calatayud J, Borreani S, Colado JC, Martin F, Rogers ME. Muscle activity levels in upper-body push exercises with different loads and stability conditions. *Phys Sportsmed*. 2014;42:106-119.

51. Lehman GJ, MacMillan B, MacIntyre I, Chivers M, Fluter M. Shoulder muscle EMG activity during push up variations on and off a Swiss ball. *Dyn Med*. 2006;5:7.

52. Marshall PW, Murphy BA. Increased deltoid and abdominal muscle activity during Swiss ball bench press. *J Strength Cond Res*. 2006;20:745-750.

53. Norwood JT, Anderson GS, Gaetz MB, Twist PW. Electromyographic activity of the trunk stabilizers during stable and unstable bench press. *J Strength Cond Res*. 2007;21:343-347.

54. Paz G, Maia M, Santiago F, Lima V, Miranda H. Muscle activity of the erector spinae during Pilates isometric exercises on and off Swiss Ball. *J Sports Med Phys Fitness*. 2014;54:575-580.

55. Workman JC, Docherty D, Parfrey KC, Behm DG. Influence of pelvis position on the activation of abdominal and hip flexor muscles. *J Strength Cond Res*. 2008;22:1563-1569.

56. McGill S, Juker D, Kropf P. Appropriately placed surface EMG electrodes reflect deep muscle activity (psoas, quadratus lumborum, abdominal wall) in the lumbar spine. *J Biomech*. 1996;29:1503-1507.

57. Juker D, McGill S, Kropf P, Steffen T. Quantitative intramuscular myoelectric activity of lumbar portions of psoas and the abdominal wall during a wide variety of tasks. *Med Sci Sports Exerc*. 1998;30:301-310.

58. Sinaki M. Exercise for patients with osteoporosis: management of vertebral compression fractures and trunk strengthening for fall prevention. *PM R*. 2012;4:882-888.

59. Yoon JS, Lee JH, Kim JS. The effect of swiss ball stabilization exercise on pain and bone mineral density of patients with chronic low back pain. *J Phys Ther Sci*. 2013;25:953-956.

60. Halpern AA, Bleck EE. Sit-up exercises: an electromyographic study. *Clin Orthop Relat Res*. 1979:172-178.

61. Willett GM, Hyde JE, Uhrlaub MB, Wendel CL, Karst GM. Relative activity of abdominal muscles during commonly prescribed strengthening exercises. *J Strength Cond Res*. 2001;15:480-485.

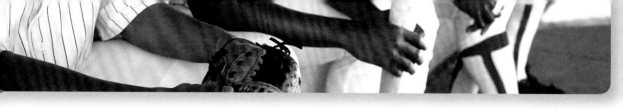

CHAPTER **42**

Spine Injury Prevention and Rehabilitation

AJ Yenchak, PT, DPT, CSCS | Joseph L. Ciccone, PT, DPT, FAAOMPT, CSCS, OCS, SCS, Cert. DN/SMT, CIMT

As a ballplayer, I would be delighted to do it again. As an individual, I doubt if I could possibly go through it again.

—*Roger Maris*

INTRODUCTION

The throwing and batting motion in baseball are a sequential, violent transfer of coordinated, forceful movements between the upper and lower extremity. The energy that is required and created to throw or hit a baseball stems from additive force production in the presence of structural joint stability, motion, soft tissue mobility, muscular endurance/strength, and fine motor control. The legs and trunk work sequentially to deliver energies to the upper extremity in preparation for ball release.[1,2] Measured strong ground reaction forces correlate with higher pitch velocities.[3] Kibler and Livingston[4] explained how the lower extremity and spine provide the foundation for arm motion. The summation of force output (arm acceleration) between the upper and lower extremity is the direct result of kinetic linkage via the spine and lumbopelvic musculature that serve as an epicenter for energy production and a conduit for energy transfer. Optimal baseball throwing/hitting mechanics are predicated on proper sequencing of force, spinal motion, and dynamic muscular control.[156] Lumbopelvic muscular control is the ability to grade and disperse force to dynamically stabilize or create motion within the lumbopelvic region in response to intrinsic/extrinsic force application.[7] There are multiple studies that have investigated the role of the lumbopelvic region to identify correlates in throwing velocity pertaining to the shoulder and elbow. Early pelvic rotation (opening toward home plate),[8-10] forward trunk tilt at ball release,[11] and increased contralateral trunk tilt[12] were all associated with higher pitch velocity with the latter two substantially increasing shoulder axial rotation and elbow valgus load.[5,12-13] Before foot contact, the trunk rotates 55° ± 6° with a mean angular acceleration of 3100°/s.[15] Lumbar paraspinals have been shown to increase their activity by up to 400% during this transition.[16] Strong gluteal muscular components were also recognized by Campbell[17] as a driving force in the transition of the body forward during throwing. The gluteals act as an integral component to controlling pelvic rotation during pitching patterns of drive.[17-19] These biomechanical studies demonstrate the necessary grading, calibration, and output of energies between the lumbopelvic region and the upper and lower extremity during the pitching motion. Any change or resistance to energy transfer among the upper and lower extremity kinetic link can increase the propensity toward developing injury at more distal segments, namely the elbow or throwing shoulder.

The hitting motion also involves a vital interplay of trunk motion, synchronous muscle firing and lumbopelvic stability to generate the forces necessary to reach angular accelerations of 7200 ± 2800 just after contact.[15] The hip complex and spine are responsible for synchronization of shoulder/hip rotation from the initial trigger of the swing through ball contact. The lumbar spine and trunk play an integral role in creating the foundation for axial rotation, torso speed, and proper neuromuscular facilitation for drive off of the back leg during the baseball swing.[20,21] Any deviation throughout the kinetic chain can potentially predispose a hitter to injury, especially to the oblique region. To date, there are no studies that correlate lumbopelvic control with injury rates in baseball pitchers. There is 1 study investigating the relationship between spinal motion and baseball players. The information contained in this chapter will provide insight into the assessment and rehabilitation necessary to prevent injury in this unique athletic population.

SPINE INJURIES IN BASEBALL

There are a multitude of injuries that can occur to the spine and hip complex resulting from the excessive forces produced during hitting, pitching, throwing, and running. At any given moment, the spine can flex, extend, rotate, laterally bend, or combine (couple) motions to produce an athletic positioning of the body, preparing the athlete to execute movement patterns that place profound demand on the musculoskeletal system. Table 42.1 represents the most prevalent spine injuries observed in baseball. [22] The majority of these injuries are classified as "mechanical," which are attributed to an acute traumatic event or cumulative trauma where pain is potentially present in spinal joints, disks, vertebrae, or soft tissues. Athletes that perform repetitive lumbar extension/rotation are more susceptible to stress reaction/fracture in the pars interarticularis, pedicle, or articular process.[23] Facet joint pain results from acute trauma, chronic repetitive trauma, and/or inflammation from cyclic rotation with the spine extended. Athletes often have pain with active extension/rotation (coupled motions) on testing. Sacroiliac (SI) joint pain can arise from trauma, poor lumbopelvic control, hip myofascial hypomobility, and predisposing inflammatory diseases such as ankylosing spondylitis.[24,25]

Radicular pain is generally associated with compression, inflammation, or injury to the spinal nerve root as seen in herniated disks, foraminal stenosis, and peridural fibrosis.[26] There is often a component of severe pain, sensation loss, and/or muscle weakness that radiates into the lower extremity along the course of the corresponding spinal nerve. Annular tears and disk herniations occur from repetitive compressive/rotatory forces within the lumbar spine that eventually lead to vulnerabilities in the annulus fibrosis of the lumbar disk. Pain is generally severe and accompanied by muscular spasm and radiating pain into the lower extremity. Stenosis develops from chronic disk protrusion, facet hypertrophy, or ligament ossification that is accompanied by radicular symptoms and/or neurogenic claudication.[22]

The most common form of spinal injury with or without low-back pain (LBP) is soft tissue trauma/myofascial strain. The pitching and hitting motions require a critical balance of stability, mobility, and endurance to withstand cyclic loading to the axial spine. The muscles involved within this aspect of the kinetic chain are most susceptible to injury owing to increasing imposed demands. Factors such as deconditioning, poor flexibility, decreased abdominal endurance, and overtraining have previously been described by Conte[27] to understand the nature of myofascial vulnerability. According to Camp,[22] 54% of Major League Baseball (MLB) abdominal injuries occurred between March and May between 2011 and 2015. Athletes who report to spring training lacking flexibility, strength from off-season inactivity pose the biggest risk to developing this type of injury. The injuries generally occur in an acute incidence with a definitive mechanism of injury. On clinical examination, these athletes have difficulty moving through full spinal range of motion (ROM)

TABLE 42.1 Prevalent Lumbar Injuries in Baseball

Condition	Features
Stress fracture/spondylolysis	Common in athletes undergoing repetitive spine extension Present in up to one-third of athletes with low-back pain Bone scan is the preferred method of diagnostic testing
Muscle injury	Acute event May have history of prior, similar injuries
Annular tears/disc herniation	Combined compressive/rotatory forces Pain often severe/potential radiating component Disk protrusion progression can lead to radicular symptoms
Facet joint pain	Facet joints are typically injured during rotation of the extended spine Pain often reproduced by active range of motion (AROM) back extension
Sacroiliac joint pain	Presents with deep pain localized to sacroiliac joint
Stenosis	Often presents with slowly progressive pain ± radicular symptoms Congenital stenosis may be predisposing factor for increased injury risk

and have focal, superficial tenderness along the muscle in question. A previous injury of similar course can also be present in this athletic population.[27]

BASEBALL INJURY PREVALENCE

Recent comprehensive advancements in training, strength/conditioning, rehabilitation, diagnostic testing, and surgical procedure have not provided full insight into the spectrum of injuries that can occur to the baseball athlete during the length of a competitive season. Despite a plethora of literature pertaining to orthopedic-related injuries relating to the baseball athletes' shoulder and elbow, spine and core injuries continue to occur with more frequency, especially in MLB.[22] Back injuries constituted 1016 disabled list days per season from 1995 to 1999.[27,28] Disabled list reports in MLB from 1989 to 2010 demonstrated that abdominal strains accounted for 4.5% of all injuries. Of those injuries, 92% were internal/external oblique or intercostal muscle strains. Spine and core injuries were responsible for 359 disabled list designations from 2002 to 2008, representing 11.7% of all injuries resulting in lost playing time.[29] During that same time period, the prevalence of spine/core injuries ranked sixth among 17 body parts reported with position players and pitchers being equally affected (7.8% and 7.4%, respectively). An upward trend was seen in MLB with injury rates 22% higher in the 2000s than the 1990s. According to Camp and colleagues,[22] MLB and Minor League Baseball players missed on average 22.2 days per abdominal injury from 2011 to 2015. During that time interval, batting injuries accounted for 45.7%, pitching 34.9%, and throwing (nonpitching) 5.8%. McFarland and Wasik[30] were the first to report epidemiologic data for collegiate baseball injury rates over 3 seasons. Their data largely coincided with the data presented by Conte[28] in that upper extremity injuries accounted for 58% of all injuries reported while 15% (trunk/back) and 27% lower extremity constituted the remaining injury groups. There is currently no literature pertaining to youth baseball spine injury prevalence.

ASSESSMENT

Identification of the musculoskeletal complaint is initiated with a thorough history pertaining to current concomitant morbidity, psychosocial factoring, and the ruling out of more severe neurologic impairments that would require immediate hospitalization (paralysis/neoplasm/infection). Additional information involving timing, severity, exacerbating factors, current symptomology, and any previous treatments should be discussed and prioritized to establish a definitive diagnosis and treatment algorithm for the proposed condition. A complete list of factors pertaining to the history outlined by McGill[31] can be found in Table 42.2. Proper imaging considerations can also be defined during this time to expedite care within the acute setting. Not all conditions will warrant further diagnostic testing initially, so it is imperative to gather all relevant information to determine additional steps within the initial plan of care and to set the framework for a structured, directed, physical examination.

Physical Examination

The physical examination will begin with observation of the athlete in stance. The spine should be visualized and assessed for abnormal posturing that would rule in adaptive compensatory strategies to limit pain. Optimal baseball throwing and batting mechanics require a significant contribution of thoracolumbar motion, particularly in the sagittal and transverse planes.[32] Active range of motion (AROM) is assessed during this time to gain understanding of the patient's readiness to perform movements that could potentially aggravate symptoms and to gain objective information as a foundational marker for tracking progress. AROM within the lumbar spine (Table 42.3) is a summation of motion

TABLE 42.2 Evaluation Checklist

- Identify the rehabilitation objectives (specific health or performance objective)
- Consider patient age and general condition
- Consider the mechanism of injury
- Describe the perceived exacerbators of pain and symptoms
- Have the patient describe the type of pain, its location, whether it is radiating, and specific dermatomes and myotomes
- Identify potential dermatomal and myotomal implications

TABLE 42.3 Active Movements of the Lumbar Spine

- Forward flexion (40°-60°)
- Extension (20°-35°)
- Side (lateral) flexion, left and right (15°-20°)
- Rotation, left and right (3°-18°)
- Sustained postures (if necessary)
- Repetitive motion (if necessary)
- Combined movements (if necessary)

Reprinted from Magee DJ. Orthopedic Physical Assessment. 5th ed. St. Louis: Saunders; 2008:533. Copyright © 2008 Elsevier. With permission.

of all segments within the axial spine including the hip complex. There is minimal lumbar segmental motion observed owing to the size of the vertebral bodies, presence of intervertebral disks, tautness of capsuloligamentous structures, and the orientation of the facet joints.[33] The priority of motion testing will be determined based on painful motions, with those motions performed last. If the problem is mechanical, at least 1 or more of the motion tests will trigger the athlete's pain.[34,35] Although active motion testing is being performed, it is important for the examiner to document specific causes of aberrant motion and or motion loss (spasm, pain, stiffness, mechanical block). Forward flexion is generally 40° to 60° and can be observed simply by observation of the lumbar lordotic curve transition into the forward bend. The lumbar spine should assume a flat or slightly flexed positioning at end-range flexion with normal kinematic motion. If this posturing is not observed, there could potentially be hypomobility present from underlying structure or soft tissue restriction[33] (Figure 42.1). Muscle twitching with complaints of "slipping out" may be an underlying sign of lumbar instability with active motion testing.[36] Special attention is given to knee position on forward bending with a loss of extension signifying potential hamstring tightness or nerve root pathology. Additional special tests may be required to differentiate between the 2 presentations if observed. On returning to the upright position, the hip/pelvis will rotate first to 45° of flexion, with the lumbar spine assuming its normal lordotic curve during the last 45° to upright. Extension AROM is normally limited to 20° to 35° within the lumbar spine. Hands are placed on the waist while performing the desired motion while the athlete describes the quality of the motion (Figure 42.2). Lateral flexion or side bending is 15° to 20° in the lumbar spine. The examiner can objectively measure with a tape the distance the athlete is able to slide

the fingertips down the lateral aspect of the leg without flexing or extending the trunk (Figure 42.3). Rotation in the lumbar spine is between 3° and 18°. The test is

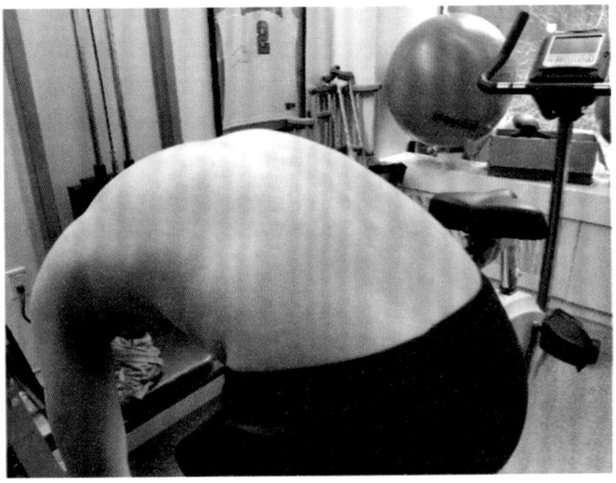

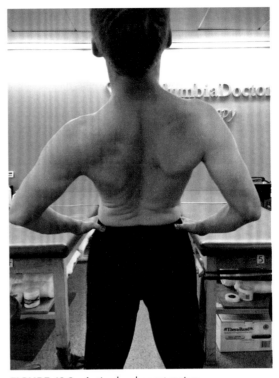

FIGURE 42.2 • Active lumbar extension.

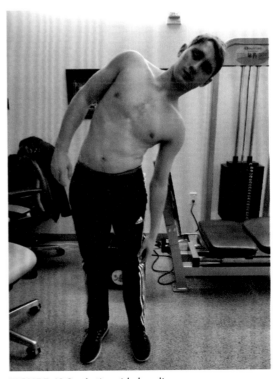

FIGURE 42.3 • Active side bending.

FIGURE 42.1 • Normal curvature of lumbar spine in forward flexion.

performed in the seated position with the arms crossed over the shoulders to eliminate extraneous motion in the pelvis and upper quarter (Figure 42.4). Baseball injuries related to the spine will most likely occur owing to combined (coupled) movements rather than uniplanar isolated motion. The examiner will most likely want to further their understanding of potential pathology within the spine by observing lateral flexion in flexion, lateral flexion in extension, flexion and rotation, and extension and rotation. These motions may create a different presentation of symptoms and are indicated if the athlete previously performed a combined motion that created their primary complaint (concordant sign) (Figure 42.5). Table 42.4 illustrates average ROM within the lumbar spine.

Resisted Isometric Strength/Dynamic Motion Testing

Resisted isometric muscle strength is tested in the neutral position with the patient seated. Movement is minimized when testing flexion, extension, lateral flexion, and rotation. The lumbar spine should maintain a neutral position for all tests administered throughout the duration of the hold. The hold should be maintained for 5 seconds. McGill and colleagues[37] showed that the relationship of endurance between the anterior, lateral, and posterior

musculature is impaired once spine injury occurs. Testing is considered normal if the patient is able to maintain static postures without pain or minimal pain for the respective time duration. The examiner can transition testing procedure toward higher level postural positions that will elicit more load demand to the lumbopelvic complex in the form of dynamic endurance testing. Biering-Sorensen's initial research on decreased torso extensor endurance concluded strong predictive values for future development of LBP.[38,39] Recently, McGill[31,40] demonstrated that the balance of endurance between the flexors, extensors, and lateral musculature was a better determinant for predicting those that would develop LBP. Being that these grouping of muscles are activated for nearly all athletic motions pertaining to baseball, the endurance of these muscles are paramount to the preventative strategies currently in place to evaluate, rehabilitate, and further condition baseball athletes for optimal performance. The testing protocol is derived by McGill,[40] which has shown high reliability coefficients (0.98 or higher) when repeated over 5 consecutive days. It is important to note that extensor endurance is decreased relative to both flexors and lateral musculature in patients with a history of spine injury.[31,41] Table 42.5 defines ratios that place the athlete at most risk for the development of spine-related injury resulting from unbalanced muscular effort.

Lateral musculature test (Figure 42.6)

Flexor endurance test (Figure 42.7)

Back extensor test (Figure 42.8)

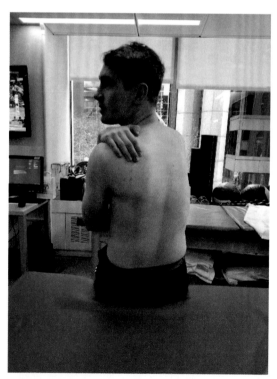

FIGURE 42.4 • Active lumbar rotation.

TRIP TO THE MOUND

Endurance Testing Interpretation

Endurance times recorded from young healthy individuals suggest that the relationship in endurance between the anterior, posterior, and lateral musculature is disrupted once injury occurs. The imbalance in endurance within the lumbopelvic region can also persist long after symptoms have normalized. Extensor endurance deficit is generally present in those athletes who continue to have chronic lumbopelvic deficiencies/injury. Endurance testing remains a critical component of the evaluation process to identify and target proper rehabilitation strategies that address these problems in baseball players.

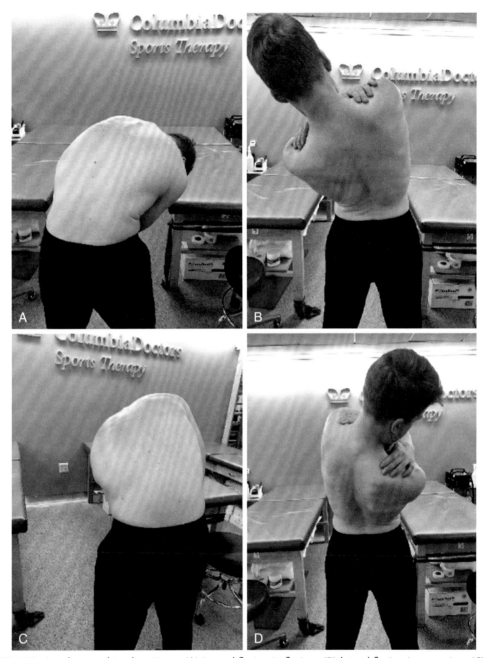

FIGURE 42.5 • Lumbar combined motions: (A) Lateral flexion in flexion; (B) lateral flexion in extension; (C) flexion and rotation; and (D) extension and rotation.

Differentiating between hip pain and back pain can be challenging. Radicular pain has been shown to potentially generate from more than 1 source.[26] If the athlete describes symptoms that emanate down the leg or are focal to the buttock region, a slump test (Figure 42.9) can be performed to stress the lumbar nerve roots and sciatic nerve. The hallmark of this test is the component of cervical flexion, which is added last in the sequence of positional changes of the head/lower extremity (LE). If cervical flexion does not recreate

the athlete's symptom, the test can be progressed to further evaluate structures such as the SI joint, piriformis, hamstrings, and hip complex. Typically, anteromedial thigh pain, groin pain, and discomfort around the inguinal crease are hallmark indicators of hip pathology.[42] Hip flexion and rotation tests are used to determine intra-articular pathology pertaining to impingement, muscle length discrepancy, and ROM of the lumbopelvic region.[42,43] The lateral step-down test (Figure 42.10) is also implemented in the

TABLE 42.4 Lumbar Spine Range of Motion (ROM)

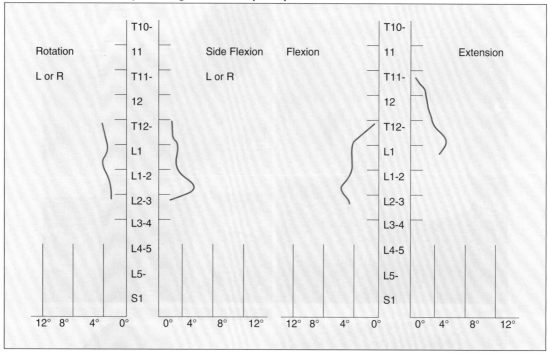

TABLE 42.5 Interpreting Endurance Scores (RISK)

Right side bridge/left side bridge endurance	>0.05
Flexion/extension endurance	>1.0
Side Bridge (either side)/extension endurance	>0.75
Extensor strength (Nm)/extensor endurance (s)	>4.0

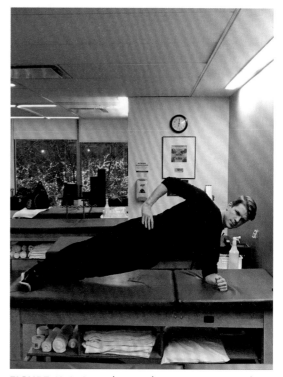

FIGURE 42.6 • Lateral musculature test. Reprinted with permission from McGill SM. *Low Back Disorders: Evidence-Based Prevention and Rehabilitation*. 3rd ed. Champaign, IL: Human Kinetics; 2016:288. Copyright © 2016 by Backfitpro, Inc.

dynamic assessment to further understand the role of the lateral hip stabilizers to lumbopelvic control. The premise of this test (pelvic obliquity) has been previously described by Chaudhari[44] during dynamic single leg stance observation. Hip drop greater than 7° can increase the likelihood of developing injuries to pitchers according to the author. This test is relatively easy to implement in any clinical/performance setting and provides valuable information to the examiner regarding proper identification of athletes who are at risk for injury/performance decline. Important information gained from these assessments will determine

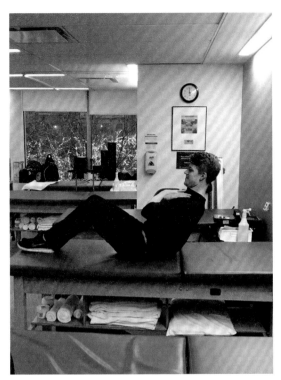

FIGURE 42.7 • Flexor endurance test.

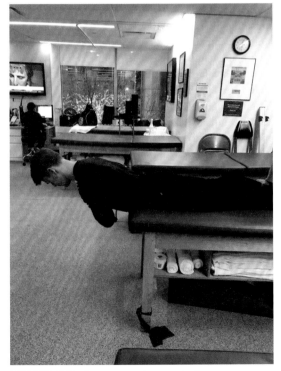

FIGURE 42.8 • Extensor endurance test.

primary or contributing factors to the athlete's pain presentation that will further define the treatment algorithm.

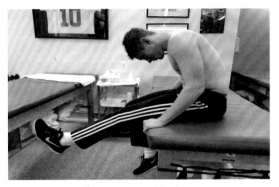

FIGURE 42.9 • Slump test positioning.

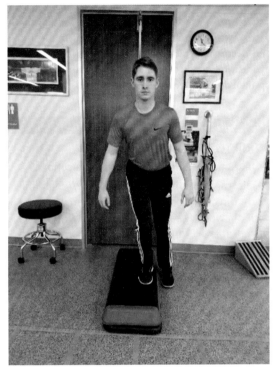

FIGURE 42.10 • Lateral step-down test.

TREATMENT/REHABILITATION

There are still a plethora of sports medicine experts who continue to believe that abdominal strength and a stronger back are most protective to the prevention of spinal injury when Luoto and colleagues[45,46] demonstrated that muscle endurance is the key determinant to spine health in the early 1980s. Surface and intramuscular electromyography (EMG) studies performed by McGill and colleagues[47] have shown that virtually all muscles within the torso have a role in spinal stabilization. Muscles including the multifidus, quadratus lumborum, iliocostalis, longissimus, and the intertransversarii produce critical stabilizing forces to the axial spine that largely go unnoticed when defining primary pathways toward this function. The "Big 3" previously described by McGill[48] include the rectus abdominis, lateral torso musculature (quadratus lumborum, lateral oblique, transverse abdominis), and back extensors form the foundation for the rehabilitation principles that will be discussed in this section. McGill previously demonstrated that there is no 1 single abdominal exercise that can be performed to challenge all abdominal musculature while sufficiently sparing the spine of deleterious load. In 1981, the National Institute for Safety and Health (NIOSH) published guidelines for maximal compressive loading of the lumbar spine with an action limit of 3400 N (750 lbs).[49-51] Subsequent studies by Marras et al[52] and Norman[53] have validated the NIOSH approach to restricting cumulative compression on the spine and decreasing the overall risk of lower spine injury by identifying postures and lifting techniques that are optimal during specific functional tasks.

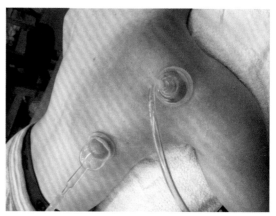

FIGURE 42.11 • Cupping modality.

TRIP TO THE MOUND

Quantifiable Efficacy in Exercise Selection

Determining exercise prescription/rehabilitation direction requires a multifactorial assessment involving the severity of injury, individual fitness level, and previous history of lumbopelvic dysfunction of the baseball athlete. NIOSH guidelines provide insight toward the effects of certain physical movements, as they pertain to functional recovery protocols. The action limits set forth by NIOSH give sports medicine specialists specific direction when referencing load penalty on the spine, as they generate exercise prescriptions. Exercises now have a quantifiable efficacy that cultivates proper exercise progression/specific tissue loading to promote more efficient recovery patterns in baseball athletes.

Exercise design, as it pertains to rehabilitation and injury prevention, is in a state of transition when describing methods to promote lumbopelvic stability. EMG activity of the conventional and highly recommended sit-up demonstrates spinal loading of over 3000 N through a flexed lumbar spine. Superman exercises that involve both upper and lower extremity extension lying in prone elicits over 6000 N of compression, which is well beyond the action limits set forth by NIOSH. The use of more objective data pertaining to specific exercise and spinal compression give specialists an evidence-based route toward progressive

tissue loading that challenges muscle, decreases overall load penalty to the spine, and provides sufficient, comprehensive stability to the lumbopelvic region during baseball activity. A rehabilitation program will follow a multiphased approach that incorporates principles of restorative myofascial lengthening, endurance-based therapeutic exercise, labile surface training, cable/free weight-resistance training, torsional conditioning, and exercise with elevated breathing patterns.[8,40,48,54]

The initial phase of rehabilitation begins with restoring ROM, decreasing pain associated with injury, and addressing musculoskeletal soft tissue irritability/mobility impairment. Treatments include manual soft tissue manipulation via ischemic compression to decrease myofascial sensitivity superficially within the target area. Modalities such as laser, iontophoresis, cupping (Figure 42.11), and ultrasound can be used to decrease inflammation, desensitize nerves, modulate pain, and stimulate blood flow. Manual trigger point massage as well as foam rolling can be initiated to the anterior/lateral/posterior pelvis to decrease superficial fascial irritation along the lumbopelvic region. Athletes can perform gentle exercise to the lumbopelvic/thoracic complex in the form of pelvic tilts and cat/camel exercises in the prone position to reduce spinal viscosity. McGill has shown that 5 to 6 cycles of each exercise are sufficient to improve motion within the axial spine.[48] Aerobic exercise when tolerable is advocated to promote mild but prolonged activation of the abdominal musculature in the presence of lower spinal load.[55,56] Walking is an excellent form of cardiovascular training. Research has demonstrated that exercise programs that combine cardiovascular components are more effective in enhancing rehabilitation programs and preventing injury.[57]

According to McGill,[58] grooving patterns of spinal stability are performed early in the rehabilitation course and are generally emphasized at the beginning of each treatment session. The spine has a particular loading memory that can modulate positioning of the spine in subsequent activity.[8,41] Engaging the "Big 3" (anterior/lateral/posterior torso) ensure a stable spine, as activities are appropriated within the athlete's program design. Exercise such as the curl up (Figure 42.12) challenges the rectus abdominis/abdominal wall under low-compression penalty to the spine (24-2800 N).[48] Variations of the side bridge (Figure 42.13) have demonstrated adequate recruitment of the quadratus lumborum (50% maximal voluntary contraction [MVC]), transverse abdominis, and abdominal obliques without load penalty (2500 N).[48] Activating the back extensors (longissimus, iliocostalis, and multifidi) is achieved by prone single leg extension holds, which activated the unilateral lumbar extensors to 18% MVC with spinal loading below 2500 N (Figure 42.14). The exercise can be further challenged to incorporate a contralateral arm raise (Figure 42.15) that imposes a load penalty of 3000 N.[55] The athlete should refrain from raising the arm or leg past parallel. Neutral spine posturing is of paramount importance when performing this exercise series. Isometric holds performed within

the 3 exercises should be maintained for no more than 7 to 8 seconds owing to rapid loss of oxygen of the contracting torso musculature.[54] At the beginning stages of the rehabilitation program 20 to 30 repetitions is recommended, progressing to 45 to 60 as the athlete gains familiarity with the program. These exercises are performed on a daily basis and are sufficient to maintain day-to-day spine health as an athlete recovers from injury. The clinician/specialist will determine the progression toward higher spinal demand as the athlete transitions to more intermediate challenges to the lumbopelvic complex. Table 42.6 demonstrates optimal endurance ratios described by McGill.

Labile surface training is performed once sufficient spinal stabilization is achieved in the beginning phases of rehabilitation. Vera-Garcia and colleagues[59,60] were able to quantify spinal load during the curl up exercise on a stability ball and showed that muscle coactivation and load penalty nearly doubled with the introduction of an uneven surface! McGill advocates for introducing this form of exercise judiciously. Labile surfaces challenge the motor system to calibrate and adapt to

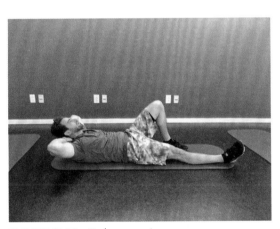

FIGURE 42.12 • Curl up exercise.

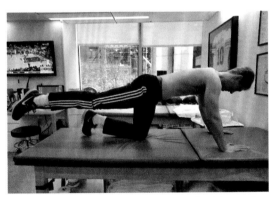

FIGURE 42.14 • Back extensor exercise bird dog (LE component).

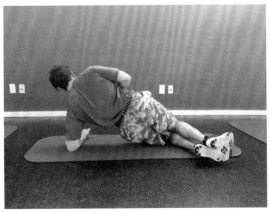

FIGURE 42.13 • Side bridge exercise.

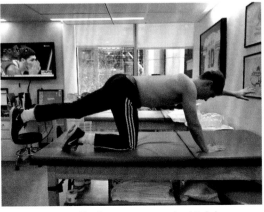

FIGURE 42.15 • Back extensor exercise bird dog (upper extremity/LE component).

TABLE 42.6 Mean Endurance Times (s)

	Men		
	Mean	SD	Ratio
Extension	161	61	1.0
Flexion	136	66	0.84
RSB	95	32	0.59
LSB	99	37	0.61
Flexion/extension ration	0.84		
RSB/LSB ration	0.96		
RSB/extension	0.58		
LSB/extension	0.61		

LSB, left side bridge; RSB, right side bridge; SD, standard deviation.

From McGill SM. Low Back Disorders, Evidence-Based Prevention and Rehabilitation. Windsor: Human Kinetics; 2002:227.

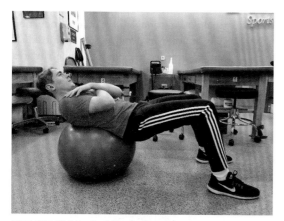

FIGURE 42.16 • Stability ball curl up.

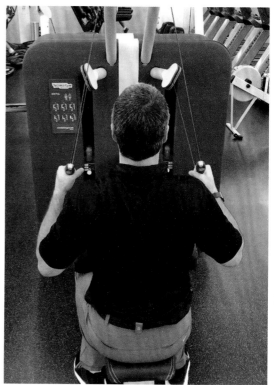

FIGURE 42.18 • Cable latissimus pulldown.

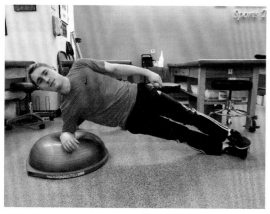

FIGURE 42.17 • Bosu side bridge.

higher level demands that coincide with dynamic tasks performed in baseball. Exercises such as the stability ball curl up (Figure 42.16) and bosu side bridge (Figure 42.17) create an unstable environment that requires additional muscle coactivation to achieve a neutral spine, thus introducing a higher level of effort necessary to maintain position. These exercises are performed for 2 to 3 sets of 10 repetitions with no more than a 7 to 8 second isometric hold at end range.

Cable and free weight exercises can be prescribed during the transition from intermediate to more performance-based strategies within the rehabilitation program. Exercises such as the cable pulldown (Figure 42.18) incorporate latissimus activation and a direct tightening of the thoracodorsal fascia that aids in spinal stabilization. Cable and free weights do not isolate to 1 specific joint and therefore are advocated when promoting whole body dynamic motion patterns. Cable push/pulls (Figure 42.19) and cable hip abductor kick outs (Figure 42.20) demand a higher level of lumbopelvic control in the presence of upper and lower extremity combined efforts.

Torsional training is addressed at the end of the rehabilitation course owing to excessive torques generated about the body's rotational axis. McGill[8] has shown that the torque generated by twisting motions about the transverse plane is 4 times greater than that of torque generated in the sagittal plane. Therefore, exercises pertaining to rotatory motion induce the highest load penalty to the spine for any given exercise and are implemented at the final stages as the athlete prepares for a return to baseball activity. High pull/low pull, cable rotation (Figure 42.21) can be performed to impart torsional stress within the lumbopelvic complex in the presence of a neutral spine. Exercises are performed for 2 to 3 sets of 10 with special attention to maintaining spine angle. According to McGill,[54] the neutral spine position is the most robust position to endure increasing spinal load and transfers optimally to other activities that require torsional stress with the least risk for spine damage. The speed at which these exercises are performed can be further challenged and progressed to simulate transitions similar to the rotatory components of pitching and hitting. Eventual baseball tee work and sock drills for simulating the pitching motion further the athlete's abilities to tolerate functional load.

Elevated breathing rates can compromise the athlete's ability to sufficiently stabilize the spine during high-level athletic activity. During deep, elevated lung ventilation, the abdominal wall musculature relaxes and can alter spinal stabilization particularly in the presence of external stress.[61] McGill cites a trend toward repeated injury after initial injury to the spine, especially under these conditions. Specific motor patterns that address increasing physiologic work rates must be addressed at the rehabilitations programs end to simulate an athlete's spinal response to fatigue. Exercises that can be performed include transitions from high-intensity stationary bike where breathing rates are elevated to a side bridge, bird dog, or curl up exercise. This sequence stimulates cocontraction of the diaphragm and upper thoracic muscles that aid in deep breathing/lung function. Exercises are to be performed for 20 to 30 repetitions at 5 to 8 second holds for bridge/curl up. Bird dog is performed for 20 to 30 repetitions maintaining a neutral spine.

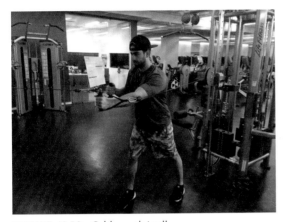

FIGURE 42.19 • Cable push/pull.

MANAGER'S TIPS

- It is still common in the sports medicine community to believe that stronger back and abdominal muscles decrease lower back injury despite a growing body of literature advocating *muscle endurance*, not strength, as a determining factor in lumbopelvic injury prevention

- A thorough history, physical examination, and functional assessment are critical components within the spinal/abdominal injury medical

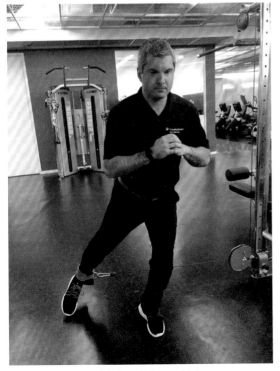

FIGURE 42.20 • Cable hip abductor kick out.

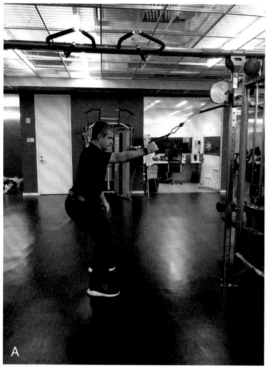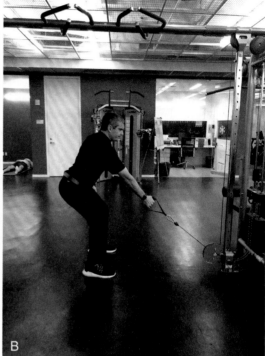

FIGURE 42.21 • Cable high pull (A)/low pull (B).

algorithm that determine proper rehabilitation strategies/return to sport performance training for the baseball athlete

- The general recommendation that the isometric holds performed in sit-up, bridge, and bird dog be no longer than 8 seconds in duration after recent evidence (infrared spectroscopy) suggests a rapid decline in available oxygen in trunk musculature contracting at those levels. Progressions are based on a building of repetition not the duration of each isometric hold

- Torsional moments about the spine along the transverse plane create 4 times the compressional stress as an equal torque in the sagittal plane (flexion/extension). Rotational exercise and the initiation of hitting/throwing programs are generally implemented during end-phase rehabilitation/return to sport advanced protocols when the sports medicine specialist is confident that all previous strategies have been appropriately completed

REFERENCES

1. Hirashima M, Yamane K, Nakamura Y, Ohtsuki T. Kinetic chain of overarm throwing in terms of joint rotations revealed by induced acceleration analysis. *J Biomech*. 2008;41(13):2874-2883.

2. Kibler WB, Press J, Sciascia A. The role of core stability in athletic function. *Sports Med*. 2006;36(3):189-198.

3. MacWilliams BA, Choi T, Perezous MK, Chao EY, McFarland EG. Characteristic ground-reaction forces in baseball pitching. *Am J Sports Med*. 1998;26(1):66-71.

4. Kibler WB, Livingston B. Closed-chain rehabilitation for upper and lower extremities. *J Am Acad Orthop Surg*. 2001;9(6):412-421.

5. Aguinaldo AL, Buttermore J, Chambers H. Effects of upper trunk rotation on shoulder joint torque among baseball pitchers of various levels. *J Appl Biomech*. 2007;23(1):42-51.

6. Fleisig G, Chu Y, Weber A, Andrews J. Variability in baseball pitching biomechanics among various levels of competition. *Sports BioMech*. 2009;8(1):10-21.

7. Chaudhari AM, McKenzie CS, Pan X, Oñate JA. Lumbopelvic control and days missed because of injury in professional baseball pitchers. *Am J Sports Med*. 2014;42(11):2734-2740.

8. McGill SM, Grenier S, Kavcic N, Cholewicki J. Coordination of muscle activity to assure stability of the lumbar spine. *J Electromyogr Kinesiol*. 2003;13(4):353-359.

9. Stodden DF, Campbell BM, Moyer TM. Comparison of trunk kinematics in trunk training exercises and throwing. *J Strength Cond Res*. 2008;22(1):112-118.

10. Stodden DF, Fleisig GS, McLean SP, Andrews JR. Relationship of biomechanical factors to baseball pitching velocity: within pitcher variation. *J Appl Biomech*. 2005;21(1):44-56.

11. Matsuo T, Fleisig GS. Influence of shoulder abduction and lateral trunk tilt on peak elbow varus torque for college baseball pitchers during simulated pitching. *J Appl Biomech.* 2006;22(2):93-102.

12. Oyama S, Waldhelm AG, Sosa AR, Patel RR, Kalinowski DL. Trunk muscle function deficit in youth baseball pitchers with excessive contralateral trunk tilt during pitching. *Clin J Sport Med.* 2017;27(5):475-480.

13. Aguinaldo AL, Chambers H. Correlation of throwing mechanics with elbow valgus load in adult baseball pitchers. *Am J Sports Med.* 2009;37(10):2043-2048.

14. Oyama S, Yu B, Blackburn JT, Padua DA, Li L, Myers JB. Effect of excessive contralateral trunk tilt on pitching biomechanics and performance in high school baseball pitchers. *Am J Sports Med.* 2013;41(10):2430-2438.

15. Fleisig GS, Hsu WK, Fortenbaugh D, Cordover A, Press JM. Trunk axial rotation in baseball pitching and batting. *Sports BioMech.* 2013;12(4):324-333.

16. Watkins RG, Dennis S, Dillin WH. Dynamic EMG analysis of torque transfer in professional baseball pitchers. *Spine (Phila Pa 1976).* 1989;14(4):404-408.

17. Campbell BM, Stodden DF, Nixon MK. Lower extremity muscle activation during baseball pitching. *J Strength Cond Res.* 2010;24(4):964-971.

18. Oliver GD, Keeley. Pelvis and torso kinematics and their relationship to shoulder kinematics in high-school baseball pitchers. *J Strength Cond Res.* 2010;24(12):3241-3246.

19. Oliver GD, Keeley DW. Gluteal muscle group activation and its relationship with pelvis and torso kinematics in high-school baseball pitchers. *J Strength Cond Res.* 2010;24(11):3015-3022.

20. Laudner K, Wong R, Onuki T, Lynall R, Meister K. The relationship between clinically measured hip rotational motion and shoulder biomechanics during the pitching motion. *J Sci Med Sport.* 2015;18(5):581-584.

21. Laudner KG, Moore SD, Sipes RC, Meister K. Functional hip characteristics of baseball pitchers and position players. *Am J Sports Med.* 2010;38(2):383-387.

22. Camp CL, Conte S, Cohen SB. Epidemiology and impact of abdominal oblique injuries in major and minor league baseball. *Orthop J Sports Med.* 2017;5(3):2325967117694025.

23. Micheli LJ. Back injuries in gymnastics. *Clin Sports Med.* 1985;4(1):85-93.

24. Prather H. Sacroiliac joint pain: practical management. *Clin J Sport Med.* 2003;13(4):252-255.

25. Prather H, Hunt D. Conservative management of low back pain, part I. Sacroiliac joint pain. *Dis Mon.* 2004;50(12):670-683.

26. Miller KJ. Physical assessment of lower extremity radiculopathy and sciatica. *J Chiropr Med.* 2007;6(2):75-82.

27. Conte SA, Thompson MM, Marks MA, Dines JS. Abdominal muscle strains in professional baseball: 1991-2010. *Am J Sports Med.* 2012;40(3):650-656.

28. Conte S, Requa RK, Garrick JG. Disability days in major league baseball. *Am J Sports Med.* 2001;29(4):431-436.

29. Posner M, Cameron KL, Wolf JM, Belmont PJ Jr, Owens BD. Epidemiology of major league baseball injuries. *Am J Sports Med.* 2011;39(8):1676-1680.

30. McFarland EG, Wasik M. Epidemiology of collegiate baseball injuries. *Clin J Sport Med.* 1998;8(1):10-13.

31. McGill SM. Linking latest knowledge of injury mechanisms and spine function to the prevention of low back disorders. *J Electromyogr Kinesiol.* 2004;14(1):43-47.

32. Laudner K, Lynall R, Williams JG, Wong R, Onuki T, Meister K. Thoracolumbar range of motion in baseball pitchers and position players. *Int J Sports Phys Ther.* 2013;8(6):777-783.

33. Okawa A, Shinomiya K, Komori H, Muneta T, Arai Y, Nakai O. Dynamic motion study of the whole lumbar spine by videofluoroscopy. *Spine (Phila Pa 1976).* 1998;23(16):1743-1749.

34. Leboeuf-Yde C, Kyvik KO. Is it possible to differentiate people with or without low-back pain on the basis of test of lumbopelvic dysfunction? *J Manip Physiol Ther.* 2000;23(3):160-167.

35. Leboeuf-Yde C, van Dijk J, Franz C, et al. Motion palpation findings and self-reported low back pain in a population-based study sample. *J Manip Physiol Ther.* 2002;25(2):80-87.

36. Paris SV. Physical signs of instability. *Spine.* 1985;10(3):277-279.

37. Axler CT, McGill SM. Low back loads over a variety of abdominal exercises: searching for the safest abdominal challenge. *Med Sci Sports Exerc.* 1997;29(6):804-811.

38. Biering-Sorensen F. Physical measurements as risk indicators for low-back trouble over a one-year period. *Spine (Phila Pa 1976).* 1984;9(2):106-119.

39. Biering-Sorensen F, Thomsen CE, Hilden J. Risk indicators for low back trouble. *Scand J Rehabil Med.* 1989;21(3):151-157.

40. McGill SM, Childs A, Liebenson C. Endurance times for low back stabilization exercises: clinical targets for testing and training from a normal database. *Arch Phys Med Rehabil.* 1999;80(8):941-944.

41. McGill SM, Cholewicki J. Biomechanical basis for stability: an explanation to enhance clinical utility. *J Orthop Sports Phys Ther.* 2001;31(2):96-100.

42. Byrd JW. Evaluation of the hip: history and physical examination. *N Am J Sports Phys Ther.* 2007;2(4):231-240.

43. Byrd JW, Jones KS. Hip arthroscopy in high-level baseball players. *Arthroscopy.* 2015;31(8):1507-1510.

44. Chaudhari AM, McKenzie CS, Borchers JR, Best TM. Lumbopelvic control and pitching performance of professional baseball pitchers. *J Strength Cond Res.* 2011;25(8):2127-2132.

45. Alaranta H, Luoto S, Heliövaara M, Hurri H. Static back endurance and the risk of low-back pain. *Clin Biomech*. 1995;10(6):323-324.

46. Taimela S, Kankaanpaa M, Luoto S. The effect of lumbar fatigue on the ability to sense a change in lumbar position. A controlled study. *Spine (Phila Pa 1976)*. 1999;24(13):1322-1327.

47. McGill S, Juker D, Kropf P. Quantitative intramuscular myoelectric activity of quadratus lumborum during a wide variety of tasks. *Clin Biomech*. 1996;11(3):170-172.

48. McGill SM. Low back exercises: evidence for improving exercise regimens. *Phys Ther*. 1998;78(7):754-765.

49. Dempsey PG. Usability of the revised NIOSH lifting equation. *Ergonomics*. 2002;45(12):817-828.

50. Stambough J, Genaidy A, Guo L. A mathematical lifting model of the lumbar spine. *J Spinal Disord*. 1995;8(4):264-277.

51. Waters TR, Putz-Anderson V, Garg A, Fine LJ. Revised NIOSH equation for the design and evaluation of manual lifting tasks. *Ergonomics*. 1993;36(7):749-776.

52. Marras WS, Fine LJ, Ferguson SA, Waters TR. The effectiveness of commonly used lifting assessment methods to identify industrial jobs associated with elevated risk of low-back disorders. *Ergonomics*. 1999;42(1):229-245.

53. Norman R, Wells R, Neumann P, Frank J, Shannon H, Kerr M. A comparison of peak vs cumulative physical work exposure risk factors for the reporting of low back pain in the automotive industry. *Clin Biomech (Bristol, Avon)*. 1998;13(8):561-573.

54. McGill SM. Low back stability: from formal description to issues for performance and rehabilitation. *Exerc Sport Sci Rev*. 2001;29(1):26-31.

55. Callaghan JP, Gunning JL, McGill SM. The relationship between lumbar spine load and muscle activity during extensor exercises. *Phys Ther*. 1998;78(1):8-18.

56. Callaghan JP, Patla AE, McGill SM. Low back three-dimensional joint forces, kinematics, and kinetics during walking. *Clin Biomech (Bristol, Avon)*. 1999;14(3):203-216.

57. Nutter P. Aerobic exercise in the treatment and prevention of low back pain. *Occup Med*. 1988;3(1):137-145.

58. Grenier SG, McGill SM. Quantification of lumbar stability by using 2 different abdominal activation strategies. *Arch Phys Med Rehabil*. 2007;88(1):54-62.

59. Vera-Garcia FJ, Grenier SG, McGill SM. Abdominal muscle response during curl-ups on both stable and labile surfaces. *Phys Ther*. 2000;80(6):564-569.

60. Vera-Garcia FJ, Moreside JM, McGill SM. Abdominal muscle activation changes if the purpose is to control pelvis motion or thorax motion. *J Electromyogr Kinesiol*. 2011;21(6):893-903.

61. Grenier SG, McGill SM. When exposed to challenged ventilation, those with a history of LBP increase spine stability relatively more than healthy individuals. *Clin Biomech*. 2008;23(9):1105-1111.

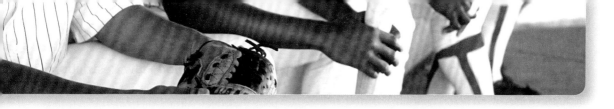

CHAPTER 43

Future Directions in Strength and Conditioning, Periodization, and Use of New Modalities and Technologies

Michael Schuk, PT, DPT, ATC | Timothy Lentych, MS, ATC/L | David Colvin, PT, DPT, MS, ATC

There may be people who have more talent than you, but there is no excuse for anyone to work harder than you.

—Derek Jeter

INTRODUCTION

The sports medicine model has consistently changed over the past 30+ years with a trend toward a further structured and integrated multidisciplinary team approach specific to the athletes' needs in mind. Strength and conditioning coaches (S&C), sport scientists, dieticians, mental skills coaches, and physical therapists are now a staple of the sports medicine team in most if not all of professional sports, including baseball. There is now a closer working dynamic between the athletic trainers, rehabilitation specialists, and the strength and conditioning coaches with shared duties for keeping athletes at peak optimal performance. The ideal progression for the athlete returning from injury involves the completion of specific strengthening and functional exercises with the rehab specialist before transitioning to a higher level and more sport-specific workload with the athletic trainers and S&C coaches before being cleared for full activity.

A great deal of importance is now focused on the strengthening and conditioning of athletes year-round, with an emphasis placed on periodization training to allow for peak athletic performance at the most important period in time for the athlete. In baseball, the macrocycle of seasons include the off-season, preseason (spring training), in-season, and postseason with each phase signifying a particular role.[1] The training program is monitored closely by the sports medicine team in conjunction with the strength and conditioning coaches and has recently migrated toward a focus of multiplanar movement and functional exercises versus one-dimensional, machine-based lifts.

REACTIVE VERSUS PROACTIVE

Along with a transition to the multidisciplinary team and the roles of the strength and conditioning coaches migration from an adjunct service to a highly emphasized and structured mainstay, the roles of the athletic trainers and rehab specialists have also adapted; the athletic training profession has transitioned from highly reactionary following injury to a more proactive approach with emphasis on the prevention of injury. Similarly, postinjury or surgical rehabilitation has transitioned to a swifter return to tissue normalization, mobility, and strengthening versus pain-guided local treatments consisting of ice, rest, and immobilization. With this transition has come the advancement of newer technologies that allow for strengthening to continue almost immediately after injury. One of these technologies gaining steam and demonstrating good initial results is blood flow restriction training.

BLOOD FLOW RESTRICTION

Blood flow restriction (BFR) rehabilitation enables strengthening and hypertrophy gains while exercising at significantly lower resistance loads than traditional strengthening guidelines suggest with the use of a tourniquet that briefly and intermittently occludes venous blood flow.[2] Typically, a flexible cuff is placed proximally around a limb and pressurized to an appropriate level to maintain arterial inflow to the muscle group while occluding venous return during exercise.[3] With personalized blood flow restriction training, a hypoxic environment is created within the muscle that allows for anaerobic metabolism to take place, even under low loads, which recruits larger/fast-twitch motor units.[2] This constrictive device selectively restricts venous outflow, thereby leading to accumulation of the metabolites, such as lactic acid, in the surrounding capillary network.[4-6] Typically, this result is only generated with high-intensity resistance exercises. By creating a hypoxic environment, anaerobic metabolism will increase resulting in fast-twitch motor unit recruitment, leading to increased protein synthesis and subsequently gains in muscle mass and strength.

Evidence

Low-resistance training with BFR has been shown to increase muscle strength, endurance, and cross-section area.[7-9] Yamanaka et al demonstrated with Division 1A football players whom had at least a 5-year history of resistance training that the group performing low-load training with BFR significantly increased their 1-repetition max (1 RM) in bench press and squats compared with the group that did not incorporate BFR.[9] The same BFR group increased their chest girth size significantly.

Much of the literature supports the notion that BFR training alone is not enough to see strength and hypertrophy gains without high-load resistance training. Instead, for maximal benefit in strength and hypertrophy, low-load BFR training should be combined with traditional high-load resistance training.[10-12] Neuromuscular adaptations require high-resistance loads and therefore signify the importance of combining the training types. Leubbers et al had collegiate football players train 4 days each week for 7 weeks in 1 of 4 groups: (1) traditional high-load training, (2) traditional high-load training supplemented with low-load training, (3) traditional high-load training supplemented with low-load BFR training, and (4) modified traditional training supplemented with low-load BFR training.[10] The group to demonstrate the largest increase in squatting 1-rep max was the third group, the high-load training group who supplemented with low-load BFR training.

Practical Uses of Blood Flow Restriction

BFR training can be practically utilized in several ways. First, a rehabbing player can begin strengthening almost immediately after injury or surgery. Secondly, a player with certain degenerative joint conditions such as arthritis can continue strengthening without loading the affected joint with high-resistance, which may ultimately lead to more pain, degeneration, and potentially ending an athlete's season. Lastly, it can be implemented with a healthy player during in-season to limit the load on joints while also allowing the athlete to maintain their off-season strength gains and in-season physical demands.

Blood Flow Restriction—Postinjury

After injury or surgery, muscles of the affected limb will immediately begin to atrophy with immobilization. It is important to regain strength and normalize the muscle girth as quickly as possible to allow for a quick return to play. In patients recovering from anterior cruciate ligament reconstruction, BFR training can attenuate muscle atrophy and enhance muscle development.[13] Loenneke et al has proposed a progressive model for incorporating BFR training from the early phases of rehabilitation through to the resumption of high-load sport-specific training: (1) BFR alone during periods of immobilization, (2) BFR during low-work rate walking, (3) BFR during low-load resistance exercise, and (4) low-load BFR training combined with normal high-load training.[14] For instance, an athlete with a lower limb injury can immediately begin doing quad sets (Figure 43.1) and hip muscular strengthening exercises with BFR training. Progression should continue once they are weight bearing to allow for ambulation with BFR and transition into functional exercises.

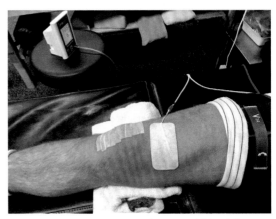

FIGURE 43.1 • Russian stimulation and blood flow restriction (BFR) utilized while athlete simultaneously contracts his quadriceps.

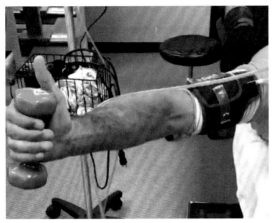

FIGURE 43.2 • Prone shoulder "Y" with blood flow restriction (BFR).

For an upper body injury, the same can be performed by doing isometric exercises at different arm angles in the early phases of rehab. A pitcher recovering from ulnar collateral ligament (UCL) reconstruction of his elbow can benefit from doing rotator cuff exercises while BFR training (Figure 43.2) in the middle phases of rehab with emphasis placed on proper form by utilizing lighter resistance.

Blood Flow Restriction—Chronic and Degenerative Diseases

An athlete with degenerative joint disease in the knee, for example, may want to limit heavy loading of the joint. Instead of performing numerous sessions a week of squats or leg press with heavy weights, the athlete can now perform the same or similar exercises with 20% to 30% of 1 RM and continue to see strength gains. Incorporating BFR training into one of the strengthening days by replacing a heavy-resistance lifting day has the potential to prolong a career by limiting impact on an already damaged joint. This same athlete may benefit from decreased volume of weight bearing cardiovascular training and instead substitute with stationary cycling with the use of BFR on bilateral lower limbs. Abe at al demonstrated that low-intensity, short-duration cycling exercise combined with BFR improves both muscle hypertrophy and aerobic capacity concurrently in young men.[15]

Blood Flow Restriction—Healthy Player

Finally, for the healthy athlete (ie, baseball pitcher) who performs postpitching strengthening exercises, benefits can be achieved from blood flow restriction training. Instead of consistently lifting the same weight for shoulder exercises time and time again, they can switch up their routine with a program consisting of BFR. This can be done with shoulder manual resistance exercises or with a shoulder program, however, using notably lighter resistance.

We like to utilize BFR training with pitchers performing upper extremity manual resistance exercises. After careful consideration as to who would be safe and appropriate to benefit from this training, we prepare the DELFI personalized tourniquet system for BFR unit to calibrate the limb occlusion pressure (LOP) of the athlete's upper limb. From there, the personalized training pressure (PTP) is preset at 50% of LOP, which will be the amount of pressure consistently monitored during the session, which typically will last less than 8 minutes with a 30-second rest between sets.[2] If more time is needed, a 1-minute break from occlusion will occur by deflating the tourniquet. The amount of manual resistance will be determined by the athlete's prior use of this training along with their pitching workload encountered that day (or week) and as discussed earlier, what cycle of the season (periodization) they are in. For a first-time user, we will begin with no external resistance. The athlete will simply complete active range of motion of the prescribed exercise positions while training with BFR. They may perform 1 to 2 sets at 10 to 15 reps of an 8 to 10 position round. After approximately 2 to 4 sessions over the course of a few weeks, we will begin using light external resistance by a qualified and trained clinician. Measured resistance can be calculated by using finger resistance beginning with 1 finger, until the whole hand is used. At that point, the trained clinician will use their judgment to dictate the amount of resistance necessary.

For use with weighted resistance, we follow guidelines set forth by Owens Recovery Science. "The standard and recommended set and repetition protocol to follow while performing Personalized Blood Flow Restriction Training is 4 sets of 30/15/15/15."[2] The first set is higher as an attempt to transition muscle metabolism from aerobic to anaerobic.[2] Sequentially, as the number of sets progresses, the workload will be harder to the athlete.

Safety and Precautions

As true with any training session and new exercise equipment, the amounts of reps and sets completed should be closely monitored by the treating clinician. Before using BFR training, it is important to have the medical clearance of the treating physician along with proper training per educational offerings of the device you opt to use. An expert understanding of the indications, contraindications, precautions, and parameters is of paramount significance just as with the use of any other modality.

TRIP TO THE MOUND

Currently, there are a number of different BFR devices, most notably Kaatsu and the DELFI unit through Owens Recovery Science. BFR should not be applied at an absolute pressure but instead should vary relative to each individual.[14,16] As it stands, the DELFI unit is the only company currently offering a device that is FDA approved and allows for a specific personalized training pressure (occlusion) dictated by a Doppler that remains connected to the athlete while exercising. Owens Recovery Science also offer 3 different cuff sizes to allow for proper selection depending on the patient's limb girth. Loenneke et al state that wide cuffs (13.5 cm) restrict arterial blood flow at lower levels than narrow cuffs (5.0 cm).[17] For further information and before using with an athlete, make sure to have completed a comprehensive patient history and examination to determine its safety for a given athlete, and you should always receive the proper training before using a BFR device.

REFERENCES

1. Gillett J, O'Brien L, Ryan M. Strategic exercise prescription for baseball: bridging the gap between injury prevention and power production. *Strength Cond J.* 2009;31:81-88.

2. Owens J. *Personalized Blood Flow Restriction Rehabilitation: Clinic Quick User Guide.* Owens Recovery Science; 2015

3. Scott BR, Loenneke JP, Slattery KM, et al. Blood flow restricted exercise for athletes: a review of available evidence. *J Sci Med Sport.* 2016;19(5):360-367.

4. Spranger MD, Krishnan AC, Levy PD, et al. Blood flow restriction training and the exercise pressor reflex: a call for concern. *Am J Physiol Hear Circ Physiol.* 2015;309(9):H1440-H1452.

5. Fujita S, Abe T, Drummond MJ, et al. Blood flow restriction during low-intensity resistance exercise increases S6K1 phosphorylation and muscle protein synthesis. *J Appl Physiol.* 2007;103(3):903-910.

6. Kawada S, Ishii N. Changes in skeletal muscle size, fibre-type composition and capillary supply after chronic venous occlusion in rats. *Acta Physiol (Oxf).* 2008;192(4):541-549.

7. Manimmanakorn A, Manimmanakorn N, Taylor R, et al. Effects of resistance training combined with vascular occlusion or hypoxia on neuromuscular function in athletes. *Eur J Appl Physiol.* 2013;113(7):1767-1774.

8. Manimmanakorn A, Hamlin MJ, Ross JJ, et al. Effects of low-load resistance training combined with blood flow restriction or hypoxia on muscle function and performance in netball athletes. *J Sci Med Sport.* 2013;16(4):337-342.

9. Yamanaka T, Farley RS, Caputo JL. Occlusion training increases muscular strength in division 1A football players. *J Strength Cond Res.* 2012;26(9):2523-2329.

10. Luebbers PE, Fry AC, Kriley LM, et al. The effects of a seven-week practical blood flow restriction program on well-trained collegiate athletes. *J Strength Cond Res.* 2014;46(5):608-611

11. Martin-Hernandez J, Marin PJ, Menendez J, et al. Muscular adaptations after two different volumes of blood flow restricted training. *Scand J Med Sci Sport.* 2013;23(2).

12. Yasuda T, Ogasawara R, Sakamaki M, et al. Combined effects of low-intensity blood flow restriction training and high-intensity resistance training on muscle strength and size. *Eur J Appl Physiol.* 2011;111(10):2525-2533.

13. Ohta H, Kurosawa H, Ikeda H, et al. Low-load resistance training muscular training with moderate restriction of blood flow after anterior cruciate ligament reconstruction. *Acta Orthop Scan.* 2003;74(1):62-68.

14. Loenneke JP, Fahs CA, Rossow LM, et al. Blood flow restriction pressure recommendations: a tale of two cuffs. *Front Physiol.* 2013;4.

15. Abe T, Fujita S, Nakajima T, et al. Effects of low-intensity cycle training with restricted leg blood flow on thigh muscle volume and VO2 max in young men. 2010;9(3):452-458.

16. Scott BR, Loenneke JP, Slattery KM, et al. Exercise with blood flow restriction: an updated evidence-based approach for enhanced muscular development. *Sports Med.* 2015;45:313-325.

17. Loenneke JP, Fahs CA, Rossow LM, et al. Effects of cuff width on arterial occlusion: implications for blood flow restricted exercise. *Eur J Appl Physiol.* 2012;112(8):2903-2912.

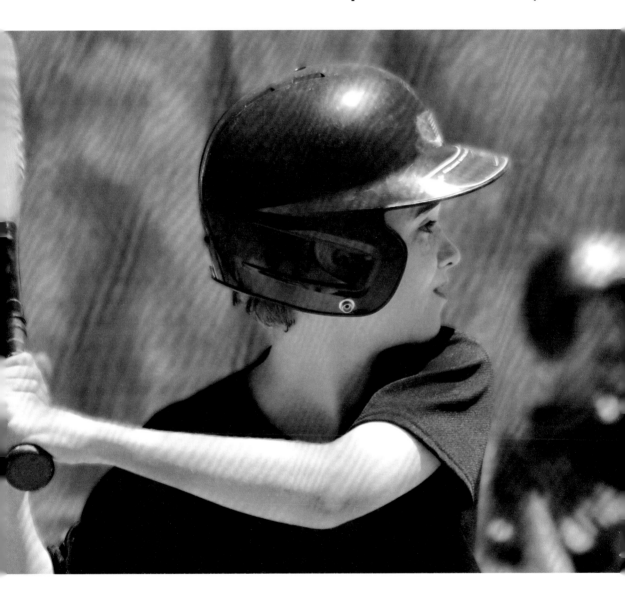

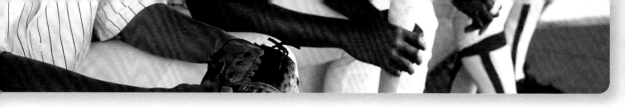

CHAPTER 44

Youth Baseball Injury Epidemiology and Baseball Specialization

Michael C. Ciccotti, MD | Patrick S. Buckley, MD | Michael G. Ciccotti, MD

You could be a kid for as long as you want when you play baseball.

—*Cal Ripken Jr*

INTRODUCTION

Baseball remains one of the most popular sports for youth athletes both in the United States and abroad. Since its founding in 1939, Little League Baseball, Inc. has grown to an organized sport that is played in over 80 countries and by 2.4 million youth athletes annually.[32] Within the United States, the Sports and Fitness Industry Association has estimated that 6.7 million American youths from 6 to 17 years of age played baseball in 2014.[50] The National Federation of State High School Associations reports that baseball is the third most popular sport among US high schools (HSs) by the number of schools with programs and is played by 490,105 HS athletes annually.[49] Furthermore, consistent with the trend toward early specialization seen in many other youth sports, baseball has become a year-round sport in many regions of the United States, with many athletes competing for school teams, travel teams, and other tournaments/showcases.

Many potential benefits exist for a young athlete who participates in baseball. Youth sports, including baseball, help athletes to engage in an active lifestyle in their community, build social relationships with teammates, and to foster a healthy self-image. In addition to theoretically allowing the athlete to improve in his or her sport, participation in youth sports can also help athletes learn important values such as teamwork, dedication to a common goal, and work ethic. However, early specialization to play baseball year-round at a young age brings potentially negative consequences.

Many in both the medical and lay communities have raised concerns about the rising trend of single-sport specialization seen in baseball and other sports. The reasons behind the rise in early single-sport specialization are varied, but it is hypothesized that many parents, coaches, and athletes believe that focusing on only 1 sport at an early age may result in a higher chance of advancing to play at a more elite level. Such advancement may result in scholarships or even ultimately the potential fame and financial rewards associated with professional play. This viewpoint has led many parents, coaches, and peers to pressure any promising athlete toward early specialization. This trend may be driven by the anecdotal stories of early single-sport specialization success by athletes such as Tiger Woods or Lionel Messi. Moreover, there has been a dramatically increased media focus on youth sports and youth athletes. Furthermore, youth sports have grown into a vast business with respect to equipment, leagues, coaching, and training facilities. However, these widely held beliefs on early single-sport specialization are not supported by existing research. In 2017, data from the National Collegiate Athletic Association (NCAA) suggest that the likelihood of a HS baseball athlete playing at a Division 1 level is 2.1%.[40] Similarly, the probability of an NCAA athlete playing professional baseball is 9.1%, although these data include both minor and major league play.[40] The likelihood of a US HS athlete playing his sport professionally is 0.2% to 0.5%, including baseball.[40]

In 2017, the long-term medical, psychological, and societal implications of early single-sport specialization remain incompletely defined. Mounting evidence in the medical literature has suggested associations between early single-sport specialization and overuse injuries, psychological burnout, and decreased involvement and participation in sports.[4,28,29] As a result, multiple medical associations and societies have issued consensus statements urging parents, coaches, and clinicians to guide children to engage in multiple sporting activities and to avoid early specialization in a single sport.[2,3,27,31] In this chapter, we will address the injury epidemiology in baseball as well as describe the trend toward and potential consequences of single-sport specialization.

BASEBALL INJURY EPIDEMIOLOGY

With millions of Americans participating in baseball annually, several studies have investigated the epidemiology of injury at various levels of play, from Little League Baseball to Major League Baseball (MLB). Although baseball may be considered relatively safe in comparison with some higher risk contact sports, notable injury rates have been identified.

At the youth and HS baseball levels, a number of authors have investigated the epidemiology of injuries. In 2000, Powell et al reported a low overall rate of injury in comparison with some other HS sports, but youth baseball had the second largest proportion of injuries resulting in time loss greater than 7 days.[45] Collins and Comstock reviewed data from the voluntary Reporting Information Online (RIO) internet-based surveillance system to report epidemiologic features of HS baseball injuries.[16] Their study was based on 341,883 athlete exposures (A-E) for HS baseball players in the 2005 to 2006 and 2006 to 2007 seasons. They reported an overall injury rate of 1.26 per 1000 A-E, although this was significantly higher for competition compared with practice (1.89 vs 0.85, respectively, $P < .001$). The most commonly injured body sites were the shoulder (17.6%), ankle (13.6%), head/face (12.3%), hand/finger (8.5%), and thigh/upper leg (8.2%). The most common diagnoses were ligament sprains (incomplete tears) (21.0%), muscle strains (incomplete tears) (20.1%), contusions (16.1%), and fractures (14.2%). The most common mechanism for baseball-related injuries was contact with a ball/bat/base (31.8%), noncontact (30.4%), and contact with the playing surface (16.2%). The most common phase of play that resulted in injury was fielding (21.6%), running bases (14.4%), and pitching (13.2%). Most concerning, a majority (50.3%) of injuries resulted in a time loss of 7 days, with 6.7% resulting in 21 days of lost time, and an additional 9.7% resulting in medical disqualification for the season. In 2002, Lyman et al reported on 298 youth baseball players (ages 9-12 years), following them over 2 consecutive seasons.[33] They reported 32% and 26% incidence of

shoulder and elbow pain, respectively. In their analysis, shoulder pain was associated with pitches thrown per season and pitches thrown per game, whereas elbow pain was associated with increasing age, arm fatigue experienced during a game, and pitches per season. Similarly, Matsuure et al reported on 1563 Japanese youth baseball players aged 7 to 12 years.[36] In their cohort, 15.9% of players reported episodes of shoulder pain and 29.2% reported episodes of elbow pain. Shoulder pain was associated with increasing age (10-12 years old), whereas elbow pain was associated with several factors including increasing age (10-12 years old), increased years of baseball experience, and playing catcher. Yang et al surveyed 754 youth pitchers aged 9-18 years to identify behaviors associated with arm pain and arm injury.[51] In their sample, 43.4% of youth pitchers pitched on consecutive days, 30.7% pitched on multiple overlapping teams, and 19% pitched multiple games in a day over the prior year. In their study, these behaviors were associated with an increased risk of reporting pitching-related arm pain and pitching with tiredness; arm pain was also associated with a greater risk of pitching-related injuries. Pytiak et al prospectively followed 26 Little League players with a pre- and postseason MRI, identifying abnormal postseason findings in 48% of their cohort.[46] These abnormalities were significantly associated with year-round play ($P < .05$), although in their study significant associations with pitch counts, player position, and types of pitches thrown were not found. Makhni et al reported on 203 youth baseball players aged 8 to 18 years, among whom 23% reported a prior overuse injury.[35] In this series, only 26% and 20% reported no pain during the day and after throwing, respectively. Thirty percent of players reported that arm pain resulted in appreciable psychosocial consequences (ie, having less fun playing). Furthermore, 46% reported being encouraged to play through despite arm pain on at least 1 occasion.

At the collegiate level, Dick et al reviewed the NCAA Injury Surveillance System over a 16-year period (1988-2004) to produce epidemiologic data for collegiate baseball.[19] Similar to the youth/HS level of play, the injury rate was low in comparison with other collegiate sports. However, the authors classified 25% of these injuries as "severe", requiring 10 or more days lost to sport. As in youth baseball, the rate of injury was significantly higher in games than in practice (5.78 vs 1.85 per 1000 A-E). The most common anatomic location of injury was the upper extremity (44.6% in game; 46.4% in practice). Furthermore, shoulder injuries accounted for a majority of severe time-loss injuries overall.

A number of authors have investigated injury epidemiology at the professional level in MLB, using data from the MLB disabled list (DL) and, more recently, the MLB Health Injury and Tracking System (HITS) injury surveillance system.[14,17,44] In 2001, Conte et al reported an 11-year analysis of MLB DL data representing seasons from 1989 to 1999, finding an increase over time in the number of players listed on the DL as well as the overall number of DL days.[17] Unfortunately, the DL data available lacked the detail necessary for further analysis, but the authors speculated that athletes who would have previously been out of baseball entirely owing to injury were now remaining in the league but spending a greater amount of time on the DL. In 2011, Posner et al reported on this topic using MLB DL data from 2002 to 2008.[44] Based on an average of 438.9 players per year placed on the DL, they calculated the risk of being placed on DL as 3.61 per 1000 A-E, with the rate highest in April (5.73) and lowest in September (0.54). Pitchers were found to have a 34% higher incidence rate for injury compared with fielders. As at other levels of play, the majority of injuries involved the upper extremity (51.4%). As one might expect, a significant association existed between position played and anatomic region of injury, with pitchers more likely to injure the upper extremity and fielders more likely to injure the lower extremity. Overall, pitchers accounted for 62.4% of DL days.

A number of more recent baseball injury epidemiologic studies performed at the professional level have taken advantage of the recently instituted MLB HITS, with an MLB-supported, targeted approach to specific injuries.[1,14,15,18] Ahmad et al reported on hamstring injuries based on analysis of MLB HIT data from 2011, calculating an injury rate of 0.7 per 1000 A-E in both the major and minor leagues with an average of 24 and 27 days missed to sport in the major and minor leagues, respectively.[1] Two-thirds of hamstring injuries were associated with base running (typically to first base). Two-thirds of injuries kept players out for at least a week, and 25% required more than a month before return to play. Hamstring injuries were statistically more common in May. Coleman et al reported on hip and groin injuries based on MLB HITS data from 2011 to 2014.[15] These represented approximately 5% of all injuries sustained by professional baseball players, and 96% were extra-articular in nature. Overall, 96.2% were treated nonoperatively and on average resulted in 12 days missed. However, intra-articular injures more often required surgery and resulted in an average of 123 days missed. Similarly, Dahm et al reported on knee injuries based on MLB HITS data from 2011 to 2014.[18] They calculated a risk of knee injury as 1.2 per 1000 A-E in

both the major and minor leagues, associated with an average of 16.2 days lost. Most recently, Ciccotti et al reported on elbow injuries using the MLB HITS data from 2011 to 2014.[14] They found an overall risk of elbow injury as 1.7 per 1000 A-E (1.0 in the majors vs 1.8 in the minors). Pitchers accounted for 40% of all professional players with elbow injuries. The mean number of days missed was 27.2, excluding those requiring surgery. Overall 29.2% of elbow injuries were season ending and 20.4% required surgery. The most common subtype of elbow injury requiring surgery was ligament injuries, and, of the 905 documented ligament injuries, 89.4% were injuries to the ulnar collateral ligament.

These epidemiologic studies have documented an increasing incidence of injury amongst baseball players at all levels of play.[9,10,14,21,22,41] Furthermore, they have documented a substantial increase in the number of surgeries performed on HS and collegiate pitchers for serious injuries.[41] Even with the resources available at the professional level, these injuries represent a substantial source of days lost to sport.[14] These epidemiologic studies have sought to more precisely define those injury rates, to identify mechanisms of injury and to establish potential risk factors, all to guide resources toward preventing and treating the most common baseball injuries.

SINGLE-SPORT SPECIALIZATION

Although a growing amount of epidemiologic data identifies significant injury risk in baseball at all levels, particularly youth, enthusiasm persists with respect to early specialization in this sport. The most widely used definition of single-sport specialization in the literature was reported by Jaynathi et al who define single-sport specialization as intensive, year-round (8+ months/year) training and competition in a single sport to the exclusion of all other organized sports[28,29] (see Table 44.1). It remains unclear what factors are most critical for inclusion in such a definition and where the tipping point lies for an individual athlete to become "over specialized". The elusive goal remains balancing the benefits of sports participation noted above with the risks of injury, psychological burnout, and social isolation that may result from specialization.

In 2017, many unanswered questions remain pertaining to the topic of single-sport specialization. Questions include the following: How many months per year playing the sport should qualify as "specialized"? Should we count training time, competition time, or both? Does the physiologic age or psychosocial maturity of the athlete play a role? Does the strength, flexibility, conditioning, or endurance of the

TABLE 44.1 Stratification of Sport Specialization From Low to High and the Accompanying Risk of Injury as Reported by Jayanthi et al[28]

Degree of Specialization	Risk of Injury	Risk of Serious Overuse Injury	Risk of Acute Injury
Low Specialization (0 or 1 of the following): Year-round training (>8 mo per year), chooses a single main sport, and quit all sports to focus on 1 sport.	Low	Low	Moderate
Moderate Specialization (2 of the following): Year-round training (>8 mo per year), chooses a single main sport, and quit all sports to focus on 1 sport.	Moderate	Moderate	Low
High Specialization (All 3 of the following): Year-round training (>8 mo per year), chooses a single main sport, and quit all sports to focus on 1 sport.	High	High	Low

Reprinted with permission from Jayanthi NA, LaBella CR, Fischer D, et al. *Sports-specialized intensive training and the risk of injury in young athletes: a clinical case-control study. Am J Sports Med.* 2015;43(4):794-801. Copyright © 2015 SAGE Publications.

athlete contribute to their injury risk? Does the type of sport (ie, team vs individual) play a role? How much rest time away from sport is appropriate? These questions remain integral to investigating the impact of single-sport specialization on youth athletes.

Furthermore, sports researchers have questioned whether early specialization actually results in enhanced performance and reliable progression to the most elite levels of competition. The existing literature examining the relationship between early specialization and achieving professional status has actually shown that elite athletes specialized later in their sport, not earlier.[5,11,25,39] Although the majority of these data were collected in Olympic level athletes, similar data have been obtained in professional athletes as well.[7] Currently, there is no evidence that indicates that early sport specialization enhances performance or increases the likelihood of progression to an elite level.

In the minds of most clinicians', the greatest unanswered question is the relationship between early single-sport specialization and injury risk. Indeed, in 2015, Jayanthi et al showed that single-sport specialization was an independent risk factor for overuse injury.[28] In 2015, Hall et al showed increased anterior knee pain in single-sport female basketball athletes.[26] In 2017, Pasulka et al showed that single-sport–specialized athletes in individual sports accounted for a higher proportion of overuse injuries and serious overuse injuries, but a lower proportion of acute injuries compared with single-sport–specialized athletes involved in team sports.[42] Moreover, in 2017, McGuine et al prospectively examined lower extremity injury rates in HS athletes and found that athletes who were classified as high or moderate on the sport specialization scale had a higher incidence of lower extremity injuries than HS athletes classified as low on the sport specialization scale.[37]

Fortunately, baseball benefits from a more robust literature on specialization than many other sports, and a substantial proportion of this literature focuses on youth and HS athletes. As much of the epidemiologic literature has shown a majority of injuries sustained in baseball are upper extremity injuries, a great deal of the specialization literature has focused on throwing and, more specifically, the pitcher position. These studies have identified a multitude of potential risk factors for injury amongst youth pitchers, including pitch velocity, pitch counts per game and per year, number of warm-up pitches, months played per year, games played per year, innings played per year, taller and heavier stature, playing pitcher and catcher, pitching with fatigue, pitching showcases, pitching on consecutive days, and pitching on multiple teams with overlapping seasons.[9,13,20,23,33,43,51] Fleisig et al showed that pitchers who threw more than 100 innings in a single calendar year had an increased risk for ulnar collateral ligament injury and recommended against playing baseball year round.[23] An epidemiologic study sponsored by the USA Baseball Medical/Safety Advisory Committee demonstrated that pitch counts correlated to both shoulder and elbow pain in youth pitchers.[34] We are beginning to understand that 1 way to possibly prevent injury in MLB pitchers is to turn our attention to the cumulative effect that repetitive throwing has on a young pitcher's arm and his future throwing career. Many youth pitchers develop adaptive changes to their immature anatomy from the impact of overhead throwing at a young age. These changes have been well described and include an alteration in the total arc of motion, increase in external rotation, decrease of internal rotation at the shoulder, and humeral retroversion.[6,12,24,38,47,48] Although some of those changes are considered adaptive and may allow heightened performance, they may also cumulatively lead to injury.

Our own institution has studied single-sport specialization in baseball by evaluating over 1750 HS, collegiate, and professional baseball players.[8] A precise survey was distributed at preparticipation evaluation by the certified training staff of each team. The survey consisted of questions on demographics, current sports commitment, injury history, future athletic plans, and perspectives on specialization. We found that a statistically higher percentage of current HS and collegiate baseball players were specializing to play 1 sport, solely baseball, when compared with their current professional athlete counterparts when they were in HS and college (60.0% of HS athletes, 73.3% of collegiate athletes, and 44.5% of professional athletes, $P < .001$). Additionally, current HS athletes who chose to specialize did so at a statistically earlier age (approximately 2 years earlier) than current collegiate or professional athletes (12.25 ± 2.30 years old vs 15.36 ± 1.87 years old and 14.09 ± 2.79 years old, $P < .001$). These data argue against the notion that specializing early is necessary to achieve elite status in the sport of baseball.

Given the diverse background of many MLB players who grew up outside the United States, we also analyzed the topic of sport specialization based on the country of origin.[8] There were no differences in the percent of athletes that specialized between US- and non-US-raised players (44.7% vs 44.1%, $P = .829$). However, of those who did specialize, non-US-raised players specialized on average more than 2 years earlier than those MLB athletes raised in the United States (12.3 ± 3.07 years of age vs 14.89 ± 2.24 years of age). Additionally, MLB players raised in America recalled a significantly higher incidence of sustaining an injury attributed to specializing in baseball than MLB athletes raised outside the United States (27.7% vs 20.6%, $P = .05$). With regard to injury, it is critical to emphasize that these data reflect the ability of each athlete to recall an injury and that injury may have been remote depending on the age of that particular athlete. These findings could reflect the socioeconomic differences between the United States and the predominantly Caribbean and Latin American countries from which non-US players originate. Additionally, this could reflect a limited number of alternative organized youth sports available in the native countries of non-US-born players compared with the variety of youth sports present for youth today in America.

When the position of pitcher was analyzed, we found that MLB pitchers raised in the United States started throwing off-speed pitches at a significantly earlier age (13.41 ± 2.22 years of age vs 13.85 ± 2.63 years of age, $P < .001$) and focused solely on pitching at a later age (16.89 ± 1.82 years of age vs 14.28 ± 2.87 years of age, $P < .001$) than MLB pitchers raised outside of the United States.[8] Non-US-born players started focusing on only pitching (rather than fielding positions) at a significantly earlier age than US-born players (14.28 ± 2.87 years of age vs 16.89 ± 1.82 years of age, $P < .001$). There was no significant difference between the percentage of athletes that specialized and the age of specialization when comparing pitchers, infielders, outfielders, and catchers. Additionally, over half of non-US-born MLB players would want their children to specialize to play 1 sport; however, less than 10% of US-born MLB players want their children to specialize (55.4% vs 7.1%, $P < .001$). We believe that this highlights the reality that specialization does not mean the same thing in all places. Climate, societal perceptions, and socioeconomic forces all likely influence the pressures felt by youth athletes and their families toward single-sport specialization.

CLINICAL EVALUATION OF THE YOUTH BASEBALL ATHLETE

Appropriate assessment of the youth baseball athlete who presents for orthopedic evaluation is critical and begins with a thorough history and physical examination. In addition to the usual history pertaining to the reason for the visit, the athlete and their parents should be asked about specifics pertaining to their involvement with the sport of baseball. Is the injury acute or chronic? If the symptoms have happened before, what treatment has been attempted? Is baseball the only sport the athlete plays? Does the athlete play baseball year round? Does the athlete play for multiple teams? If so, do the seasons overlap? How many months per year is the athlete playing baseball? What position does the athlete play? If the athlete is a pitcher, does he throw on a pitch count? Does he throw off-speed pitches? Does the athlete participate in showcases/ tournaments? If so, do they require pitching for a prolonged period of time or for a higher volume of pitches? What period of rest is planned and implemented in between pitching?

It is our experience that all too often the "treatment" the injured athlete has tried did not actually stop the causative movement (ie, pitching) and often was not pursued for a sufficient period of time. We feel appropriate rehab for a youth baseball athlete with a chronic injury from repetitive throwing involves "shutting down" the athlete from baseball activities until asymptomatic. During that time a supervised overall body, kinetic chain rehabilitation program should be carried out. Once the athlete is pain free, then a closely moni-tored, progressive short toss, long toss, and mound (if pitcher) program should be initiated.[30]

CONCLUSION

Participation in youth baseball can form the foun-dation for lifelong success both on and off the field. An increasing amount of epidemiologic data at all levels of baseball indicates that there are substantial injury risks, particularly in the upper extremity of these athletes. These overuse injuries, especially from the cumulative effect of overhead throwing, can have a substantial impact on the immature anatomy of youth baseball players. With a growing body of evi-dence that specialization often imparts an increased risk of injury and a limited amount of evidence for its tangible benefit, avoiding or altering perspective on early sport specialization may reduce the injury bur-den amongst youth baseball players. Further research focused on the biomechanical evaluations of specific sport techniques and the basic science of tissue heal-ing, comparing youth and adult athletes, is necessary. Standardized sports specialization survey tools and methods should be developed. Moreover, prospective evaluations should be carried out to collect longitu-dinal data on age of sport specialization, incidence of sport-related injury, and likelihood of progression to elite competition. In this way, the true impact of early single-sport specialization can be determined, and safe, common sense guidelines pertaining to spe-cialization can be developed for our youth athletes to remain healthy and on the field.

MANAGER'S TIPS

- The rates of single-sport specialization are on the rise in youth baseball
- Early data suggest that specialization is not neces-sary for advancement to an elite level in one's sport
- Specialization appears to be a risk factor for over-use injury, especially for pitchers
- Well-rounded sport participation should be encouraged for youth athletes, and year-round par-ticipation in a single sport should be discouraged

REFERENCES

1. Ahmad CS, Dick RW, Snell E, et al. Major and minor league baseball hamstring injuries: epidemiologic find-ings from the major league baseball injury surveillance system. *Am J Sports Med.* 2014;42(6):1464-1470.

2. American Academy of Pediatrics, Council on sports medicine and fitness. policy statement: baseball and softball. *Pediatrics.* 2012;129:842-856.

3. American Academy of Family Physicians, Academy of Orthopaedic Surgeons, American College of Sports Medicine, American Medical Society for Sports Medicine, American Orthopaedic Society for Sports Medicine, American Osteopathic Academy of Sports Medicine. Selected issues for the adolescent ath-lete and the team physician: a consensus statement. *Med Sci Sports Exerc.* 2008;40:1997-2012.

4. Andrews J, Yaeger D. *Any Given Monday: Sports Injuries and How to Prevent Them for Athletes, Parents, and Coaches - Based on My Life in Sports Medicine.* New York: Scribner; 2013.

5. Barynina I, Vaitsekhovskii S. The aftermath of early sports specialization for highly qualified swimmers. *Fitness Sports Rev Int.* 1992;27:132-133.

6. Bigliani LU, Codd TP, Connor PM, Levine WN, Littlefield MA, Hershon SJ. Shoulder motion and laxity in the professional baseball player. *Am J Sports Med.* 1997;25(5):609-613. doi:10.1177/036354659702500504.

7. Buckley PS, Bishop ME, Kane PW, et al. Early single sport specialization: a survey of 3090 high school, col-legiate, and professional athletes. *Orthop J Sports Med.* 2017;5(7):1-7.

8. Buckley PS, Ciccotti MC, Bishop ME, et al. From high school to the big leagues: single sport specialization in baseball. 2017. Unpublished Data. Manuscript in progress.

9. Bushnell BD, Anz AW, Noonan TJ, Torry MR, Hawkins RJ. Association of maximum pitch veloc-ity and elbow injury in professional baseball pitchers. *Am J Sports Med.* 2010;38(4):728-732. doi:10.1177/0363546509350067.

10. Cain EL, Andrews JR, Dugas JR, et al. Outcome of ulnar collateral ligament reconstruction of the elbow in 1281 athletes. *Am J Sports Med.* 2010;38(12):2426-2434. doi:10.1177/0363546510378100.

11. Carlson R. The socialization of elite tennis players in Sweden: an analysis of the players' backgrounds and development. *Sociol Sport J.* 1988;5(3):241-256. doi:10.1123/ssj.5.3.241.

12. Carson WG, Gasser SI. Little leaguer's shoulder. *Am J Sports Med.* 1998;26(4):575-580. doi:10.1177/03635465980260041901.

13. Chalmers PN, Sgroi T, Riff AJ, et al. Correlates with history of injury in youth and adolescent pitchers. *Arthrosc J Arthrosc Relat Surg.* 2015;31(7):1349-1357. doi:10.1016/j.arthro.2015.03.017.

14. Ciccotti MG, Pollack KM, Ciccotti MC, et al. Elbow injuries in professional baseball: epidemiological find-ings from the major league baseball injury surveillance system. *Am J Sports Med.* 2017;45(10):2319-2328. doi:10.1177/0363546517706964.

15. Coleman SH, Mayer SW, Tyson JJ, Pollack KM, Curriero FC. The epidemiology of hip and groin inju-ries in professional baseball players. *Am J Orthop.* 2016;45(3):168-175.

16. Collins CL, Comstock CD. Epidemiological features of high school baseball injuries in the United States, 2005 – 2007. *Pediatrics*. 2008;121(6):1181-1187.

17. Conte S, Regua RK, Garrick JG. Disability days in major league baseball. *Am J Sports Med*. 2001;29(4): 431-436.

18. Dahm DL, Curriero FC, Camp CL, et al. Epidemiology and impact of knee injuries in major and minor league baseball players. *Am J Orthop*. 2016;45(3):E54-E62.

19. Dick R, Sauers EL, Agel J, et al. Descriptive epidemiology of collegiate men's baseball injuries: national collegiate athletic association injury surveillance system, 1988-1989 through 2003-2004. *J Athl Train*. 2007;42(2):183-193.

20. Dun S, Flesig GS, Loftice K, Kingsley D, Andrews JR. The relationship between age and baseball pitching kinematics in professional baseball pitchers. *J Biomech*. 2007;40(2):265-270.

21. Erickson BJ, Nwachukwu BU, Rosas S, et al. Trends in medial ulnar collateral ligament reconstruction in the United States. *Am J Sports Med*. 2015;43(7):1770-1774. doi:10.1177/0363546515580304.

22. Erickson BJ, Chalmers PN, Axe MJ, Romeo AA. Exceeding pitch count recommendations in little league baseball increases chance of requiring Tommy John surgery as a professional baseball pitcher. *Orthop J Sports Med*. 2017;5(3):2325967117695085. doi:10.1177/2325967117695085.

23. Flesig GS, Andrews JR, Cutter GR, et al. Risk of serious injury for young baseball pitchers: a 10-year prospective study. *Am J Sports Med*. 2010;39(2):253-257.

24. Greenberg EM, Lawrence JT, Fernandez-Fernandez A, McClure P. Humeral retroversion and glenohumeral motion in youth baseball players compared with age-matched nonthrowing athletes. *Am J Sports Med*. 2017;45(2):454-461. doi:10.1177/0363546516676075.

25. Gullich A, Emrich E. Evaluation of the support of young athletes in the elite sports system. *Eur J Sport Sci*. 2006;13(3):85-108.

26. Hall RR. Sport specialization's association with an increased risk of developing anterior knee pain in adolescent female athletes. *J Sport Rehabil*. 2015;24(1):31-35. doi:10.1123/jsr.2013-0101.

27. Intensive training and sports specialization in young athletes. *Pediatrics*. 2000;106(1):154.

28. Jayanthi NAN. Sports-specialized intensive training and the risk of injury in young athletes: a clinical case-control study. *Am J Sports Med*. 2015;43(4):794-801. doi:10.1177/0363546514567298.

29. Jayanthi NN. Sports specialization in young athletes: evidence-based recommendations. *Sports Health*. 2013;5(3):251-257. doi:10.1177/1941738112464626.

30. Kibler WB, Thomas SJ. Pathomechanics of the throwing shoulder. *Sports Med Arthrosc*. 2012;20(1):22-29. doi:10.1097/JSA.0b013e3182432cf2.

31. LaPrade RF, Agel J, Baker J, et al. AOSSM early sport specialization consensus statement. *Orthop J Sports Med*. 2016;4(4). doi:10.1177/2325967116644241.

32. Little League Baseball and Softball. http://www.little-league.org/Little_League_Big_Legacy/About_Little_League/Who_We_Are.htm.

33. Lyman S, Flesig GS, Andrews JR, Osinski ED. Effect of pitch type, pitch count, and pitching mechanics on risk of elbow and shoulder pain in youth baseball pitchers. *Am J Sports Med*. 2002;30(4):463-468.

34. Lyman SS. Longitudinal study of elbow and shoulder pain in youth baseball pitchers. *Med Sci Sports Exerc*. 2001;33(11):1803-1810.

35. Makhni EC, Morrow ZS, Luchetti TJ, et al. Arm pain in youth baseball players: a survey of healthy players. *Am J Sports Med*. 2015;43(1):41-46. doi:10.1177/0363546514555506.

36. Matsuure T, Suzue N, Iwama T, Arisawa K, Fukuta S, Sairyo K. Epidemiology of shoulder and elbow pain in youth baseball players. *Phys Sportsmed*. 2016;44(2):97-100. doi:10.1080/00913847.2016.1149422.

37. McGuine TA, Post EG, Hetzel SJ, Brooks MA, Trigsted S, Bell DR. A prospective study on the effect of sport specialization on lower extremity injury rates in high school athletes. *Am J Sports Med*. 2017:363546517710213. doi:10.1177/0363546517710213.

38. Meister K, Day T, Horodyski M, Kaminski TW, Wasik MP, Tillman S. Rotational motion changes in the glenohumeral joint of the adolescent/little league baseball player. *Am J Sports Med*. 2005;33(5):693-698. doi:10.1177/0363546504269936.

39. Moesch KK. Late specialization: the key to success in centimeters, grams, or seconds (cgs) sports. *Scand J Med Sci Sports*. 2011;21(6):e282-e290. doi:10.1111/j.1600-0838.2010.01280.x.

40. National Collegiate Athletic Association Research. Available at http://www.ncaa.org/about/resources/research/baseball. Accessed August 12, 2017.

41. Olsen SJ, Fleisig GS, Dun S, Loftice J, Andrews JR. Risk factors for shoulder and elbow injuries in adolescent baseball pitchers. *Am J Sports Med*. 2006;34(6):905-912. doi:10.1177/0363546505284188.

42. Pasulka J, Jayanthi N, McCann A, Dugas LR, LaBella C. Specialization patterns across various youth sports and relationship to injury risk. *Phys Sportsmed*. 2017;45(3):344-352. doi:10.1080/00913847.2017.1313077.

43. Petty DH, Andrews JR, Fleisig GS, Cain EL. Ulnar collateral ligament reconstruction in high school baseball players. *Am J Sports Med*. 2004;32(5):1158-1164. doi:10.1177/0363546503262166.

44. Posner M, Cameron KL, Wolf JM, Belmont PJ Jr, Owens BD. Epidemiology of major league baseball injuries. *Am J Sports Med*. 2011;39(8):1676-1680.

45. Powell JW, Barber-Foss KD. Sex-related injury patterns among selected high school sports. *Am J Sports Med*. 2000;28(3):385-391.

46. Pytiak AV, Stearns P, Bastrom TP, et al. Are the current little league pitching guidelines adequate? A single-season prospective MRI study. *Orthop J Sports Med.* 2017;5(5):2325967117704851. doi:10.1177/2325967117704851.

47. Reagan KM, Meister K, Horodyski MB, Werner DW, Carruthers C, Wilk K. Humeral retroversion and its relationship to glenohumeral rotation in the shoulder of college baseball players. *Am J Sports Med.* 2002;30(3):354-360. doi:10.1177/03635465020300030901.

48. Sabick MB, Kim Y-K, Torry MR, Keirns MA, Hawkins RJ. Biomechanics of the shoulder in youth baseball pitchers. *Am J Sports Med.* 2005;33(11):1716-1722. doi:10.1177/0363546505275347.

49. The National Federation of State High School Associations. *2015-16 High School Athletics Participation Survey Results.* 2016. Available at http://www.nfhs.org/ParticipationStatistics/ParticipationStatistics. Accessed August 12, 2017.

50. The Sports & Fitness Industry Association. *2014 Sports, Fitness, and Leisure Activities Topline Participation Report.* 2014. Available at https://www.sfia.org/reports/.

51. Yang J, Mann BJ, Guettler JH, et al. Risk-prone pitching activities and injuries in youth baseball: findings from a national sample. *Am J Sports Med.* 2014;42(6):1456-1463.

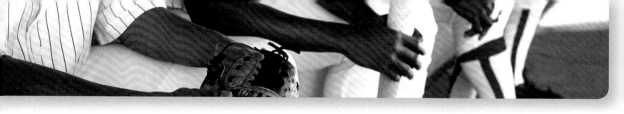

CHAPTER 45

Adolescent Pitching Mechanics and Pitch Counts

Peter N. Chalmers, MD | Brandon J. Erickson, MD

That's baseball. Anything can happen, and it happened today.

—*Mariano Rivera*

INTRODUCTION

Baseball is one of the most popular sports for adolescents in the United States and around the world. In the United States alone, an estimated 5 million children between the ages of 6 and 17 years are involved in various baseball leagues each year.[35] Although contact injuries in baseball are rare, shoulder and elbow pain from overuse, as well as overuse injuries, specifically to pitchers, are becoming more common.[15] Studies have found that elbow and shoulder pain in adolescent baseball pitchers is very common, with rates of 30% to 50% and 23%, respectively.[21,22] In a recent study, 36% of adolescent baseball pitchers admitted to elbow pain during pitching and 32% stated they continued to pitch through the pain.[12] This mentality of playing through pain, although encouraged by coaches, is not safe. Pitching while fatigued increases a pitcher's risk of shoulder and elbow injury.[24,35] In an effort to prevent injuries and pain in this population, guidelines regarding pitch counts have been put forth in various baseball leagues. The objective of these guidelines is to allow adolescents to continue to compete but mitigate the risk of injury. Similarly, coaches have attempted to focus on proper pitching mechanics in their adolescent pitchers to ensure that they are not overstressing any 1 part of their body during their pitching motion.

PITCHING MECHANICS

The overhand baseball pitch is among the fastest human motions to have been measured and comprehensively studied.[32] To achieve the high ball velocity necessary to deny the batter the decision time to understand the likely trajectory of the pitch, the pitcher must perform a highly coordinated full body motion in which the force generated by the large, strong muscles of the lower extremity and trunk is leveraged through the upper extremity.[13,16,17,26,32] As youth and adolescent pitchers learn this motion and develop from a muscular and skeletal perspective, the mechanics of this motion change.[8,14,27] Advancement in progression of muscular strength and mechanics with a concomitant increase in velocity before skeletal development predictably leads to a characteristic series of injuries, such as Little Leaguer's shoulder and Little Leaguer's elbow.[18,19,30] Those who care for youth and adolescent pitchers must thus have an understanding for the normal development of pitch mechanics so that abnormalities can be identified and addressed.

Full pitch mechanics are addressed in chapter 2. To briefly review, the pitch is most commonly divided into 6 phases: (1) the windup phase, (2) the stride phase, (3) the cocking phase, (4) the acceleration phase, (5) the deceleration phase, and (6) the follow-through phase, with the phases defined based on kinematic events (Figure 45.1).[9,16,17,31] During the windup phase the body prepares for force generation by bringing the hands to the chest and by lifting the lead leg.[9,16,17,31] During the stride phase, the back foot remains stable while the front foot strides down the mound; the pelvis also rotates forward.[9,16,17,31] During the cocking phase, the hands separate, the torso rotates forward, and the throwing shoulder is brought into abduction and external rotation.[9,16,17,31] During the acceleration phase, the arm internally rotates, the elbow extends, and the wrist flexes, ending with ball release.[9,16,17,25,31] During the deceleration phase, the arm slows but continues

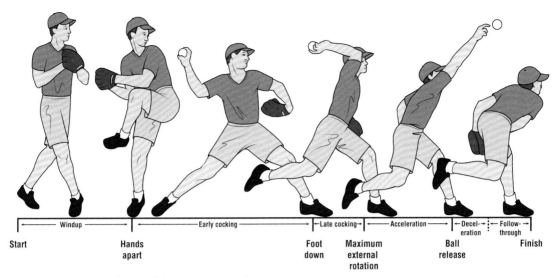

FIGURE 45.1 • The 6 phases of the overhand pitch.

to internally rotate as the biceps acts to decelerate the arm.[9,16,17,31] During the follow-through phase, the body moves into a fielding position.[9,16,17,25,31] The entire motion can be conceptualized as a kinetic chain in which the force generated by the lower extremity and trunk is transferred to the shoulder and elbow during cocking. The late cocking portion of the pitch thus has the highest shoulder and elbow torques, as all of the energy of the pitch is stored at this moment in stretch of the soft tissues of the shoulder and elbow.[1,2,16,23]

Several studies have been conducted to compare pitching mechanics across level of play. In an early study performed in 1999 at the American Sports Medicine Institute, kinematics (ie, angles and velocities but not torques or forces) were examined in a variety of pitchers, and no differences were found between youth, high school, collegiate, and professional pitchers.[17] A subsequent study performed at the Kerlan Jobe Orthopedic Clinic examined qualitative mechanics in 169 youth and adolescent pitchers did demonstrate changes with age.[8] This study specifically examined 5 qualitative motion factors considered by most pitching coaches to be associated with "good" mechanics, including leading with the hips, having the hand on top of the ball during early cocking, having the arm in the throwing position in early cocking, having proper separation of rotation of the hips and shoulders, and having the stride foot pointed toward home plate. Of these factors, adolescent pitchers were more likely than youth pitchers to have their hand on top of the ball during early cocking (66% vs 92%, P = .001) and tended to be more likely to have proper separation of hips and shoulders (23% vs 37%, P = .065). Adolescent pitchers were more likely to have more than 3 correct factors than youth pitchers

(64% vs 81%, P = .017). In addition, these factors were associated with decreased shoulder and elbow torques and improved pitch efficiency (torque per velocity). Overall, this study suggests that as pitchers age, their mechanics improve and that with these improvements, strain on the arm and pitching efficiency also improve.[8] In a subsequent study performed at the American Sports Medicine Institute, pitchers in high levels of play were demonstrated to have more pitch-to-pitch consistency in mechanics than those in lower levels of play, with sequential improvements seen from youth to adolescent to college to minor and then to major league pitchers.[14] This further speaks to the importance of proper pitching mechanics to allow effective, reproducible pitches.

In the largest study performed to date, at Rush University Medical Center, over 400 pitchers of age 9 to 22 years were examined with biplanar video.[27] This study redemonstrated the previous findings of the Kerlan Jobe Orthopedic Clinic's study, with improvement in qualitative mechanics with level of play, such as having the throwing hand on top of the ball in early cocking (P < .001) and having proper hip and shoulder separation (P < .001). However, several differences were also demonstrated in kinematics. Older pitchers had a higher maximum knee height, improving from 63% of pitcher height in 9 to 12-year-olds to 67% of pitcher height in 16 to 17-year-olds with a P value of .001. Older pitchers also had longer stride length, improving from 73% to 80% of pitcher height in the same age-groups with a p value of less than .001. Older pitchers had more knee flexion at front foot contact, improving from 39° to 47° in the same age-groups with a P value of <.001. These 3 findings suggest that as pitchers age, their ability to get the most force from their lower extremity improves, as during the early phases of the pitch they stride farther and deeper. Ball release mechanics were also significantly changed, with more lead hip flexion at ball release and more lead knee flexion at ball release, both of which also suggest a longer, more leveraged stride. These changes were largely seen between the ages of 9 and 17 years, with few changes seen after skeletal maturity. Interestingly, few changes were seen in arm position at any point during the pitch between levels of play. These findings suggest that much of the development in pitching mechanics may occur via improved lower extremity and core strength to allow balance into a longer, deeper stride (Figure 45.2).[27]

One specific biomechanical factor that changes with age in a nearly linear fashion was adequate separation of the hips and shoulders, ie, proper timing of thoracic rotation. Previous studies have also demonstrated this variable to be the best correlate with a history of injury, to be the best correlate with fatigue, and to be the best motion correlate with velocity.[7,12,29] These data further suggest that core strength may be a key area of improvement as pitchers develop.

One final factor that changes in a predictable manner as pitchers age is an increase in pitch velocity.[3,7] Between ages 8 and 14 years, pitch velocity increases from a mean of 40 mph to a mean of 60 to 65 mph, and between ages 14 and 18 years, pitch velocity increases from a mean of 60 to 65 to 75 mph (Figure 45.3). Understanding these norms can help those who help care for pitchers to identify those at risk for injury, as pitch velocity has been demonstrated to strongly correlate with injury.[6,7]

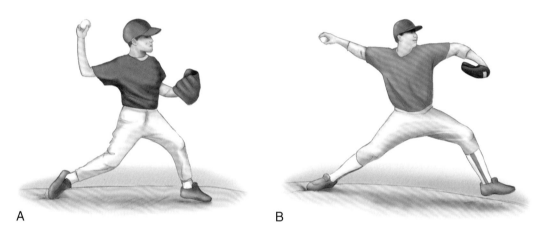

FIGURE 45.2 • These 2 schematics demonstrate a youth pitcher with a shorter, shallower stride (A) and an older adolescent pitcher with a longer, deeper stride (B).

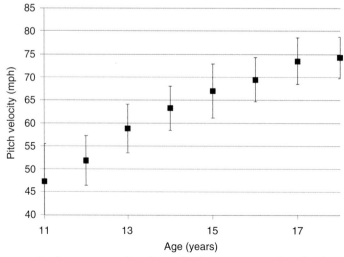

FIGURE 45.3 • This scatterplot demonstrates the relationship between age and pitch velocity in miles per hour (mph). Squares demonstrate mean values, while error bars demonstrate 1 standard deviation.

RISK FACTORS FOR INJURY

There are numerous risk factors for injury in baseball pitchers. These risk factors include pitching while fatigued, high pitch counts, pitching on consecutive days, pitching more than 100 innings per year, pitching for multiple teams, pitching with higher velocity, pitching with supraspinatus weakness, geography (growing up in warmer weather climates), pitching with a glenohumeral internal rotation deficit (GIRD), and, most recently, pitching with a loss of total arc of motion.[4-6,11,15,24,33,34]

Fatigue

As mentioned, arm fatigue is a common finding in adolescent pitchers. Unfortunately, this has been linked to an increase in injuries in these pitchers. Yang et al evaluated 754 youth pitchers (ages 9-18 years) to determine pitching-related risk factors for arm pain and injuries.[35] The authors found that adolescent pitchers who often pitched with arm tiredness and arm pain had 7.88 and 7.50 greater odds of sustaining a pitching-related injury, respectively. Similarly, Olsen et al found that pitchers who frequently pitched with arm fatigue and who continued to pitch despite arm pain were significantly more likely to sustain a shoulder or elbow injury than those who never pitched with arm fatigue or pain.[24] It is somewhat difficult to quantify fatigue and is therefore difficult to counsel pitchers on when to come out of games to prevent injuries.

One recent study evaluated the effect of fatigue on pitching mechanics in adolescent pitchers to determine if there was an objective parameter (such as elbow flexion angle at ball release) coaches and parents could use to determine when their child was becoming fatigued so that they could be removed from a game before sustaining an injury.[12] The authors did not find any specific kinematic parameter that changed as the adolescent pitchers became fatigued. However, as pitchers fatigued, the authors found a change in a qualitative metric: hip to shoulder separation. As pitchers fatigued, their hip to shoulder separation significantly decreased, meaning they were throwing with more of an open shoulder position than a closed position. This likely was indicative of core weakness that manifested as a change in shoulder position. Hence, a core strengthening program may prove beneficial in decreasing shoulder/elbow pain and injures in adolescents, although further work on this subject must be done.

Pitch Counts

One of the easiest risk factors to modify and control is a player's pitch count. Previous long-term studies have found that high pitch counts, as well as throwing more than 100 innings in a single year, place pitchers at an increased risk for shoulder and elbow injury.[15,24] Pitchers now are often competing on more than 1 team at a time (recent evidence has shown that 46% of adolescent pitchers play on more than 1 team).[12] Unfortunately, a coach can only keep track of their pitchers when they pitching for his or her team, and as pitchers often play for multiple teams under multiple coaches, it can be difficult for coaches to maintain an accurate pitch count on these athletes. Therefore, it is the responsibility of the parents, as well as the athlete, to be honest about their pitch counts, so the proper recommendations can be followed.

There has been a significant push in the last 10 years to attempt to prevent shoulder and elbow injuries in adolescent pitchers through the institution of age-specific pitch counts. In 2007, Little League Baseball changed their regulations from an inning limit to a pitch count limit to better control the number of pitches players were throwing in games.[15,21,28] Once recent study attempted to determine the efficacy of this change, as it related to injuries in these Little League pitchers who went on to pitch professionally. The authors found that significantly more pitchers who pitched in the Little League World Series before the regulations changed from an inning limit to a pitch count limit underwent an ulnar collateral ligament reconstruction (UCLR) when they reached Major League Baseball (MLB) and Minor League Baseball.[10] This indicates that the pitch count limits have been effective in preventing long-term ulnar collateral ligament (UCL) injuries in these athletes. However, little is known about the efficacy of these pitch count limits on preventing injuries in the short term. The current pitch count recommendations set forth by Little League Baseball and MLB Pitch Smart program (http://m.mlb.com/pitchsmart/pitching-guidelines/) can be found in Table 45.1. Coaches, parents, and players of all levels should familiarize themselves with these guidelines to ensure proper compliance.

Velocity

Via simple physics, a higher maximum velocity places a high valgus stress on the elbow compared with a slower pitch. However, the ability of a pitcher to throw a fastball over 90 mph is predictive of their ability to play at the collegiate and major league level. Thus, while many pitchers strive to increase their fastball speed to increase their competitiveness, they are also increasing their risk for shoulder and elbow

TABLE 45.1 Current Adolescent Pitch Count Recommendations Set Forth by Little League Baseball and Major League Baseball's Pitch Smart Program (http://m.mlb.com/pitchsmart/pitching-guidelines/)

Age (y)	Daily Max (Pitches in Game)	Required Rest (Pitches)				
		0 d	1 d	2 d	3 d	4 d
7-8	50	1-20	21-35	36-50	N/A	N/A
9-10	75	1-20	21-35	36-50	51-65	66+
11-12	85	1-20	21-35	36-50	51-65	66+
13-14	95	1-20	21-35	36-50	51-65	66+
15-16	95	1-30	31-45	46-60	61-75	76+
17-18	105	1-30	31-45	46-60	61-75	76+
19-22	120	1-30	31-45	46-60	61-75	76+

injuries. Olsen et al surveyed 95 adolescent pitchers who had a history of shoulder or elbow surgery and 45 healthy controls to determine risk factors for necessitating surgery.[24] The authors found that the control pitchers had a statistically significantly slower average fastball speed of 82.7 mph while those with a history of a shoulder or elbow injury averaged 88.6 and 88.1 mph on their fastballs, respectively. Similarly, Chalmers et al recently evaluated pitch velocity on the risk of UCL injuries in MLB pitchers and found that pitchers who underwent UCLR had significantly higher preinjury peak pitch velocity than control pitchers without a history of a UCLR (93.3 vs 92.1 mph).[6]

It was once believed that throwing breaking pitches at an early age was a risk factor for injury, as many thought the torque needed to throw these pitches was detrimental to the developing elbow. Some made recommendations that pitchers should not be allowed to throw a curveball or breaking ball until they had facial hair. This theory has since been disproven in several well-done studies showing no increase in shoulder or elbow injury rates in pitchers who threw breaking balls and curveballs.[15,24] Interestingly, evidence has emerged that has linked throwing a higher percentage of fastballs compared with other pitches to risk of UCL injury.[20] Hence, an ability to throw off-speed pitches may actually be protective for adolescent pitchers, as this allows them to throw at a much lower velocity than just throwing fastballs every pitch.

Height/Weight

Although the previously listed risk factors have all been modifiable, a pitcher's height is not. Height and weight have been a subject of interest in regard to shoulder and elbow injuries in recent years, as pitchers have become bigger and stronger over this period of time. Olsen et al in their survey study found that pitchers with a history of elbow injuries were more likely to be taller and heavier than healthy, uninjured controls (185.5 vs 181.3 cm for height, 86.5 vs 80.6 kg for weight).[24] Similarly, Chalmers et al found weight to be an independent risk factor for sustaining a UCL injury in MLB pitchers.[6] While a pitchers height cannot be modified, a pitcher's weight can be managed. Therefore, it is imperative for pitchers to maintain a reasonable weight to decrease their risk of sustaining a UCL injury. It remains unclear exactly how height relates to injury; it may be that taller pitchers have longer forearms that exert more torque on the elbow.

MANAGER'S TIPS

- Teaching adolescent baseball pitchers proper throwing mechanics can help decrease the risk of injury over time
- Pitchers who throw at a high velocity should be warned that this puts them at an increased risk of injury. Mixing up their pitching repertoire to include off-speed pitches may help decrease the risk of injury
- Risk factors for injury include pitching while fatigued, high pitch counts, pitching on consecutive days, pitching more than 100 innings per year, pitching for multiple teams, pitching with higher velocity, pitching with supraspinatus weakness, geography (growing up in warmer weather climates), pitching with a GIRD, and, most recently, pitching with a loss of total arc of motion
- It is imperative that adolescent pitchers adhere to the current pitch count limits. Further studies are needed to assess the efficacy of the current pitch count recommendations

REFERENCES

1. Aguinaldo AL, Chambers H. Correlation of throwing mechanics with elbow valgus load in adult baseball pitchers. *Am J Sports Med.* 2009;37(10):2043-2048.

2. Anz AW, Bushnell BD, Griffin LP, Noonan TJ, Torry MR, Hawkins RJ. Correlation of torque and elbow injury in professional baseball pitchers. *Am J Sports Med.* 2010;38(7):1368-1374.

3. Axe MJ, Strube M, Osinski D, Andrews JR, Snyder-Mackler L. A speed distance-based classification system for injury prevention and research in international and domestic youth baseball players. *Int J Sports Phys Ther.* 2014;9(3):346-355.

4. Bushnell BD, Anz AW, Noonan TJ, Torry MR, Hawkins RJ. Association of maximum pitch velocity and elbow injury in professional baseball pitchers. *Am J Sports Med.* 2010;38(4):728-732.

5. Byram IR, Bushnell BD, Dugger K, Charron K, Harrell FE Jr, Noonan TJ. Preseason shoulder strength measurements in professional baseball pitchers: identifying players at risk for injury. *Am J Sports Med.* 2010;38(7):1375-1382.

6. Chalmers PN, Erickson BJ, Ball B, Romeo AA, Verma NN. Fastball pitch velocity helps predict ulnar collateral ligament reconstruction in major league baseball pitchers. *Am J Sports Med.* 2016;44(8):2130-2135.

7. Chalmers PN, Sgroi T, Riff AJ, et al. Correlates with history of injury in youth and adolescent pitchers. *Arthroscopy.* 2015;31(7):1349-1357.

8. Davis JT, Limpisvasti O, Fluhme D, et al. The effect of pitching biomechanics on the upper extremity in youth and adolescent baseball pitchers. *Am J Sports Med.* 2009;37(8):1484-1491.

9. Dillman CJ, Fleisig GS, Andrews JR. Biomechanics of pitching with emphasis upon shoulder kinematics. *J Orthop Sports Phys Ther.* 1993;18(2):402-408.

10. Erickson BJ CP, Axe MJ, Romeo AA. Exceeding pitch count recommendations in little league baseball increases the chance of requiring Tommy John surgery as a professional baseball pitcher. *Orthop J Sports Med.* 2017;5(3).

11. Erickson BJ, Harris J, Tetreault M, Bush-Joseph C, Cohen MS, Romeo AA. Is Tommy John surgery performed more frequently in major league baseball pitchers from warm weather areas? *Orthop J Sports Med.* 2014;2(10).

12. Erickson BJ, Sgori T, Chalmers PN, et al. The impact of fatigue on baseball pitching mechanics in adolescent male pitchers. *Arthroscopy.* 2016;32(5):762-771.

13. Feltner GS, Dapena J. Three-dimensional interactions in a two-segment kinetic chain. Part 1: general model. *Int J Sports Biomech.* 1989;5:403-419.

14. Fleisig G, Chu Y, Weber A, Andrews J. Variability in baseball pitching biomechanics among various levels of competition. *Sports BioMech.* 2009;8(1):10-21.

15. Fleisig GS, Andrews JR, Cutter GR, et al. Risk of serious injury for young baseball pitchers: a 10-year prospective study. *Am J Sports Med.* 2011;39(2):253-257.

16. Fleisig GS, Andrews JR, Dillman CJ, Escamilla RF. Kinetics of baseball pitching with implications about injury mechanisms. *Am J Sports Med.* 1995;23(2):233-239.

17. Fleisig GS, Barrentine SW, Escamilla RF, Andrews JR. Biomechanics of overhand throwing with implications for injuries. *Sports Med.* 1996;21(6):421-437.

18. Frank RM, Lenart BA, Cohen MS. Olecranon physeal nonunion in the adolescent athlete: identification of two patterns. *J Shoulder Elbow Surg.* 2017;26(6):1044-1051.

19. Heyworth BE, Kramer DE, Martin DJ, Micheli LJ, Kocher MS, Bae DS. Trends in the presentation, management, and outcomes of little league shoulder. *Am J Sports Med.* 2016;44(6):1431-1438.

20. Keller RA, Marshall NE, Guest JM, Okoroha KR, Jung EK, Moutzouros V. Major league baseball pitch velocity and pitch type associated with risk of ulnar collateral ligament injury. *J Shoulder Elbow Surg.* 2016;25(4):671-675.

21. Lyman S, Fleisig GS, Andrews JR, Osinski ED. Effect of pitch type, pitch count, and pitching mechanics on risk of elbow and shoulder pain in youth baseball pitchers. *Am J Sports Med.* 2002;30(4):463-468.

22. Makhni EC, Morrow ZS, Luchetti TJ, et al. Arm pain in youth baseball players: a survey of healthy players. *Am J Sports Med.* 2015;43(1):41-46.

23. Nissen CW, Westwell M, Ounpuu S, Patel M, Solomito M, Tate J. A biomechanical comparison of the fastball and curveball in adolescent baseball pitchers. *Am J Sports Med.* 2009;37(8):1492-1498.

24. Olsen SJ II, Fleisig GS, Dun S, Loftice J, Andrews JR. Risk factors for shoulder and elbow injuries in adolescent baseball pitchers. *Am J Sports Med.* 2006;34(6):905-912.

25. Pappas AM, Zawacki RM, Sullivan TJ. Biomechanics of baseball pitching. A preliminary report. *Am J Sports Med.* 1985;13(4):216-222.

26. Putnam CA. Sequential motions of body segments in striking and throwing skills: descriptions and explanations. *J Biomech.* 1993;26(suppl 1):125-135.

27. Riff AJ, Chalmers PN, Sgroi T, et al. Epidemiologic comparison of pitching mechanics, pitch type, and pitch counts among healthy pitchers at various levels of youth competition. *Arthroscopy.* 2016;32(8):1559-1568.

28. Series LLBW. *2015 Little League Baseball World Series.* Available at: http://www.llbws.org. Accessed February 4, 2016.

29. Sgroi T, Chalmers PN, Riff AJ, et al. Predictors of throwing velocity in youth and adolescent pitchers. *J Shoulder Elbow Surg.* 2015;24(9):1339-1345.

30. Shanley E, Thigpen C. Throwing injuries in the adolescent athlete. *Int J Sports Phys Ther.* 2013;8(5):630-640.

31. Werner SL, Fleisig GS, Dillman CJ, Andrews JR. Biomechanics of the elbow during baseball pitching. *J Orthop Sports Phys Ther*. 1993;17(6):274-278.

32. Werner SL, Gill TJ, Murray TA, Cook TD, Hawkins RJ. Relationships between throwing mechanics and shoulder distraction in professional baseball pitchers. *Am J Sports Med*. 2001;29(3):354-358.

33. Wilk KE, Arrigo CA, Hooks TR, Andrews JR. Rehabilitation of the overhead throwing athlete: there is more to it than just external rotation/internal rotation strengthening. *PM R*. 2016;8(3 suppl):S78-S90.

34. Wilk KE, Macrina LC, Fleisig GS, et al. Deficits in glenohumeral passive range of motion increase risk of shoulder injury in professional baseball pitchers: a prospective study. *Am J Sports Med*. 2015;43(10):2379-2385.

35. Yang J, Mann BJ, Guettler JH, et al. Risk-prone pitching activities and injuries in youth baseball: findings from a national sample. *Am J Sports Med*. 2014;42(6):1456-1463.

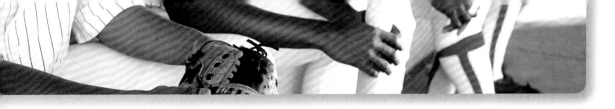

CHAPTER 46

Little Leaguer's Shoulder

Peter N. Chalmers, MD | Timothy Kahn, MD

A team is where a boy can prove his courage on his own. A gang is where a coward goes to hide.

—*Mickey Mantle*

INTRODUCTION

First described by Dotter in 1953,[1] Little Leaguer's shoulder (LLS) is an increasingly common and well-recognized condition affecting young overhead athletes, particularly adolescent pitchers.[2,3] Initially described as a Salter-Harris I fracture of the epiphyseal plate, it is now generally considered to be a form of epiphysiolysis affecting the proximal humerus. Although the etiology of the disease is not fully known, the prevailing thought process is that LLS is an overuse injury due to prolonged, recurrent microtrauma.[3,4] Fundamental to our understanding of LLS is the knowledge gained regarding growth plate biomechanics, throwing mechanics, and training habits of adolescent baseball players, particularly pitching schedules.

CLINICAL EVALUATION

History

Although LLS likely has the potential to affect any overhead athlete population, the vast majority of described cases have been in adolescent baseball players, particularly pitchers. In a recent study by Heyworth et al, of the 95 reported cases, 97% involved baseball players, of which 86% were primarily pitchers. However, their series also included 3 tennis players who were affected as well.[3]

The age of those afflicted with LLS ranges from 8 to 16 years old, with an average age of 13 to 14 years.[3,5] The reason that this particular age range is most affected is likely due to a combination of factors unique to adolescent baseball pitchers. First, there is a general increase in volume of pitches thrown by these players, particularly if they are participating in

showcases or year-round play.[6,7] As players begin to develop shoulder musculature, there are also physiologic changes in shoulder mechanics that take place. These changes include a substantial decrease in shoulder rotational range of motion. Decreased rotational range of motion may then lead to increased stress at the physis during throwing.[8] Likewise, the rapid growth at the proximal humeral physis leads to weakening of its overall structural stability. These changes particularly occur at the zone of hypertrophy. Biomechanically the shear strength of the physis plateaus and can decrease between ages 10 and 13 years old.[9] These physiologic changes occur simultaneous to increasing pitch velocity as players age. As shown by Gainor et al, the internal torque experienced around the proximal humerus during an average baseball pitch can reach up to 14,000 inch-lb before ball release.[10] This excessive force across the physis is thought to lead to repetitive microtrauma and the pathologic changes seen with LLS.[4,11] Therefore, the pathophysiology of LLS is similar to other well-described disease processes involving the physis in adolescent athletes, such as Little Leaguer's elbow, Osgood-Schlatter, or Sever disease, which all involve excessive force causing repetitive injury to the physis in other locations.

During the pitching motion, the proximal humerus experiences its highest torsional forces at maximum external rotation during late arm cocking. The highest distraction forces are observed just subsequent to the time of ball release during deceleration.[12,13] Both these kinetic parameters are thought to be contributing factors in the development of LLS.

Patients presenting with LLS may report symptoms of shoulder pain with throwing, particularly with high-velocity pitches. In a case report of 23 patients by

Carson et al, the most common presenting complaint was pain localized to the proximal humerus during throwing.[5] Patients generally describe a pattern of gradual onset and progressive worsening, rather than developing symptoms after a specific pitch or action, although this has been described.[5] These progressive symptoms are usually associated with an increase in pitching volume.

In the largest case series to date, Heyworth et al studied the association of LLS with glenohumeral internal rotation deficit (GIRD) and found that 30% of patients with LLS were found to have GIRD on physical examination. In this study, GIRD was defined as a 10° side-to-side loss in internal rotation. It is unclear from this study whether GIRD itself is specifically associated with LLS, as the study did not contain a control population. These authors treated all patients with physical therapy focused on addressing the GIRD in addition to rest from throwing.[3] In another study by Nakamizo et al of 25 asymptomatic baseball players of the ages 10 to 12 years old, 10 players were found to have GIRD, which was defined as 20° side-to-side loss in internal rotation. Certainly, these findings suggest that GIRD may not be pathologic in adolescent baseball players.[14]

Although some authors have suggested that poor throwing mechanics may contribute to the development of LLS and have therefore suggested that mechanical adjustment should be a portion of treatment,[3] no study has demonstrated such an association.

Physical Examination

The most common physical finding associated with LLS is tenderness to palpation over the lateral proximal humerus.[3,5] This finding is reported in 74% to 87% of patients with LLS. Weakness of external rotation has been noted as well in some patients,[3,5] although this is generally considered to be secondary to pain. Provocative maneuvers include eliciting pain with resisted external rotation.[15] Bilateral abducted rotational range of motion should also be elicited on every patient, although it is unclear whether glenohumeral rotational range of motion is directly associated with LLS. Finally, the senior author also routinely tests core strength in his evaluation of youth and adolescent throwers, as alterations in trunk rotation timing during the pitch have been linked to fatigue and possibly to injury in this population, although not specifically to LLS.[16-18]

Imaging

In any patient where LLS is suspected, anteroposterior (AP) and external/internal rotation views of the shoulder should be obtained. These views are generally sufficient to establish a diagnosis of LLS.[3,5] However, if clinical suspicion remains high after equivocal radiographs, magnetic resonance imaging (MRI) may provide further diagnostic information.[3,19]

To fully understand the radiographic presentation of LLS, it is important to note the anatomy of the proximal humeral physis, which is a wavy, cone-shaped structure. The morphology of the physis and the strong posteromedial periosteum both confer a great deal of stability to the proximal humerus physis.[20] It has been postulated that the strong posteromedial periosteum may contribute to the greater lateral than medial widening seen in the physis in LLS.[5]

Radiographic findings in LLS include widening of the proximal humeral physis, particularly in the lateral portion—this finding has been reported to have a sensitivity of nearly 100% in patients with symptoms for more than 3 weeks (Figure 46.1).[15] Fragmentation of the lateral aspect of the proximal humeral metaphysis, sclerosis of the proximal humeral metaphysis, demineralization, and cystic changes have also all been noted.[21] MRI may redemonstrate these findings (Figure 46.2). Medial shift of the humeral head compared with the shaft has been described as well, although findings of this severity are rare.[22]

In a recent study of 41 youth baseball players with pain in their throwing shoulder, Kanematsu et al described a classification system for LLS radiographic findings (Figure 46.3). Grade I constitutes widening of the epiphyseal plate in the lateral portion; grade II describes widening at all portions of the epiphyseal plate; and grade III refers to a slipped epiphysis. Of the 15 patients with LLS in the study, 9 had grade I changes, 5 had grade II changes, and only 1 had grade III changes.[23]

In another study by Kanematsu et al, 19 patients with LLS were followed radiographically through symptom resolution. The mean time required for radiographic evidence of healing was 4.7 months. Interval radiographs demonstrated that healing generally progresses from medially to laterally.[24]

Mair et al evaluated 79 youth baseball players and demonstrated that some proximal humeral physeal widening may be a normal adaptive change in adolescent baseball players. Widening of the proximal humeral physis in the dominant arm as compared with the nondominant arm was visualized in 62% of symptomatic players and 55% of asymptomatic players.[25] These findings call into question the importance of these radiographic findings. This suggests that isolated

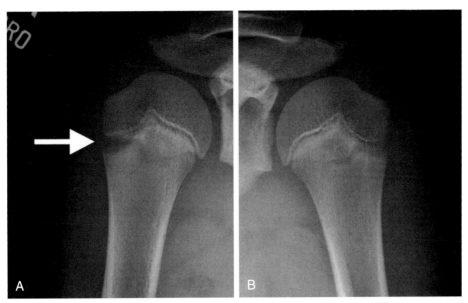

FIGURE 46.1 • This anteroposterior radiograph in external rotation demonstrates proximal humeral epiphyseal widening consistent with Little Leaguer's shoulder. A, The symptomatic shoulder with arrow indicating lateral widening. B, Contralateral shoulder. (Courtesy Christopher S. Ahmad, MD.)

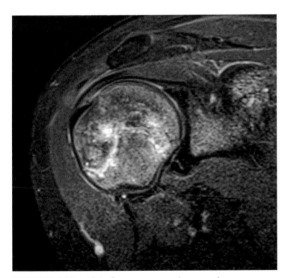

FIGURE 46.2 • This fat-suppressed coronal T2-weighted magnetic resonance image demonstrates increased signal at the proximal humeral epiphysis consistent with Little Leaguer's shoulder. (Courtesy Christopher S. Ahmad, MD.)

radiographic physeal widening is not sufficient for diagnosis of LLS and that treatment should be based on clinical findings.

Like radiographic findings, MRI will demonstrate widening of the proximal humeral physis, particularly on the lateral aspect.[19,26] Subtle periosteal elevation and edema may be noted as well. T1- and T2-weighted sequences may show increased signal within the physis with associated periphyseal marrow edema.[19,27] To

date, there are no MRI studies of asymptomatic pitchers, and thus it remains unclear whether these findings may also be adaptive.

TREATMENT

Nonoperative

The treatment of LLS is essentially always nonoperative, conservative measures. This generally consists of a 3-month cessation of throwing rest period, with or without accompanying physical therapy with a home exercise program.[3,5] Of note, rest from throwing should be strict, not just rest from competition play. Affected players should be advised against any throwing in practice or throwing recreationally until cleared by their physician.

Physical therapy (whether formal or patient directed) should focus on stretching of glenohumeral soft tissue structures to increase glenohumeral internal rotation, strengthening of scapular stabilizers, rotator cuff, and core. Patients should be encouraged to work with their coaching staff to improve throwing mechanics as they gradually return to play. Furthermore, some players could consider a temporary position change to decrease recurrent stress to the physis.

Operative

At this point, there is essentially no role for surgical intervention in patients with uncomplicated LLS owing to the very high success rates with conservative treatment.

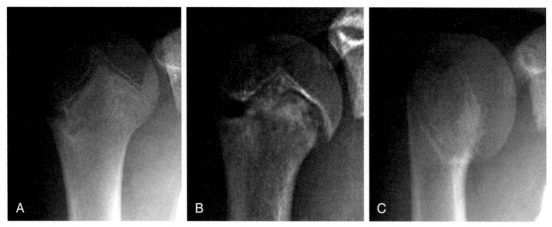

FIGURE 46.3 ● These anteroposterior radiographs demonstrate Kanematsu's classification system for Little Leaguer's shoulder. A, Grade I had lateral epiphyseal widening. B, Grade II has widening of the entire epiphysis. C, Grade III has a slipped epiphysis. (Reproduced, with permission from Kanematsu Y, Matsuura T, Kashiwaguchi S, et al. Epidemiology of shoulder injuries in young baseball players and grading of radiologic findings of little leaguer's shoulder. *J Med Invest.* 2015;62(3-4):123-125. Copyright © 2015 by The University of Tokushima Faculty of Medicine.)

REHABILITATION

As stated earlier, the most universally accepted treatment protocol involves strict avoidance of throwing and/or pitching for approximately 3 months, although no comparison between length of rest and resolution of symptoms has been studied yet. The currently accepted time line of 3 months can be derived from the 2 largest case series to date which both demonstrated low recurrence rates with this rest period.[3,5]

The benefits of physical therapy in the treatment of LLS are not well established. In the case series by Heyworth, 79% of patients underwent formal physical therapy, although no difference in recurrence rate, time to symptom resolution, or time to return to play was found between patients who did or did not participate in physical therapy. In the same study, all patients with documented GIRD were prescribed physical therapy.[3] The role of GIRD in the pathogenesis of this and other pitching-related injuries remains unclear.

Whether or not patients participate in formal physical therapy, stretching to decrease GIRD as well as strengthening of shoulder girdle musculature should be encouraged. Patients should participate in a gradual return to play as long as they remain symptom free. Some patients may need to consider a temporary position change if symptoms recur.[3]

RESULTS

Fortunately, the expected prognosis of LLS treated with adequate rest and gradual return to play is very favorable, with most adolescents returning to play

without pain or recurrence. In the study by Heyworth et al, after an average 4.2 months of cessation of throwing in 64 patients, only 7% of patients had recurrence of LLS symptoms at follow-up. Of those with recurrence, there was an average of 7.6 months from primary diagnosis to recurrence. No other complications were reported in the study. There were no differences in recurrence rate or time to resolution between patients who did and did not undergo formal physical therapy. The average time to symptom resolution was 2.4 months, and the average time to return to play was 4.2 months.[3]

Carson and Gasser demonstrated that of the 23 patients with LLS treated with 3 months of throwing cessation, 21 were able to return to play without recurrence during the follow-up time. The other 2 patients in the study were still in the 3-month rehabilitation phase at the time of study conclusion.[5]

Yanematsu et al demonstrated radiographic resolution at 4.7 months. This time is significantly longer than which would be expected with a simple Salter-Harris I fracture. The increased length of time for resolution may be because of the chronicity of the injury.[24]

COMPLICATIONS

Although complications of LLS are rare when treated with adequate rest and rehabilitation, there have been reports of epiphyseal complications, including a possible Salter-Harris III fracture of the epiphysis and premature closure of the proximal humeral physis.[5] Because 80% of the length of the humerus arises from the proximal physis, a premature closure could theoretically affect overall arm length. In the single reported premature physeal closure, the patient was asymptomatic and had no limb length discrepancy during the study follow-up period.[5]

TRIP TO THE MOUND

Our preferred treatment for Little Leaguer's shoulder includes cessation of throwing, core and leg strengthening, rehabilitation of the upper extremity including stretching and strengthening of the rotator cuff, and strengthening of the periscapular stabilizers. Once all pain has resolved, the pitcher then begins a progressive throwing program with a focus on mechanics. We also recommend players consider playing a position other than pitcher for their first season back. On initial evaluation, athletes should know that it may take a year for their symptoms to completely resolve.

MANAGERS' TIPS

- As the number of reported cases of LLS has increased substantially during the past few decades, there should be an increased vigilance among coaching staff regarding symptoms of LLS

- Prompt evaluation should be undertaken in players who develop symptoms (particularly proximal humerus pain with throwing) to decrease risk of complications as well as to facilitate a quicker return to asymptomatic play

- Increased volume of play without adequate rest, exceeding recommended pitch counts, and playing with pain all likely increase the risk of developing LLS, as well as other upper extremity injury, and should be avoided[6]

REFERENCES

1. Dotter WE. Little leaguer's shoulder: a fracture of the proximal epiphysial cartilage of the humerus due to baseball pitching. *Guthrie Clin Bull.* 1953;23(1):68-72.
2. Osbahr DC, Kim HJ, Dugas JR. Little league shoulder. *Curr Opin Pediatr.* 2010;22(1):35-40.
3. Heyworth BE, Kramer DE, Martin DJ, Micheli LJ, Kocher MS, Bae DS. Trends in the presentation, management, and outcomes of little league shoulder. *Am J Sports Med.* 2016;44(6):1431-1438.
4. Cahill BR, Tullos HS, Fain RH. Little league shoulder: lesions of the proximal humeral epiphyseal plate. *J Sports Med.* 1974;2(3):150-152.
5. Carson WG, Gasser SI. Little leaguer's shoulder. A report of 23 cases. *Am J Sports Med.* 1998;26(4):575-580.
6. Fleisig GS, Andrews JR, Cutter GR, et al. Risk of serious injury for young baseball pitchers: a 10-year prospective study. *Am J Sports Med.* 2011;39(2):253-257.
7. Olsen SJ, Fleisig GS, Dun S, Loftice J, Andrews JR. Risk factors for shoulder and elbow injuries in adolescent baseball pitchers. *Am J Sports Med.* 2006;34(6):905-912.
8. Meister K, Day T, Horodyski M, Kaminski TW, Wasik MP, Tillman S. Rotational motion changes in the glenohumeral joint of the adolescent/little league baseball player. *Am J Sports Med.* 2005;33(5):693-698.
9. Chung SM, Batterman SC, Brighton CT. Shear strength of the human femoral capital epiphyseal plate. *J Bone Joint Surg Am.* 1976;58(1):94-103.
10. Gainor BJ, Piotrowski G, Puhl J, Allen WC, Hagen R. The throw: biomechanics and acute injury. *Am J Sports Med.* 1980;8(2):114-118.
11. Tisano BK, Estes AR. Overuse injuries of the pediatric and adolescent throwing athlete. *Med Sci Sports Exerc.* 2016;48(10):1898-1905.
12. Keeley DW, Hackett T, Keirns M, Sabick MB, Torry MR. A biomechanical analysis of youth pitching mechanics. *J Pediatr Orthop.* 2008;28(4):452-459.
13. Fleisig GS, Andrews JR, Dillman CJ, Escamilla RF. Kinetics of baseball pitching with implications about injury mechanisms. *Am J Sports Med.* 1995;23(2):233-239.
14. Nakamizo H, Nakamura Y, Nobuhara K, Yamamoto T. Loss of glenohumeral internal rotation in little league pitchers: a biomechanical study. *J Shoulder Elbow Surg.* 2008;17(5):795-801.
15. Fleming JL, Hollingsworth CL, Squire DL, Bisset GS. Little leaguer's shoulder. *Skeletal Radiol.* 2004;33(6):352-354.
16. Sgroi T, Chalmers PN, Riff AJ, et al. Predictors of throwing velocity in youth and adolescent pitchers. *J Shoulder Elbow Surg.* 2015;24(9):1339-1345.
17. Chalmers PN, Sgroi T, Riff AJ, et al. Correlates with history of injury in youth and adolescent pitchers. *Arthroscopy.* 2015;31(7):1349-1357.
18. Erickson BJ, Sgroi T, Chalmers PN, et al. The impact of fatigue on baseball pitching mechanics in adolescent male pitchers. *Arthroscopy.* 2016;32(5):762-771.
19. Popkin CA, Posada A, Clifford PD. Little leaguer's shoulder. *Clin Imaging.* 2006;30(5):365-367.
20. Dameron TB Jr, Rockwood CA Jr. Fractures and dislocations of the shoulder. In: Rockwood CA Jr, Wilkins KE, King RE, eds. *Fractures in Children.* Philadelphia: JB Lippincott Co.; 1984:577-607
21. Barnett LS. Little league shoulder syndrome: proximal humeral epiphyseolysis in adolescent baseball pitchers. A case report. *J Bone Joint Surg Am.* 1985;67(3):495-496.

22. Torg JS, Pollack H, Sweterlitsch P. The effect of competitive pitching on the shoulders and elbows of preadolescent baseball players. *Pediatrics*. 1972;49(2):267-272.

23. Kanematsu Y, Matsuura T, Kashiwaguchi S, et al. Epidemiology of shoulder injuries in young baseball players and grading of radiologic findings of little leaguer's shoulder. *J Med Invest*. 2015;62(3-4):123-125.

24. Kanematsu Y, Matsuura T, Kashiwaguchi S, et al. Radiographic follow-up study of Little Leaguer's shoulder. *Skeletal Radiol*. 2015;44(1):73-76.

25. Mair SD, Uhl TL, Robbe RG, Brindle KA. Physeal changes and range-of-motion differences in the dominant shoulders of skeletally immature baseball players. *J Shoulder Elbow Surg*. 2004;13(5):487-491.

26. Song JC, Lazarus ML, Song AP. MRI findings in little leaguer's shoulder. *Skeletal Radiol*. 2006;35(2):107-109.

27. Obembe OO, Gaskin CM, Taffoni MJ, Anderson MW. Little Leaguer's shoulder (proximal humeral epiphysiolysis): MRI findings in four boys. *Pediatr Radiol*. 2007;37(9):885-889.

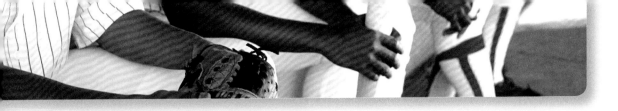

CHAPTER 47

Little Leaguer's Elbow and Medial Epicondyle Epiphyseal Avulsion

Fiona E. Nugent, NP | David P. Trofa, MD | Christopher S. Ahmad, MD

There is always some kid who may be seeing me for the first time. I owe him my best.

—*Joe DiMaggio*

INTRODUCTION

Youth athletes are being exposed to extreme performance demands that have led to high rates of early sports specialization. Although early specialization has not been proven to increase chances of future professional-level play, it has been shown to increase the rates of overuse injuries, burnout, and psychological stress.[1-3] This is especially true in baseball. In fact, 20% to 30% of baseball players between the ages of 9 to 12 years will be diagnosed with an overuse injury each year.[4] Furthermore, Makhni et al found that as many as 70% of youth throwers may develop pain in their throwing arm at some point and still be encouraged to play through that pain.[5] These results are troubling, as Yang et al found in a national survey of 754 youth pitchers that those who threw through pain and fatigue had greater than 7 times the odds of sustaining a pitching-related injury.[6]

During throwing, the medial structures of the elbow are placed under tension during late cocking and early acceleration. While older athletes may be more at risk of ulnar collateral ligament (UCL) pathology because of this repetitive valgus stress, the medial epicondylar physis is more susceptible to overuse injury in skeletally immature athletes. The medial epicondyle is the humeral origin of the flexor-pronator mass as well as the UCL, and it is the last ossification center of the elbow to fuse, usually between the ages of 15 to 16 years in males.[4,7] Before fusion, the physis is a weak link in the kinetic chain, which may be injured when coupled with improper throwing mechanics, overuse, and inadequate rest.

There is a spectrum of disease severity related to pathology of the medial epicondyle physis that ranges from apophysitis or Little Leaguer's elbow to an avulsion fracture that requires operative fixation. Below we review the clinical features and treatment of both these pathologies. While treatment of these injuries is vital for athletes' return to play, it is important to remember that they also represent overuse injuries and treatment prevention is of the utmost importance in adolescent throwers. As such, in 2010 Little League Baseball updated pitching guidelines to minimize the risk of youth baseball injuries.[8] These guidelines set pitch count recommendations, call for avoidance of breaking pitches until skeletal maturity, and promote good throwing mechanics and rest.

LITTLE LEAGUE ELBOW— CLINICAL EVALUATION

History

Patients with Little League elbow are typically between 10 and 14 years of age and present with progressively worsening medial-sided elbow pain associated with throwing that results in decreased velocity, accuracy, and distance.[4,9,10] On history, these patients have often recently increased their throwing demand or velocity or experienced a growth spurt in the past year.[10,11] These young athletes also often have a history of overuse, play on multiple teams, attend showcases, and play year round.[12,13] The examiner should inquire about the duration of symptoms, as this is an indicator of severity with more chronic injuries taking longer to heal. Finally, the examiner should also inquire about any tingling experienced in the fourth and fifth digits, as concomitant ulnar neuritis is not uncommon.

Physical Examination

Physical examination will demonstrate tenderness of the medial epicondylar apophysis with palpation and possible edema over the epicondyle. Pain is often reproduced with resisted pronation of the forearm, which activates the flexor-pronator mass, placing tension on the apophysis. Assessing for valgus instability using the *moving valgus stress test* can indicate more severe apophysitis or an avulsion injury. In this test, the examiner applies valgus stress while moving the elbow from flexion to extension. A positive test elicits pain by reproducing traction force on the epicondyle. Given that the UCL is typically uninjured, it is not usually tender in midsubstance fibers or distal attachment to sublime tubercle. Occasionally, these athletes will present with flexion contractures. The ulnar nerve should also be assessed for subluxation or concurrent neuritis using the *Tinel* test at the cubital tunnel. Finally, given that the radiocapitellar joint may become a significant secondary stabilizer to valgus stress of the elbow, it is important to rule out a concurrent osteochondritis dissecans lesion in the joint. This can be performed by palpating the radiocapitellar joint for tenderness, crepitus, or edema and assessing forearm pronation and supination.

General muscle strength should be assessed, including a core and lower extremity strength assessment. Studies show that strength deficits in these areas can have an effect on the kinetic chain resulting in poor throwing mechanics.[9,14] Often these athletes have weak muscles, which can be corrected with rehabilitation programs.

Imaging

Although largely a clinical diagnosis based on history and physical examination, patients with a presumed diagnosis of medial apophysitis should obtain standard elbow radiographs with anteroposterior (AP), lateral, and oblique views. Although these images may be normal,[15] positive findings typically demonstrate physeal widening (Figure 47.1). The radiocapitellar joint should also be evaluated for a compression injury owing to chronic valgus stress placed on the joint. Magnetic resonance imaging (MRI) can be used to evaluate for bony edema and soft tissue injury and assess the integrity of the UCL, but this is not routinely necessary.[16]

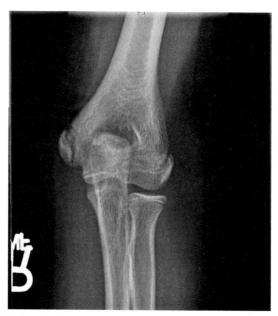

FIGURE 47.1 • Anteroposterior (AP) radiograph of a symptomatic 15-year-old male baseball pitcher demonstrating medial epicondylar physeal widening consistent with Little Leaguer's elbow.

TREATMENT

Nonoperative

Little League elbow responds well to nonoperative management. A period of rest from all throwing for 4 to 6 weeks and activity modification will allow the physis to heal.[4,9,11,16,17] Ice and nonsteroidal anti-inflammatory drugs (NSAIDS) can be used as an analgesic and to improve edema. Casting can cause elbow stiffness and should be avoided. Bracing with range of motion can increase compliance with avoidance of throwing. If there is stiffness, range of motion exercises with a physical therapist can restore motion and address underlying muscle weaknesses in the kinetic chain.

After a period of rest, a progressive throwing program for 6 weeks can return an athlete to throwing. Identifying errors in pitching mechanics can also help decrease stress on the medial epicondylar physis.[9,13,17] If pain reoccurs, immediate cessation of throwing is important. Generally, it is recommended to return to baseball as a position player for the upcoming season and then the following season return to baseball as a pitcher. Sport diversification is recommended through the winter months. On rare occasion, the medial apophysis will fail to fuse and remain symptomatic, indicating surgery with fixation similar to medial apophyseal avulsion as described in the next section.

MEDIAL APOPHYSEAL AVULSION FRACTURE

Medial epicondyle fractures represent 10% to 20% of all elbow fractures and are most commonly sustained by male patients at a peak age of 11 to 12 years.[7,18] Medial epicondyle fractures can be caused by a wide variety of mechanisms, and the approach for treatment is not necessarily the same. For example, a medial epicondyle fracture can be sustained with an elbow dislocation, a simple fall, a direct blow to the medial aspect of the elbow, or an avulsion force from repetitive valgus stress (aka throwing).

The specific subset of medial epicondyle fractures caused by avulsion of the apophysis is part of the same pathologic continuum as Little Leaguer's elbow. As both static and dynamic medial stabilizers attach to the medical epicondyle, valgus overload stress caused by throwing is transferred to the weaker more susceptible medial epicondylar physis, which can lead to fracture. This fracture fragment may be displaced anteriorly and distally by the attachment of flexor-pronator mass and can cause pain, instability, and inability to throw. As discussed further below, this is a unique fracture pattern in a very specific subset of patients whom strongly depend on the medial epicondyle to withstand the significant valgus stress associated with throwing. As such, this is an injury many authors would opt to treat surgically in their high-performance athletes.

CLINICAL EVALUATION

History

Chief complaints for patients presenting with a medial apophyseal avulsion fracture will include acute medial elbow pain, swelling, and ecchymosis, typically after a discrete throwing event. They may recall hearing an audible pop while throwing with inability to continue to play after. They may also recount a history of apophysitis-like symptoms before the acute onset of increased pain. As in any patient with medial elbow pain, the examiner should inquire about ulnar nerve symptoms such as tingling in the ulnar digits. Furthermore, the examiner should obtain a full throwing history inclusive of the patient's workout regimen, changes in performance levels or training, the number of teams played for, maximum throwing velocity, and the types of pitches thrown.

Physical Examination

Examination reveals exquisite tenderness to palpation over the medial epicondyle, soft tissue edema, loss of motion compared with the contralateral side, and ecchymosis. As previously described, the moving valgus stress test will likely be positive owing to incompetence of the medial stabilizers, but it will be difficult to perform in the acutely injured patient. Tests to assess ulnar nerve mobility and neuritis as previously described should also be performed.

Imaging

Plain radiographs including AP, oblique, and lateral views should be obtained to visualize the avulsed fracture fragment with or without displacement (Figure 47.2).[5] Studies have shown that there is poor inter- and intrareliability in assessing displacement on AP and lateral radiographs.[19] Furthermore, recent investigations have shown that fractures classified as nondisplaced on AP and lateral radiographs may actually have >1 cm of anterior displacement as determined by advanced imaging.[20] Alternatively, 45° internal oblique and distal humeral axial view radiographs are better imaging choices to assess fracture displacement.[21,22] Valgus stress radiographs can also be obtained and provide information regarding instability.[5] Finally, while advanced imaging is not routinely necessary for most primary cases, it can provide invaluable information. For example, MRI can be attained if there is concern for concomitant injury to the UCL and/or flexor-pronator mass while a computed topography (CT) scan can be attained to better characterize bony anatomy in the revision setting.

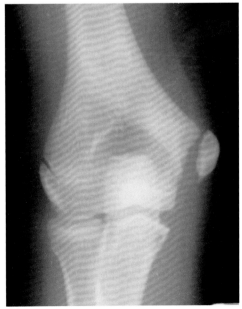

FIGURE 47.2 • Anteroposterior (AP) radiograph of a displaced medial apophyseal avulsion fracture.

TREATMENT

There is no consensus in the literature regarding nonoperative versus operative management of medial epicondyle fractures in adolescents. Commonly accepted indications for surgery include an irreducible elbow dislocation where the medial epicondyle fracture fragment has become incarcerated in the joint, significant fracture displacement greater than 5 to 15 mm, open fractures, ulnar nerve involvement/entrapment, and gross instability.[5,7,18] Long-term data provided by Farsetti et al has shown similar outcomes of conservative and surgical management of medial epicondyle fracture with displacement of 5 to 15 mm at a mean follow-up of 30 years.[23] However, the authors did note that most patients treated nonoperatively via cast immobilization developed a nonunion. A more recent systematic review also found that conservative management resulted in higher nonunion rates and concluded that as the functional demands of pediatric patients continue to increase, stable fixation to ensure bony union may be desirable.[24]

While the optimal treatment for medial epicondyle fractures in the general population continues to be debated, the threshold for surgical intervention in the setting of an apophyseal avulsion fracture is lower in an adolescent thrower wishing to return to high-level play. In fact, some authors advocate for operative intervention in a competitive overhead thrower even in the setting of minimal displacement to ensure anatomic reduction and to avoid a nonunion incapable of withstanding significant valgus stress.[7,11,25-28] Nonetheless, if after a discussion of the risks and benefits of conservative versus surgical treatment the patient and parents opt for a nonoperative treatment plan, the extremity is placed in a long arm cast in 70° to 90° of flexion and neutral forearm rotation for 2 to 4 weeks.[29] After cast removal, passive range of motion in a hinged elbow brace can be initiated to prevent stiffness and protect the elbow from valgus instability. Active range of motion should not be initiated until there is no tenderness to palpation about the medial epicondyle. Possible complications with nonoperative treatment include delayed apophyseal closure, loss of elbow range of motion, nonunion, and malunion. Nonunion and/or malunion should be of particular concerns to the adolescent thrower, as healing of the medial epicondyle in a displaced position may functionally lengthen the UCL, leading to valgus instability.[25,30] Furthermore, some authors suggest that a fibrous union may be associated with chronic pain and dysfunction in high-level throwers.[14]

If surgical intervention is desired, the goals are anatomic reduction and stable fracture fixation. This will allow early range of motion to avoid postoperative stiffness and rapid return to play while avoiding the complications associated with prolonged casting. Surgical options that have been described include Kirschner (K) wire fixation, screw fixation, suture fixation, and excision of the avulsion fragment with a soft tissue repair. The author's preferred surgical technique includes open reduction internal fixation (ORIF) with a single screw with a washer if the size of the fracture fragment can accommodate it.

Authors' Preferred Surgical Technique

Preoperative Planning

A preoperative elbow examination should be performed on the day of surgery. The surgeon should also carefully evaluate for ulnar nerve symptoms and any concomitant pathology.

Equipment Needed

- Hand table
- Nonsterile tourniquet
- Mini C-arm fluoroscopy
- 3.5 and 4.0 mm partially threaded cannulated screw set
- Curved curettes
- #2 nonabsorbable suture

Technique, Step by Step

- The patient is positioned supine with the operative extremity on a hand table
- Anesthesia is established according to surgeon preference
- A nonsterile tourniquet is placed as far proximal on the upper arm as possible, and the patient is prepped and draped in standard surgical fashion
- Anatomic landmarks are appropriately marked, and the location of the ulnar nerve is confirmed
- The limb is exsanguinated, and the tourniquet is elevated to 250 mm Hg
- A 3 to 4 cm incision is made just posterior to the medial epicondyle and dissection is carried down to soft tissue. Minimal dissection is often necessary, as the displaced fracture fragment is usually subcutaneous
- The ulnar nerve should be visualized and protected with vessel loops. Transposition is not recommended or required
- The fracture site is identified and mobilized. A #2 nonabsorbable suture may be placed in the tendinous portion of the flexor-pronator mass to help

mobilize the fragment (Figure 47.3A) and expose the fracture site (Figure 47.3B). The fracture hematoma should be evacuated and any soft tissue preventing anatomic reduction of the fracture should be debrided. Curettage of the apophyseal cartilage may also be performed to stimulate healing and enhance bony union

- With the fragment reduced, a guidewire for a 3.5 or 4.0 mm cannulated screw is placed. Alternatively, this guidewire may be placed in the distal fragment before anatomic reduction (Figure 47.4). The guidewire should be directed proximally in a slight posterior to anterior direction into the medial column of the humerus. Placement in the olecranon fossa should be avoided. A second wire may be placed for rotational control but is not always necessary

- Fluoroscopy is used to assess fracture reduction and confirm wire positioning

- A soft tissue protector is used, and a drill hole is created taking care that the ulnar nerve is not incarcerated in the fracture fragment

- An appropriate length 3.5 or 4.0 mm partially threaded cannulated screw is placed over the guidewire (Figure 47.5) and under fluoroscopic guidance (Figure 47.6A and B). If possible, a washer can be placed to provide a wide surface area of compression. Care should be taken to not splinter the fracture fragment

- The sutures controlling the flexor-pronator mass can be tied around the screw to enhance stability during fracture healing (Figure 47.7)

- Fluoroscopy is used to confirm reduction and screw placement

- A postoperative image showing bony union at follow-up can be seen in Figure 47.8

Postsurgical Rehabilitation

Postoperatively, patients are immobilized in a posterior splint set in 70° to 90° of flexion and neutral forearm rotation for 7 to 10 days allowing for soft tissue rest. After splint removal, a hinged elbow brace is applied for 5 weeks. This allows for the initiation of passive flexion

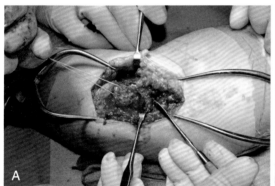
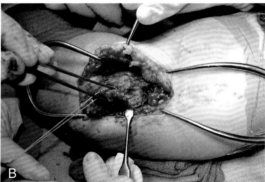

FIGURE 47.3 • Intraoperative image illustrating placement of a #2 nonabsorbable suture in the tendinous portion of the flexor-pronator mass (A) to help mobilize the fragment and expose the fracture site (B).

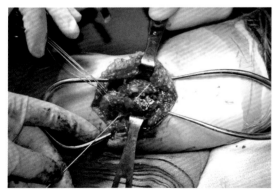

FIGURE 47.4 • Intraoperative image showing placement of a guidewire for a 3.5 or 4.0 mm cannulated screw into the distal fracture fragment before anatomic reduction.

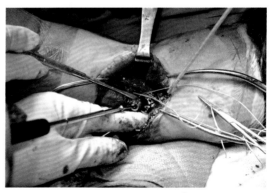

FIGURE 47.5 • Intraoperative image illustrating screw and washer placement over the guidewire for final fixation.

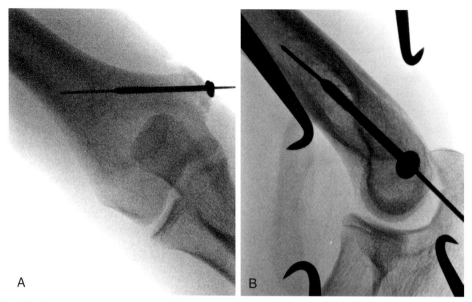

FIGURE 47.6 • Anteroposterior (AP) (A) and lateral (B) intraoperative fluoroscopic images showing cannulated screw fixation over a guidewire.

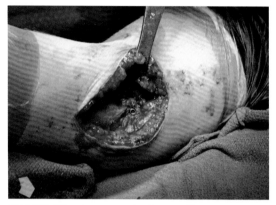

FIGURE 47.7 • Intraoperative image after screw fixation of a medial epicondyle avulsion fracture with the #2 nonabsorbable suture in the flexor-pronator mass tied around the screw to enhance stability during fracture healing.

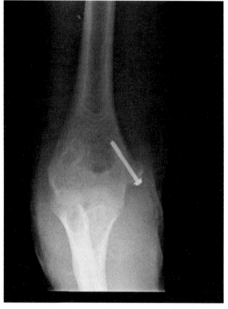

FIGURE 47.8 • Postoperative anteroposterior (AP) radiograph after cannulated screw fixation of a medial apophyseal avulsion fracture illustrating bony union.

and extension range of motion but will protect the elbow from valgus stress. Active range of motion is avoided until patients have no tenderness to palpation about the medial epicondyle. On obtaining full range of motion, patients gradually progress into flexor-pronator strengthening exercises, isokinetic training, a throwing program, and sport-specific functional drills. Players can expect to return to sports and throwing 3 months postoperatively.

RESULTS

Although a number of small case series have published results on ORIF of medial epicondyle fractures, few have specifically examined avulsion fracture treatment

in throwers. Nonetheless, reported outcomes for surgical management of medial epicondyle fractures with screw fixation are generally excellent. For example, Case et al reported outcomes in 8 athletes (3 baseball players) after ORIF with screw fixation of a medial epicondyle fracture.[26] All fractures united at an average 6 weeks postoperatively, and all patients were reported to have pain-free range of motion, stability to valgus stress, and return to their previous levels of athletic activities. Pace et al also recently found 100% union rates in a series of 16 patients who underwent ORIF for displaced medial epicondyle fractures.[25] The authors reported that 15 of the patients were competitive athletes but did not specify what sports were played or their ability to return to play.

It should also be mentioned that some authors have found equivalent results with nonoperative and operative treatment in adolescent athletes. For example, Lawrence et al compared outcomes in 20 athletes with medial epicondyle fractures, in which 14 underwent ORIF and 6 were treated conservatively.[31] Both groups had 100% bony union rate and successful return to sports at their previous level of play. This included 7 baseball pitchers, 4 of whom underwent ORIF and 3 of whom were treated nonoperatively. The authors concluded that even in overhead throwers nonoperative management may be appropriate in the setting of minimal displacement. Although these data are promising, the study is limited by the low number of athletes treated in their nonoperative cohort.

COMPLICATIONS

Although ORIF of medial epicondyle fractures is largely a successful procedure, complications may include painful hardware necessitating removal, ulnar nerve injury, and loss of motion. In 1 series, 58% of fractures treated with a screw and washer required hardware removal compared with 0% of cases treated with a screw alone.[25] Regarding ulnar nerve symptoms, Lawrence et al found that 6 of 14 patients treated via ORIF reported occasional episodic numbness with prolonged elbow flexion.[31] In the same study, 1 patient required a surgical capsular release owing to postoperative stiffness.

MANAGER'S TIPS

- As Little Leaguer's elbow remains prevalent, coaches and parents should continue to monitor for fatigue, high pitch counts, and good pitching mechanics. Prompt diagnosis of medial apophysitis can respond well to nonoperative management
- Patients should return to play as a position player for a full season before returning to the mound
- Surgical indications vary across the literature for medial epicondyle fractures. Although the concept of displacement guiding operative management of medial epicondyle fracture is appropriate for acute traumatic medial epicondyle fractures in the general population, it may not be the most ideal guide for treatment in elite throwers with avulsion-type injuries

- The authors recommend ORIF for both displaced and nondisplaced avulsion fractures of the medial epicondyle apophysis in elite throwing athletes hoping for return to play at high levels to ensure bony union, valgus stability, and early motion
- Use of a washer increases the surface area for compression, improves stability, and may prevent fragmentation of the avulsion fracture; however, it may lead to hardware irritation necessitating removal
- While athletes are recovering from their elbow injury, they can work on the rest of their kinetic chain

REFERENCES

1. DiFiori JP, Benjamin HJ, Brenner JS, et al. Overuse injuries and burnout in youth sports: a position statement from the American Medical Society for Sports Medicine. *Br J Sports Med*. 2014;48(4):287-288.
2. Jayanthi NA, LaBella CR, Fischer D, et al. Sports-specialized intensive training and the risk of injury in young athletes: a clinical case-control study. *Am J Sports Med*. 2015;43(4):794-801.
3. LaPrade RF, Agel J, Baker J, et al. AOSSM early sport specialization consensus statement. *Orthop J Sport Med*. 2016;4(4):232596711664424.
4. Benjamin HJ, Briner WW. Little league elbow. *Clin J Sport Med*. 2005;15(1):37-40.
5. Makhni EC, Jegede KA, Ahmad CS. Pediatric elbow injuries in athletes. *Sports Med Arthrosc*. 2014;22(3):e16-e24.
6. Yang J, Mann BJ, Guettler JH, et al. Risk-prone pitching activities and injuries in youth baseball: findings from a national sample. *Am J Sports Med*. 2014;42(6):1456-1463.
7. Redler LH, Dines JS. Elbow trauma in the athlete. *Hand Clin*. 2015;31(4):663-681.
8. *Pitchsmart*. Available at www.pitchsmart.org. Accessed November 3, 2017 [mlb website].
9. Shanley E, Thigpen C. Throwing injuries in the adolescent athlete. *Int J Sports Phys Ther*. 2013;8(5):630-640.
10. Yukutake T, Nagai K, Yamada M, et al. Risk factors for elbow pain in little league baseball players: a cross-sectional study focusing on developmental factors. *J Sports Med Phys Fitness*. 2015;55(9):962-968.
11. Crowther M. Elbow pain in pediatrics. *Curr Rev Musculoskelet Med*. 2009;2(2):83-87. doi:10.1007/s12178-009-9049-4.
12. Fleisig GS, Andrews JR, Cutter GR, et al. Risk of serious injury for young baseball pitchers. *Am J Sports Med*. 2011;39(2):253-257.
13. Lyman S, Fleisig GS, Andrews JR, et al. Effect of pitch type, pitch count, and pitching mechanics on risk of elbow and shoulder pain in youth baseball pitchers. *Am J Sports Med*. 2002;30(4):463-468.

14. Hutchinson MR, Ireland ML. Overuse and throwing injuries in the skeletally immature athlete. *Instr Course Lect.* 2003;52:25-36.

15. Hang DW, Chao CM, Hang Y-S. A clinical and roentgenographic study of little league elbow. *Am J Sports Med.* 2004;32(1):79-84.

16. Kijowski R, Tuite M. Pediatric throwing injuries of the elbow. *Semin Musculoskelet Radiol.* 2010;14(4):419-429.

17. Ray TR. Youth baseball injuries: recognition, treatment, and prevention. *Curr Sports Med Rep.* 2010;9(5):294-298.

18. Gottschalk HP, Eisner E, Hosalkar HS. Medial epicondyle fractures in the pediatric population. *J Am Acad Orthop Surg.* 2012;20(4):223-232.

19. Pappas N, Lawrence JT, Donegan D, et al. Intraobserver and interobserver agreement in the measurement of displaced humeral medial epicondyle fractures in children. *J Bone Joint Surg Am.* 2010;92(2):322-327.

20. Edmonds EW. How displaced are "nondisplaced" fractures of the medial humeral epicondyle in children? Results of a three-dimensional computed tomography analysis. *J Bone Joint Surg Am.* 2010;92(17): 2785-2791.

21. Gottschalk HP, Bastrom TP, Edmonds EW. Reliability of internal oblique elbow radiographs for measuring displacement of medial epicondyle humerus fractures: a cadaveric study. *J Pediatr Orthop.* 2013;33(1):26-31.

22. Souder CD, Farnsworth CL, McNeil NP, et al. The distal humerus axial view. *J Pediatr Orthop.* 2015;35(5):449-454.

23. Farsetti P, Potenza V, Caterini R, et al. Long-term results of treatment of fractures of the medial humeral epicondyle in children. *J Bone Joint Surg Am.* 2001;83-A(9):1299-1305.

24. Kamath AF, Baldwin K, Horneff J, et al. Operative versus non-operative management of pediatric medial epicondyle fractures: a systematic review. *J Child Orthop.* 2009;3(5):345-357.

25. Pace GI, Hennrikus WL. Fixation of displaced medial epicondyle fractures in adolescents. *J Pediatr Orthop.* 2017;37(2):e80-e82.

26. Case SL, Hennrikus WL. Surgical treatment of displaced medial epicondyle fractures in adolescent athletes. *Am J Sports Med.* 1997;25(5):682-686.

27. Cain EL, Dugas JR, Wolf RS, et al. Elbow injuries in throwing athletes: a current concepts review. *Am J Sports Med.* 2003;31(4):621-635.

28. Woods GW, Tullos HS. Elbow instability and medial epicondyle fractures. *Am J Sports Med.* 1977;5(1):23-30.

29. Cruz AI, Steere JT, Lawrence JTR. Medial epicondyle fractures in the pediatric overhead athlete. *J Pediatr Orthop.* 2016;36:S56-S62.

30. Gilchrist AD, McKee MD. Valgus instability of the elbow due to medial epicondyle nonunion: treatment by fragment excision and ligament repair—a report of 5 cases. *J Shoulder Elbow Surg.* 2002;11(5):493-497.

31. Lawrence JTR, Patel NM, Macknin J, et al. Return to competitive sports after medial epicondyle fractures in adolescent athletes: results of operative and nonoperative treatment. *Am J Sports Med.* 2013;41(5):1152-1157.

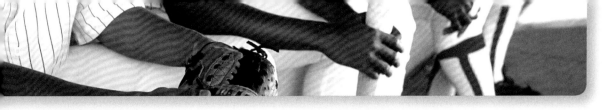

CHAPTER 48

Capitellar Osteochondritis Dissecans

Donald S. Bae, MD

> Little League baseball is a very good thing because it keeps the parents off the streets.
>
> —*Yogi Berra*

INTRODUCTION

With the rise in youth baseball participation, the incidence of overuse injuries to the elbow may be rising.[1,2] Younger age at first participation, earlier specialization, and year-round play—in addition to increased awareness—may all contribute to higher reported rates of overuse conditions. Risk factors for elbow injuries in the skeletally immature throwing athlete include high pitch counts, year-round baseball participation, and suboptimal biomechanics.[3,4] Indeed, high valgus forces across the elbow may lead to compression injuries to the lateral compartment of the elbow and, in particular, osteochondritis dissecans (OCD) of the capitellum.[5]

Currently, capitellar OCD is thought to be due to repetitive microtrauma to the developing capitellum, which is particularly vulnerable owing to its mechanical properties and limited vascularity.[6-10] Typically affecting throwing, overhead, or upper extremity weight bearing athletes between 10 and 14 years of age, OCD results in subchondral bone necrosis, articular cartilage failure, and ultimately loose body formation.

OCD is fairly common among pediatric and adolescent baseball players, affecting 2% to 4% of participating athletes. Kida et al detected OCD by ultrasonography in 3.4% of 2433 adolescent baseball players.[11] In a similar ultrasonographic prevalence study of 4249 Japanese baseball players, OCD was noted in approximately 2% of all athletes between the ages of 9 and 16 years.[12] In addition to elbow pain, functional limitations, and time out of sport, up to half of patients with capitellar OCD may ultimately progress to surgical treatment.[13,14]

Most concerning, perhaps, is that the natural history of OCD is one of persistent impairment and progressive joint degeneration. Bauer et al published long-term outcomes on 31 patients with OCD at a mean follow-up of 23 years.[15] Over a third of patients reported noticeable elbow stiffness, and 16% had persistent elbow pain. Radiographic degenerative joint changes were seen in 19 patients (61%). In another study of 53 patients with a mean follow-up 12.6 years, Takahara et al reported that half of patients with OCD had poor functional outcomes, characterized by pain and stiffness with activities of daily living or even at rest.[16] As a result, great efforts have been made to improve nonoperative and surgical treatment of capitellar OCD.

CLINICAL EVALUATION

History

Patients with capitellar OCD typically present with elbow pain, often poorly localized to the lateral aspect of the elbow. Pain is often insidious in onset, and unlike other throwing injuries (eg, medial epicondylar apophyseal fracture, ulnar collateral ligament rupture), there is often no inciting event. Patients will typically describe a long history of throwing, often with recent increase in frequency, duration, or intensity.[11,13] Further clarity about pitching loads and participation will provide insights into both potential contributing factors as well as opportunities for future activity modification. Up to a third of symptomatic patients will endorse mechanical symptoms of locking, catching, or giving way, and many athletes will not seek medical attention until mechanical symptoms develop. These mechanical symptoms develop in setting of osteochondral fragment instability and loose body formation.

Further query will often yield a history of shoulder discomfort during or after throwing. Given our understanding of the prevalence of posterior capsular contracture or changes in glenoid and humeral version in young throwing athletes, this shoulder pain may arise from internal impingement and resultant rotator cuff tendinosis.[17-19]

Physical Examination

Inspection of the elbow in patients with capitellar OCD will rarely demonstrate swelling over the radiocapitellar joint and posterolateral gutter; in advanced cases, prominence of the radial head and/or radiocapitellar subluxation may be seen.

Careful evaluation of range of motion should be performed, both of the flexion-extension and pronation-supination arcs. Flexion contractures are not uncommon, and when >20°, may indicate more advanced OCD and portend a less favorable prognosis.[20]

Cursory palpation along the lateral column of the distal humerus may not elicit tenderness, and it is imperative that specific palpation of the capitellum be performed in young throwing or overhead athletes presenting with lateral elbow pain. With elbow flexion, the radial head moves anterosuperiorly, uncovering the capitellum and allowing direct palpation of the capitellum by the examiner. Palpation of the capitellum in this position will elicit characteristic tenderness (Figure 48.1).

Lateral compression injuries may sometimes be accompanied by medial traction injuries. The medial epicondyle should be palpated to assess for tenderness, and valgus stress testing should be performed to assess the competency of the ulnar collateral ligament complex.

As noted above, altered throwing mechanics (reduced arm-trunk angle) may increase compressive forces across the capitellum. For this reason, careful examination of shoulder range of motion and strength is imperative to identify possible internal rotation deficits, rotator cuff tendinosis, and/or scapulothoracic dyskinesis.

Although capitellar OCD is rarely associated with neuritis, nerve compression, or vascular insufficiency, a thorough distal neurovascular examination is always advised in the initial assessment of the throwing athlete.

Imaging

Plain radiographs of the affected elbow are indicated in young throwers with elbow pain and reproducible capitellar tenderness. Standard anteroposterior (AP) and lateral radiographs provide important information regarding physeal status and may rule out other sources of pain, including olecranon or medial epicondylar apophyseal stress injuries or radial head stress fractures. In advanced OCD, plain radiographs may demonstrate a lucency within the capitellum and occasionally opacities consistent with in situ or intra-articular loose bodies (Figure 48.2).

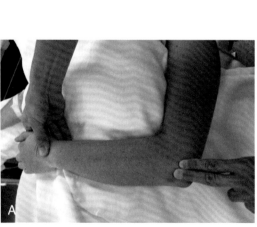
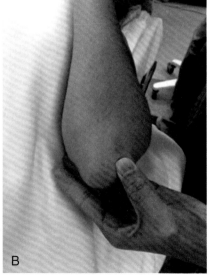

FIGURE 48.1 • A, During clinical examination, tenderness is not typically elicited with palpation along the lateral elbow, as the capitellar osteochondritis dissecans (OCD) is covered by the radial head. B, With the elbow in hyperflexion, the capitellum is unroofed and tenderness may be noted with direct palpation of the capitellum. (Courtesy of Children's Orthopedic Surgery Foundation.)

As OCD lesions of the capitellum are not located at the most inferior aspect of the distal humerus, standard views of the elbow do not always depict the OCD lesion. Flexion oblique radiographs—taken with the elbow flexed 45°—may be used to bring the OCD

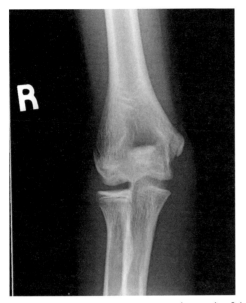

FIGURE 48.2 • Anteroposterior (AP) radiograph of the right elbow demonstrates cystic and sclerotic changes within the capitellum, consistent with osteochondritis dissecans (OCD). (Courtesy of Children's Orthopedic Surgery Foundation.)

lesion into profile.[20] Others have advocated a 30° external rotation oblique for improved visualization and diagnostic accuracy.

Although plain radiographs may provide diagnostic information, magnetic resonance imaging (MRI) provides greater characterization of the OCD lesion, thus providing prognostic information and guiding treatment. Furthermore, MRI is useful in high-risk patients in whom a high clinical suspicion for OCD exists despite negative plain radiographs. MRI should be carefully inspected for OCD size, location, articular cartilage integrity, and status of the underlying subchondral bone (Figure 48.3). Careful analysis of coronal and sagittal T2 sequences will provide insight into articular cartilage integrity and potential fragment instability. MRI signs of OCD instability include[1] the following: high signal line beneath the lesion[2]; a focal defect in the articular cartilage[3]; a fracture of the articular cartilage; and[4] the presence of subchondral cysts.[21] T1 images will provide qualitative insights into the extent of subchondral necrosis. Additional sequences may be used to characterize the extent of bony involvement with greater detail and clarity, including double-echo steady state (DESS) and multiecho in steady-state acquisition (MENSA) sequences.

Computed tomography (CT) is advocated by some authors in the assessment of capitellar OCD. Although helpful in assessing location and size of the OCD lesion, CT may not provide information regarding the

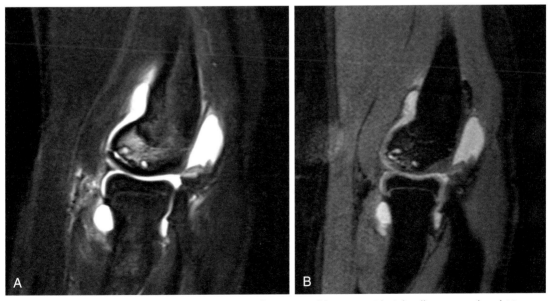

FIGURE 48.3 • Magnetic resonance imaging (MRI) of a 13-year-old patient with right elbow osteochondritis dissecans (OCD). A, Sagittal T2 and (B) double-echo steady state (DESS) sequences demonstrate a breach of the articular cartilage, subchondral cysts, and underlying subchondral bone disease. (Courtesy of Children's Orthopedic Surgery Foundation.)

status of the overlying cartilage or presence of a predominantly cartilaginous loose body.[22] Furthermore, CT does involve additional radiation exposure to the growing elbow.

CLASSIFICATION

A host of classification systems have been proposed for capitellar OCD; many are applications or derivations from prior attempts at classifying OCD lesions of the knee.[23-26] Some classification schemes are based purely on radiographic findings, while others are predicated on arthroscopic or intraoperative appearance of the lesion (Tables 48.1 and 48.2). All fundamentally characterize articular cartilage integrity and fragment stability, in hopes of providing prognostic information and guiding treatment. While subtle differences exist among the various proposed classifications, the author's preference is to utilize the International Cartilage Repair Society (ICRS) and Nelson classification schemes.

TREATMENT

There are host of treatment options for capitellar OCD, ranging from simple rest to complex osteoarticular reconstruction. Little long-term prospective data are available, and comparative analysis of the existing published literature is difficult owing to variable indications, classifications, and outcomes assessments of treatment modalities. In general, the goals are to achieve subchondral bone healing, preservation of articular congruity and joint stability, resolution of pain, and return to activities, including baseball or other sporting activities.

Nonoperative

Nonoperative treatment is typically reserved for stable OCD lesions in which the articular surface is preserved/congruent and there is a capacity for subchondral bone healing (ICRS grade I and II). Nonoperative treatment consists of rest, with cessation of throwing and avoidance of functional loading of the elbow. Bracing has been used by some providers, although there is no evidence-based information to inform clinicians regarding ideal brace type, duration, or realistic expectations regarding relative efficacy over rest alone. Variable clinical and/or radiographic healing rates have been reported following nonoperative treatment. Matsuura performed a retrospective review of 101 adolescent male baseball players treated with rest and cessation of throwing/batting for minimum of 6 months (no bracing was used in these patients).[27] Healing was seen in 76 of 84 patients with stage I OCD (90.5%) after a mean of 14.9 months. Radiographic and clinical healing was seen in only 9 of 17 patients (52.9%) with stage II lesions. Interestingly, patients with stage I and II OCD who did not rest but chose to change positions had lower healing rates of 70% and 50%, respectively; patients who did not rest uniformly failed to heal.

Mihara reported on 30 adolescent baseball players treated nonoperatively for capitellar OCD.[28] Of 26 early stage (Iwase I) lesions, 23 demonstrated healing.[29] Only 2 of 4 Iwase stage IIA lesions healed, and only 1 of 10 Iwase stage IIB and III injuries healed radiographically. Interestingly, 16 of 17 patients with open physes healed, whereas only 11 of 22 patients with closed physes healed.

Takahara et al further evaluated the influence of physeal status on healing potential in their retrospective analysis of 109 patients with elbow OCD.[20] All 10 patients with stable lesions, and open physes went on to successful healing with rest; 7 of 10 patients with closed physes similarly healed with nonoperative treatment. Statistically significant improvements in healing, comfort, radiographic findings, and return to sports were seen in patients with open physes compared with skeletally mature patients.

In summary, patients with early (ICRS stage I or II) OCD may heal with nonoperative treatment, although healing may take 6 to 15 months and is more likely in

TABLE 48.1 International Cartilage Repair Society (ICRS) Classification of Osteochondritis Dissecans (OCD)[25]

Grade	Features
I	Softened but intact articular cartilage
II	Partial cartilage disruption but stable
III	Complete discontinuity; unstable in situ
IV	Displaced loose body

TABLE 48.2 Nelson MRI Classification of Osteochondritis Dissecans (OCD)[23]

Grade	MRI Features
0	Normal
1	Intact articular cartilage; subchondral signal changes
2	Breech in articular cartilage; nondisplaced fragment
3	Thin, high-signal rim behind OCD fragment (unstable in situ); attached by flap of articular cartilage
4	Displaced intra-articular loose body

younger patients with open physes. Given the more guarded prognosis and lower healing rates, surgical intervention may be considered in older patients and those with stage II disease for healing and expedited return to sports, although further investigation is needed to characterize prognostic factors in stage II OCD.

Operative

Indications

Surgical treatment is indicated for patients with pain and functional limitations in the setting of unstable OCD lesions (ICRS grade III and IV) or those who fail nonoperative treatment. The presence of unstable in situ or intra-articular loose bodies is an indication for surgery. As noted above, there is limited natural history and prognostic information regarding ICRS grade II lesions (ie, which grade II lesions will predictably go on to healing with nonsurgical care); for this reason, surgical indications for grade II lesions continue to evolve, and shared decision-making is needed to determine if immediate surgical intervention is warranted in these cases. While there are no absolute contraindications to surgical treatment, patients with advanced radial head changes (articular surface degeneration, radial head enlargement) and radiocapitellar joint subluxation have a more guarded prognosis following surgical treatment.

Surgical Options

A host of surgical treatment options are available, and no single procedure is appropriate for every patient. Individualized decision-making should be made based on patient expectations, preoperative examination and radiographic findings, size and location of the OCD lesion, and surgeon comfort with available techniques. The author's current preferred treatment algorithm is presented in Figure 48.4.

Drilling

Drilling may be performed for persistent OCD lesions failing rest and nonoperative treatment. Conceptually, transarticular or retroarticular drilling with small diameter Kirschner (K-) wires may stimulate healing through creation of vascular channels and/or inflammatory response within the diseased subchondral bone.[30,31] Drilling may be performed arthroscopically or via small arthrotomy. Given the location of the typical capitellar OCD, accessory lateral working portals may need to be created to achieve the appropriate access and trajectory to drill under direct visualization.[32,33]

Fixation

Internal fixation is a conceptually appealing surgical option. Restoration of articular congruity by osteochondral fragment reduction, followed by stable internal fixation, may provide bony healing and joint preservation. Like any reduction and fixation procedure, however, rigid stabilization alone may not be sufficient to achieve healing/union. The vascularity of the affected capitellar bone—progeny and donor site—likely influences healing potential. At present, assessment of the health of the subchondral bone is challenging, and future investigation is needed to elucidate prognostic factors conducive to fixation.

Fixation may be achieved using a number of different surgical methods. Following surgical reduction, bone pegs, transosseous wires or sutures, dynamic staples, headless variable pitch screws, and bioabsorbable implants have all been used to stabilize the OCD fragment to the underlying capitellum[34-38] (Figure 48.5). Many authors advocate elevation of overlying osteochondral fragment and debridement of the fibrous tissue and necrotic bone beneath, with or without bone grafting, before fixation to achieve maximal healing.

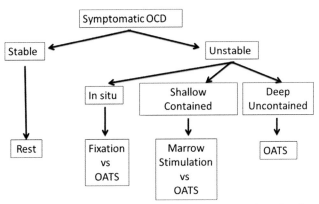

FIGURE 48.4 ● Schematic representation of the author's current treatment algorithm for elbow osteochondritis dissecans (OCD). OATS, osteochondral autologous transplantation surgery. (Courtesy of Children's Orthopedic Surgery Foundation.)

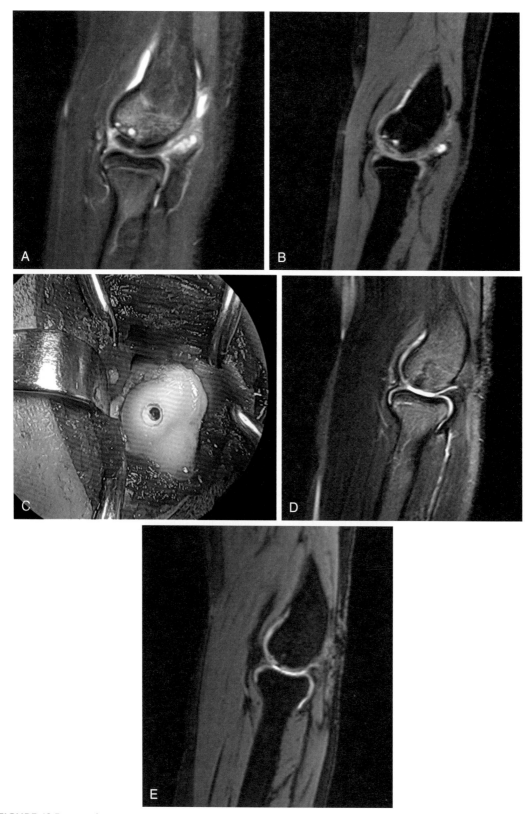

FIGURE 48.5 • A and B, Preoperative T2 and double-echo steady state (DESS) MRI sequences depicting an ICRS (International Cartilage Repair Society) grade III osteochondritis dissecans (OCD), unstable in situ. C, Intraoperative photograph following fixation with a bioabsorbable tack. D and E, MRI images obtained 6 months postoperatively depicting healing. The implant has not yet absorbed and is seen as the linear low-intensity signal within the prior OCD lesion. (Courtesy of Children's Orthopedic Surgery Foundation.)

Microfracture

Microfracture or marrow stimulation techniques are often chosen in patients with ICRS IV OCD, in which there is a loss of the hyaline cartilage surface of the capitellum. In theory, creation of channels within the healthy underlying subchondral bone allows for bleeding and ultimately fibrocartilaginous fill of the defect. This may be best performed in "shallow" OCD lesions in which there is a preserved subchondral plate and viable subchondral bone. While the biomechanical properties of fibrocartilage are different than native hyaline cartilage, restoration of a smooth, congruent articular surface may result in pain relief and functional improvement.[39,40]

Microfracture may be performed using commercially available picks, awls, or smooth K-wires. If an entirely arthroscopic procedure is to be performed, chondroplasty picks may be inserted through the direct lateral or anterolateral portals. The varying angles of these picks will allow for precise placement of microfracture holes orthogonal to the bony surface of the capitellum. Alternatively, 0.035 inches smooth K-wires may be used to drill the lesion until bleeding is seen. Treating the residual OCD defect is important, as fragment removal alone has been associated with poor long-term outcomes.

Osteochondral Grafting

Osteochondral autologous transplantation surgery (OATS) confers the theoretical advantages of replacing the diseased osteochondral lesion with both healthy hyaline cartilage and subchondral bone. OATS may provide a better reconstructive solution for large defects and may give clinically superior results for lateral or uncontained lesions.[41-44] Early published reports are promising, and, to date, donor site morbidity appears to be minimal.[45]

AUTHORS' PREFERRED SURGICAL TECHNIQUE OF OSTEOCHONDRAL GRAFTING

Preoperative Planning

Once the decision has been made to proceed with osteochondral grafting, little additional preoperative planning is needed. Radiographs and MRI are carefully evaluated to measure the size of the OCD lesion and identify the presence and location of any associated loose bodies. The author does not routinely obtain knee radiographs in patients undergoing osteochondral grafting, as the donor osteochondral plug is taken under direct visualization distal to the femoral physis and superior to the weight bearing surface of the femoral condyle.

Equipment Needed

The author's preference is to perform these procedures in the supine position, facilitating exposure of both the elbow as well as the ipsilateral knee for osteochondral donor graft harvest. In addition to a standard small joint arthroscope, commercially available systems are available for cylindrical osteochondral graft harvest and recipient site preparation. Intraoperative fluoroscopy is not used during the procedure.

Surgical Technique

In the supine position, diagnostic arthroscopy is performed in the standard fashion and the capitellar OCD is assessed; intra-articular loose bodies, if present, may be removed (Figure 48.6A). Although osteochondral grafting may be performed arthroscopically, the author's preference is to perform this via an arthrotomy.[46-48] Under tourniquet control and with the elbow hyperflexed, a longitudinal or oblique incision is created directly over the capitellum (Figure 48.6B). The anconeus fascia is incised in-line with the skin incision, and the anconeus muscle fibers are spread in split bluntly. With careful retraction of the anconeus muscle, the capsule overlying the capitellum is carefully incised, providing excellent exposure of the affected articular surface (Figure 48.6C and D). This anconeus-splitting approach is ligament sparing and provides direct, orthogonal access to the cartilaginous surface of the capitellum.

The OCD lesion is inspected and sized, with careful correlation to preoperative imaging. In cases in which loose body removal is performed, the dimensions of the hyaline cartilage defect and integrity of the underlying bone are easily quantified. With in situ lesions, careful probing is performed to identify the transition from injured to healthy tissue. A cylindrical core of injured cartilage and subchondral bone is removed using an appropriately sized cylindrical chisel (Recipient Harvester, OATS Single Use Kit, Arthrex, Inc., Naples, FL); this is typically 10 mm in diameter and 10 to 12 mm in depth. Care is taken to stay perpendicular to the articular surface and prepare the recipient site deep enough to remove all the diseased subchondral bone, avoiding cortical breakout posteriorly or laterally. Although many authors espouse mosaicplasty technique, the author's preference is to reconstruct the OCD lesion with a single large osteochondral graft. Prior investigations have demonstrated adequate anatomic restoration with a single-plug technique, and a single large graft is technically more straightforward.[49] Currently, the author reserves multiple-plug mosaicplasty for lesions greater than 12 mm in diameter, which are not amenable to single-plug reconstruction.

The author's preference is to harvest donor osteochondral graft from the lateral femoral condyle via a small lateral parapatellar arthrotomy (Figure 48.6E). Given the location of the distal femoral physis in skeletally immature patients, care is taken to harvest the osteochondral graft distally while remaining superior to the sulcus terminalis and weight bearing portion of the lateral condyle. A size-appropriate osteochondral plug is obtained from the lateral femoral condyle (Donor Harvester, OATS Single Use Kit, Arthrex, Inc., Naples, FL). The chisel is oriented to produce a matching contour to the recipient site. After successful plug harvest, the knee wound is closed in layers, tourniquet deflated, and a sterile bandage applied.

The donor osteochondral plug is brought to the elbow and press fit into the previously prepared recipient site (Figure 48.6F). Care is made to restore a congruent articular surface, ensuring that the donor graft is flush (or slightly countersunk) with the adjacent capitellar surface; overzealous impaction with a mallet is avoided to preserve chondrocyte viability and mechanical integrity. The elbow is ranged to confirm full flexion-extension, and forearm rotation motion can be achieved without graft instability or joint crepitus. The capsule and anconeus fascia are reapproximated with absorbable sutures and the skin closed. A sterile bandage is applied, followed by a long-arm bivalved cast. Full unrestricted weight bearing on the lower extremity is allowed immediately.

Postsurgical Rehabilitation

The cast is removed at 2 weeks postoperatively, and gentle elbow range of motion exercises are begun. Patients are restricted for heavy lifting for the first 6 postoperative weeks. Physical therapy is initiated at 6 weeks postoperatively for elbow range of motion and gentle closed chain strengthening. Although uncommon, supervised therapy for the knee may also be performed if there are issues regarding knee motion, quadriceps strength, or patellar tracking. During this time, additional work is done for posterior capsular stretching as well as periscapular and cuff strengthening of the throwing shoulder. As recent published literature suggests that complete healing of the osteochondral plug is not achieved for up to 6 months postoperatively, the author's current preference is to allow patients to initiate an interval throwing program and return to sports at 6 months postoperatively[50] (Figure 48.6G and H).

RESULTS

A recent meta-analysis by Westermann and colleagues identified 24 studies on surgical treatment of OCD with data on 492 patients of a mean age of 14.3 years.[51] With microfracture and debridement, 71% of patients returned to prior level of sports participation compared with 64% of those who underwent fixation. Notably, OATS yielded a 94% rate of return to primary sport participation ($P < .01$). This meta-analysis did not find a significant difference in either elbow range of motion or Timmerman scores between surgical interventions. These findings are consistent with the authors own experience and were corroborated by a second systematic review of the OATS literature, also noting a 94% return to primary sports.[38,40,43,44,52] While these authors have highlighted prior hypotheses that having fewer plugs may lead to faster osseous union, they concluded that this supposition could not be reliably evaluated given the available data. Indeed, none of the studies included in either of these systematic reviews were exclusively evaluating single-plug OATS from a lateral femoral condyle donor site.

COMPLICATIONS

Complications of nonoperative treatment include failure of healing and progression to fragment instability and loose body formation. Serial clinical and radiographic evaluations are essential in patients treated with rest for stable OCD lesions, and healing cannot be assumed from the absence of pain alone. Persistent or progressive disease may similarly be seen after drilling of early stage OCD, resulting in the need for additional surgical care.

Although fixation of unstable in situ OCD lesions (ICRS grade III) leads to healing and return to play in most patients, up to a third of patients fail fixation and have persistent symptoms. Again, careful clinical and radiographic follow-up is needed to confirm resolution before return to throwing.

Specific complications of osteochondral grafting, although rare, include early failure due to suboptimal graft placement. Prior biomechanical studies have demonstrated increased contact pressures and strains when osteochondral plugs are left 0.5 to 1 mm proud, potentially leading to pain, limitations in elbow motion, and premature graft failure.[53,54] Every effort should be made, therefore, to ensure that the osteochondral plug is press fit flush to the adjacent intact cartilage surface. Furthermore, during osteochondral grafting, failure to replace all the abnormal bone may result in persistent disease around the margin of osteochondral grafts. Careful preoperative

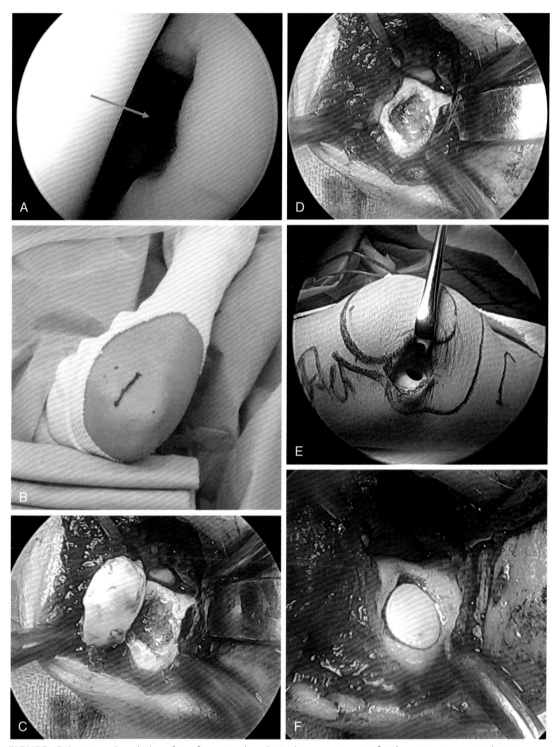

FIGURE 48.6 • Osteochondral grafting for osteochondritis dissecans (OCD) for the patient presented in Figure 48.3. A, During arthroscopy, the OCD lesion is seen of the capitellum (arrow). B, Surgical incision is created over the capitellum with the elbow hyperflexed. C, After anconeus split and capsulotomy, direct access to the OCD lesion is obtained. In this case, there is a large unstable fragment. D, After osteochondral loose body removal, the capitellar recipient site is seen. Preparations were made for a single-plug osteochondral graft. E, Via a lateral parapatellar arthrotomy, a donor cylindrical osteochondral plug is harvested. F, The donor osteochondral plug is press fit into the recipient site, restoring articular surface congruity. G and H, T2 and double-echo steady state (DESS) MRI sequences obtained 6 months postoperatively demonstrate graft incorporation and restoration of a congruent capitellar articular surface. (Courtesy of Children's Orthopedic Surgery Foundation.)

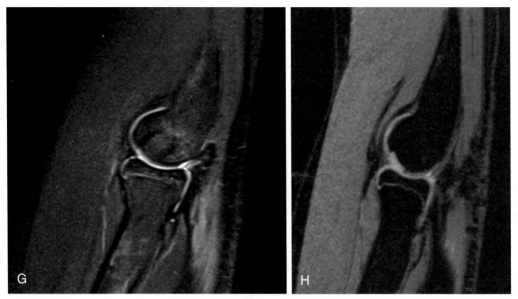

FIGURE 48.6—CONT'D

radiographic evaluation and thorough intraoperative inspection is needed to ensure appropriate recipient site preparation.

The greatest long-term concern is the development of degenerative changes of the radiocapitellar joint. Persistent radiocapitellar incongruity may lead to radial head enlargement, joint instability, and arthrosis. Although osteochondral grafting theoretically restores subchondral bone and hyaline articular cartilage, there are no long-term data regarding the longevity and durability of these surgical reconstructions, particularly in young growing athletes who return to baseball. Continued investigation—including multicenter prospective longitudinal studies—is needed to determine if current treatments are effective in alleviating pain and maximizing functional outcomes in patients with elbow OCD.

MANAGER'S TIPS

Clinical Evaluation

- Tenderness is best elicited with direct palpation of the capitellum with the elbow hyperflexed
- Clinical evaluation should include careful examination of the shoulder girdle to assess for glenohumeral contracture, scapulothoracic motion, and rotator cuff function
- Careful radiographic evaluation—including use of T1, T2, and DESS sequences on MRI—is needed to classify capitellar OCD and guide treatment

Surgical Treatment

- Articular cartilage integrity and the depth of subchondral bony involvement, rather than the surface area of the capitellum involved, should guide surgical decision-making
- An anconeus-splitting approach provides safe and direct access to the capitellum and may be effectively used for drilling, microfracture, fixation, or osteochondral grafting
- Osteochondral grafting—via single-plug or mosaicplasty techniques—provides higher healing and return to sports rates than drilling, microfracture, or fixation for capitellar OCD

Postoperative care

- Owing to the time required for osteochondral graft healing, patients do not initiate a return to throwing program until 6 months postoperatively
- Rehabilitation of all elements of the kinetic chain—including scapulothoracic and glenohumeral motion and strength—and careful analysis of throwing mechanics should be considered in patients with elbow OCD

REFERENCES

1. Heyworth BE, Kramer DE, Martin DJ, Micheli LJ, Kocher MS, Bae DS. Trends in the presentation, management, and outcomes of little league shoulder. *Am J Sports Med.* 2016;44:1431-1438.

2. Okamoto Y, Maehara K, Kanahori T, Hiyama T, Kawamura T, Minami M. Incidence of elbow injuries in adolescent baseball players: screening by a low field magnetic resonance imaging system specialized for small joints. *Jpn J Radiol.* 2016;34:300-306.

3. Fleisig GS, Andrews JR, Cutter GR, et al. Risk of serious injury for young baseball pitchers: a 10-year prospective study. *Am J Sports Med.* 2011;39:253-257.

4. Fleisig GS, Andrews JR. Prevention of elbow injuries in youth baseball pitchers. *Sports Health.* 2012;4:419-424.

5. Ruchelsman DE, Hall MP, Youm T. Osteochondritis dissecans of the capitellum: current concepts. *J Am Acad Orthop Surg.* 2010;18:557-567.

6. Haraldsson S. On osteochondrosis deformans juvenilis capituli humeri including investigation of intra-osseous vasculature in distal humerus. *Acta Orthop Scand.* 1959;30(suppl 38):5-232.

7. Konig F. Ueber freie Korper in den Gelenken [On loose bodies in the joint]. *Dtsch Z Chir.* 1887;27:90-109.

8. Schenck RC Jr, Athanasiou KA, Constantinides G, Gomez E. A biomechanical analysis of articular cartilage of the human elbow and a potential relationship to osteochondritis dissecans. *Clin Orthop Relat Res.* 1994;299:305-312.

9. Schenck RC Jr, Goodnight JM. Osteochondritis dissecans. *J Bone Joint Surg Am.* 1996;78:439-456.

10. Yang Z, Wang Y, Gilula LA, Yamaguchi K. Microcirculation of the distal humeral epiphyseal cartilage: implications for post-traumatic growth deformities. *J Hand Surg Am.* 1998;23:165-172.

11. Kida Y, Morihara T, Kotoura Y, et al. Prevalence and clinical characteristics of osteochondritis dissecans of the humeral capitellum among adolescent baseball players. *Am J Sports Med.* 2014;42:1963-1971.

12. Otoshi K, Kikuchi S, Kato K, Sato R, Igari T, Kaga T, Konno S. Age-specific prevalence and clinical characteristics of humeral medial epicondyle apophysitis and osteochondritis dissecans: ultrasonographic assessment of 4249 players. *Orthop J Sports Med.* 2017;5:2325967117707703 [eCollection May 2017].

13. Iwame T, Matsuura T, Suzue N, et al. Outcome of an elbow check-up system for child and adolescent baseball players. *J Med Invest.* 2016;63:171-174.

14. Weiss JM, Nikizad H, Shea KG, et al. The incidence of surgery in osteochondritis dissecans in children and adolescents. *Orthop J Sports Med.* 2016;4:2325967116635515 [eCollection March 2016].

15. Bauer M, Jonsson K, Josefsson PO, Linden B. Osteochondritis dissecans of the elbow. A long-term followup study. *Clin Orthop Relat Res.* 1992;284:156-160.

16. Takahara M, Ogino T, Sasaki I, Kato H, Minami A, Kaneda K. Long term outcome of osteochondritis dissecans of the humeral capitellum. *Clin Orthop Relat Res.* 1999;363:108-115.

17. Hibberd EE, Oyama S, Myers JB. Increase in humeral retrotorsion accounts for age-related increase in glenohumeral rotation deficit in youth and adolescent baseball players. *Am J Sports Med.* 2014;42:851-858.

18. Kibler WB, Sciascia A, Thomas SJ. Glenohumeral internal rotation deficit: pathogenesis and response to acute throwing. *Sports Med Arthrosc.* 2012;20:34-38.

19. Meister K, Day T, Horodyski M, Kaminski TW, Wasik MP, Tillman S. Rotational motion changes in the glenohumeral joint of the adolescent/little league baseball player. *Am J Sports Med.* 2005;33:693-698.

20. Takahara M, Mura N, Sasaki J, Harada M, Ogino T. Classification, treatment, and outcome of osteochondritis dissecans of the humeral capitellum. *J Bone Joint Surg Am.* 2007;89:1205-1214.

21. De Smet AA, Ilahi OA, Graf BK. Reassessment of the MR criteria for stability of osteochondritis dissecans in the knee and ankle. *Skeletal Radiol.* 1996;25:159-163.

22. Bexkens R, Oosterhoff JH, Tsai TY, et al. Osteochondritis dissecans of the capitellum: lesion size and pattern analysis using quantitative 3-dimensional computed tomography and mapping technique. *J Shoulder Elbow Surg.* 2017;26:1629-1635.

23. Nelson DW, DiPaola J, Colville M, Schmidgall J. Osteochondritis dissecans of the talus and knee: prospective comparison of MR and arthroscopic classifications. *J Comput Assist Tomogr.* 1990;14:804-808.

24. Jacobs JC, Archibald-Seiffer N, Grimm NL, Carey JL, Shea KG. A review of arthroscopic classification systems for osteochondritis dissecans of the knee. *Orthop Clin N Am.* 2015;46:133-139.

25. Brittberg M, Winalski CS. Evaluation of cartilage injuries and repair. *J Bone Joint Surg Am.* 2003;85(suppl 2):58-69.

26. Difelice GS, Meunier MJ, Paletta GA Jr. Elbow injury in the adolescent athlete. In: Altchek DW, Andrews JR, eds. *The Athlete's Elbow.* Philadelphia, PA: Lippincott Williams & Wilkins; 2001:231-248.

27. Matsuura T, Kashiwaguchi S, Iwase T, Takeda Y, Yasui N. Conservative treatment for osteochondrosis of the humeral capitellum. *Am J Sports Med.* 2008;36:868-872.

28. Mihara K, Tsutsui H, Nishinaka N, Yamaguchi K. Nonoperative treatment for osteochondritis dissecans of the capitellum. *Am J Sports Med.* 2009;37:298-304.

29. Iwase T, Igata T. Osteochondrosis of the humeral capitellum [in Japanese]. *Seikeigeka Mook.* 1988;54:26-44.

30. Edmonds EW, Albright J, Bastrom T, Chambers HG. Outcomes of extra-articular, intra-epiphyseal drilling for osteochondritis dissecans of the knee. *J Pediatr Orthop.* 2010;30:870-878.

31. Chambers HG, Shea KG, Carey JL. AAOS Clinical Practice Guideline: diagnosis and treatment of osteochondritis dissecans. *J Am Acad Orthop Surg.* 2011;19:307-309.

32. van den Ende KI, McIntosh AL, Adams JE, Steinmann SP. Osteochondritis dissecans of the capitellum: a review of the literature and a distal ulnar portal. *Arthroscopy.* 2011;27:122-128.

33. Trofa DP, Gancarczyk SM, Lombardi JM, Makhni EC, Popkin CA, Ahmad CS. Visualization of the capitellum during elbow arthroscopy: a comparison of 3 portal techniques. *Orthop J Sports Med.* 2017;5(6):2325967117712228.

34. Nobuta S, Ogawa K, Sato K, Nakagawa T, Hatori H, Itoi E. Clinical outcome of fragment fixation for osteochondritis dissecans of the elbow. *Ups J Med Sci* 2008;113:201-208.

35. Oka Y, Ohta K, Fukuda H. Bone-peg grafting for osteochondritis dissecans of the elbow. *SICOT.* 1999;23:53-57.

36. Inoue G. Bilateral osteochondritis dissecans treated by Herbert screw fixation. *Br J Sports Med.* 1991;25:142-144.

37. Harada M, Ogino T, Takahara M, Ishigaki D, Kashiwa H, Kanauchi Y. Fragment fixation with a bone graft and dynamic stables for osteochondritis dissecans of the humeral capitellum. *J Shoulder Elbow Surg.* 2002;11:368-372.

38. Hennrikus WP, Miller PE, Micheli LJ, Waters PM, Bae DS. Internal fixation of unstable in situ osteochondritis dissecans lesions of the capitellum. *J Pediatr Orthop.* 2015;35:467-473.

39. Bedi A, Feeley BT, Williams RJ III. Management of articular cartilage defects of the knee. *J Bone Joint Surg Am.* 2010;92:994-1009.

40. Lewine EB, Miller PE, Micheli LJ, Waters PM, Bae DS. Early results of drilling and/or microfracture for grade IV osteochondritis dissecans of the capitellum. *J Pediatr Orthop.* 2016;36:803-809.

41. Yamamoto Y, Ishibashi Y, Tsuda E, et al. Osteochondral autograft transplantation for osteochondritis dissecans of the elbow in juvenile baseball players: minimum 2-year follow- up. *Am J Sports Med.* 2006;34:714-720.

42. Iwasaki N, Kato H, Ishikawa J, et al. Autologous osteochondral mosaicplasty for capitellar osteochondritis dissecans in teenaged patients. *Am J Sports Med.* 2006;34:1233-1239.

43. Zlotolow DA, Bae DS. Osteochondral autograft transplantation in the elbow. *J Hand Surg Am.* 2014;39:368-372.

44. Kirsch JM, Thomas JR, Khan M, Townsend WA, Lawton JN, Bedi A. Return to play after osteochondral autograft transplantation of the capitellum: a systematic review. *Arthroscopy.* 2017;33:1412-1420.

45. Iwasaki N, Kato H, Kamishima T, et al. Donor site evaluation after autologous osteochondral mosaicplasty for cartilaginous lesions of the elbow joint. *Am J Sports Med.* 2007;35:2096-2100.

46. Gancarczyk SM, Makhni EC, Lombardi JM, Popkin CA, Ahmad CS. Arthroscopic articular reconstruction of capitellar osteochondral defects. *Am J Sports Med.* 2015;43:2452-2458.

47. Churchill RW, Munoz J, Ahmad CS. Osteochondritis dissecans of the elbow. *Curr Rev Musculoskelet Med.* 2016;9:232-239.

48. Takahara M, Mura N, Sasaki J, Harada M, Ogino T. Classification, treatment, and outcome of osteochondritis dissecans of the humeral capitellum. Surgical technique. *J Bone Joint Surg Am.* 2008;90(suppl 2 pt 1):47-62.

49. Vezeridis AM, Bae DS. Evaluation of knee donor and elbow recipient sites for osteochondral autologous transplantation surgery in capitellar osteochondritis dissecans. *Am J Sports Med.* 2016;44:511-520.

50. Iwasaki N, Kato H, Kamishima T, Minami A. Sequential alterations in magnetic resonance imaging findings after autologous osteochondral mosaicplasty for young athletes with osteochondritis dissecans of the humeral capitellum. *Am J Sports Med.* 2009;37:2349-2354.

51. Westermann RW, Hancock KJ, Buckwalter JA, Kopp B, Glass N, Wolf BR. Return to sport after operative management of osteochondritis dissecans of the capitellum: a systematic review and meta-analysis. *Orthop J Sports Med.* 2016;4(6):2325967116654651.

52. Bae DS, Ingall EM, Miller PE, Lewine EB. Early results of single-plug autologous osteochondral grafting for osteochondritis dissecans of the capitellum in adolescents. *J Pediatr Orthop;* 2018.

53. D'Lima DD, Chen PC, Colwell CC. Osteochondral grafting: effect of graft alignment, material properties, and articular geometry. *Open Orthop J.* 2009;3:61-68.

54. Koh JL, Wirsing K, Lautenschlager E, Zhang LO. The effect of graft height mismatch on contact pressure following osteochondral grafting: a biomechanical study. *Am J Sports Med.* 2004;32:317-320.

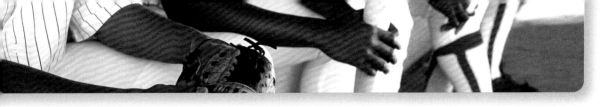

CHAPTER 49

Injury Prevention in Youth Baseball

Brandon J. Erickson, MD | Peter N. Chalmers, MD | Christopher S. Ahmad, MD | James R. Andrews, MD

The future ain't what it used to be.

—*Yogi Berra*

INTRODUCTION

Despite a great deal of attention being paid to the increasing injury rates of professional baseball players, injury rates in youth and adolescent baseball players have been significantly increasing over the past decade.[9,13,16,19] These injuries in youth players have received less media attention than the injuries in professional baseball players. Many risk factors for injury have recently been identified including high pitch counts, high pitch velocity, high overall pitching workload, pitching year round, pitching while fatigued, a more southern geographic location allowing more year-round play, loss of shoulder motion (including forward flexion, internal rotation, and total arc of motion), loss of hip motion, increased elbow torque, early sports specialization, and others.[1-3,5-7,11,12,15,19,20,22,24-27,32-34] Interestingly, although there were early data suggesting that throwing a curveball or breaking ball earlier in a player's career led to an increased risk of shoulder and elbow injury, subsequent studies have found this not to be the case.[8,21,28] In fact, varying pitch types may be protective of shoulder and elbow injury, as studies have found throwing a higher percentage of fastballs and throwing fastballs with a higher velocity are risk factors for sustaining an injury.[6,23,29] The purpose of this chapter is to review the current injury prevention programs and to provide a framework for future directions in injury prevention in youth baseball players.

CURRENT INJURY PREVENTION PROGRAMS

The topic of risk factors for shoulder and elbow injuries has been covered in chapter 45 and therefore will not be restated here. It is important to understand the multitude of risk factors for sustaining an injury that exist for youth and adolescent baseball players, as our current understanding for the risk factors has been the basis for the injury prevention programs that have been developed.[14,32] Please refer to chapter 45 for a list of these risk factors. As the number of risk factors for injury has increased, the number of injury prevention strategies has also increased. There are many injury prevention programs that exist, including pitch count limits, mandated days of rest, decreasing sport specialization, and maintaining hip and shoulder range of motion (ROM).

Pitch Counts

The first important topic in current injury prevention programs is pitch counts. Using pitch counts as a marker for workload in youth baseball is a relatively new concept. Before 2007, pitch count limits did not exits in Little League Baseball, rather inning limits were put in place to decrease injury risk by limiting a pitcher's workload in a given game.[10,31] However, as the number of pitches thrown by a single pitcher in a single inning can vary dramatically, inning limits are a less precise method to control workload. Pitch counts have been linked to injury rates in adolescent baseball pitchers in several large, prospective studies.[18,19] Therefore, to mitigate the risk of injury from throwing too many pitches, a task force on injury prevention in youth athletes has made recommendations for pitch count limits based on age.[32] These recommendations take several factors into account and provide guidelines as to the number of pitches a player can throw in a given game based on their age. The task force recommends a pitch count limit of 50 for those aged 7 to 8 years, which increases age up to 120 pitches at age 19 to 22 years.[32] Although pitch counts are important and should be closely monitored, the number of innings that these players pitch in a season should also be recorded. A 10-year prospective study by Fleisig et al found that pitching >100 innings in a single season was a risk factor for sustaining a shoulder and/or elbow injury in youth baseball players aged 9 to 14 years.[19]

Days of Rest in Between Pitching Outings

Although pitch counts limits are important in youth baseball, the amount of time of rest in between pitching outings has also been shown to be important in injury prevention. Studies have found that pitching on consecutive days is a risk factor for injury in youth baseball players.[19] Hence, to mitigate this risk the Major League Baseball (MLB), task force on injury prevention has also set guidelines on the proper number of days of rest between pitching outings.[32] These guidelines are not solely based on age but are also based on the number of pitches thrown in the previous game. For example, if an 11-year-old throws 55 pitches in a game, that player should have 3 days of rest before their next pitching outing. Conversely, if an 18-year-old throws 55 pitches in a game, that player should have 2 days of rest before their next pitching outing.[32] In addition, youth baseball players who pitch should not play catcher on the days they are not pitching, as this can increase their risk of injury.[18]

Participate in Multiple Sports

There has been a recent push by parents to have their children specialize in a specific sport with the hopes that this specialization will give them a competitive advantage and help them succeed.[26,27] Sport specialization can be defined as intensive year-round training in a single sport at the exclusion of other sports.[26] Previous authors have elaborated on this definition to include athletes who choose 1 main sport, participate for greater than 8 months per year in their main sport, and quit all other sports to focus on 1 sport.[26] Unfortunately, sport specialization and year-round participation in baseball leads to an increased risk of injury.[19,26,27] Therefore, to prevent injury, the task force has recommended that these athletes take at least 4 months off from throwing each year, ensuring 2 to 3 of those months off are consecutive.[32] This recommendation varies slightly by age but has the same take-home message: do not participate in year-round baseball/throwing.

Maintaining Adequate Shoulder and Hip Range of Motion and Strength

Wilk et al performed 2 studies, both looking at the relationship between shoulder ROM and risk of shoulder and elbow injuries.[33,34] The aim of the first study was to determine whether passive ROM of the glenohumeral joint was predictive of shoulder injury or shoulder surgery in professional baseball pitchers, while the aim of the second study was to determine whether decreased ROM of the throwing shoulder was correlated with the onset of elbow injuries in professional baseball pitchers. Both studies were conducted with the same group of players over 8 consecutive seasons (2005-2012). All of the preseason measurements were obtained at spring training, and these pitchers were followed throughout the season to see if they sustained an injury/underwent surgery. In total, 296 pitchers participated in the study (74% right handed). At spring training a goniometer was used to measure shoulder external and internal rotations at 90° of abduction and in the scapular plane. Total arc of shoulder motion was calculated by adding together shoulder external and internal rotation. Average follow-up time for all players was 48.4 months and ranged from 5.5 to 89.5 months. Fifty-one pitchers (17%) suffered a total of 75 shoulder injuries that placed them on the disabled list (DL) at some point during the study period. Of these, 20 (7%) required surgery. 46% of pitchers (133/288) had insufficient shoulder external rotation (defined as >5° from side to side), 23% of whom were placed on the DL for a shoulder injury. This was significantly more than the 12% of pitchers who were placed on the DL who did not have an external rotation deficit ($P = .019$). Pitchers with insufficient external rotation were also more likely to undergo shoulder surgery (13% vs 4%; $P = .009$). Hence, pitchers with insufficient external rotation were 2.2 times more likely be placed on the DL for a shoulder injury and 4.0 times more likely to undergo shoulder surgery than pitchers without an external rotation deficit. Among pitchers with a total shoulder rotation deficit (defined as >5° from side to side), significantly more (19%) suffered elbow injuries compared with those without deficits (8%) ($P = 0.007$). Players with total shoulder rotation deficits were 2.6 times more likely to be placed on the DL for elbow injuries. Furthermore, 18% of players (52/287) had shoulder flexion deficits (defined as >5° from side to side), of which 25% sustained elbow injuries. This was significantly more compared with only 11% of players without flexion deficits ($P = .008$). Players with shoulder flexion deficits were 2.8 times more likely to be placed on the DL for elbow injuries.

Li et al evaluated 201 MLB players (93 pitchers, 22 catchers, and 86 position players) during the 2010 to 2011 season to determine if hip ROM was a significant risk factor for sustaining hip, hamstring, and groin injuries.[25] Hip internal and external rotation measurements were taken in spring training and all players were followed throughout the season to see if they sustained a hip, hamstring, or groin injury. Position players had the greatest hip ROM compared with pitchers and catchers. Twenty nine players suffered in-season hip, hamstring, or groin injuries. When comparing players that had in-season injury relating to the hip region with players that did not have any injury, the overall arc of motion on both right and left sides was decreased (right hip arc 73° vs 77° and left hip arc 75° vs 78°, respectively). Additionally, in the group of players who had hip injuries, when comparing them to the no-injury group, both internal rotation (right hip internal rotation [IR] 29° vs 35° and left hip IR 34° vs 36°) and overall arc of hip motion (right hip arc 70° vs 77° and left hip arc 73° vs 78°) were decreased. Hence, there was a correlation between decreased hip internal rotation and total arc of hip motion with hip, hamstring, and groin injuries. Based on the results of these 3 studies, programs have been instituted to achieve and maintain hip and shoulder ROM in these players throughout the season to decrease risk of injury.

Sakata et al performed a prospective study on youth baseball players aged 8 to 11 years to determine if a routing strengthening and stretching program decreased injury rates.[30] The players were allocated to the intervention group (n = 136) or control group (n = 169). The intervention group performed an injury prevention program, which consisted of 9 stretching and 9 strengthening exercises during warm-up or at home, ideally 1 or more times per week (this is how they defined "high compliance"). In regard to compliance, 78 players (57.4%) in the intervention group were highly compliant and averaged performing the program 1.3 times per week, while 58 players (42.6%) were less compliant, averaging performing the program only 0.3 times per week. The control group had no intervention. The incidence of medial elbow injury was significantly lower in the intervention group (0.8/1000 athlete exposures) than the control group (1.7/1000 athlete exposures) ($P = .016$). In regard to ROM, the program improved total shoulder arc of motion, hip internal rotation, shoulder internal rotation, lower trapezius muscle strength, and thoracic kyphosis angle. The authors also found that improvements in total shoulder arc of motion, hip internal rotation of the nondominant side, and less thoracic kyphosis angle were predictive of a lower rate of medial elbow injury. This study indicates a simple program.

> **TRIP TO THE MOUND**
> **Motion is Lotion**
> These several studies have shown that loss of shoulder and hip motion place pitchers at increased risk for both upper and lower extremity injuries. While these studies were done in adult baseball players, the results can be applied to youth baseball players. Maintaining proper shoulder and hip ROM is an essential step in injury prevention.

FUTURE DIRECTIONS

Although several injury prevention strategies have recently been implemented, there is still a long road ahead to ensure the safety of these adolescent athletes. Although the recommendations set forth previously should be followed, there is still substantial room for improvement to keep these players healthy.

Core Strength

One of the more interesting findings from several studies has been that as pitchers fatigue, their core weakness becomes more evident as their hip to shoulder separation changes (they open up more).[7,17] This weakness likely leads to a greater amount of stress placed on the shoulder and elbow during the throwing motion, thereby increasing a player's risk of injury. Hence, there are 2 future directions that can be taken based on this finding; core-strengthening programs and removing pitchers from games when they begin to show signs of core weakness. Unfortunately, no study to date has been able to describe how to measure core strength. It is therefore difficult to conduct a study in which a core-strengthening program is instituted to determine if this decreases injury risk, as there is no way to prove that the core-strengthening program was effective in strengthening the player's core. It may be worthwhile to institute a core-strengthening program and follow youth players prospectively during a season to see if injury rates decrease, but it would be difficult to prove this decrease was a result of the added core-strengthening program. However, the second direction of removing a pitcher from a game when his hip to shoulder separation increases to a critical amount is feasible. Many games use video technology to evaluate pitchers and hitters throughout the entire course of the game. This video technology could be used to determine when a pitcher begins to exhibit signs of increasing hip to shoulder separation so that they can be removed from the game. The increasing hip to shoulder separation essentially would be used as an objective marker of increasing fatigue (as youth players cannot be counted on to reliably tell their coaches when they are fatigued), which studies have shown to be a risk factor for injury.[17-19]

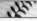

TRIP TO THE MOUND
Put It in the Books!
While core strength is difficult to quantify, core weakness may be a significant risk factor for shoulder and elbow injury. Furthermore, using hip to shoulder separation as a proxy for fatigue may allow coaches to remove players from games when they start to fatigue to prevent injury.

Wearable Technology

Wearable technology is another possible method whereby the force placed on a pitcher's shoulder and elbow can be measured in real time while they are pitching. There are rules against wearing sensors while pitching in professional baseball, but these rules are less stringent at lower levels of competition.[4] These wearable sensors may have the ability to measure overall workload for an individual player. This workload can be tracked over time. Several centers are currently conducting studies to determine the appropriate limits for workload measured using these wearable sensors. Furthermore, these sensors allow the promise that pitchers could be compared with their previous workload, allowing more personalized guidelines for fatigue.

Limiting the Number of Fastballs

One possible future direction in injury prevention is to limit the number of fastballs a pitcher can throw in an inning or in a game. Several studies have found that players who undergo ulnar collateral ligament reconstruction (UCLR) throw a higher percentage of fastballs and throw fastballs with a higher velocity. These studies have been performed in MLB pitchers, but the results can be extrapolated to youth pitchers. Prodromo et al evaluated 114 MLB pitchers who underwent UCLR between 2002 and 2015 and compared them with 3780 MLB pitchers who did not undergo UCLR (control group) to determine if pitchers who underwent UCLR threw a greater percentage of fastballs and had higher pitch velocities compared with age-matched controls in the season before their injury.[29] The authors found that for each 1-mph increase in fastball velocity, the odds

of undergoing UCLR increased 15%, and for a 5-mph increase in fastball velocity, the odds of injury increased by 98%. Pitchers with greater changeup velocity also had an increased risk, but their increased risk was 9% per 1-mph increase. Throwing higher velocity fastballs, sliders, curveballs, changeups, and split-fingers were all correlated with increased risk of UCLR. However, the strongest risk factor for undergoing UCLR was fastball velocity (higher fastball velocity correlated with undergoing UCLR).

Similarly, Chalmers et al performed a retrospective case control study where they reviewed 1327 professional baseball players in an effort to determine the risk factors for undergoing UCLR among MLB pitchers.[6] The authors collected demographic data and data on pitch velocity and pitch type for all included pitchers between 2007 and 2015. They separated pitchers out based on whether they underwent UCLR and then matched the pitchers who underwent UCLR to pitchers who had no history of UCLR. Of the 1327 included pitchers, 309 pitchers (26.8%) had undergone UCLR while 1018 had no history of UCLR and were thus the control group. The results showed that preinjury peak pitch velocity was significantly higher among the pitchers that underwent UCLR compared with controls (93.3 vs 92.1 mph; $P < .001$). Interestingly, in the group of pitchers who required a UCLR, 20% of pitchers with a peak velocity >95.7 mph needed a revision UCLR, while only 7.8% of pitchers with a peak velocity <86.9 mph required a second UCLR. Furthermore, higher mean pitch velocity ($P = .013$), higher body mass index (BMI) ($P = .010$), and younger age ($P = .006$) were correlated with increased risk of undergoing UCLR. Hence, based on these 2 studies, it may be worthwhile to explore the possibility of limiting the number of fastballs thrown in a game or in each inning. Although it would be impractical to limit a pitcher's velocity, youth pitchers should focus on mechanics, technique, command, and control instead of purely on pitch velocity to reduce injury rates.

TRIP TO THE MOUND
It's Outta Here!
Although there was a growing sentiment that throwing curveballs and breaking balls at an early age increased a players risk of injury, the data now clearly show that fastballs, and specifically high-velocity fastballs, are the most significant risk factor for injury. Hence, limiting the number of fastballs and increasing a players' repertoire of pitches may decrease their risk of injury.

MANAGER'S TIPS

- The number of injuries in youth baseball players is continuing to increase
- There are several injury prevention programs in place including pitch counts, mandated days of rest in-between starts, mandated number of months off from throwing each year, and maintaining hip and shoulder ROM
- There are several future directions of injury prevention including improving core strength, wearable technology, and limiting the number/percentage of fastballs a player can throw in a given outing

REFERENCES

1. Anz AW, Bushnell BD, Griffin LP, Noonan TJ, Torry MR, Hawkins RJ. Correlation of torque and elbow injury in professional baseball pitchers. *Am J Sports Med*. 2010;38(7):1368-1374.

2. Axe MJ, Strube M, Osinski D, Andrews JR, Snyder-Mackler L. A speed distance-based classification system for injury prevention and research in international and domestic youth baseball players. *Int J Sports Phys Ther*. 2014;9(3):346-355.

3. Bushnell BD, Anz AW, Noonan TJ, Torry MR, Hawkins RJ. Association of maximum pitch velocity and elbow injury in professional baseball pitchers. *Am J Sports Med*. 2010;38(4):728-732.

4. Camp CL, Tubbs TG, Fleisig GS, et al. The relationship of throwing arm mechanics and elbow varus torque: within-subject variation for professional baseball pitchers across 82,000 throws. *Am J Sports Med*. 2017;45(13):3030-3035.

5. Camp CL, Zajac JM, Pearson DB, et al. Decreased shoulder external rotation and flexion are greater predictors of injury than internal rotation deficits: analysis of 132 pitcher-seasons in professional baseball. *Arthroscopy*. 2017;33(9):1629-1636.

6. Chalmers PN, Erickson BJ, Ball B, Romeo AA, Verma NN. Fastball pitch velocity helps predict ulnar collateral ligament reconstruction in major league baseball pitchers. *Am J Sports Med*. 2016;44(8):2130-2135.

7. Chalmers PN, Sgroi T, Riff AJ, et al. Correlates with history of injury in youth and adolescent pitchers. *Arthroscopy*. 2015;31(7):1349-1357.

8. Dun S, Loftice J, Fleisig GS, Kingsley D, Andrews JR. A biomechanical comparison of youth baseball pitches: is the curveball potentially harmful? *Am J Sports Med*. 2008;36(4):686-692.

9. Erickson BJ, Bach BR Jr, Bush-Joseph CA, Verma NN, Romeo AA. Medial ulnar collateral ligament reconstruction of the elbow in major league baseball players: where do we stand? *World J Orthop*. 2016;7(6):355-360.

10. Erickson BJ, Chalmers PN, Axe MJ, Romeo AA. Exceeding pitch count recommendations in little league baseball increases the chance of requiring Tommy John surgery as a professional baseball pitcher. *Orthop J Sports Med*. 2017;5(3):2325967117695085.

11. Erickson BJ, Chalmers PN, Bach BR Jr, et al. Length of time between surgery and return to sport after ulnar collateral ligament reconstruction in major league baseball pitchers does not predict need for revision surgery. *J Shoulder Elbow Surg*. 2017;26(4):699-703.

12. Erickson BJ, Cvetanovich GL, Bach BR Jr, Bush-Joseph CA, Verma NN, Romeo AA. Should we limit innings pitched after ulnar collateral ligament reconstruction in major league baseball pitchers? *Am J Sports Med*. 2016;44(9):2210-2213.

13. Erickson BJ, Gupta AK, Harris JD, et al. Rate of return to pitching and performance after Tommy John surgery in major league baseball pitchers. *Am J Sports Med*. 2014;42(3):536-543.

14. Erickson BJ, Harris JD, Chalmers PN, et al. Ulnar collateral ligament reconstruction: anatomy, indications, techniques, and outcomes. *Sports Health*. 2015;7(6):511-517.

15. Erickson BJ HJ, Tetreault M, Bush-Joseph C, Cohen MS, Romeo AA. Is Tommy John surgery performed more frequently in major league baseball pitchers from warm weather areas? *Orthop J Sports Med*. 2014;2(10).

16. Erickson BJ, Nwachukwu BU, Rosas S, et al. Trends in medial ulnar collateral ligament reconstruction in the United States: a retrospective review of a large private-payer database from 2007 to 2011. *Am J Sports Med*. 2015;43(7):1770-1774.

17. Erickson BJ, Sgori T, Chalmers PN, et al. The impact of fatigue on baseball pitching mechanics in adolescent male pitchers. *Arthroscopy*. 2016;32(5):762-771.

18. Fleisig GS, Andrews JR. Prevention of elbow injuries in youth baseball pitchers. *Sports Health*. 2012;4(5):419-424.

19. Fleisig GS, Andrews JR, Cutter GR, et al. Risk of serious injury for young baseball pitchers: a 10-year prospective study. *Am J Sports Med*. 2011;39(2):253-257.

20. Fleisig GS, Andrews JR, Dillman CJ, Escamilla RF. Kinetics of baseball pitching with implications about injury mechanisms. *Am J Sports Med*. 1995;23(2):233-239.

21. Fleisig GS, Bolt B, Fortenbaugh D, Wilk KE, Andrews JR. Biomechanical comparison of baseball pitching and long-toss: implications for training and rehabilitation. *J Orthop Sports Phys Ther*. 2011;41(5):296-303.

22. Fortenbaugh D, Fleisig GS, Andrews JR. Baseball pitching biomechanics in relation to injury risk and performance. *Sports Health*. 2009;1(4):314-320.

23. Keller RA, Marshall NE, Guest JM, Okoroha KR, Jung EK, Moutzouros V. Major League Baseball pitch velocity and pitch type associated with risk of ulnar collateral ligament injury. *J Shoulder Elbow Surg*. 2016;25(4):671-675.

24. Keller RA, Mehran N, Khalil LS, Ahmad CS, ElAttrache N. Relative individual workload changes may be a risk factor for rerupture of ulnar collateral ligament reconstruction. *J Shoulder Elbow Surg*. 2017;26(3): 369-375.

25. Li X, Ma R, Zhou H, et al. Evaluation of hip internal and external rotation range of motion as an injury risk factor for hip, abdominal and groin injuries in professional baseball players. *Orthop Rev*. 2015; 7(4):6142.

26. Myer GD, Jayanthi N, Difiori JP, et al. Sport specialization, Part I: does early sports specialization increase negative outcomes and reduce the opportunity for success in young athletes? *Sports Health*. 2015;7(5):437-442.

27. Myer GD, Jayanthi N, DiFiori JP, et al. Sports specialization, Part II: alternative solutions to early sport specialization in youth athletes. *Sports Health*. 2016;8(1):65-73.

28. Nissen CW, Westwell M, Ounpuu S, Patel M, Solomito M, Tate J. A biomechanical comparison of the fastball and curveball in adolescent baseball pitchers. *Am J Sports Med*. 2009;37(8):1492-1498.

29. Prodromo J, Patel N, Kumar N, Denehy K, Tabb LP, Tom J. Pitch characteristics before ulnar collateral ligament reconstruction in major league pitchers compared with age-matched controls. *Orthop J Sports Med*. 2016;4(6):2325967116653946.

30. Sakata J, Nakamura E, Suzuki T, et al. Efficacy of a prevention program for medial elbow injuries in youth baseball players. *Am J Sports Med*. 2018;46(2):460-469.

31. *Series LLBW. 2015 Little league baseball World Series*. Available at http://www.llbws.org. Accessed February 4, 2016.

32. Smart MP. *Guidelines for Youth and Adolescent Pitchers*. Available at http://m.mlb.com/pitchsmart/pitching-guidelines/. Accessed January 3, 2016.

33. Wilk KE, Macrina LC, Fleisig GS, et al. Deficits in glenohumeral passive range of motion increase risk of elbow injury in professional baseball pitchers: a prospective study. *Am J Sports Med*. 2014;42(9):2075-2081.

34. Wilk KE, Macrina LC, Fleisig GS, et al. Deficits in glenohumeral passive range of motion increase risk of shoulder injury in professional baseball pitchers: a prospective study. *Am J Sports Med*. 2015;43(10):2379-2385.

Index

Note: Page numbers followed by "f" indicate figures, "t" indicate tables and "b" indicate boxes.